Traditional Chinese Veterinary Medicine for Neurological Diseases

Proceedings of
The 13th Annual International TCVM Conference

Traditional Chinese Veterinary Medicine for Neurological Diseases

Proceedings of
The 13th Annual International TCVM Conference

Edited by: Huisheng Xie, Cheryl Chrisman and Lisa Trevisanello

Jing Tang Publishing

Edition first published 2011

© 2011 Jing Tang Publishing

The publisher, editors, and authors are not responsible (as a matter of product liability, negligence, or otherwise) for any injury resulting from any material contained herein. This publication contains information relating to general principles of medical care which should not be construed as specific instructions for individual patients. Manufacturers' product information and package inserts should be reviewed for current information, including contraindications, dosages, and precautions.

ISBN: 978-1-934786-28-4

Published and distributed by
   Jing Tang Publishing
   9700 West Hwy 318
   Reddick, FL 32686
   www.tcvm.com
   Tel: 352.591. 2141
   Fax: 352.591.2854

Printed by Tianjin Huanheng Color Printing Technology Development Co., Ltd. Intersection of 13th Rd and Jintang Rd, Hedong District, Tianjin, China

All rights reserved. This book is protected by copyright. No part of this publication may be reproduced in any form or by any means, electronic or mechanical, including photocopying, recording, or any information storage and retrieval system without written permission from the copyright owner.

TABLE OF CONTENTS

ABOUT THE EDITORS ix

CONTRIBUTORS x

INTRODUCTION 1

    Traditional Chinese Veterinary Medicine for Neurological Disorders 3
        Cheryl L Chrisman DVM, MS, EdS, DACVIM-Neurology, CVA

CHAPTER 1: The Integrated Neurological Evaluation and Research on Neurological Disorders

    Integrated Neurological Evaluation 11
        Cheryl L Chrisman DVM, MS, EdS, DACVIM-Neurology, CVA

    Recent Research on Acupuncture for Neurological Disorders 31
        Songhua Hu, DVM, PhD, MS

CHAPTER 2: Cerebral Disorders

    Dementia, Stupor and Coma Disorders 41
        Cheryl L Chrisman DVM, MS, EdS, DACVIM-Neurology, CVA

    Seizure Disorders 71
        Cheryl L Chrisman DVM, MS, EdS, DACVIM-Neurology, CVA

    Tremor Disorders 95
        Cheryl L Chrisman DVM, MS, EdS, DACVIM-Neurology, CVA

    Seizures in a 20 Year Old Quarter Horse Mare 107
        Joan D Winter, DVM

    How I Treat Cognitive Dysfunction Syndrome 113
        Huisheng Xie DVM, MS, PhD

    How I Treat Hydrocephalus 117
        Roger M Clemmons, DVM, PhD, CVA, CVFT

    How I Treat CNS Neoplasia 121
        Roger M Clemmons, DVM, PhD, CVA, CVFT

    TCVM for Treatment of an Intracranial Lesion in a Dog 129
        Heidi Woog, DVM, CVA, CVCH

    Right Retrobulbar Squamous Cell Carcinoma in a Dog 135
        Joan D Winter, DVM, CVA, CVCH, CVTP

Granulomatous Meningoencephalomyelitis and Other Immune-mediated CNS Diseases 139

 Bruce Ferguson, DVM, MS, CVA, CVCH, CVTP, CVFT

CHAPTER 3: Cranial Nerve Disorders

Peripheral Cranial Nerve Disorders 149

 Cheryl L Chrisman DVM, MS, EdS, DACVIM-Neurology, CVA

Treatment of Head Tilt/Vestibular Disease with Acupuncture and Chinese Herbal Medicine in a Chinese Pug 211

 Daniel King, DVM, CVA, CVCH, CVTP

TCVM Treatment of Severe Canine Geriatric Vestibular Disease 217

 Margaret Fowler, DVM, CVA, CVCH, CVTP, CVFT

CHAPTER 4: Spinal Cord Disorders

Spinal Cord Disorders... 225

 Cheryl L Chrisman DVM, MS, EdS, DACVIM-Neurology, CVA

Acupuncture Helps Dog With Vertebral Fracture Return to Near Normal Function 323

 Elisa Katz, DVM, CVA

Canine Intervertebral Disk Disease Treated with Aquapuncture and Chinese Herbal and Western Medicine 331

 Chi Hsien Chien, DVM, PhD

An Effective and Simple Protocol to Treat Intervertebral Disk Disease Associated with a *Qi*-Deficient/Stagnation Pattern... 333

 Bruce Ferguson, DVM, MS, CVA, CVCH, CVTP, CVFT

Acupuncture for the Treatment of Spinal Cord Injuries 337

 Weerapongse Tangjitjaroen DVM, PhD

How I Treat Degenerative Myelopathy 347

 Roger M Clemmons, DVM, PhD, CVA, CVFT

CHAPTER 5: Neuromuscular Disorders

Generalized Neuromuscular Disorders... 355

 Cheryl L Chrisman DVM, MS, EdS, DACVIM-Neurology, CVA

Acupuncture and *Tui-na* Treatment of Generalized Tetanus in a Dog 387

 Margaret Fowler, DVM, CVA CVCH, CVTP, CVTFT

Idiopathic Phrenic Neuropathy in a Cria 391

 Joan D Winter, DVM, CVA, CVCH, CVTP

CHAPTER 6: Peripheral Nerve Injuries

Peripheral Spinal Nerve Injuries 399
 Cheryl L Chrisman DVM, MS, EdS, DACVIM-Neurology, CVA

Neurological Case Studies Associated with Trauma 417
 Han Wen Cheng, DVM

CHAPTER 7: Equine Neurological Disorders

TCVM for Treatment of Equine Neurological Diseases 431
 Huisheng Xie, DVM, MS, PhD

TCVM Treatment of Suprascrapular Nerve Injury in a Dutch Warmblood Filly 447
 Margaret Fowler, DVM, CVA, CVCH, CVTP, CVFT

CHAPTER 8: *Wei* Syndrome, *Tan-Huan* Syndrome and Others

How I Treat *Wei* Syndrome 455
 Bruce Ferguson, DVM, MS, CVA, CVCH, CVTP, CVFT and Linda Boggie, DVM, CVA

How to Use Acupuncture to Treat Downer Cow Syndrome 467
 Huisheng Xie, DVM PhD

Suggested Changes in Location and Function and Pairing of Eight Distal Limb Acupoints in Dogs and Cats 469
 Bruce Ferguson, DVM, MS, CVA, CVCH, CVTP, CVFT

INDEX 477

ABOUT THE EDITORS

Huisheng Xie has taught and practiced Traditional Chinese Veterinary Medicine in both small and large animals since 1983. He is the founder of the Chi Institute, in Reddick, Florida, which is dedicated to train veterinarians in veterinary acupuncture, herbal medicine, food therapy and tui-na. His textbooks include *Traditional Chinese Veterinary Medicine-Fundamental Principles, Xie's Veterinary Acupuncture, Xie's Veterinary Herbology,* and *Application of Tui-na in Veterinary Medicine.* He had been the assistant and associate professor of College of Veterinary Medicine, Beijing China Agriculture from 1983 to 1994. He is currenly a clinical associate professor of College of Veterinary Medicine University of Florida.

Cheryl L Chrisman received her DVM from Michigan State University in 1968 and became a Diplomate of the ACVIM Specialty of Neurology in 1975. She practiced and taught neurology at the Ohio State University and University of Florida for 37 years. As a graduate of Chi Institute, she became certified in veterinary acupuncture and also practiced acupuncture at University of Florida as a faculty member of the Acupuncutre Service. She is currently on the faculty of Chi Institute and Editor-in-Chief of the American Journal of Tradtional Chinese Veterinary Medicine.

Lisa Trevisanello received her DVM from the University of Padua, Italy in 2003. As a graduate of the Chi Institute, she became certified in veterinary acupuncture. She incorporated acupuncture into her practice of small animal medicine. Currently, she is working on her Master Degree of TCVM from the Southwest University, China. She co-authored chapters of *Xie's Veterinary Acupuncture,* Equine Acupoints CD and *Xie's Chinese Veterinary Herbology*.

CONTRIBUTORS

Chi Hsien Chen DVM, PhD
National PingTung University of Science and Technology,
Taiwan, CHINA

Han Wen Cheng DVM
Taibei, Taiwan, CHINA

Cheryl L Chrisman DVM, MS, EdS, DACVIM-Neurology, CVA
University of Florida, FL, USA

Roger M Clemmons DVM, PhD, CVA, CVFT
University of Florida, FL, USA

Bruce Ferguson DVM, MS, CVA, CVCH, CVTP, CVFT
Murdoch University, AUSTRALIA

Margaret Fowler DVM, CVA, CVCH, CVTP, CVFT
Panama City Beach, FL, USA

Songhua Hu DVM, PhD
Hanzhou, Zhejiang, CHINA

Elisa Katz DVM, CVA
Wallingford, CT, USA

Daniel King DVM, CVA, CVCH, CVTP
Tolono, IL, USA

Weerapongse Tangjitjaroen DVM, PhD
Chiang Mai University, THAILAND

Joan D Winter DVM, CVA, CVCH, CVTP
Simi Valley, CA, USA

Heidi Woog DVM, CVA, CVCH
Ketchum, ID, USA

Huisheng Xie DVM, MS, PhD
University of Florida, FL, USA

INTRODUCTION

Traditional Chinese Veterinary Medicine for Neurological Disorders

Cheryl L Chrisman DVM, MS, EdS, DACVIM-Neurology, CVA

In the Chinese medical classic text, *Huang Di Nei Ching* (Yellow Emperor's Classic of Internal Medicine or Canon of Medicine), written during the Warring States period (401–250 BC), the brain was not viewed as one of the important five *Zang* organs (e.g. Liver, Heart, Spleen, Lung, Kidney).[1] The Kidney was considered the center for vigor and strength. The brain was viewed more as a reservoir of the Kidney system, because when full, the body felt strong and light, but when it was Deficient, dizziness, tinnitus, blurred vision, aching limbs and tiredness resulted.[1] Since the brain resided within the bony skull, it was considered a reservoir of bone marrow and came to be known as the "Sea of Marrow". The spinal cord was considered bone marrow within the vertebral canal. Peripheral nerves were not mentioned in early records. Marrow from a traditional Chinese medicine (TCM) perspective thus includes brain, spinal cord and bone marrow.

The ideas of *Yin* and *Yang* and the Five Elements as well as the treatments used in TCM and traditional Chinese veterinary medicine (TCVM) originated with the *Daoists*, ancient Chinese philosophers, whose ideas coalesced around 500 BC. The *Daoists* had an advanced view of the brain as an organ.[1] They considered the brain as the palace of *Ni Huan*, a Chinese translation of the Sanskrit word for "nirvana." The brain was considered the source of seminal Essence. The spinal cord was the Channel linking the cavity of the "Sea of Marrow" with *Ming Men* (the gate of life) situated between the Kidneys. As the idea of Extraordinary *Fu* organs evolved in TCM, the Brain became recognized as one of these special organs and became not only the "Sea of the Marrow", but also the "House of the Mind and Spirit" similar to the earlier *Daoists* perception.[2]

In TCVM, the correct *Bian Zheng* or pattern identification is paramount to achieve the optimum treatment outcome.[2] Although there are several useful diagnostic systems and theories in TCVM, the ones most useful to describe TCVM patterns of neurological diseases are a combination of the theories of *Yin/Yang*, Eight Principles, TCVM Pathogens, Five Elements, Five Treasures and *Zang-Fu* physiology and pathology. The six roots of the Eight Principles are extensively used to describe neurological problems as External or Internal, Excess or Deficiency and Hot or Cold. The location of the neurological disorder can be External and involve the Channels, peripheral nerves and muscles or Internal affecting the Extraordinary *Fu* organs (Brain and Spinal cord) of the Kidney system often with concurrent imbalances in the Spleen, Liver or Heart systems according to their Five Element theory relationships. Excess neurological patterns often involve invasion of a TCVM pathogen like Wind-Heat, Wind-Cold or Damp-Heat or Stagnation of *Qi* or Blood or both (*Qi*/Blood Stagnation). Deficiency patterns often involve the Elements and *Zang* organs of the Kidney, Liver, Spleen and Heart. Further, the most common Deficiency patterns of neurological diseases include Deficiencies of *Jing, Qi, Yin, Yang* and Blood. *Qi* Deficiency may be primarily localized to one or more Channels (Exterior) and result in neurological deficits related to the specific cranial or spinal nerves and muscles involved (e.g. facial nerve paralysis or masticatory myositis). When *Qi* Deficiency involves the spinal cord, it has an Interior location and is associated with Kidney *Qi* Deficiency causing paresis or paralysis of the pelvic limbs or all four limbs.

As a review from the conventional anatomic perspective, the nervous system of dogs and cats consists of central and peripheral components.[3-6] The central nervous system (CNS) is the brain and the spinal cord and the peripheral nervous system (PNS) is the cranial and spinal nerves. The brain is further divided into the cerebrum and brainstem and the brainstem consists of four sections from rostral to caudal: 1) the diencephalon containing the thalamus, hypothalamus and other structures, 2) midbrain, 3) pons and 4) medulla oblongata. The cranial nerves and spinal nerves of the PNS enter and/or exit specific brain stem and spinal cord segments respectively.

The spinal cord is divided into five sections that relate to the thoracic and pelvic limbs.[3-6] The cranial cervical spinal cord (C1-C5) is caudal to the medulla oblongata, but just cranial to the thoracic limbs. The caudal cervical spinal cord (C6-T2) is located in the thoracic limb region and motor and sensory peripheral spinal nerves of the limb form the brachial plexus. The thoracic and cranial lumbar spinal cord (T3-L3) is located between the thoracic and pelvic limbs. The caudal lumbar and sacral spinal cord (L4-S2) is located in the region of the pelvic limbs and the femoral nerves (L4-L5) and sciatic nerves (L6-S2) enter and exit to form the lumbosacral plexus. The sacrocaudal spinal cord (S2-Cd5+) is located caudal to the nerves of the pelvic limbs. In dogs, the spinal cord is shorter than the vertebral column in the caudal lumbar region and terminates at vertebrae L6 or L7. The nerve roots L6-Cd5+ continue in the spinal canal to form the cauda equina and each one exits immediately behind the vertebra of the same number. Most discussions of neurological disorders also include primary muscle diseases, because muscles have a symbiotic relationship with peripheral nerves.

Conventional veterinary medicine and traditional Chinese veterinary medicine (TCVM) differ in their approach to the diagnosis and treatment of neurological diseases. However, when integrated, the two medical paradigms can lead to a deeper understanding of dysfunction and more effective therapeutic options for neurological patients. Understanding the disease process from a conventional perspective can deepen the understanding and application of TCVM theories and disease patterns and lead to better TCVM treatments. Understanding TCVM theories and disease patterns can deepen the understanding of the conventional disease and offer treatment when there are no conventional treatments. The conventional neurological examination is needed for accurate lesion location so that correct local acupoints or acupoints on Channels that traverse the lesion can be treated. Most common conventional neurological diagnoses are associated with one to seven different TCVM patterns that require different treatments.

The TCVM patterns and suggested acupuncture, Chinese herbal medicine, *Tui-na* and Food therapy treatments will presented in the subsequent chapters for the following conventional neurological disorders: 1) head injury, 2) cognitive dysfunction, 3) meningoencephalitis, 4) brain tumor, 5) idiopathic epilepsy, 6) congenital hydrocephalus, 7) idiopathic tremors, 8) geriatric tremors, 9) optic neuritis, 10) trigeminal neuritis, 11) facial paralysis, 12) vestibular disease, 13) deafness, 14) laryngeal paralysis, 15) masticatory myopathy, 16) intervertebral disk disease, 17) spinal cord trauma, 18) cervical spondylomyelopathy (wobbler syndrome), 19) fibrocartilaginous embolism, 20) diskospondylitis, 21) degenerative myelopathy, 22) atlantoaxial malformation, 23) meningomyelitis, 24) spinal cord tumor, 25) brachial plexus injury, 26) sciatic nerve injury, 27) lumbosacral degeneration 28) cauda equina injury, 29) polyneuropathy, 30) myasthenia gravis and 31) polymyositis. There is increasing research support that confirms practitioners' experiences that integration of TCVM treatments can result in less conventional medications with adverse side effects, fewer invasive neurosurgical procedures, faster recovery, improved degree of recovery, less disease recurrence and overall improved quality of life for neurological patients.

References:
1. Chu NS. Neurology and Traditional Chinese Medicine. In Finger S, Boller F, Tyler KL, (eds). Handbook of Clinical Neurology. Cambridge, MA: Elsevier 2010:755-767.
2. Xie H, Priest V. Traditional Chinese Veterinary Medicine. Reddick, FL: Jing Tang Publishing 2002:209-293,307-380,409-419.
3. De Lahunta A, Glass E. Veterinary Neuroanatomy and Clinical Neurology 3nd Ed. Philadelphia, PA:WB Saunders 2008:95-113,14.
4. Chrisman C, Mariani C, Platt S, Clemmons R. Neurology for the Small Animal Practitioner. Jackson Wy: Teton NewMedia 2003:125-167.
5. Platt S, Olby N (ed). BSAVA Manual of Canine and Feline Neurology 5th Ed. Gloucester, UK:BSAVA Publications 2011:1-500.
6. Kline KL, Caplan ER, Joseph RJ. Acupuncture for neurological disorders. In Schoen AM (ed) Veterinary Acupuncture 2nd Ed. St Louis, Mo: Mosby Publishing 2001:179-192.

INTRODUCTION 7

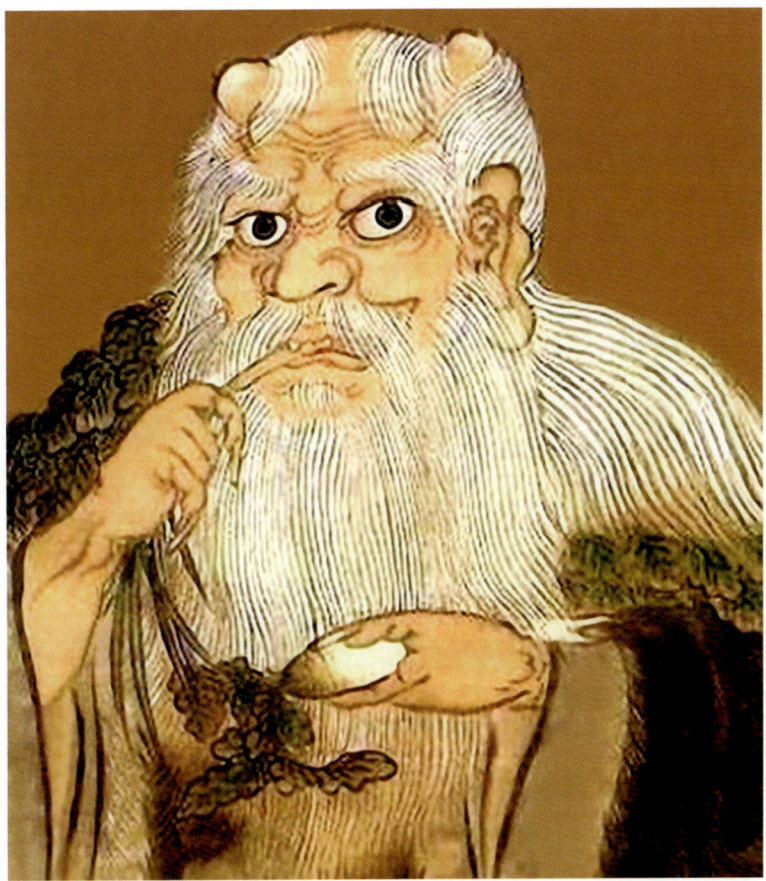

SHEN NONG 神农氏

Shen Nong, also known as Yan Di, was a ruler of China about 5,000 years ago. He taught the ancient Chinese to clear land with fire, plow fields with oxen and cultivate crops as food instead of hunting and gathering. His name literally means "*the Divine Farmer*". It is he that established a stable agricultural society in China. In addition, *Shi Ji* (The *Records of the Grand Historian*), the first systematic Chinese historical text, written by Sima Qian, states that "Shen Nong tasted hundreds of herbs and started Chinese medicines". Shen Nong discovered that some herbs were effective to relieve signs of illness and eliminate certain diseases. In order to evaluate more plants and confirm these effects, he taught ancient healers to taste and test herbs for their medicinal properties. Since Shen Nong's era, the rich knowledge of Chinese herbs including their medical actions, localities of production, harvesting, processing, natures and flavors, toxicity and safety, dosage and administration has accumulated from generation to generation.

A collection of information on 365 medicinal herbs discovered before the Han dynasty (206 BCE–220 CE) was compiled into the text *Shen Nong Ben Cao Jing* (Shen Nong's Book of Medical Herbs). To honor his contribution to Chinese herbal medicine, Shen Nong was used as part of the title of the book. This book was written between 100 BCE and 100 CE and became the earliest Chinese herbal materia medica. These 365 herbs are still used on a daily basis in modern Traditional Chinese Medicine (TCM) and Traditional Chinese Veterinary Medicine (TCVM) practice.

CHAPTER 1

The Integrated Neurological Evaluation and Research on Neurological Disorders

Integrated Neurological Evaluation

Cheryl L Chrisman DVM, MS, EdS, DACVIM-Neurology, CVA

Integration of the conventional history, physical and neurological examinations and the TCVM evaluation *Si Zhen* or Four Diagnostic Methods can lead to a more complete evaluation and deeper understanding of disease processes causing neurological disorders in animals.[1-5] Both approaches will be reviewed and an integration of the two will be presented.

The purpose of the conventional history and physical and neurological examinations is to determine:
1. If the animal has a neurological disorder
2. If so, where it is localized within the nervous system
3. How severe the disorder is
4. Clues about disease etiology
5. The need to do further diagnostic tests
6. The appropriate conventional therapy
7. Most likely prognosis

The purpose of the TCVM history and physical examination (*Si Zhen*) is to determine:
1. The basic constitution of the animal
2. If there is an imbalance in the body causing specific clinical signs
3. Which one or more of the Five Elements are affected
4. The relationship between Elements when two or more are affected
5. If the disease process is External or Internal or has aspects of both
6. If an Excess or Deficiency pattern or combination pattern is present
7. If the disease process is Hot or Cold
8. The current TCVM disease pattern(s)
9. The appropriate TCVM therapy
10. Most likely prognosis

SIGNALMENT AND PRIMARY COMPLAINTS FROM CONVENTIONAL AND TCVM PERSPECTIVES

Clues to the disease etiology, from both conventional and TCVM perspectives can be obtained from the signalment (age, breed and sex) of the animal.[1-5] From the conventional perspective, young animals are more likely to have neurological signs from congenital problems, infections and trauma, while older animals are more likely to have degenerative and neoplastic diseases. From the TCVM perspective young animals are more likely to have a neurological disorder from Kidney *Jing* Deficiency or an Excess pattern such as Excess Damp Heat in the brain (meningoencephalitis) or *Qi*/Blood Stagnation from injury.[1] Old animals are more likely to have a Deficiency or combination of Excess and Deficiency patterns (e.g. Spinal cord *Qi*/Blood Stagnation associated with an underlying Kidney *Yang* Deficiency pattern as occurs in some animals with intervertebral disk disease). From a TCVM perspective dogs and cats may also have a predisposition for certain diseases based on their primary constitution type (Wood, Fire, Earth,

Metal or Water) and an underlying prenatal Kidney *Jing* Deficiency that causes genetic, congenital and breed specific disorders and premature neural degeneration.

The first clue to determine the presence and location of a neurological disease from both conventional and TCVM perspectives is the primary complaint.[3] Based on the primary complaint from a conventional perspective, a disease may be localized to either above or below the foramen magnum (the opening in the skull between the caudal medulla oblongata and 1st cervical vertebra). The brain and cranial nerves are located above the level of the foramen magnum and common primary complaints typical of disease here include: stupor, coma, dementia, seizures, tremors and cranial nerve deficits. The spinal cord and spinal nerves reside below the foramen magnum and common complaints include: neck or back pain and limb ataxia, paresis or paralysis.

From a TCVM perspective, the primary complaint and signalment can provide clues to the Five Element system(s) involved and the underlying process. Dementia is a *Shen* disturbance associated with imbalances (disharmonies) of the Heart system that are often associated with Liver and Kidney imbalances in neurological disorders.[1] Seizures and tremors are Internal Wind disorders that reflect imbalances of the Liver. Focal cranial nerve disorders and generalized peripheral nerve and muscle disorders are often associated with the Wind-Heat or Wind-Cold invasions of different Channels on the head, body and limbs. The result is focal or multifocal *Qi*/Blood Stagnation with *Qi* Deficiency that cause dysfunction of the nerves or muscles.

CONVENTIONAL AND TCVM HISTORICAL FINDINGS

The history is similar from the conventional and TCVM perspectives and consists of a series of questions to determine the most likely etiology of the primary complaint and to assist in making a final diagnosis, treatment plan and an accurate prognosis.[1-5] The onset and progression of the primary neurological complaint may be neonatal non-progressive, acute non-progressive, acute progressive, chronic progressive or episodic (Table 1). Neonatal non-progressive disorders become apparent shortly after birth and remain unchanged (e.g. cerebellar hypoplasia). Animals with acute non-progressive disorders develop neurological signs immediately or within 72 hours and then remain unchanged or improve (e.g. spinal cord injury or fibrocartilaginous embolism). Animals with acute progressive disorders develop signs immediately or within 72 hours that progressively worsen (e.g. meningoencephalitis). Animals with chronic progressive disorders develop signs over several days, weeks or months that continue to worsen (e.g. degenerative myelopathy). Animals with episodic disorders are normal in-between the clinical signs (e.g. intermittent seizures from idiopathic epilepsy). The duration of the signs may have an impact on TCVM treatment frequency. Acute disorders may initially need treatment daily or every 3-5 days. Chronic disorders may initially need treatment every 1-2 weeks. A thorough investigation of other neurological signs, concurrent or previous illness, vaccination status, the possibility of trauma or exposure to toxins, similar familial problems, current medications and supplements, environment and lifestyle are essential to accurately determine the etiology of the primary complaint and develop effective conventional and TCVM treatment strategies.

Table 1: The signalment, onset and progression of disease and other findings associated with conventional etiologies of neurological disease[3,4]

	Conventional Etiology	Signalment (Age, Breed, Gender)	Onset and Progression of Clinical Signs	Other Helpful Information or Diagnostic Tests	Common Neurologic Deficits and Symmetry or Asymmetry of Deficits
D	Degenerative	Adult, often a breed predilection (DM, IVDD), either gender	Chronic progressive	History of previous neck or back pain or diagnosis of IVDD	Cognitive dysfunction, deafness, symmetrical or asymmetrical paresis/paralysis
A	Anomalous (Congenital)	Young, often a breed predilection, either gender	Neonatal non-progressive or chronic progressive	Family history, other littermates affected	Symmetrical seizures, deafness, ataxia, symmetrical or asymmetrical paresis/paralysis
M	Metabolic	Any age and breed, either gender	Acute or chronic progressive	Serum biochemistry profile and bile acids	Dementia, stupor, coma, symmetrical seizures
N	Nutritional	Any age and breed, either gender	Acute or chronic progressive	History of a diet deficient in thiamine	Dementia, stupor, coma, symmetrical seizures
N	Neoplastic	Adult, breed predilection, either gender	Usually chronic progressive	History of previous known neoplasia; thoracic and abdominal radiographs and ultrasound	Dementia, stupor, coma, seizures often asymmetrical, paresis/paralysis often asymmetrical
I	Inflammatory or Infectious	Any age and breed, either gender	Acute or chronic progressive	Depression, may be anorexic or febrile, other animals sick	Dementia, stupor, coma, seizures often asymmetrical, paresis/paralysis often asymmetrical
I	Idiopathic	Varies with the syndrome	Acute or episodic	Specific syndromes:	Symmetrical or asymmetrical seizures, unilateral or bilateral facial paresis/paralysis, vestibular deficits, laryngeal paresis/paralysis

T	Toxic	Any age and breed, either gender	Acute progressive	Possible or known exposure to toxic substances or plants	Dementia, stupor, coma, symmetrical seizures
T	Traumatic	Any age and breed, either gender	Acute non-progressive	Known or possibility of trauma, physical evidence of trauma	Stupor, coma, cranial nerve deficits, paresis/paralysis, symmetrical or asymmetrical
V	Vascular	Any age, large breed dogs most common, either gender (CVA, FCE)	Acute non-progressive	No known or possible trauma	Stupor, coma, often asymmetrical paresis/paralysis

DM= degenerative myelopathy common in German Shepherd, Boxer and Welsh Corgi dogs; IVDD= intervertebral disk disease common in Dachshund, Beagles, Miniature Poodles, Cocker Spaniels and many other dog breeds; CVA cerebrovascular accidents (brain); FCE= fibrocartilaginous embolism (spinal cord)

The DAMNITV scheme of the ten conventional etiologies of neurological disease is easy to remember so consideration can be given for the possibility of each, when formulating the conventional differential diagnosis for the neurological signs (Table 1).[3,4] The D= degenerative processes (e.g. degenerative intervertebral disk disease and degenerative myelopathy in dogs causing paresis or paralysis or geriatric cognitive dysfunction causing dementia). The A= anomalous or congenital disorders (e.g. congenital hydrocephalus, causing seizures or atlantoaxial malformations and cervical spondylomyelopathy of young dogs causing ataxia, paresis or paralysis). The M= metabolic disorders (e.g. hypoglycemia and hepatoencephalopathy, causing seizures). The N= nutritional and neoplastic disease. The I= inflammatory and idiopathic disorders (e.g. meningoencephalitis and idiopathic epilepsy causing seizures). The T= traumatic and toxic etiologies (e.g. automobile accidents and toxic substances causing stupor and seizures) and V= vascular disorders (e.g. fibrocartilaginous embolism causing hemiplegia or paraplegia). Details of questions concerning each etiology are beyond the scope of this text, but a brief outline of typical clinical findings associated with each disease mechanism is outlined in Table 1. With a thorough history, neurological examination and knowledge about the frequency of occurrence of different disorders, the conventional differential diagnosis can often be narrowed to 2-3 possibilities, which may reduce the necessity for invasive diagnostic tests.

During the TCVM evaluation, *Wen* is the history or inquiry part of *Si Zhen* (Four Diagnostic Methods).[1] *Wen* is very important and besides the typical history, other questions are asked, regarding personality traits, to determine the animal's basic Five Element constitution. Typically Wood animals are bossy and like to be in charge. Fire animals are hyperactive and like to be petted and loved. Earth animals are easy going, laid-back and sweet natured. Metal animals are confident and aloof. Water animals tend to be timid and fear biters. Questions regarding spontaneous episodes of panting, cool seeking and heat seeking behavior are also very important to determine if a Hot or Cold TCVM pattern is present. The types of food and medications consumed may contribute to the Hot or Cold signs and should be questioned as well. The typical TCVM pattern etiologies associated with each DAMNITV conventional etiology are outlined in Table 2. As can be seen, for many of the conventional etiologies, there can be different TCVM patterns with very different treatments. That is why when acupuncture, Chinese herbal medicine, *Tui-na* and Food Therapy are to be integrated with conventional therapy or used as a sole treatment, the TCVM pattern diagnoses must be known. Only in this way can the treatments be most effective and not cause harm, especially when Chinese herbal medicines are administered.

Table 2: TCVM patterns and clinical findings associated with conventional etiologies[1,3-5,8,9]

Conventional Etiology	TCVM Patterns	Clinical Findings	Tongue	Pulses
D — Degenerative (DM, IVDD)	Kidney *Jing* Deficiency (Combined with one of the patterns below)	Paresis/paralysis Breed predilection	Pale, wet, swollen	Deep, weak both sides
	Spleen *Qi* Deficiency	Pelvic limb weakness on rising, muscle atrophy	Pale, wet, swollen	Deep, weak, right weaker than left
	Kidney *Qi* Deficiency (*Tan-Huan* syndrome)	Paresis/paralysis Older dog	Pale, wet	Deep, weak, right weaker than left
	Kidney *Yang* Deficiency	Paresis/paralysis Older dog Seeks Heat Cold ears, feet and back	Pale, purple, wet, swollen	Deep, weak, right weaker than left, slow
	Kidney *Qi* and *Yin* Deficiencies	Paresis/paralysis Older dog Seeks Cool Panting Warm ears, feet and back	Pale, wet or red, dry, cracked	Deep, weak both sides, may be rapid and thready
	Kidney *Yang* and *Yin* Deficiencies	Paresis/paralysis Older dog Seeks Heat Cold ears, feet and back Panting Warm ears, feet and back Often Warm front, Cold rear	Pale, purple, wet, swollen or red, dry, cracked	Deep, weak both sides, may be rapid and thready
	Qi/Blood Stagnation (combined with one of the above patterns)	Neck or back pain Acute paresis/paralysis	Purple	Wiry

A	Anomalous (Congenital)	Kidney *Jing* Deficiency	Signs vary with each disorder, neonatal non-progressive or chronic progressive	Pale	Deep, weak both sides
M	Metabolic	Kidney *Jing* Deficiency with Liver *Qi* Stagnation	Seizures, dementia (portosystemic shunt, hepatoencephalopathy)	Pale or red	Deep, weak both sides or wiry
		Spleen *Qi* Deficiency with Liver *Yang* Rising	Seizures, dementia, stupor, coma (hypoglycemia)	Pale or red	Deep, weak worse on right or wiry
N	Nutritional	Liver *Yin* Deficiency	Seizures, dementia, stupor, coma (thiamine Deficiency)	Red, dry	Wiry or weak worse left, rapid, thready
		Liver Blood Deficiency	Seizures (thiamine Deficiency)	Pale, dry	Wiry or weak worse left
N	Neoplastic	Focal Brain or Spinal Cord Phlegm or Blood Stagnation	Seizures, head pain, progressive dementia or stupor, progressive paresis	Purple	Wiry
I	Inflammatory or infectious	Damp-Heat in the Brain or Spinal Cord or Heat in the *Ying* Stage (CNS)	Dementia, seizures, paresis or paralysis, may or not have fever, increased WBC and/or protein in the CSF	Red, dry, yellow coating	Superficial, forceful, rapid
		Obstruction by Wind Phlegm	Dementia, confusion, seizures, paresis, paralysis, increased WBC and/or protein in the CSF	Pale or purple with a white greasy coating	Wiry, slippery
I	Idiopathic	May involve Wind-Heat or Wind-Cold invasion of Channels or Deficiencies affecting Kidney, Liver and/or Spleen	Seizures, facial paresis/paralysis, vestibular signs, laryngeal paresis/paralysis	Vary depending on type of Excess or Deficiency pattern	Vary depending on type of Excess or Deficiency pattern
T	Toxic (substances or plants)	Liver *Yin* Deficiency with Heat Toxin	Seizures, tremors	Red, dry	Wiry
T	Traumatic	Brain *Qi*/Blood Stagnation	Stupor, coma, head pain, fractured skull	Purple	Wiry
		Spinal Cord *Qi*/Blood Stagnation	Acute paresis/paralysis, may be painful	Purple	Wiry
V	Vascular	Brain *Qi*/Blood Stagnation	Acute stupor or coma	Pale or purple	Weak or wiry

| | | (Wind-Stroke) | | | |
| | | Spinal Cord *Qi*/Blood Stagnation | Acute paresis/paralysis, not painful | Purple or purple | Weak or wiry |

CNS= central nervous system; WBC= white blood cells; CSF= cerebrospinal fluid

THE CONVENTIONAL PHYSICAL AND NEUROLOGICAL AND TCVM EXAMINATIONS

The routine physical examination is always performed to evaluate the other body systems.[3] Most veterinarians have the same physical examination routine they perform on all animals and usually obtain a complete blood count and serum biochemistry profile as well. Other clinicopathological tests may be warranted for some primary complaints, but will be described below in each conventional diagnosis discussion. If cardiopulmonary disease or neoplasia is suspected, thoracic and abdominal radiographs should also be obtained.

In order to properly evaluate the nervous system and localize lesions, a conventional neurological examination must also be performed.[2-4] Like the physical examination, the neurological examination can become routine and be completed within 7-10 minutes. The neurological examination consists of: 1) evaluation of the brain and cranial nerves 2) evaluation of the gait, 3) evaluation of tests of subtle dysfunction (e.g. hemistanding, hemiwalking, wheelbarrowing, hopping and conscious proprioception) 4) evaluation of spinal reflexes 7) examination for muscle atrophy 6) evaluation of superficial and deep sensations. A description of how to perform a neurological examination is beyond the scope of this text, but can be found elsewhere.[2-4]

If there is clinical evidence of a lesion above the level of the foramen magnum (the brain and cranial nerves), an attempt should be made to explain any abnormalities found on the rest of the neurological examination, as being associated with the brain lesion. If that is impossible, then a multifocal disease process must be present, but this is less common than a focal disease process. If the brain is normal, then a lesion, if present, is most likely below the foramen magnum affecting the spinal cord, spinal nerves or muscles. Lesions can usually be localized to one of the brain or spinal cord subdivisions, spinal nerves or muscles based on the neurological findings. An overview of the neurological examination findings with lesions at different locations can be found in Tables 3-5.

Besides assigning special meaning to conventional routine physical examination findings, the TCVM examination includes unique special observations such as: 1) ear, feet and body surface temperature, 2) skin, hair coat and dandruff changes 3) sensitivity along the Channels, 3) sensitivity at specific acupoints like the Back *Shu* Association points, Front *Mu* Alarm points, *Ah-shi* points or Trigger points, 4) tongue color, moisture level and coating and 5) pulse characteristics.[1,6,7] Typical clinical findings associated with TCVM patterns of neurological disorders by conventional etiology are outlined in Table 2. Ear, nose, body and feet temperatures are increased in Excess Heat patterns like Invasion of Wind-Heat or Damp-Heat (True Heat) and also with *Yin* Deficiency patterns (False Heat) like Kidney and Liver *Yin* Deficiency.[1] Reduced ear, nose, body and feet temperatures are common with Excess Cold patterns like Invasion of Wind-Cold (True Cold) and also with *Yang* Deficiency patterns (False Cold) like Kidney *Yang* Deficiency. Dry skin and small dandruff flakes are common in Heart, Liver and Kidney *Yin* Deficiencies causing neurological diseases. Extremely dry and burned appearing hair coat, large flakes of dandruff and cracked pads are common in animals with seizures associated with Liver Blood Deficiency.

Table 3: Localizing neurological signs, gait, tests of subtle dysfunction and spinal cord reflex changes with lesions of the central nervous system above the foramen magnum[2-4]

Lesion Location	Localizing Neurological Signs	Gait Coordination and Strength	Tests of Subtle Limb Dysfunction*	Spinal Cord Reflexes
Cerebrum Diencephalon	Pacing, circling, head pressing, dementia, stupor, coma, seizures, loss of smell (CN1) and blind with dilated pupils (CN2)	Transient quadriparesis or hemiparesis (acute lesions), normal (chronic lesions)	May be normal or decreased in one or more limbs	Normal or increased in all four limbs
Midbrain	Stupor, coma, dilated pupils (CN3), midrange fixed pupils, ventrolateral strabismus (CN3), deviation of vertical pupil in cats (CN4)	Quadriparesis or hemiparesis	Decreased or absent in one or more limbs	Normal or increased reflexes in all four limbs
Pons	Normal mentation, stupor or coma, atrophy of the temporal and masseter muscles, decreased or increased facial sensation (CN5)	Normal, hemiparesis or quadriparesis	Decreased or absent in one or more limbs	Normal or increased reflexes in all four limbs
Rostral Medulla Oblongata	Normal or depressed mentation, medial strabismus (CN6), facial paresis/paralysis (CN7), head tilt, nystagmus and/or disequilibrium (CN8)	Normal, hypermetria, hemiparesis, quadriparesis	Decreased or absent in one or more limbs	Normal or increased reflexes in all four limbs
Caudal Medulla Oblongata	Normal or depressed mentation, dysphagia megaesophagus laryngeal paresis/paralysis (CN 9/10/11), tongue paresis/paralysis, atrophy (CN12)	Normal, hemiparesis or quadriparesis	Decreased or absent in one or more limbs	Normal or increased reflexes in all four limbs

Cerebellum	Intention tremors and ataxia of the head, head tilt away from lesion, nystagmus, loss of menace response	Unilateral or bilateral ataxia, hypermetria or hypometria with normal limb strength	Ataxia, normal strength and conscious proprioception	Normal in all four limbs

*Tests of subtle dysfunction = hemistanding, hemiwalking, wheelbarrowing, hopping and conscious proprioception; May have one or more clinical signs; neurological deficits are on the side opposite the lesion in the cerebrum, diencephalon and upper midbrain; deficits are on the same side as the lesion in the lower midbrain, pons and medulla oblongata; CN =cranial nerves; CN deficits are on the same side as the lesion (except CN4); CN1 olfactory nerves, CN2 optic nerves, CN3 oculomotor nerves, CN4 trochlear nerves, CN5 trigeminal nerves, CN6 abducens nerves, CN7 facial nerves, CN8 vestibulocochlear nerves, CN9 glossopharyngeal nerves, CN10 vagus nerves, CN11 spinal accessory nerves and CN12 hypoglossal nerves.

Table 4: Neurological signs, gait, tests of subtle dysfunction and spinal cord reflex and sensation changes with lesions of the spinal cord and cauda equina nerve roots[2-4]

Lesion Location	Neurological Signs	Gait Coordination and Strength	Tests of Subtle Limb Dysfunction*	Spinal Cord Reflexes and Sensation
Spinal Cord C1- C5 Vertebrae C1- C4 -dog	+/- Horner's syndrome Normal brain and cranial nerves, fecal and/or urinary incontinence, +/- neck pain	Ataxia, hemiparesis, paraparesis, quadriparesis, quadriplegia (respiratory paralysis)	Normal, decreased or absent in one or more limbs	Normal or increased reflexes in all four limbs
Spinal Cord C6-T2 Vertebrae C5-T2 dog	+/- Horner's syndrome Normal brain and cranial nerves, fecal and/or urinary incontinence, +/- neck pain, atrophy of scapular muscles,	Ataxia, hemiparesis, paraparesis, quadriparesis, quadriplegia (respiratory paralysis)	Normal, decreased or absent in one or more limbs	Normal, decreased or absent reflexes in thoracic limbs, normal or increased reflexes in pelvic limbs
Spinal Cord T3-L3 Vertebrae T3-L2 dog	Normal brain and cranial nerves and thoracic limbs, fecal and urinary incontinence, +/- back pain	Pelvic limb ataxia, paraparesis/ paraplegia	Normal thoracic limbs, decreased or absent in one or both pelvic limbs	Normal reflexes in thoracic limbs, normal or increased reflexes in pelvic limbs, depressed or absent cutaneous trunci response from lesion site caudally, +/- deep pain
Spinal Cord and cauda equina nerve	Normal brain and cranial nerves and thoracic limbs, fecal	Pelvic limb ataxia, paraparesis/par	Normal thoracic limbs, decreased or	Normal reflexes in thoracic limbs Decreased or absent

roots L4-S2 Vertebrae L3- L7 dog	and urinary incontinence, pelvic limb muscle atrophy, +/- back pain	aplegia	absent in one or both pelvic limbs	patellar reflex with lesions at L4-5 (vertebrae L3-5)
				Decreased or absent flexor, gastrocnemius, and cranial tibial reflexes with lesions at L6-S2 (vertebrae L5-7)
				Decreased or absent anal reflex with lesions at S1-3 (vertebrae L5-S3)
				+/- deep pain
Cauda Equina nerve roots S1- Cd5 Vertebrae L5-S3 dog	Normal brain and cranial nerves and thoracic and pelvic limbs, mild pelvic limb ataxia and mild paraparesis, tail paralysis, fecal and urinary incontinence +/- sacrocaudal pain	Normal or may have mild pelvic limb ataxia or paresis	Normal thoracic and pelvic limbs or slightly decreased in one or both pelvic limbs	Normal reflexes in thoracic and pelvic limbs, decreased/absent anal reflex with S1-3 (vertebrae L5-S3) lesions, decreased or absent tail reflex with lesions at Cd1-5 (vertebrae L6-Cd)

*Tests of subtle dysfunction = hemistanding, hemiwalking, wheelbarrowing, hopping and conscious proprioception; May have one or more clinical signs; Clinical signs are always on the same side as the lesion; Horner's syndrome= ptosis, miosis, enophthalmos due to loss of sympathetic innervation to the eye

Table 5: Localizing clinical signs, gait, tests of subtle dysfunction, spinal cord reflex and sensation changes with lesions of the peripheral nervous system and muscles[2-4]

SIGNS OF COMMON PERIPHERAL CRANIAL NERVES AND MUSCLES LESIONS

Lesion Location	Localizing Clinical Signs	Gait Coordination and Strength	Tests of Subtle Limb Dysfunction*	Spinal Cord Reflexes and Limb Sensation
Optic nerves CN2	Blindness with dilated pupils unresponsive to light	Normal	Normal	Normal
Trigeminal nerves CN 5 (Motor nerves)	Inability to close the mouth or chew; atrophy of temporalis and masseter muscles	Normal	Normal	Normal

Lesion Location	Localizing Clinical Signs	Gait Strength and Coordination	Tests of Subtle Limb Dysfunction*	Spinal Cord Reflexes and Limb Sensation
Temporalis and masseter muscles	Pain and atrophy of the temporalis and masseter muscles, inability to open the mouth due to muscle fibrosis	Normal	Normal	Normal
Trigeminal nerves CN 5 (Sensory nerves)	Increased, reduced or absent sensation of the same side of the head	Normal	Normal	Normal
Facial nerves CN 7	Inability to close the eyelid, move the lips or ears on one or both sides	Normal	Normal	Normal
Vestibular nerves CN 8	Head tilt, nystagmus, swinging of the head from side to side (bilateral lesions)	Circling, falling, rolling toward side of lesion or generalized disequilibrium	Normal	Normal
Cochlear nerves CN 8	Deafness	Normal	Normal	Normal
Glossopharyngeal and Vagus nerves CN9 and CN10	Dysphagia, laryngeal paresis or paralysis, megaesophagus (bilateral nerve, neuromuscular junction or muscle lesion)	Normal	Normal	Normal

SIGNS OF COMMON PERIPHERAL SPINAL NERVES AND MUSCLE LESIONS

Lesion Location	Localizing Clinical Signs	Gait Strength and Coordination	Tests of Subtle Limb Dysfunction*	Spinal Cord Reflexes and Limb Sensation
Brachial plexus	Partial paresis or paralysis of the thoracic limb Horner's syndrome	Normal except for one thoracic limb	Abnormal in the affected limb but normal in the other limbs	Decreased/absent flexor, triceps and biceps reflexes, decreased/absent sensation, muscle atrophy
Sciatic nerve	Knuckling of the pelvic limb and inability to flex the stifle or flex and extend the hock and digits	Normal except for one pelvic limb	Abnormal in the affected limb but normal in the other limbs	Decreased/absent flexor, cranial tibial and gastrocnemius reflexes, decreased/absent sensation on all, but medial side of limb

Cauda equina	Dilated anus with fecal incontinence, flaccid bladder with urinary incontinence and tail paresis or paralysis	Often normal, but may have mild pelvic limb weakness similar to partial bilateral sciatic nerve dysfunction	Often normal	Decreased/absent anal reflex, decreased/absent sensation in the perineal area
Polyneuropathy	Normal brain and cranial nerves or one or more CN deficits, quadriparesis or quadriplegia with depressed or absent spinal reflexes	Paraparesis, quadriparesis, quadriplegia with respiratory paralysis and death	Decreased/absent in pelvic limbs or all four limbs	Decreased/absent patellar reflexes only, decreased/absent spinal reflexes in all four limbs, generalized muscle atrophy, increased or decreased/absent sensation
Polymyopathy	Normal brain and cranial nerves or may have temporalis and masseter muscle atrophy, Quadriparesis or quadriplegia with generalized muscle atrophy	Paraparesis, quadriparesis, quadriplegia with respiratory paralysis and death	Weak hemistanding, hemiwalking, wheelbarrowing and hopping, but conscious proprioception is normal	Spinal reflexes normal (except in severe cases), generalized muscle atrophy, normal sensation or muscle pain

*Tests of subtle dysfunction = hemistanding, hemiwalking, wheelbarrowing, hopping and conscious proprioception; Clinical signs are always on the same side as the lesion in peripheral nerve and muscle lesions

If increased sensitivity is found along a Channel, it usually means blocked *Qi*/Blood flow somewhere along that Channel.[1] Increased sensitivity of Back *Shu* Association points and Front *Mu* Alarm points may be associated with an imbalance in the associated *Zang* organ.[1] *Ah-shi* points and Trigger points may be due to local *Qi*/Blood Stagnation near the site of the painful point, but may also be referred from some distant somatic or visceral imbalance.[1,6,7] *Ah-shi* points are painful acupoints or other non-specific points that reflect pain in some part of the body. Trigger points may develop around muscle motor points (where motor nerve endings branch out to connect to muscle fibers) and result in a painful "knot" in the muscle.[7] Many Trigger points are also acupoints and some authors suggest that hypersensitive acupoints, *Ah-shi* points and Trigger points all have the same neural mechanism and acupuncture of these points results in pain relief.[1,6,7] In general, *Ah-shi* and Trigger points are associated with *Qi* and/or Blood Stagnation in the local area or the Channel that courses through the region.

Observation of the tongue color, moisture and coating and palpation of the femoral artery pulses are often most helpful to determine the TCVM pattern, causing the neurological signs (Table 2).[1] The tongue is red and dry and the pulses superficial, strong and forceful in the Excess patterns of Wind-Heat and Damp Heat invasion (e.g. idiopathic cranial neuropathies and meningoencephalitis respectively). The tongue is purple and the pulses are strong, but slow with the Excess pattern of Wind-Cold invasion (e.g. idiopathic cranial neuropathies). The pulses are usually wiry (taut like guitar string) in most TCVM patterns resulting in Internal Wind (seizures, tremors) or *Qi*/Blood Stagnation (pain, brain or spinal cord injury, vascular disorders or blood related tumors).

The tongue is typically pale and wet with Kidney, Spleen and Heart *Qi* Deficiency patterns. The pulses are deep and weak, worse on the right side and especially in the right Kidney position (most distal position) in Kidney *Qi* Deficiency. The tongue is typically red and dry and the pulses are deep, rapid and thready (thin), weaker on the left in *Yin* Deficiency. The pulses may be weaker in the Heart position (upper left) in Heart *Yin* Deficiency, weaker in the Liver position (left middle) in Liver *Yin* Deficiency and weaker in the Kidney position (left distal) in Kidney *Yin* Deficiency. The tongue is pale and dry with Blood Deficiency and the pulses are deep and weak, often weaker on the left side (e.g. Liver Blood Deficiency, resulting in seizures).

The specific clinical manifestation of a TCVM pattern will vary in an individual animal based on the following factors: 1) Constitution, 2) Prenatal *Jing* (e.g. Breed predisposition and genetic factors), 3) post-natal *Jing* levels (e.g. diet and function of the Spleen), 4) life style (e.g. balanced activity and rest periods, sedentary or excessive activity and training), 5) environmental stressors (e.g. household human and animal interaction stress levels, climate, pollution and pesticide and radiation exposure) and 6) concurrent chronic illness (imbalances) in other TCVM systems (e.g. creating a pathological cycle according to the Five Element *Zang* organ relationships). The same TCVM pattern can have many different neurological disease manifestations (one pattern many diseases), as listed in Table 6. Several different individual TCVM patterns or combinations of TCVM patterns may be associated with a single conventional diagnosis (one disease many patterns), as outlined in Table 6. A combination of Excess and Deficiency patterns involving several Channels and/or one or more *Zang* organs is typically found in most neurological disorders and each TCVM pattern must be treated for optimum results.

Table 6: Overview of TCVM Patterns associated with common conventional neurological diagnoses at different anatomic locations

Excess Patterns and Conventional Neurological Disorders by Anatomic Region				
TCVM pattern	**Brain**	**Cranial Nerves and Muscles**	**Spinal Cord**	**Spinal Nerves and Muscles**
Wind-Heat Invasion	Idiopathic tremors of adult dogs	Optic neuritis, Idiopathic trigeminal neuritis, Idiopathic facial paralysis, Idiopathic laryngeal paresis or paralysis, Masticatory myopathy	*	Polyradiculoneuritis Polymyositis
Wind-Cold Invasion	*	Idiopathic facial paresis/paralysis, Idiopathic vestibular disease, May find others with more experience	*	Polyradiculoneuritis

Damp-Heat	Meningoencephalitis Encephalitis	Facial paresis or paralysis (otitis media) Vestibular signs (otitis interna) Deafness (bilateral otitis media/interna)	Diskospondylitis Meningitis, Meningomyelitis, Myelitis	*
Qi/Blood Stagnation (Associated with a TCVM pathogen or underlying Deficiency)	Idiopathic tremors of adult dogs	Optic neuritis Idiopathic trigeminal neuritis Idiopathic facial paralysis Idiopathic laryngeal paresis or paralysis Masticatory myopathy	Intervertebral disk disease, Cervical spondylomyelopathy, Fibrocartilaginous embolism, Atlantoaxial malformation	Polyradiculoneuritis Polyneuritis Polymyositis
Qi Blood Stagnation (Associated with trauma)	Head Injury	Facial nerve injury Vestibular nerve injury Laryngeal nerve injury	Spinal cord injury	Brachial plexus injury Sciatic nerve injury Cauda equina injury
Phlegm or Blood Stagnation	Brain tumors	Cranial nerve tumors	Spinal cord tumors	Peripheral nerve tumors

Deficiency Patterns and Conventional Neurological Disorders by Region

TCVM Pattern	Brain	Cranial Nerves	Spinal Cord	Spinal Nerves and Muscles
Kidney *Jing* Deficiency	Inherited epilepsy, congenital hydrocephalus	Idiopathic vestibular syndrome, congenital deafness, laryngeal paresis	Cervical spondylomyelopathy, degenerative myelopathy, atlantoaxial malformation	Muscular dystrophy and other inherited polymyopathies and polyneuropathies
Kidney *Yin* Deficiency	Idiopathic epilepsy	*	Intervertebral disk disease, cervical spondylomyelopathy, degenerative myelopathy	Diabetic polyneuropathy
Kidney *Qi* Deficiency	Geriatric pelvic limb tremors	Deafness	Intervertebral disk disease, cervical spondylomyelopathy degenerative myelopathy, spinal cord tumors	Polyneuropathy, myasthenia gravis, polymyositis
Kidney *Yang* Deficiency	*	*	Intervertebral disk disease, cervical spondylomyelopathy, degenerative myelopathy	*

Liver *Yin* Deficiency	Idiopathic epilepsy	*	Degenerative myelopathy	*
Liver Blood Deficiency	Idiopathic epilepsy	*	*	*
Spleen *Qi* Deficiency	Hypoglycemia, geriatric cognitive dysfunction, congenital hydrocephalus, geriatric pelvic limb tremors	Idiopathic vestibular syndrome	Degenerative myelopathy	Idiopathic polyneuropathy, myasthenia gravis, polymyositis
Heart *Qi* Deficiency	Geriatric cognitive dysfunction	*	*	*
Heart *Yin* Deficiency	Geriatric cognitive dysfunction	*	*	*
Heart Blood Deficiency	Geriatric cognitive dysfunction	*	*	*

* Neurological disorders in this region not found for this pattern; Note: the same TCVM pattern can have many different conventional neurological disease manifestations (one pattern many diseases); each conventional neurological disease may also be caused by several different individual TCVM patterns or combinations of TCVM patterns (one disease many patterns).

Combining the information gained from the signalment, history and physical, neurological and TCVM examinations, the correct TCVM pattern(s) can be identified (*Bian Zheng*) and an effective TCVM treatment strategy planned to treat the clinical signs, TCVM pattern and constitution of the animal. The appropriate acupuncture technique and acupoints can be selected and Chinese herbal medicines prescribed. Further, Food to treat the TCVM disease pattern and *Tui-na* techniques to further relieve *Qi*/Blood Stagnation and tonify Deficiencies can also be added to the treatment regime to restore homeostasis and normal neurological function (Tables 7 and 8). The integration of knowledge from both conventional medicine and TCVM can ultimately result in more effective treatments with fewer side effects and improved patient care and quality of life. The TCVM patterns and suggested treatment associated with thirty-one conventional neurological diagnoses are outlined below. With more documented clinical experience and experimental studies of the TCVM treatment of neurological disorders, other disease patterns will most likely be identified and the current patterns and treatments suggested modified, so this chapter represents an initial attempt to integrate TCVM patterns and specific conventional diagnoses for neurological diseases.

Table 7: Food Therapy for TCVM Deficiency and Excess patterns associated with neurological disorders[10]

Foods for Deficiency Patterns	
Food Attributes and TCVM Patterns Treated	**Foods to Supplement**
Food that tonify *Jing* to to treat Kidney *Jing* Deficiency	Liver, kidneys, fish, bone and bone marrow, millet, quinoa, spelt, wheat, almonds, black sesame, microalgae (e.g. chlorella, spirulina, wild blue-green algae), barley, wheat grass, black soy beans, black beans, kidney beans, seaweed, sea salt, mulberries, raspberries, strawberries, almonds, black sesame, clarified butter (ghee), royal jelly, bee pollen
Foods that tonify Blood to treat Heart Blood and Liver Blood Deficiencies	Beef, bone marrow, eggs, liver, heart, pheasant, oysters, salmon, sardines, barley, corn, oats, short grain (glutinous rice), wheat, adzuki, black kidney beans, beet root, carrots, dark leafy greens, kelp, microalgae, cherries, dates, figs, longan, molasses
Foods that tonify *Qi* to treat Kidney *Qi*, Heart *Qi* and Spleen *Qi* Deficiencies and local *Qi* Deficiencies	Beef, chicken, sardines, egg, potato, yam, sweet potato, rice, oats, millet, lentils, carrots, squash, microalgae, dates, figs, molasses, royal jelly
Foods that clear false Heat and tonify *Yin* to treat Liver *Yin* and Kidney *Yin* Deficiencies	Turkey, pork, duck, clams, crab, eggs, rice, wheat, wheat germ, wheat berries, Belgian endive, string beans, peas, kidney beans, sweet potatoes, yams, tomato, spinach, tofu, kiwi, lemons, rhubarb, pears, bananas, watermelon, sesame, seaweed
Foods that clear false Cold and tonify *Yang* to treat Kidney *Yang* Deficiency	Chicken, lamb, corn fed beef, corn, millet, oats, brown rice, microalgae, pumpkin, squash, rutabaga, shiitake mushrooms, yams, sweet potatoes, winter squash, cherries, dates, figs, hawthorn fruit, lychees, molasses, royal jelly

Foods for Excess Patterns	
Food Attributes and TCVM Patterns Treated	**Foods to Supplement**
Foods that promote *Qi*/Blood circulation to treat *Qi*/Blood Stagnation	Chicken eggs, crab, sweet rice, peaches, carrots, coriander, squash, turnips
Foods that drain Damp to treat Excess Damp	Eel, mackerel, quail, corn, barley, rye, blueberries, celery, mushrooms

Foods that create Damp to <u>avoid</u> in Damp patterns	<u>Avoid</u> in Damp patterns and <u>do not supplement</u>: Pork, eggs, milk, cheese, yoghurt, ghee, bananas, sugar
Foods that soothe Liver *Qi* and calm *Shen* to treat Liver *Qi* Stagnation with Liver *Yang* Rising and Internal Profusion of Phlegm-Fire	Crayfish, duck, shrimp, brown rice, oats, spelt, wheat, wheat germ, Belgian endive hearts, celery, cucumbers, kohlrabi, lettuce, legumes, mung beans and sprouts, mushrooms, radishes, rhubarb, seaweed, spinach, sprouts, lemons, apples, mangos, mulberries, schisandra berries, jujube seeds, basil, chamomile, catnip, coriander, dill, ginger in small amount, garlic in small amount, marjoram, skullcap, valerian, vinegar (small amount)
Foods that soothe the Liver and dispel Internal Wind to generally treat Seizures and Tremors (Avoid Hot foods in *Yin* Deficiencies)	Chicken, lamb, carrot, chestnut, hawthorn berry, tangerine peel, parsley, radish, chive, coriander, dill seed, ginger, turmeric, vinegar
Foods that Clear Fire and reduce Phlegm to treat Internal Profusion of Phlegm-Fire	Grass fed beef, clams, duck, sardines, turkey, deep ocean fish, barley, brown rice, alfalfa sprouts, asparagus, avocado, bok choy, broccoli, celery, Chinese cabbage (Napa cabbage), cucumbers, dandelion greens, mushrooms, potatoes, seaweed, spinach, tofu, tomatoes, bananas, lemons, rhubarb, watermelon
Cold foods to Clear Wind-Heat and Heat toxin to treat Invasion of Wind-Heat, Heat or Heat Toxin	Turkey, duck, duck eggs, conch, clams, mussels, yogurt, millet, barley, spinach, broccoli, celery, egg plant, kelp, alfalfa, cucumbers, pears, bananas, white radishes, watermelon
Hot foods to Clear Wind-Cold for Invasion of Wind-Cold	Lamb, shrimp, corn-fed beef, chicken, trout, squash, turnips, sweet rice, basal, caraway, cherries, chilies, cinnamon, ginger, rosemary, sage
Foods that tonify the Spleen to transform Phlegm	Chicken, oats, glutinous rice, brown rice, pumpkin, squash, sweet potato, almond, garlic, ginger, pear, radish, seaweed, thyme

Food therapy is most important for Deficiency patterns, but can be useful for Excess patterns too

Table 8: Descriptions, actions and indications of *Tui-na* techniques useful to treat neurological disorders[11]

Name	Description of Technique	Actions and Indications
An-fa Pressing	Applying gentle pressure to acupoints and *Ah-shi* points and other areas with the finger or palm (see *Dian-fa*)	Invigorates *Qi* and Blood and relieves Stagnation
Ba-shen-fa Stretching	While holding and supporting, gently stretch the neck, tail, limbs or digits straight, forward and backward	Regulates *Qi* flow in the Channels
Ban-fa Wrenching	Bending joints to increase range of motion	Corrects malposition and increases smooth joint movements
Ca-fa Rubbing	Rapid, linear and mildly forceful rubbing firmly touching the skin using the palms of the hands	Heats the underlying tissue and is especially good for

	for larger areas and the thumb for smaller areas	Kidney *Yang* Deficiency
Cuo-fa Kneading	With the palms of both hands hold the neck and rub forward and back	Invigorates *Qi* and Blood, regulates the Channels
Dian-fa Knocking	Applying deeper pressure on acupoints and *Ah-Shi* points than *An-fa*, using the finger tips, knuckle or elbow; also called acupressure or *shiatsu*	Invigorates Blood, relieves pain, balances *Zang-fu* functions
Dou-fa Shaking	Gently shake the limb, while holding it out stretched	Invigorates *Qi* and Blood flow and relaxes the joints
Gun-fa Rolling	Using the back of the hand, proximal to the fifth metatarsal, perform a cyclical rotary movement on the skin and deeper tissues	Invigorates the Blood, relaxes the tendons and joints, reduces pain in back and neck
Mo-fa Touching and rubbing	Touching or rubbing in a circular motion with the palm of the hand or one or more fingers	Improves Blood and *Qi* circulation in subcutaneous tissues
Moo-fa Massaging/Daubing	Up and down or side to side motion with the thumbs or fingers	Calms the spirit, benefits the eyes
Na-fa Pulling	Similar to *Nie-fa* (below) except involves grasping the muscle, along with the epidermis and dermis, between the thumb and fingers and lifting and holding	Improves Blood and *Qi* circulation in the Channels
Nian-fa Holding and kneading	The digits are grasped between the thumb and forefinger and light traction is applied, while kneading the digit from side to side	Invigorates Blood and *Qi* circulation in the Channels
Nie-fa Pinching and squeezing	Pinching and squeezing the epidermis and dermis with the fingers going up and down the neck and back or at acupoints; easy for clients to do at home	Invigorates the *Qi* and Blood, regulates the Spleen and Stomach
Rou-fa Rotary Kneading	Rotary kneading using the heel of the palm on the superficial dermal tissues	Soothing and calming, reduces pain
Tui-fa Pushing	Strong pushing movement using the finger, palm, thumb or elbow; push deeply in one direction along the vertebral column and other areas to lengthen, soften and divide the connective tissue	Powerful myofascial bodywork, improves Blood circulation, relaxes tendons, dissipates nodules and masses
Yao-fa Rocking	Similar to performing range of motion manipulation, gently flex and extend joints limbs, neck and back	Unblocks *Qi* Stagnation in the Channels
Yi-zhi-chan Single thumb	Using the thumb pressed on the acupoint or other area, rapidly push in and out (120 times/minute)	Promotes *Qi* and Blood circulation in the Channels

References:
1. Xie H, Priest V. Traditional Chinese Veterinary Medicine. Reddick, FL: Jing Tang Publishing 2002:209-293,307-380,409-419.
2. De Lahunta A, Glass E. Veterinary Neuroanatomy and Clinical Neurology 3nd Ed. Philadelphia, PA:WB Saunders 2008:95-113,14.

3. Chrisman C, Mariani C, Platt S, Clemmons R. Neurology for the Small Animal Practitioner. Jackson Wy: Teton NewMedia 2003:125-167.
4. Platt S, Olby N (ed). BSAVA Manual of Canine and Feline Neurology 5th Ed. Gloucester, UK:BSAVA Publications 2012:1-500.
5. Kline KL, Caplan ER, Joseph RJ. Acupuncture for neurological disorders. In Schoen AM (ed) Veterinary Acupuncture 2nd Ed. St Louis, Mo: Mosby Publishing 2001:179-192.
6. Hwang YC, Egerbacher M. Anatomy and classification of acupoints. In Schoen AM (ed). Veterinary Acupuncture 2nd Ed. St. Louis, MO: Mosby 2001:33,21-22.
7. Janssens LA. Trigger point therapy. In Schoen AM (ed). Veterinary Acupuncture 2nd Ed. St. Louis, MO:Mosby 2001:201-203.
8. Xie H, Priest V. Xie's Veterinary Acupuncture. Ames, Iowa:Blackwell Publishing 2007:585.
9. Xie H, Preast V. Chinese Veterinary Herbal Handbook 2nd Ed. Reddick, FL: Chi Institute of Chinese Medicine 2008:305-585.
10. Leggett D. Helping Ourselves: A Guide to Traditional Chinese Food Energetics. Totnes, England: Meridian Press 2005:21-36.
11. Xie H, Ferguson B, Deng X. Application of *Tui-na* in Veterinary Medicine 2nd Ed. Reddick, FL:Chi Institute 2007:1-94,129-132.

Recent Research on Acupuncture for Neurological Disorders

Songhua Hu, DVM, PhD, MS

ABSTRACT:
Acupuncture treatment is useful for relief of neurological disorders such as the pain found in diabetic peripheral neuropathy. The mechanisms underlying the acupuncture treatment remain unclear. Recent investigations indicate that the spinal GABA receptors and the opioid receptors mediate the acupuncture effects. Although the brain and spinal cord are surrounded by strong membranes, enclosed in the bones of the skull and spinal vertebrae, and isolated by the so-called blood-brain barrier, they are very susceptible if compromised. Peripheral nerves are inclined to lie deep under the skin but are also still relatively exposed to damage. The specific causes vary by disorder and sometimes by individual case, but can include genetic disorders, congenital abnormalities, infections, malnutrition and brain injury, spinal cord injury or nerve injury. The problem may start in another body system that interacts with the nervous system; for example cerebrovascular disorders involve brain injury due to problems with the blood vessels (cardiovascular system) supplying the brain, and autoimmune disorders involve damage caused by the body's own immune system. A neurological disorder is an illness of the body's nervous system. Structural, biochemical or electrical malfunction in the brain, spinal cord, or in the nerves can result in symptoms such as paralysis, muscle weakness, loss of sensation, seizures, pain and altered levels of consciousness. Interventions include preventative measures, lifestyle changes, physiotherapy or other therapy, neurorehabilitation, pain management, medication, or operations performed by neurosurgeons.

Peripheral nerve injury often causes chronic neuropathic pain characterized by a spontaneous burning sensation, hyperalgesia, and allodynia.[1] It has been shown that neuropathic pain is often poorly responsive to common analgesics like morphine.[2] Therefore, alternative medicine, such as acupuncture, is usually used in patients who cannot find suitable ways to treat. Acupuncture is an approach to stimulate skin regions called acupoints by a variety of techniques, including insertion of small, thin needles through the skin surface followed by manual or electrical manipulation.[3] Acupuncture has long been used as a therapeutic treatment in Chinese medicine and is known to be effective in relieving chronic pain.[4-8] In addition to the clinical observations on the effectiveness of acupuncture therapy, recent research has paid much attention to the mechanisms of acupuncture treatment.

1. Acupuncture treatment relieves diabetic peripheral neuropathy in humans

Diabetic peripheral neuropathy (DPN) is the most common late complication of diabetes, often associated with its morbidity and mortality.[9] It is estimated that 12–50% of people with diabetes have some level of DPN.[10] About 15% of people with diabetes develop at least one foot ulcer during their lifetime.[11-12] While vascular disease leading to ischemia is certainly a factor in the pathogenesis, 60–70% of diabetic foot ulcers primarily originates from neuropathy.[12] Symptoms include loss of sensation, strength, prickling or pain.[13] The patients have reduced nerve conduction velocity, decreased temperature sensation, decreased tendon reflex response, and a decreased ability to detect vibration and touch.

Although many trials have shown that strictly glycemic control diminishes the incidence and progression of diabetes-related complications,[14,15] this method alone does not entirely get rid of complications. Thus development of new therapy to manage diabetes complications is needed. Acupuncture, one of the most commonly used forms of alternative medicine, has been practiced for more than 2500 years in China. In traditional acupuncture, needles are inserted into precisely defined, specific points on the body, each of which has distinct therapeutic actions.[16] According to traditional Chinese medicine (TCM), when an acupoint is stimulated, treatment effects have a tendency to occur on the specific parts of the body along a particular meridian that contains this specific acupoint. As a safe form of treatment, acupuncture offers clear clinical advantages in reduction of symptoms related to nervous disorders. Paul et al.[17] reported that two of the total three patients showed increased benefit when a series of six acupuncture sessions was added to the ongoing nefazodone therapy for the treatment of DPN. In a randomized controlled trial in China, Chen et al.[18] concluded that the point through point method of acupuncture was superior to mecobalamin for the improvement of motor nerve conduction velocity (MNCV) of the common peroneal nerve. The results of another randomized trial showed that acupuncture lowered the pain in DPN.[19]

Tong et al.[20] compared 42 cases treated with acupuncture and 21 cases exposed to sham acupuncture. Three of the six measures of motor nerves, and two measures of sensory function, demonstrated significant improvement over the 15-day treatment period in the acupuncture group, while no motor or sensory function significantly improved in the sham acupuncture group. There were also significant differences in vibration perception threshold between the groups and when compared to the baseline levels in the acupuncture group. Acupuncture was significantly more effective than sham for treatment of numbness of the lower extremities, spontaneous pain in the lower extremities, rigidity in the upper extremities and alterations in temperature perception in the lower extremities after therapy. Therefore, acupuncture is useful for the treatment of diabetic peripheral neuropathy.

2. Spinal GABA receptors mediate the suppressive effect of electroacupuncture (EA) on cold allodynia in rats

Neuropathic pain is often caused by peripheral nerve injury, and is still one of the most complicated clinical syndromes to treat. It is characterized by spontaneous burning pain, hyperalgesia (an increased response to a stimulus which is normally painful) and allodynia (a pain as a result of a stimulus which does not normally provoke pain). The underlying mechanisms are complex and appear to involve both peripheral and central components of the nervous system.[21] Moreover, therapeutic consequence of conventional analgesics have been observed as variable. Recent animal studies by several groups demonstrated that EA significantly relieved mechanical and heat hyperalgesia,[22] mechanical allodynia[23] and cold allodynia[24] in rat models.

GABA is an important inhibitory neurotransmitter in the CNS and is involved in multiple physiological and pathological functions. In the spinal cord, GABA exerts tonic modulation of nociceptive neurotransmission between primary afferents and second-order spino-thalamic tract neurons.[25] There are three GABA receptor subtypes: $GABA_A$, $GABA_B$ and $GABA_C$[26]. It has been known that $GABA_A$ and $GABA_B$ receptors contribute to modulation of pain.[27] It has been shown that $GABA_A$ and $GABA_B$ receptors are present in the rat spinal cord[28] and $GABA_A$ and $GABA_B$ receptor agonists have antinociceptive effects in a variety of rodent models.[29]

Park et al.[30] reported that spinal GABAergic systems mediate the relieving effects of low frequency EA on cold allodynia in a rat tail model of neuropathic pain. For neuropathic surgery, the right superior caudal trunk was resected at the level between the S1 and S2 spinal nerves innervating the tail. Two weeks after the nerve injury, the intrathecal catheter was implanted. Five days after the catheterization, rats were intrathecally injected with gabazine ($GABA_A$ receptor antagonist, 0.0003, 0.001 or 0.003 µg), or saclofen ($GABA_B$ receptor antagonist, 3, 10 or 30 µg). Ten minutes after the injection, EA (2 Hz) was applied to the ST-36 acupoint for 30 min. The cold allodynia was assessed by the tail immersion test (i.e. immersing the tail in cold (4 °C) water and measuring the latency of an abrupt tail movement) before and after the EA treatment. EA stimulation at ST-36 significantly inhibited the cold allodynia sign, whereas EA at non-acupoint and plain acupuncture at ST-36 (without electrical stimulation) did not show antiallodynic effects. Intrathecal administration of gabazine or saclofen blocked the relieving effects of ST-36 EA stimulation on cold allodynia. These results suggest that spinal $GABA_A$ and $GABA_B$ receptors mediate the suppressive effect of low frequency EA on cold allodynia in the tail neuropathic rats.

3. Spinal opioid receptors mediate the effects of electroacupuncture (EA) on mechanical allodynia in rats

Neuropathic pain is characterized by combined spontaneous burning pain, hyperalgesia and allodynia. The underlying mechanisms are complex and appear to involve various peripheral and central components of sensory systems.[31] Numerous studies have attempted to elucidate pathophysiological mechanisms or drug effects for abnormal sensation in patients or these animal models.[31] A wide range of drugs or methods have been used such as systemic local anesthetics, tricyclic antidepressants, α2-adrenergic receptor agonists and sympathectomy.[32] Unfortunately, the usual therapeutic outcome has been variable.[33] Therefore it is worth searching for additional therapeutic options for the relief of neuropathic pain.

The analgesic effects of EA on acute pain are believed to be mediated by the endogenous opioids.[34] In addition, the relieving effects of electrical acupuncture (EA) on mechanical allodynia were prevented by naloxone in neuropathic rats.[35] However, the effects of opioid on neuropathic pain remain controversial.[36]

Kim et al.[37] investigated the relieving effects of EA on mechanical allodynia and its mechanism related to the spinal opioid system in a rat model of neuropathic pain. To produce neuropathic pain in the tail, the right superior caudal trunk was resected between the S1 and S2 spinal nerves. Two weeks after the surgery, EA stimulation (2 or 100 Hz, 0.3 ms, 0.2–0.3 mA) was delivered to *Zu-san-li* (ST-36) for 30 min. The degree of mechanical allodynia was evaluated quantitatively by touching the tail with von Frey hair (2.0 g) at 10 min intervals. These rats were then subjected to an i.t. injection with one of the three specific opioid agonists in successive ways: the mu agonist (DAMGO 25, 50 and 100 pmol), the delta agonist (DADELT II 0.5, 1 and 2 nmol), and the kappa agonist (U50488H 5, 10 and 20 nmol) separated by 10 min in cumulative doses. During 30 min of EA stimulation, specific opioid antagonists were subjected to i.t. injection: the mu antagonist (h-FNA 5, 10 and 20 nmol), the delta antagonist (naltrindole 5, 10 and 20 nmol), and the kappa antagonist (nor-BNI 3, 6 and 12 nmol) separated by 10 min in cumulative doses. As a result, EA reduced the behavioral signs of mechanical allodynia. Two Hz EA induced a robust and longer lasting effect than 100 Hz. All three opioid agonists also showed relieving effects on mechanical allodynia. However, nor-BNI could not block the EA effects on mechanical allodynia, whereas h-FNA or naltrindole significantly blocked EA effects. These results suggest that the mu and delta, but not kappa, opioid receptors in the spinal cord of the rat, play important roles in mediating relieving effects on mechanical allodynia induced by 2 Hz EA.

References:
1. Talmoush AJ. Causalgia: Redefinition as a clinical pain syndrome. Pain 1981;10:187-97.

2. Arner S, Meyerson BA. Lack of analgesic effect of opioids on neuropathic and idiopathic forms of pain. Pain 1988;33:11-23.
3. Vincent CA, Richardson PH. The evaluation of therapeutic acupuncture: concepts and methods. Pain 1986;24:1-13.
4. Berman BM, Singh BB, Lao L, Langenberg P, Li H, Hadhazy V, et al. A randomized trial of acupuncture as an adjunctive therapy in osteoarthritis of the knee. Rheumatology (Oxford) 1999;38:346-54.
5. Birch S, Hammerschlag R, Berman BM. Acupuncture in the treatment of pain. J Altern Complement Med 1996; 2:101-24.
6. Ezzo J, Hadhazy V, Birch S, Lao L, Kaplan G, Hochberg M, et al. Acupuncture for osteoarthritis of the knee: a systematic review. Arthritis Rheum 2001;44:819-25.
7. Koo ST, Park YI, Lim KS, Chung K, Chung JM. Acupuncture analgesia in a new rat model of ankle sprain pain. Pain 2002;99:423-31.
8. Richardson PH, Vincent CA. Acupuncture for the treatment of pain: a review of evaluative research. Pain 1986;24:15-40.
9. Vinik AI, Mehrabyan A. Diabetic neuropathies. Med Clin North Am 2004;88:947-99.
10. Nicolucci A, Carinci F, Cavaliere D, Scorpiglione N, Belfiglio M, Labbrozzi D, et al. A meta-analysis of trials on aldose reductase inhibitors in diabetic peripheral neuropathy. Diabet Med 1996;13:1017-26.
11. Kantor J, Margolis DJ. Treatment options for diabetic neuropathic foot ulcers: a cost-effectiveness analysis. Dermatol Surg 2001;27:347-51.
12. Gonzalez ER, Oley MA. The management of lower-extremity diabetic ulcers. Manag Care Interface 2000;13:80-7.
13. Melton LJ III, Dyck PJ. Diabetic polyneuropathy. In: Dyck PJ, Thomas PK, eds. Diabetic Neuropathy, 2nd ed. Philadelphia: WB Saunders, 1999:49-50.
14. Diabetes Control and Complications Trial Research Group. The effect of intensive treatment of diabetes on the development and progression of long-term complications in insulin-dependent diabetes mellitus. N Engl J Med 1993; 329:977-86.
15. UK Prospective Diabetes Study (UKPDS) Group. Intensive blood-glucose control with sulphonylureas or insulin compared with conventional treatment and risk of complications in patients with type 2 diabetes (UKPDS 33). Lancet 1998;352:837-53.
16. Hurtak JJ. An overview of acupuncture medicine. J Altern Complement Med 2002;8:535-8.
17. Paul JG, Karen B, Xue LW, Adarsh K. Acupuncture and neuropathy. Am J Psychiatry 2000;157:1342-3.
18. Chen YL, Ma XM, Hou WG, Cen J, Yu XM, Zhang L. Effects of penetrating acupuncture on peripheral nerve conduction velocity in patients with diabetic peripheral neuropathy: a randomized controlled trial. Zhong Xi Yi Jie He Xue Bao 2009;7:273-5. [In Chinese]
19. Ahn AC, Bennani T, Freeman R, Hamdy O, Kaptchuk TJ. Two styles of acupuncture for treating painful diabetic neuropathy— a pilot randomised control trial. *Acupunct Med* 2007; 25:11-7.
20. Tong YQ, Guo HY, Han B. Fifteen-day Acupuncture Treatment Relieves Diabetic Peripheral Neuropathy. J Acupunct Meridian Stud 2010;3:95−103.
21. Bridges D, Thompson SWN, Rice ASC. Mechanisms of neuropathic pain. Br. J. Anaesth. 2001; 87: 12-26.

22. Dai Y, Kondo E, Fukuoka T, Tokunaga A, Miki K, Noguchi K. The effect of electroacupuncture on pain behaviors and noxious stimulus-evoked fos expression in a rat model of neuropathic pain. J. Pain 2001; 2: 151-59.
23. Huang C, Li HT, Shi YS, Han JS, Wan Y. Ketamine potentiates the effect of electroacupuncture on mechanical allodynia in a rat model of neuropathic pain. Neurosci. Lett. 2004; 368: 327-331.
24. Kim SK, Park JH, Bae SJ, Kim JH, Hwang BG, Min BI, Park DS, Na HS. Effects of electroacupuncture on cold allodynia in a rat model of neuropathic pain: mediation by spinal adrenergic and serotonergic receptors. Exp. Neurol. 2005; 195: 430–436.
25. Lin Q, Peng YB, Willis WD. Role of GABA receptor subtypes in inhibition of primate spinothalamic tract neurons: difference between spinal and periaqueductal gray inhibition. J. Neurophysiol. 1996; 75: 109-123.
26. Malcangio M, Bowery N. GABA and its receptors in the spinal cord. Trends Pharmacol. Sci. 1996; 17: 457–462.
27. Millan MJ. The induction of pain: an integrative review. Prog. Neurobiol. 1999; 57: 1-164.
28. Price GW, Wilkin GP, Turnbull MJ, Bowery NG. Are baclofen-sensitive GABAB receptors present on primary afferent terminals of the spinal cord? Nature 1984; 307: 71-74.
29. Sawynok J. GABAergic mechanisms of analgesia: an update. Pharmacol. Biochem. Behav. 1987; 26: 463-474.
30. Parka JH, Hana JB, Kim SK, Park JH, Go DH, Sun B, Min B. Spinal GABA receptors mediate the suppressive effect of electroacupuncture on cold allodynia in rats. Brain Research 2010; 1322: 24-29
31. Fields HL, Baron R, Rowbotham MC. Peripheral neuropathic pain: an approach to management, in: P.D. Wall, R. Melzack (Eds.), Textbook of Pain, Churchill Livingstone, Edinburgh, 1999, pp. 1523-1533.
32. Arner S, Lindblom U, Meyerson BA, Molander C. Prolonged relief of neuralgia after regional anesthetic blocks: a call for further experimental and systematic clinical studies, Pain 43 (1990) 287-297.
33. Lee DH, Katner J, Iyengar S, Lodge D. The effect of lumbar sympathectomy on increased tactile sensitivity in spinal nerve ligated rats. Neurosci. Lett. 2001; 298: 99-102.
34. Han JS. Acupuncture: neuropeptide release produced by electrical stimulation of different frequencies, Trends Neurosci. 2003; 26:17-22.
35. Hwang BG, Min BI, Kim JH, Na HS, Park DS. Effects of electroacupuncture on the mechanical allodynia in the rat model of neuropathic pain, Neurosci. Lett. 2001; 320: 49-52.
36. Dellemijn P. Are opioids effective in relieving neuropathic pain? Pain 1999; 80: 453- 462.

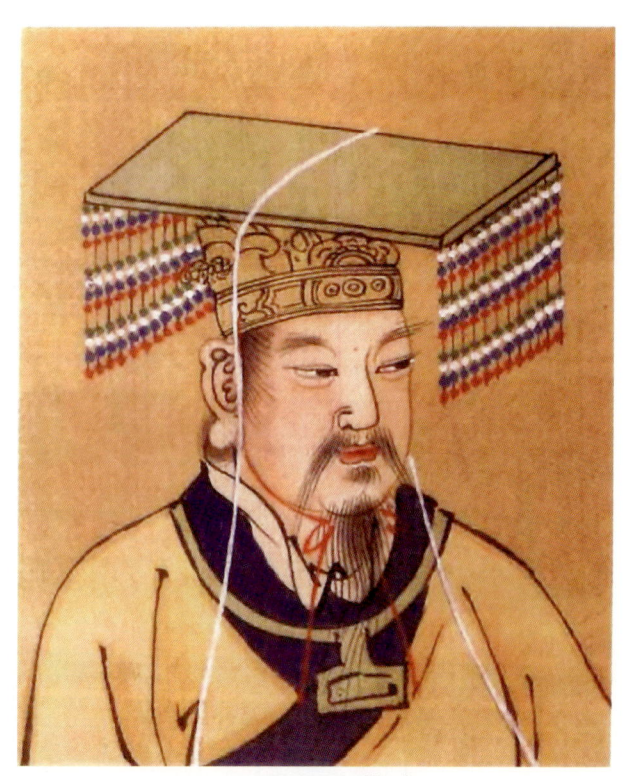

HUANG DI 黃帝

Huang Di, literally meaning Yellow Emperor, is believed to be the ancestor of all Chinese people and the founder of Chinese civilization. He was born in Qufu, Shandong Province about 4,700 years ago. His real name was Gongsun Xuanyuan. During that time, the majority of Chinese clans and tribes lived along the Yellow River and the Yangtze River. Huang Di became the most renowned tribal leader because his tribe flourished while other tribes including the one led by Yan Di (Shen Nong) began to decline. After defeating many tribes and clans, he reigned from 2,696 BCE to 2,598 BCE. Under Huang Di's leadership, palaces and boats were devised, arithmetic began to appear, people started to feed silkworms and spin thread into silk, early Chinese written characters and musical instruments were invented. Because Huang Di was the first leader to develop early Chinese civilization and due to his great moral fortitude and superior wisdom, all Chinese ethnic groups regard him as the forefather of the Chinese and call themselves the offspring of Huang Di.

In addition, Chinese medicine was developed during the Huang Di period. To honor his achievement, Huang Di was used as a part of the title of the most important Traditional Chinese Medicine (TCM) and Traditional Chinese Veterinary Medicine (TCVM) ancient textbook called *Huang Di Nei Jing* (*Yellow Emperor's Inner Canon*), written during the Warring States Period (475 to 221 BCE). This text is comparable in importance to the Hippocratic Corpus in Greek medicine. The work collects the theories and experiences of the ancient Chinese people in their struggle against disease, thereby documenting the fundamental principles, physiology, pathology, diagnosis, treatment, herbology and formulations, acupuncture, Channels and Meridians. It is composed of two texts: *Su Wen* (*Basic Questions*) and *Ling Shu* (*Spiritual Pivot*). To study *Huang Di Nei Jing* is one of the required curriculums for any TCM and TCVM education in China.

CHAPTER 2

Cerebral Disorders

Dementia, Stupor and Coma Disorders

Cheryl L Chrisman DVM, MS, EdS, DACVIM-Neurology, CVA

The reticular activating system is the central core of the brainstem that projects to the frontal region of the cerebrum to "awaken" the brain and is the location of lesions causing dementia, stupor and coma.[1-3] Dementia is usually a progressive loss of intellectual function and perception that results in changes in personality, routines, habits and normal responses to intellectual stimuli. Dementia in dogs and cats includes confusion, loss of house and obedience training, loss of recognition of the caretaker, staring off into space, getting lost in closets or corners and phobias. Dementia is usually associated with lesions of the cerebrum and diencephalon. Stupor is impaired consciousness with a reduced response to noxious and other environmental stimuli and can be mild to severe. Coma is unconsciousness with no responses to any stimulus. Stupor and coma may be associated with lesions of the brainstem reticular activating system or cerebrum. Lesions of the midbrain, pons and medulla oblongata usually have associated cranial nerve deficits that localize lesions to one of these brainstem segments. The level of consciousness may be graded on a scale from 1 to 6 (1=most severe and 6= mildest) as part of the modified Glasgow Coma Scale adapted to dogs.[4]

1= Comatose and unresponsive to repeated noxious stimuli
2= Semicomatose and responsive only to repeated noxious stimuli
3= Semicomatose and responsive to auditory and noxious stimuli
4= Semicomatose and responsive to visual, auditory and noxious stimuli
5= Depression or delirium, capable of responding, but the response may be inappropriate
6= Occasional periods of alertness and responsiveness to environment

Serial evaluations and grading of consciousness can be compared to determine the effectiveness of conventional and TCVM treatments over time.

The most common conventional causes of acute dementia, stupor and coma are head injury, toxicity, hypoglycemia, hepatic encephalopathy, meningoencephalitis and cerebrovascular disorders. The most common conventional causes of chronic progressive dementia and stupor are meningoencephalitis, geriatric cognitive dysfunction, hypoglycemia, hepatic encephalopathy, hydrocephalus and brain tumors. When an animal is presented with dementia, stupor or coma with no history of trauma or exposure to toxic substances, a thorough history, physical, neurological and TCVM examinations, complete blood count, fasting serum biochemistry profile and fasting and post-prandial bile acids are essential to rule out metabolic disorders. Referral to a neurologist for further diagnostic tests may be necessary to obtain a definitive diagnosis. A cerebrospinal fluid (CSF) analysis is needed to diagnose meningoencephalitis and a magnetic resonance imaging (MRI) or computerized axial tomography (CT) is needed to confirm hydrocephalus, meningoencephalitis or a brain tumor.[2,3] Hypoglycemia, hepatic encephalopathy and intoxications are usually treated with conventional methods and rarely referred to TCVM practitioners for treatment, but TCVM patterns and supportive treatment are outlined in Tables 1 and 2.[5-7]

Table 1: Common conventional diagnoses and traditional Chinese veterinary medicine (TCVM) patterns and examination findings associated with dementia, stupor and coma[5-7]

Conventional Diagnosis	TCVM Pattern	Clinical Findings	Tongue	Pulses
Hypoglycemia	Spleen *Qi* Deficiency with Liver *Yang* Rising	Dementia, stupor, coma, Seizures, low serum glucose	Pale or red (Liver *Yang* Rising)	Deep, weak worse on right or wiry
Portosystemic Liver shunt	Kidney *Jing* Deficiency with Liver *Qi* Stagnation	Dementia, stupor, coma, stunted growth, low blood urea nitrogen, low serum albumin, elevated bile acids, liver enzymes usually normal	Pale	Deep, weak
Head injury	Brain *Qi*/Blood Stagnation without Phlegm	History or physical evidence of trauma, dementia, stupor, coma, may have seizures immediately or up to 2 years later	Pale or purple	Wiry or weak
Head injury	Brain *Qi*/Blood Stagnation with Phlegm	History or physical evidence of trauma, dementia, stupor, coma, may have seizures immediately or up to 2 years later	Pale or purple, white greasy coat	Wiry or weak and slippery
Geriatric cognitive dysfunction	Spleen *Qi* and Heart *Qi* Deficiencies with Phlegm Misting the Mind	Cognitive decline, loss of interest in food	Pale, wet	Deep, weaker on right
Geriatric cognitive dysfunction	Heart *Yin* and Blood Deficiencies with Blood Stagnation in the Brain	Cognitive decline, barks, howls, yowls especially at night, anxious, fearful, phobias	Red or pale, dry	Deep, thready, weaker on the left
Meningoencephalitis Encephalitis	Damp Heat in the Brain (Heat In the *Ying* Stage)	Acute dementia, seizures, paresis or paralysis, may or not have fever, increased WBC in CSF	Red, yellow coating, dry	Superficial, forceful, rapid, wiry
Meningoencephalitis Encephalitis	Obstruction by Wind-Phlegm	Acute dementia, seizures, paresis or paralysis, no fever or evidence of Heat, increased WBC in CSF	Pale or purple with a white greasy coating	Wiry, slippery
Brain tumor	Brain Phlegm	Progressive dementia,	Pale, white	Slippery

		seizures, head may be painful on palpation, non-blood related tumors	greasy coat	
	Brain Blood Stagnation	Progressive dementia, seizures, head may be painful on palpation, blood related tumors	Purple	Wiry

CNS= central nervous system; WBC= white blood cells; CSF= cerebrospinal fluid; may not have all of the listed clinical signs

Table 2: Treatment strategy, acupuncture points and Chinese herbal medicine used to treat dementia, stupor and coma*[5-9]

Conventional Diagnosis	TCVM Pattern	TCVM Treatment Strategy	Acupuncture points[5]	Chinese Herbal Medicine**	Comments
Hypoglycemia	Spleen *Qi* Deficiency with Liver *Yang* Rising	Dispel Internal Wind Tonify Spleen Soothe the Liver	BL-20, BL-21, SP-3, ST-36, LI-10	*Tian Ma Bai Zhu*	May be controlled with diet alone in cases not associated with pancreatic tumors
Portosystemic shunt	Kidney *Jing* Deficiency with Liver *Qi* Stagnation	Nourish Kidney *Jing* Soothe liver *Qi*	KID-3, BL-23, LI-10, ST-36, LIV-3, BL-18, BL-19, KID-10, CV-4, CV-6	Epimedium Formula and *Xiao Yao San*	Often require surgery and long-term intermittent treatment; feed low protein diet
Head Injury	Brain *Qi*/Blood Stagnation (with or without Phlegm)	Stop bleeding Move *Qi* and Blood to resolve pain and Stagnation	EA: GV-26/GV-14, *Nao-shu/Nao-shu*, PC-6/PC-6, HT-9/HT-9, KID-1/KID-1 DN: PC-9, LU-7, ST-40 (if Phlegm present)	*Yunnan Bai Yao* red pellets Stasis in Mansion of Mind	*Yunnan Bai Yao* for 1 week. Stasis in Mansion of Mind for 1-3 months or longer if needed
Geriatric cognitive dysfunction	Spleen *Qi* and Heart *Qi* Deficiencies with Phlegm Misting the Mind	Tonify Heart and Spleen, dispel Phlegm and unblock *Shen*	EA: *Tian-men/Long-hui*, GV-20/*Nao-shu*, *Da-feng-men*/TH-23 DN: HT-7, HT-9, BL-14, BL-15, BL-20, BL-21, CV-14, CV-17, ST-40, ST-36, LI-10	*Wen Dan Tang* and Stasis in Mansion of Mind	Treat for 3-6 months then as needed for maintenance
	Heart *Yin* and Blood	Nourish *Yin* and Blood,	EA: *Tian-men/Long-hui*,	Shen Calmer and Stasis in	Treat for 3-6 months then as

Condition	Pattern	Principle	Acupuncture	Herbal Formula	Notes
	Deficiencies with Blood Stagnation in the Brain	resolve Blood Stagnation	GV-20/*Nao-shu*, *Da-feng-men*/TH-23 **DN:** HT-7, HT-9, BL-14, BL-15, BL-17, BL-43, BL-44, SP-6, SP-9, SP-10, KID-3	Mansion of Mind	needed for maintenance
Meningo-encephalitis/ Encephalitis	Damp-Heat in the Brain (Heat in the *Ying* Stage)	Clear Heat in the *Ying* Stage and Damp Heat in Brain	**EA:** avoided can induce seizures **DN:** *Tian-men, Long-hui*, GV-20, *Nao-shu, Da-feng-men*, GV-14, LI-4, LI-11, *Er-jian*, ST-44, SP-9	Damp Heat in Mind	Treat for 3-6 months or longer if needed
	Obstruction by Wind Phlegm	Dispel Wind Expel Phlegm Balance immune system	**EA:** avoided can induce seizures **DN:** *Tian-men, Long-hui*, GV-20, *Nao-shu, Da-feng-men*, BL-10, GB-20, ST-40, BL-20, BL-21, ST-36, LIV-3, GB-41	*Ding Xian Wan*	Treat 3-6 months or longer if needed
Brain tumor	Brain Phlegm	Expel Phlegm and Balance the immune system	EA: GB-34/GB-34, ST-40/ST/40, BL-20/BL-20, KID-1/KID-1, LU-7/LU-7 DN: GB-39, TH-5, LIV-3, GV-14, LI-11, ST-36, PC-9, HT-9; if seizures occur do not use EA and add DN at GV-1, GB-20, BL-18, HT-7	Stasis in Mansion of Mind and Stasis Breaker	If seizures add: *Di Tan Tang* and reduce the dose of the other formulas by half Treatment may be palliative, but could improve the clinical signs and prolong the quality of life

Brain Blood Stagnation	Resolve Blood Stagnation and Balance the immune system	EA: GB-34/GB-34, BL-17/BL-17, LI-4/LI-4, KID-1/KID-1, LU-7/LU-7	Stasis in Mansion of Mind and Stasis Breaker	If seizures add: *Di Tan Tang* 0.5 gm/10-20# twice daily orally and then reduce the dose of the other formulas by half
		DN: ST-41, GB-39, TH-5, LIV-3, GV-14, LI-11, ST-36, PC-9, HT-9; if seizures occur do not use EA and add DN at GV-1, GB-20, BL-18, HT-7		Treatment may be palliative, but could improve the clinical signs and prolong the quality of life

The number of acupoints selected and treatment frequency will vary with the animal's condition and response to treatment; Chinese herbal medicine doses are generally 0.5 gm/10-20# orally twice daily, use 0.5 gm/10# when signs are severe; EA=electro-acupuncture, DN=dry needle acupuncture; All Chinese herbal formulas available from Jing Tang herbal:www.tcvmherbal.com

    The treatment of *Chung Feng* "attacked by Wind" or *Zhong Feng* "Wind-stroke" was discussed in the early ancient texts and is treated with TCM today.[10,11] "Wind-stroke" is a sudden reduction or loss of consciousness and neurological impairment from Internal Wind and is often associated with cerebrovascular disease.[11] From a conventional perspective "Wind-stroke" is associated with a transient ischemic attack (TIA, cerebrovascular spasms) or cerebral embolism, thrombosis or hemorrhage. As early as 1997, the NIH consensus position stated that acupuncture could be useful as an adjunct treatment, an acceptable alternative or included in a comprehensive management of stroke rehabilitation in humans.[12] Cerebrovascular disease is rare in animals compared to humans, but is becoming recognized more frequently, with the increased use of MRI in animals with acute dementia, stupor, coma and seizures. The TCVM diagnosis of cerebrovascular disease is Wind-stroke causing Brain *Qi*/Blood Stagnation. On the rare occasion a TCVM practitioner may be asked to treat an animal with Wind-stroke causing Brain *Qi*/Blood Stagnation and a treatment similar to that described for the rehabilitation of animals with head injury discussed below might be useful. Currently there are no clinical reports or studies of treating animals with cerebrovascular disease with TCVM.

    The conventional diagnosis of an animal with dementia, stupor or coma is often known or strongly suspected by the time the patient is referred to the TCVM practitioner. The four most common neurological disorders, causing dementia, stupor or coma in small animals, treated with TCVM are: 1) head injury, 2) cognitive dysfunction syndrome 3) meningoencephalitis or encephalitis and 4) brain tumors and these will be the focus of this section.[2,6] Acupoints GV-26,

HT-9, PC-9 and KID-1 are useful to treat stupor or coma.[6,14] Other acupoints, Chinese herbal medicines, *Tui-na* techniques and Food therapy will vary with each associated TCVM pattern.[6-9,15,16] The response to treatment depends on the underlying conventional etiology and TCVM patterns. TCVM treatments may be used alone or integrated with conventional therapy.

HEAD INJURY

Head injury is a common cause of dementia, stupor or coma in animals and often requires emergency conventional treatment to control shock, progressive bleeding or edema that can result in death.[1-3] Dry needle acupuncture (DN) with manual pecking and rotational stimulation at GV-26, HT-9, PC-9 and KID-1 has been recommended to be integrated with conventional treatments for shock and cardiorespiratory arrest and coma.[6,14] Traumatic brain damage may include hemorrhage into or around the parenchyma with or without tearing of brain tissue by bone fractures or penetrating objects. Concussion is a temporary loss of function lasting approximately 1-3 days in animals, but brain contusion is associated with hemorrhage and edema with disruption of nerve fibers and continuing neurological deficits.

Patients are most commonly referred to TCVM practitioners for treatment, after the animal has been stabilized. The modified Glasgow Coma Scale can be useful to determine the prognosis and follow the recovery.[4] If the animal has a Grade 1 consciousness level (coma) with midrange fixed pupils, that persists after 72 hours of conventional and TCVM treatments, a midbrain contusion is suspected. The prognosis for recovery is considered grave, although affected animals may continue in a persistent vegetative state.[1-3] Although there are no reports of the outcome of acupuncture and Chinese herbal medicine in these severely affected patients, TCVM treatment should be tried for one month, since the only other option is euthanasia. There are anecdotal reports of good TCVM treatment responses in animals with less severe injuries, but no clinical research in animals has been published in english.[5,6]

The research on acupuncture for rehabilitation of humans with head injury has been very positive.[17,18] Electro-acupuncture (EA) integrated with conventional treatments has been reported to improve consciousness of head injured patients in a coma. In one study of patients in a coma for more than 3 weeks, conventional treatments plus EA at *Bai-hui* (GV-20 in animals), GV-26 and KID-1 for 30 min (then leaving needles in place without EA or other manipulation for 30 minutes) was performed once daily and resulted in faster arousal and improvement of the Glasgow coma scale compared to conventional treatment alone.[17] In another recent randomized controlled trial of 56 humans with traumatic brain injury, the arousal rate and time based on the Glasgow coma scale was significantly better ($p=<0.01$) for the group of patients receiving continuous EA at PC-6 than control groups not receiving EA.[18]

Etiology and Pathology

Applying the basic TCVM theories of *Yin/Yang*, Eight Principles, TCVM pathogens, Five Treasures, Five Elements and *Zang Fu* physiology and pathology to make a TCVM diagnosis, there are two basic TCVM patterns associated with head injuries: Brain *Qi*/Blood stagnation with or without significant Phlegm. When Phlegm is present the condition is considered more serious and the stupor and coma lasts longer and may have to be treated longer.[5] These patterns are differentiated primarily by tongue and pulse findings. Although the prognosis is different, the treatment is similar, so they will be discussed together below. An overview of the TCVM diagnosis and treatment of head injuries is in found in Tables 1 and 2.[6-9]

1. **Brain *Qi*/Blood Stagnation without and with Phlegm**
   In TCVM, concussion results in Stagnation of *Qi* flow and contusion results in Stagnation of both *Qi* and Blood flow and bleeding. In the first few hours following injury, *Qi*/Blood Stagnation is the primary pattern.[5] The *Qi* and Blood Stagnation may cause pain around the injury site. The Deficiency and Stagnation of *Qi* and bleeding depletes Blood and *Gu Qi* that nourish the neurons and other cells of the region and degeneration and demyelination of brain tissue occurs. As the *Qi* and Blood Stagnation continue depleting Blood and *Gu Qi*, Deficiency of *Qi*, Blood or *Yang* develop. When *Qi* and *Yang* Deficiency occurs, this often result sin Damp (edema) that can transform into Phlegm.

Pattern Differentiation and Treatment

1. Brain *Qi*/Blood Stagnation with or without Phlegm

Clinical Signs:
- Dementia, stupor, coma
- History or physical evidence of trauma
- May or not have seizures
- Tongue- Pale, purple; will have a white, greasy coat if Phlegm is present
- Pulses- weak, wiry; will become slippery if Phlegm is present

TCVM Diagnosis:
   The diagnosis of Brain *Qi*/Blood Stagnation with or without Phlegm is based on the clinical signs and a history or physical evidence of trauma. Initially the tongue may be pale if the animal is in shock or has had extensive bleeding. A purple tongue reflects the *Qi*/Blood Stagnation. A white, greasy tongue coating reflects the presence of Phlegm. While the animal is in shock the pulses may be weak, but wiry pulses reflects the presence of *Qi*/Blood Stagnation. If the pulses are slippery, then Phlegm is present.

Treatment Principles:
- Stop bleeding
- Move *Qi* and Blood to resolve Stagnation and pain
- Expel Phlegm

Acupuncture treatment:
   EA at 20 Hz (hertz, cycles/second) 15 minutes, then 80-120 Hz for 15 minutes is more effective to resolve *Qi*/Blood Stagnation and promote regeneration of brain tissue than DN alone. If the level of consciousness is Grades 1-4, treat everyday until consciousness improves. When the level of consciousness is between 5-6, reduce the treatment frequency to every 3-5 days, then as needed every 1-2 weeks. Do not insert acupuncture needles in areas of bruising or where suspected or known fractures have occurred. If seizures occur, do not use EA.

   Acupoints recommended
   - If no seizures EA: GV-26/GV-14, *Nao-shu/Nao-shu,* PC-6/PC-6, HT-9/HT-9, KID-1/KID-1
   - DN: PC-9, LU-7, ST-40 (if Phlegm present)

- If delirious add: GV-20, *An-shen*, SI-3, SI-19, ST-41, CV-24
- If seizures: add GV-1, GB-20, BL-17, BL-18, LIV-3, HT-7
- Aqua-AP: *Nao-shu*, if no fractures or bruising in the area

Pertinent acupoint actions
- For EA, GV-26 is connected to GV-14 to promote *Qi*/Blood flow along the Governing Vessel which passes dorsally over the brain region
- GV-26 is known to be effective for resuscitation and coma
- For EA, *Nao-shu* (in the temporalis muscle, one third the way along a line from the cranial ear base to the lateral canthus) is connected bilaterally to promote *Qi*/Blood flow across the brain region
- *Nao-shu* is the Brain Association point
- PC-6, HT-9 and KID-1 are connected bilaterally to stimulate *Qi*/Blood flow to the brain as these acupoints are known to stimulate the brain and improve consciousness
- LU-7 is the Master point of the head and neck
- ST-40 is useful to expel Phlegm
- PC-9 is also useful to improve consciousness
- GV-20, An-shen, HT-7, SI-13, SI-19, ST-41, CV-24 are acupoints known to treat mania and delirium and calm *Shen*

Herbal Medicine:
- For the first 24 hours administer *Yunnan Bai Yao* (JT)[a] red pellets (emergency pill) orally as soon as possible followed by 0.5 gm/20# orally every 6 hours (four times daily) for one week to stop bleeding
- Combine with Stasis in Mansion of Mind (JT)[a] 0.5 gm/10-20# twice daily orally for 1-3 months (up to 6 months if needed) to resolve *Qi*/Blood Stagnation
- If seizures add *Di Tan Tang* (JT)[a] 0.5 gm/10-20# twice daily orally for 1-3 months (up to 6 months or longer if needed)
- A description of all the ingredients of the Chinese herbal medicine listed is beyond the scope of this text, but can be found elsewhere.[8,9]

Food Therapy:
The purpose of Food Therapy is to further promote *Qi*/Blood flow in the brain during the months of rehabilitation. Foods that are Cold or Hot are avoided. On serial TCVM evaluations, the foods needed may vary depending on whether *Qi*, Blood or *Yang* Deficiency develops in the debilitated patient.[16]
- Foods to supplement to promote *Qi* and Blood circulation include: chicken egg, crab, sweet rice, peaches, carrots, coriander, squash, turnips
- Cold foods to avoid: Turkey, duck, duck eggs, conch, clams, mussels, yogurt, millet, barley, spinach, broccoli, celery, egg plant, kelp, alfalfa, cucumbers, pears, bananas, white radishes, watermelon
- Hot foods to avoid: Lamb, shrimp, corn-fed beef, chicken, trout, squash, turnips, sweet rice, basal, caraway, cherries, chilies, cinnamon, ginger, rosemary, sage

Tui-na Procedures:
The purpose of *Tui-na* is to further promote *Qi*/Blood flow in the brain during the months of rehabilitation. The descriptions and indications of each technique are outlined in more detail in Chapter 1 Table 8.[15]
- Performed after 72 hours when the animal is stable
- Avoid the head as there may be fractures or painful bruising
- *Moo-fa* daubing or massaging for 3-5 minutes each at HT-9 and PC-9 to awaken the brain
- Combine *Yi-zhi-chan* single thumb and *Rou-fa* rotary kneading at KID-1 to awaken brain and ST-40 to reduce Phlegm

Daily Life Style Recommendation for Owner Follow-up:
- *Moo-fa* daubing or massaging at HT-9, PC-9, GV-26 and KID-1 for 1-3 minutes each daily to awaken the brain
- Turn to opposite side every 4-6 hours, if the animal remains in lateral recumbency to avoid atelectasis and decubitus ulcers
- Keep clean of feces and urine to avoid skin lesions
- Hand feed and water if necessary
- Assist when able to walk

Comments:
Because the cerebral cortex is less important for a functional pet than a functional human, dogs and cats usually recover from brain injuries within 3-6 months, even when the initial clinical signs are severe. After 6 months when the head injury resolves, if the animal had seizures, the seizures may continue periodically and should be treated as idiopathic epilepsy (See **IDIOPATHIC EPILEPSY** in the section on **SEIZURES** in Chapter 2). It is also possible that seizures will begin 1-2 years after the head injury and should be treated as idiopathic epilepsy at that time.

COGNITIVE DYSFUNCTION SYNDROME
Cognitive dysfunction syndrome is a chronic progressive dementia seen in middle aged and geriatric dogs and cats. Affected animals not only sleep more, but become less responsive to their family and environmental stimuli and forget previous training, such as house breaking, basic obedience training and tricks. In a recent study of cats with geriatric cognitive dysfunction, 61% had excessive vocalization (31% at night) and 73% of another group had house soiling and increased marking behaviors.[19] Except for the dementia and stupor, the rest of the neurological examination is usually normal. Since signs of progressive cognitive dysfunction occur in animals with brain tumors, serial neurological examinations are important. If seizures, circling or asymmetrical conscious proprioceptive deficits develop, then a brain tumor is likely and a CT or MRI may be important to confirm the diagnosis. The TCVM patterns and treatment and response to therapy of cognitive dysfunction syndrome and brain tumors are different, so a correct treatment is essential. The side effects and sometimes ineffectiveness of the conventional treatments for cognitive dysfunction syndrome make TCVM an attractive alternative. There are no veterinary clinical studies of TCVM treatment for cognitive dysfunction syndrome, but anecdotal clinical reports are promising and warrant further investigation.[5,6]

Cognitive dysfunction syndrome in animals has two basic TCVM patterns. These patterns can be differentiated on the basis of the behavior changes and the tongue and pulse characteristics. With more experience, other TCVM patterns may be documented. Because most of the animals to be treated are old and have arthritis, a concurrent *Bi* syndrome associated with Kidney *Qi, Yin* or *Yang* Deficiencies may also be present. An overview of the TCVM clinical findings and treatment of cognitive dysfunction patterns is found in Tables 1 and 2.[5-9]

Etiology and Pathology

Since the TCVM Heart houses the mind, cognitive dysfunction is primarily related to an underlying imbalance in the Heart system and is considered a disturbance of *Shen*.[2] When Heart *Qi* or Heart *Yin* becomes Deficient, the brain function becomes affected. In TCVM, when Spleen *Qi* and Heart *Qi* become Deficient, non-substantial Phlegm can "Mist the Mind", obstruct normal mental functions and be challenging to treat.[2] Heart *Yin* is necessary to nourish the *Shen,* so when Heart *Yin* becomes Deficient, *Shen* disturbances occur, especially pacing and yowling or whining at night. In both of these instances the mind is primarily affected and although it is a function of the brain, in TCVM the imbalance is primarily in the Heart system, instead of the Kidney system. Applying the basic TCVM theories of *Yin/Yang*, Eight Principles, TCVM pathogens, Five Treasures, Five Elements and *Zang Fu* physiology and pathology to make a TCVM diagnosis, cognitive dysfunction syndrome has two common TCVM patterns:

1. **Spleen *Qi* and Heart *Qi* Deficiencies with Phlegm Misting the Mind**
   Over time poor nutrition, chronic illness or environmental stress can result in Spleen *Qi* Deficiency Reduced appetite or interest in food and loss of muscle mass are common signs of aging that are typical if Spleen *Qi* is Deficient. In animals with Spleen *Qi* Deficiency, increased Damp commonly occurs. From Five Element Theory, the Spleen is the "Child" of the Heart and when the "Child" is chronically sick, the "Mother" can also become sick and in this case, Heart *Qi* becomes Deficient. Since the Heart controls the *Shen* or mind, when Heart *Qi* becomes Deficient poor memory and sleep disturbances result. Unsubstantial Phlegm created from Damp and associated with the Spleen *Qi* Deficiency, "mists" the Mind causing *Shen* obstruction and cognitive decline.

2. **Heart *Yin* and Blood Deficiencies with Blood Stagnation in the Brain**
   Heart *Yin* and Blood nourish and support each other and when one becomes Deficient the other follows. A weak body constitution, as can occur from improper nutrition and stress, can lead to premature aging and Heart *Yin* and Blood Deficiency. Both Heart Blood and *Yin* nourish the *Shen* and when these are Deficient, *Shen* disturbances such as anxiety, fearfulness, insomnia and restlessness can occur. Blood and *Qi* also have a very close relationship. "Blood is the mother of *Qi*, but *Qi* is the commander of Blood."[2] When Blood becomes Deficient, it can no longer carry enough *Qi* and *Qi* becomes Deficient. Since *Qi* is needed to move Blood, when *Qi* is Deficient, Blood can no longer flow and in this case Blood becomes Stagnant in the Brain and further affects cognition.

CHAPTER 2

Pattern Differentiation and Treatment

1. Spleen *Qi* and Heart *Qi* Deficiencies with Phlegm Misting the Mind

Clinical Signs:
- Progressively less responsive to the caretakers
- Paces and wanders aimlessly
- May get lost in corners and closets or under furniture
- Forgets house training and other training
- Sleeps more
- Loses interest in food
- Tongue: pale, wet
- Pulses: deep, weaker in the right side

TCVM Diagnosis:
The diagnosis of Spleen *Qi* and Heart *Qi* Deficiencies with Phlegm Misting the Mind is based on the history of progressive cognitive dysfunction without much anxiety and insomnia, instead the animal often sleeps more. The tongue is usually pale and wet reflecting both the Spleen *Qi* and Heart *Qi* Deficiencies. The pulses are deep and weak and may be weaker on the right side reflecting the *Qi* Deficiency, especially in the middle Spleen area.

Treatment Principles:
- Tonify Spleen *Qi* to support Heart *Qi*
- Tonify Heart *Qi* to support *Shen*
- Dispel Phlegm to remove obstruction of *Shen*

Acupuncture treatment:
A combination of EA, DN and Aqua-AP is recommended. EA for 10 minutes at 20 Hz and 10 minutes at 80-120 Hz and DN for 20 minutes is usually performed. The practitioner may begin with a few acupoints and increase the number selected based on the animal's condition and initial response to treatment. After *Tui-na* Aqua-AP injecting 0.25-0.5 ml vitamin B12 may be performed. AP treatment is repeated every 1-2 weeks for 3 times, then the frequency can be reduced to once every 3-4 weeks for as long as needed to maintain improved cognition.

Acupoints recommended
- EA: *Tian-men/Long-hui*, GV-20/*Nao-shu*, *Da-feng-men*/TH-23
- DN: (Can do a bilateral EA connection of one or more these acupoints) HT-7, HT-9, BL-14, BL-15, BL-20, BL-21, CV-14, CV-17, ST-40, ST-36, LI-10
- Aqua-AP: BL-14, BL-15, BL-20, BL-21, ST-40

Pertinent acupoint actions
- *Tian-men* (midline at the level of the caudal edge of the ear bases) is connected to *Long-hui* (midline between the temporal fossae) during EA to

form a midline line over the brainstem and connection of the two hemispheres of the brain to unblock *Shen* and normalize brain function
- GV-20 is connected to and *Nao-shu* (in the temporalis muscle, a third of the way along a line from the cranial ear base to lateral canthus) during EA to form a line over the sensory region of the cerebrum to unblock *Shen* and normalize brain function
- *Da-feng-men* (midline at level of cranial edge of the ear bases) is connected to TH-23 during EA to form a line over the motor region of the cerebrum; these are local acupoints for the brain useful to unblock *Shen* and normalize brain function
- HT-7 is the Heart *Yuan* Source point, useful to treat *Shen* disturbances
- HT-9 is a "Mother" point useful to treat Deficiencies and also awakens the brain
- BL-14 is the Back *Shu* Association point for the Pericardium, useful to treat *Shen* disturbances
- BL-15 is the Back *Shu* Association point for the Heart, useful to treat Shen disturbances and cognitive disorders
- BL-20 is the Back *Shu* Association point for the Spleen, useful to treat Spleen *Qi* Deficiency
- BL-21 is the Back *Shu* Association point for the Stomach, useful to treat Spleen *Qi* Deficiency
- CV-14 is the Front *Mu* alarm point for the Heart useful to treat *Shen* disturbances
- CV-17 is the Front *Mu* alarm point for the Pericardium useful to treat *Shen* disturbances
- ST-40 is useful to treat Phlegm
- ST-36 and LI-10 are a general *Qi* tonics

Herbal Medicine:
- *Wen Dan Tang* (JT)[a] 0.5 gm/10-20# twice daily orally to strengthen the Spleen, transform Phlegm and move *Qi* to resolve Stagnation
- Combine with Stasis in the Mansion of Mind (JT)[a] 0.5 gm/10-20# twice daily orally to move Blood and resolve Stasis in the Brain
- Treat for 3-6 months then maintenance as needed
- A description of all the ingredients of the Chinese herbal medicine listed is beyond the scope of this text, but can be found elsewhere.[8,9]

Food Therapy:
The purpose of the Food Therapy is to tonify Spleen and Kidney *Qi* so neutral and slightly warming foods are suggested. Foods that are too Cold or too Hot are avoided.[16] Serial TCVM examinations are needed in geriatric animals as Kidney *Yin* or *Yang* Deficiency can develop and require different foods for treatment.[16]
- Food to supplement to tonify *Qi*: Beef, chicken, sardines, egg, potato, yam, sweet potato, rice, oats, millet, lentils, carrots, squash, microalgae, cherries, dates, figs, molasses, royal jelly

- Cold foods to avoid: Turkey, duck, duck eggs, conch, clams, mussels, yogurt, millet, barley, spinach, broccoli, celery, egg plant, kelp, alfalfa, cucumbers, pears, bananas, white radishes, watermelon
- Hot foods to avoid: Lamb, shrimp, corn-fed beef, chicken, trout, squash, turnips, sweet rice, basal, caraway, cherries, chilies, cinnamon, ginger, rosemary, sage

Tui-na Procedures:

The purpose of the *Tui-na* therapy is to tonify *Qi* and remove Phlegm obstruction. The descriptions and indications of each technique are outlined in more detail in Chapter 1 Table 8.[15]

- *Yi-zhi-chan* single thumb plus *Tui-fa* pushing from *Long-hui* (midline between the temporal fossae) to *Da-feng men* (midline at level of cranial edge of the ear bases) for 3-5 minutes
- *Yi-zhi-chan* single thumb plus *Tui-fa* pushing from *Da-feng men* (midline at level of cranial edge of the ear bases) to TH-23 for 3-5 minutes
- *Yi-zhi-chan* single thumb plus *Tui-fa* pushing from GV-20 to *Nao-shu* (in the temporalis muscle, a third of the way along a line from the cranial ear base to lateral canthus) for 3-5 minutes
- *Rou-fa* rotary-kneading plus *Tui-fa* pushing clockwise using the palms at CV-12 (Front *Mu* alarm point for the Stomach) for 2 to 5 minutes to stimulate appetite

Daily Life Style Recommendation for Owner Follow-up:

- *Moo-fa* massaging around the top of the head and at HT-9 and PC-9 for 3-5 minutes per day
- High quality nutrition with easily absorbable foods is important
- Add antioxidant supplementation
- Take for short walks to stimulate brain

Comments:

Expect improvement within one month after initiating treatment; treat for 3-6 months then maintenance treatment as needed.

2. Heart *Yin* and Blood Deficiency with Brain Blood Stagnation

Clinical Signs:

- Progressively less responsive to the caretakers
- Paces and wanders aimlessly
- May get lost in corners and closets or under furniture
- Forgets house training and other training
- Sleeps more during the day, but less at night
- Barks, whines, howls or yowls and paces especially at night
- May howl or yowl for no reason
- Anxious and may develop separation anxiety
- May seek cool or pant
- May have warm ears, back and feet

- Tongue: red or pale, dry
- Pulses: deep thready (thin), weaker on the left side

TCVM Diagnosis:

The diagnosis of Heart *Yin* and Blood Deficiency with Brain Blood Stagnation is based on the history of progressive cognitive decline with increasing anxiety, insomnia and restlessness at night. Cool seeking behavior, panting and warm ears, back and feet are associated with *Yin* Deficiency, but the coolness associated with Blood Deficiency may reduce the appearance of these signs. The tongue can be red reflecting Heat from *Yin* Deficiency or pale and dry because of Blood Deficiency, depending on which pattern is more prominent. The pulses are weak, often worse on the left and may be thready reflecting the *Yin* and Blood Deficiency

Treatment Principles:
- Tonify Heart *Yin*
- Tonify Heart Blood
- Resolve Brain Blood Stagnation

Acupuncture treatment:

A combination of EA, DN and Aqua-AP is recommended. EA for 10 minutes at 20 Hz and 10 minutes at 80-120 Hz and DN for 20 minutes is usually performed. The practitioner may begin with a few acupoints and increase the number selected based on the animal's condition and initial response to treatment. After *Tui-na*, Aqua-AP injecting 0.25-0.5 ml vitamin B12 can be performed. Treatment is repeated every 1-2 weeks for 3 times then the frequency can be reduced to once every 3-4 weeks for as long as needed to maintain improved cognition.

Acupoints recommended
- EA: *Tian-men/Long-hui,* GV-20/*Nao-shu,* Da-feng-men/TH-23
- DN: (Can do a bilateral EA connection of one or more these acupoints) HT-7, HT-9, BL-14, BL-15, BL-17, BL-43, BL-44, SP-6, SP-9, SP-10, KID-3
- Aqua-AP: BL-14, BL-15, BL-17

Pertinent acupoint actions
- *Tian-men* (midline at the level of the caudal edge of the ear bases) is connected to *Long-hui* (midline between the temporal fossae) during EA to form a midline line over the brainstem and connection of the two hemispheres of the brain to unblock *Shen* and normalize brain function
- GV-20 is connected to and *Nao-shu* (in the temporalis muscle, a third of the way along a line from the cranial ear base to lateral canthus) during EA to form a line over the sensory region of the cerebrum to unblock *Shen* and normalize brain function
- Da-feng-men (midline at level of cranial edge of the ear bases) is connected to TH-23 during EA to form a line over the motor region of the cerebrum; these are local acupoints for the brain useful to unblock *Shen* and normalize brain function
- HT-7 is the Heart *Yuan* Source point, useful to treat *Shen* disturbances

- HT-9 is a "Mother" point useful to treat Deficiencies and also awakens the brain
- BL-14 is the Back *Shu* Association point for the Pericardium useful to treat *Shen* disturbances and BL-43 is useful to further treat the emotional aspects
- BL-15 is the Back *Shu* Association point for the Heart useful to support the Heart and normalize *Shen* and BL-44 is useful to further treat the emotional aspects
- BL-17 is the Back *Shu* Association point to nourish Blood
- SP-6 is the crossing of three *Yin* Channels and is useful to treat *Yin* Deficiency
- SP-9 is the *He*-Sea point and useful to treat *Yin* Deficiency patterns
- SP-10 is the "Sea of Blood" and useful to treat Blood Stagnation and Blood deficiency
- KID-3 is the Kidney *Yuan* Source point to support brain ("Sea of Marrow") function
- *An-shen* calms the *Shen*

Herbal Medicine:
- Shen Calmer (JT)[a] 0.5 gm/10-20# twice daily orally to tonify Heart *Yin* and Blood and soothe Liver *Qi;* treat for 3-6 months then as needed for maintenance
- Combine with Stasis in Mansion of Mind (JT)[a] 0.5 gm/10-20# twice daily orally to move Blood and break down Stasis in the Brain
- Administer herbal formulas for 3-6 months then as needed for maintenance
- A description of all the ingredients of the Chinese herbal medicine listed is beyond the scope of this text, but can be found elsewhere.[8,9]

Food Therapy:
The purpose of the Food Therapy is to tonify *Yin* and Blood so foods that support these are added. Hot foods that further stress the *Yin* are avoided.[16]
- Foods to supplement for *Yin* Deficiency: Rabbit, duck, crab, tofu, yams, apples, tomatoes, string beans, watermelon, pear
- Foods to supplement for Blood Deficiency: Beef, bone marrow, eggs, liver, heart, pheasant, oysters, salmon, sardines, barley, corn, oats, short grain (glutinous rice), wheat, adzuki, black kidney beans, beet root, carrots, dark leafy greens, kelp, microalgae, cherries, dates, figs, longan, molasses
- Hot foods to avoid: Lamb, shrimp, corn-fed beef, chicken, trout, squash, turnips, sweet rice, basal, caraway, cherries, chilies, cinnamon, ginger, rosemary, sage

Tui-na Procedures:
The purpose of the *Tui-na* therapy is to stimulate *Qi* and Blood flow in the brain and support Heart *Yin* and Blood. The descriptions and indications of each technique are outlined in more detail in Chapter 1 Table 8.[15]
- *Yi-zhi-chan* single thumb plus *Tui-fa* pushing from *Long-hui* (midline between the temporal fossae) to *Da-feng men* (midline at level of cranial edge of the ear bases) for 3-5 minutes

- *Yi-zhi-chan* single thumb plus *Tui-fa* pushing from *Da-feng men* (midline at level of cranial edge of the ear bases) to TH-23 for 3-5 minutes
- *Yi-zhi-chan* single thumb plus *Tui-fa* pushing from GV-20 to *Nao-shu* (in the temporalis muscle, a third of the way along a line from the cranial ear base to lateral canthus) for 3-5 minutes
- *An-fa* pressing and *Rou-fa* rotary kneading at HT-9, BL-14, BL-15, BL-17, SP-6, SP-9 for 2 minutes each to support Heart *Yin* and Blood

Daily Life Style Recommendation for Owner Follow-up:
- *Moo-fa* massaging around the top of the head and at HT-9 and PC-9 for 3-5 minutes per day
- High quality nutrition with easily absorbable foods is important
- Add antioxidant supplementation
- Take for short walks to stimulate brain

Comments:
Expect improvement within one month after initiating treatment; treat for 3-6 months then maintenance treatment as needed

MENINGOENCEPHALITIS AND ENCEPHALITIS

Meningoencephalitis or encephalitis (parenchymal involvement only with no inflammation of the meninges) is on the differential diagnosis list for any dog or cat presented with acute or chronic progressive dementia, stupor or coma.[1-3] Affected dogs may also have seizures, compulsive circling or pacing, cranial nerve deficits and other asymmetrical neurological deficits found on the tests of subtle dysfunction. In some cases the primary clinical problem is seizures. From a conventional perspective, meningoencephalitis in dogs and cats may be due to organisms like canine distemper virus, feline infectious peritonitis virus, rabies virus, Toxoplasma gondii, Neospora caninum, Cryptococcus neoformans and other fungi, Erhlichia canis and other rickettsia, spirochetes and bacteria (rare). In dogs steroid responsive meningoencephalitis (SRME) and granulomatous meningoencephalitis (GME) are the most common brain inflammations, but the underlying etiology for these is unknown. An immune dysfunction or some unclassified viral infection is suspected. Although there is no specific conventional treatment for viral infections, there are conventional pharmaceutical drugs that can effectively treat many of the other organisms and TCVM can be integrated into the treatment to promote nerve regeneration and recovery. The dogs with SRME and GME are often treated with long-term corticosteroids and other immunosuppressive drugs and TCVM is integrated into the therapy to reduce conventional drug doses and treatment times to reduce adverse long-term effects on the liver, bones, muscles and other body systems. Currently there are no case or clinical studies on the treatment of meningoencephalitis with acupuncture or Chinese herbal medicine in animals or humans, but based on experimental studies of the benefit of TCVM treatments on cognitive function and the immune system, further studies of TCVM treatments for meningoencephalitis are warranted.[20-22] An overview of the clinical findings and treatment of the TCVM patterns of meningoencephalitis is found in Tables 1 and 2.[5-9]

Etiology and Pathology

When *Zheng Qi* is weakened from poor nutrition, chronic illness, environmental stress or age, the *Wei Qi* portion of *Zheng Qi* that protects the body's exterior becomes weak and external pathogens such as Wind, Heat, Damp and/or Heat Toxin gain entrance.[2] From a TCVM perspective, Heat toxin usually means invasion of a conventional organism like a virus, fungus or other infectious agent. The Heat can reduce Body Fluids and result in Stagnation of non-substantial Phlegm in the brain and cause dementia or stupor and if the Liver is affected Internal Wind (seizures) can arise.

Wind-Damp invasion can result in non-substantial Phlegm, a TCVM secondary pathogen especially in animals that may have a weak Spleen associated with their basic constitution or poor diet. Such animals may also have anorexia associated with a concurrent Spleen *Qi* Deficiency. The Phlegm obstructs the flow of *Qi*/Blood in the brain resulting in Stagnation that disrupts normal functions leading to dementia, stupor or coma. If Wind invades internally to the Liver, then Liver Wind (Internal Wind or seizures) may occur. Applying the basic TCVM theories of *Yin/Yang*, Eight Principles, TCVM pathogens, Five Treasures, Five Elements and *Zang Fu* physiology and pathology to make a TCVM diagnosis, there are currently two basic patterns associated with meningoencephalitis, but with more experience other TCVM patterns, with different diagnostic features and requiring different treatment, may be found.

1. **Damp-Heat in the Brain (Heat in the *Ying* Stage)**
   Inflammation of the brain is due to a weak *Zheng Qi* and the invasion of the exterior pathogens Wind/Damp/Heat and Heat Toxin resulting in Damp Heat in the brain. Infectious diseases may also be viewed from another diagnostic system called the Four Stages or Four levels of Disease. Based on the Four Stages the disease progresses from superficial levels to deeper levels and becomes more difficult to treat the deeper it goes. The Four Stages or Levels are: 1) the *Wei* stage (exterior level), 2) *Qi* stage (next level), 3) *Ying* stage (nutrient level, level of the CNS) and 4) *Xue* stage (Blood level) is the deepest level of all. Organisms (Heat Toxin) causing meningoencephalitis are generally located at the *Ying* stage, so have already invaded the body relatively deeply. Disease at this level may require intensive and prolong treatment to ensure recovery. Damp-Heat in the Brain can also be described as Heat in the *Ying* Stage using this diagnostic system.

   Wind-Phlegm with *Qi*/Blood Stagnation of the Brain
   Inflammation of the brain is due to a weak *Zheng Qi* and the invasion of the exterior Wind/Damp and the development of Phlegm in dogs with weak Spleen function as described above. The onset of clinical signs of dementia stupor and coma is acute and with no obvious fever or other evidence of Heat is usually associated with Phlegm. Seizures may accompany the other clinical signs or be the primary clinical sign.

Pattern Differentiation and Treatment

1. Damp-Heat in the Brain (Heat in the *Ying* Stage)

Clinical Signs:
- Acute or chronic progressive dementia, stupor and coma
- May have seizures

- May or not have head pain
- May have a low grade or high fever
- Ears, back and feet feel warm
- Animal may pant
- Tongue- red, yellow coating and dry
- Pulses- superficial, forceful and rapid

TCVM Diagnosis:

The diagnosis of Damp Heat in the Brain or Heat in the *Ying* Stage is based on the history, clinical signs localizing the disease to the brain and clinical evidence of Heat on the TCVM examination. A possible fever and warm ears, back and feet and panting as well as a red tongue with a yellow coating reflects Heat in the body. The superficial, forceful and rapid pulses are typical of Excess Heat. A wiry pulse reflects Internal Wind if the animal has seizures or can be associated with *Qi*/Blood Stagnation in the brain, if head pain is present.

Treatment Principles:
- Clear Heat in the *Ying* Stage
- Clear Damp Heat in Brain

Acupuncture treatment:

Because animals with meningoencephalitis are prone to develop seizures, EA is not recommended unless the level of consciousness is between 3-6. Instead only DN is recommended along with Aqua-AP with 0.25-0.5 ml vitamin B12. Treatment is repeated every 1-2 weeks for 3-5 times then the frequency can be reduced to once every 3-4 weeks for 6 months or more as needed.

Acupoints recommended
- EA: Avoided as can induce seizures
- DN: *Tian-men, Long-hui,* GV-20, *Nao-shu, Da-feng-men*, GV-14, LI-4, LI-11, *Er-jian*, ST-44, SP-9
- DN: If seizures add: GV-1, GB-20, BL-17, BL-18, LIV-3, HT-7

Pertinent acupoint actions
- *Tian-men* (on the midline level with the caudal ear bases), Long-hui (on the midline between the temporal fossae), GV-20 and *Da-feng-men* (on the midline level with the cranial ear bases) are local acupoints to support the Brain
- *Nao-shu* (in the temporalis muscle, a third of the way along a line from the cranial ear base to lateral canthus) is the Brain Association point
- GV-14, LI-4, LI-11, *Er-jian* (ear tip) and ST-44 are useful to clear Heat
- SP-9 is useful to clear Damp
- If consciousness level is between 3-6 add GV-26, PC-6, PC-9, HT-9 to awaken the brain and can do EA
- GV-1 is useful to treat seizures
- GB-20 is useful to treat Internal Wind (seizures)

- BL-17 is an Influential point for Blood that is useful to dispel Internal Wind
- BL-18 is the Back *Shu* Association point for the Liver to support the Liver and reduce Internal Wind)
- HT-7 is useful to treat seizures

Herbal Medicine:
- Damp Heat in Mind (JT)[a] 0.5 gm/10-20# twice daily orally to clear Damp Heat
- If seizures add: *Di Tan Tang* (JT)[a] 0.5 gm/10-20# twice daily orally to clear Internal Wind, stop seizures and eliminate Damp
- Treat for 3-6 months or longer if needed
- A description of all the ingredients of the Chinese herbal medicine listed is beyond the scope of this text, but can be found elsewhere.[8,9]

Food Therapy:
The purpose of the Food therapy is to clear Heat and Damp and promote *Qi*/Blood circulation and nerve regeneration. Cooling foods are prescribed and Damp producing and Hot foods are avoided.[16]
- Foods to supplement to clear Heat: Turkey, duck, duck eggs, conch, clams, mussels, yogurt, millet, barley, spinach, broccoli, celery, egg plant, kelp, alfalfa, cucumbers, pears, bananas, white radishes, watermelon
- Foods to supplement to Drain Damp: Eel, mackerel, quail, corn, barley, rye, blueberries, celery, mushrooms
- Foods to promote *Qi*/Blood circulation: Crab, sweet rice, peaches, carrots, coriander, turnips
- Damp producing foods to avoid: Eggs, milk, cheese, yoghurt, ghee, bananas, sugar
- Hot foods to avoid: Lamb, shrimp, corn-fed beef, chicken, trout, squash, turnips, sweet rice, basal, caraway, cherries, chilies, cinnamon, ginger, rosemary, sage

Tui-na Procedures:
The purpose of *Tui-na* therapy is to promote *Qi*/Blood flow in the Brain to reduce dementia, stupor or coma and promote regeneration of the brain tissues. A description of each technique and their actions can be found Chapter 1 Table 8.[15]
- *Yi-zhi-chan* single thumb plus *Tui-fa* pushing from *Long-hui* (midline between the temporal fossae) to *Da-feng men* (midline at level of cranial edge of the ear bases) for 3-5 minutes
- *Yi-zhi-chan* single thumb plus *Tui-fa* pushing from *Da-feng men* (midline at level of cranial edge of the ear bases) to TH-23 for 3-5 minutes
- *Yi-zhi-chan* single thumb plus *Tui-fa* pushing from GV-20 to *Nao-shu* (in the temporalis muscle a third of the way along a line from the cranial ear base to lateral cantus) for 3-5 minutes
- *An-fa* pressing and *Rou-fa* rotary kneading using the finger tips at HT-9 and PC-9

Daily Life Style Recommendation for Owner Follow-up:
- *Moo-fa* daubing or massaging at HT-9, PC-9, GV-26 and KID-1 for 3 minutes each daily to awaken the brain

- Keep in a quiet restful environment
- Avoid loud noises and over handling

Comments:

Acupuncture may have to be frequent initially and then continue for 6 months, but TCVM and supportive care may improve the outcome. When the meningoencephalitis resolves, if the animal had seizures, the seizures may continue periodically and should be treated as idiopathic epilepsy (See **IDIOPATHIC EPILEPSY** in the section on **SEIZURES**). It is also possible that seizures will begin 1-2 years after recovery and should be treated as idiopathic epilepsy at that time.

2. Wind-Phlegm with *Qi*/Blood Stagnation of the Brain

Clinical Signs:
- Acute onset of dementia and confusion
- With or without seizures
- No fever or evidence of Excess Heat
- Tongue- purple or pale with a white greasy coating
- Pulses- wiry, slippery

TCVM Diagnosis:

The diagnosis of Wind-Phlegm with *Qi*/Blood Stagnation in the Brain and obstruction of normal functions is based on the history, clinical signs and TCVM examination findings, including tongue and pulse characteristics. The acute onset is suggestive of invasion of Wind. If Wind becomes Internal and affects the Liver, the animal may have seizures. Unexplained dementia and confusion is often the result of Phlegm in TCVM. There is no evidence of Heat on the examination. A purple tongue and wiry pulses are a reflection of Wind and *Qi*/Blood Stagnation. The tongue may also be pale with a white greasy coating and the pulses slippery reflecting the Phlegm.

Treatment Principles:
- Strengthen the Spleen to expel Phlegm
- Soothe the Liver to dispel Internal Wind

Acupuncture treatment:

Because animals with meningoencephalitis are prone to develop seizures, EA is not recommended unless the level of consciousness is between 3-6. Instead only DN is recommended along with Aqua-AP with 0.25-0.5 ml vitamin B12. Treatment is repeated every 1-2 weeks for 3-5 times then the frequency can be reduced to once every 3-4 weeks for 6 months or more as needed.

Acupoints recommended
- EA: Avoided as can induce seizures
- DN: *Tian-men, Long-hui,* GV-20, *Nao-shu, Da-feng-men,* BL-10, GB-20, ST-40, BL-20, BL-21, ST-36, LIV-3, GB-41

- DN: If seizures add: GV-1, GB-20, BL-17, BL-18, LIV-3, LI-4, HT-7
- Aqua AP: BL-10, ST-40

Pertinent acupoint actions
- *Tian-men* (on the midline level with the caudal ear bases), *Long-hui* (on the midline between the temporal fossae), GV-20 and *Da-feng-men* (on the midline level with the cranial ear bases) are local acupoints to support the Brain
- *Nao-shu* (in the temporalis muscle, a third of the way along a line from the cranial ear base to lateral canthus) is the Brain Association point
- BL-10 and GB-20 is useful to dispel Internal Wind
- ST-40 is useful to expel Phlegm
- BL-20, BL-21 and ST-36 strengthen the Spleen to transform Phlegm
- LIV-3 and GB-41 soothe Liver *Qi* to dispel Internal Wind
- GV-1 is useful to treat seizures
- GB-20 is useful to treat Internal Wind (seizures)
- BL-17 is an Influential point for Blood that is useful to dispel Internal Wind
- BL-18 is the Back *Shu* Association point for the Liver (reduce Internal Wind)
- HT-7 is useful to treat seizures

Herbal Medicine:
- *Ding Xian Wan* (JT)[a] 0.5 gm/10-20# twice daily orally to expel Phlegm and extinguish Internal Wind
- If seizures continue after 2-3 weeks on *Ding Xian Wan* add: *Di Tan Tang* (JT)[a] 0.5 gm/10-20# twice daily orally to clear Internal Wind, stop seizures and eliminate Damp
- Treat for 3-6 months or longer if needed
- A description of all the ingredients of the Chinese herbal medicine listed is beyond the scope of this text, but can be found elsewhere.[8,9]

Food Therapy:
The purpose of the Food Therapy is to support the Spleen to transform Phlegm and to soothe the liver and dispel Internal Wind. Foods that are Damp producing and Hot are avoided.[16]
- Foods to supplement to strengthen the Spleen and transform Phlegm: Chicken, oats, glutinous rice, brown rice, pumpkin, squash, sweet potato, almond, garlic, ginger, pear, radish, seaweed, thyme
- Foods to soothe the Liver and dispel Internal Wind: Carrot, chestnut, hawthorn berry, tangerine peel, parsley, radish, chive, coriander, dill seed, turmeric, vinegar
- Damp producing foods to avoid: Eggs, milk, cheese, yoghurt, ghee, bananas, sugar
- Hot foods to avoid: Lamb, shrimp, corn-fed beef, chicken, trout, squash, turnips, sweet rice, basal, caraway, cherries, chilies, cinnamon, ginger, rosemary, sage

Tui-na Procedures:
The purpose of *Tui-na* therapy is to promote *Qi*/Blood flow in the Brain to reduce dementia, stupor or coma and promote regeneration of the brain tissues. A description of each technique and their actions can be found in Chapter 1 Table 8.[15]

- *Yi-zhi-chan* single thumb plus *Tui-fa* pushing from *Long-hui* (midline between the temporal fossae) to *Da-feng men* (midline at level of cranial edge of the ear bases) for 3-5 minutes
- *Yi-zhi-chan* single thumb plus *Tui-fa* pushing from *Da-feng men* (midline at level of cranial edge of the ear bases) to TH-23 for 3-5 minutes
- *Yi-zhi-chan* single thumb plus *Tui-fa* pushing from GV-20 to *Nao-shu* (in the temporalis muscle a third of the way along a line from the cranial ear base to lateral cantus) for 3-5 minutes
- *An-fa* pressing and *Rou-fa* rotary kneading using the finger tips at HT-9 and PC-9

Daily Life Style Recommendation for Owner Follow-up:
- *Moo-fa* daubing or massaging at HT-9, PC-9, GV-26 and KID-1 for 3 minutes each daily to awaken the brain
- Keep in a quiet restful environment
- Avoid loud noises and over handling

Comments:
Expect TCVM treatments to improve the clinical signs within 3-4 weeks. Resolution of meningoencephalitis may occur in 6 months After the meningoencephalitis resolves, if the animal had seizures, the seizures may continue periodically and should be treated as idiopathic epilepsy (See IDIOPATHIC EPILEPSY in the section on SEIZURES, chapter 2). It is also possible that seizures will begin 1-2 years after recovery and also should be treated as idiopathic epilepsy at that time.

BRAIN TUMORS

Genetic predisposition, chronic nutritional deficiencies and environmental stress and toxins all play a role in creating a dysfunctional immune system that manifests as a neoplastic disorder.[20] Tumors of the cerebrum and brainstem usually cause chronic progressive dementia and stupor with or without seizures.[1-3] The diagnosis of a brain tumor is often suspected based on the history and clinical findings, but CT or MRI and possible biopsy are necessary to confirm the diagnosis and determine the tumor type. Meningiomas can often be surgically removed and radiated and have the best prognosis, but for other primary brain tumors, there are few therapeutic options. Corticosteroids reduce edema secondary to the tumor and can improve the clinical signs temporarily, but have adverse long-term effects. By the time of referral to a TCVM practitioner, the diagnosis is usually known or highly suspected.

Acupuncture and Chinese herbal medicine have been shown to have positive effects on the immune system and will most likely be increasingly integrated into cancer therapies.[20] Studies of *Yuan* Source points in brain tumor patients show an imbalance in functional activities of the bilateral Channels, but what this imbalance implies for the treatment of brain tumors with TCVM is yet unknown.[21] Acupuncture has been suggested for the treatment of tumor related pain and other side effects of tumors and chemotherapy.[22] There is a growing body of research on the positive effects of Chinese herbal medicine for the treatment of all types of neoplasia, although specific clinical trials in humans and animals are still lacking.[20] An overview of the current suggested treatment of brain tumors is outlined in Tables 1 and 2.[6-9]

Etiology and Pathology

Genetic factors, chronic environmental toxins, poor nutrition and emotional stress result in a weaken Spleen and *Zheng Qi* and allow Phlegm or Blood to accumulate in the brain and create a tumor mass.[2] Some animals such as Boxers and Boston Terriers that have a high incidence of brain tumors may have an underlying prenatal Kidney *Jing* Deficiency (breed genetic predisposition for brain tumors). The masses of Phlegm or Blood obstruct normal *Qi*/Blood flow in specific areas of the brain disrupting normal function and causing dementia, stupor or coma with or without cranial nerve deficits and seizures. Applying the basic TCVM theories of *Yin/Yang*, Eight Principles, TCVM pathogens, Five Treasures, Five Elements and *Zang Fu* physiology and pathology to make a TCVM diagnosis, there are currently two basic Excess patterns associated with brain tumors:

1. **Brain Phlegm**
   Brain tumors originating from brain tissue like meningiomas, astrocytomas, oligodendroglioma, other gliomas types, ependymoma, pituitary tumors and non-blood origin metastatic tumors are an Excess pattern of Brain Phlegm.

2. **Blood Stagnation of the Brain**
   When brain tumors are associated with blood like lymphosarcoma and hemangiosarcoma they are an Excess pattern of Brain Blood Stagnation.

Pattern Differentiation and Treatment.

1. Brain Phlegm

Clinical Signs:
- Chronic progressive dementia, stupor
- May have cranial nerve deficits
- May have asymmetrical seizures
- Pain on palpation of the head
- Tongue- pale, greasy coat
- Pulses- slippery

TCVM Diagnosis:
The diagnosis of brain tumor is suspected from the clinical findings based on knowledge of tumor type and/or tongue and pulse characteristics. The pale tongue with a greasy coating and the slippery pulses are typical of Phlegm.

Treatment Principles:
- Expel Phlegm to shrink the mass
- Balance the immune system to reduce further mutation and tumor growth

Acupuncture treatment:

Acupuncture may be combined with corticosteroids to control brain edema secondary to the tumor. A combination of EA, DN and Aqua-AP is usually performed treating both sides to control pain, support the Spleen to transform Phlegm and support the immune system. EA at 20 Hz for 10-15 minutes and 80-120 Hz for 10-15 minutes is recommended. No local acupoints in the area of the tumor are treated, but instead distant acupoints on the Governing Vessel and other Channels that end or begin on the head and acupoints with specific actions can be treated bilaterally. Acupoints that help control pain and balance the immune system are also recommended. Repeat treatments every 1-2 weeks as needed to improve clinical signs and improve the quality of life.

Acupoints recommended
- EA: GB-34/GB-34, ST-40/ST/40, BL-20/BL-20, KID-1/KID-1, LU-7/LU-7
- DN: GB-39, TH-5, LIV-3, GV-14, LI-11, ST-36, PC-9, HT-9
- If seizures occur do not use EA and add DN at GV-1, GB-20, BL-18, HT-7
- Aqua-AP: BL-20, GV-14, ST-40

Pertinent acupoint actions
- GB-34 is a distal acupoint of the Gallbladder Channel that begins on the head and is also useful to treat *Qi*/Blood Stagnation
- ST-40 is a distal acupoint point on the Stomach Channel that begins on the head and is an Influential acupoint for Phlegm
- LI-4 is useful to treat pain and balance the immune system
- KID-1 is useful to treat Grade 5-2 Stupor or Grade 1 Coma
- LU-7 is a Master point of the head and neck
- GB-39 is the Influential point for Marrow to support the extraordinary Fu organ, the Brain
- TH-5 is an acupoint distal to the head on the Triple Heater Channels that ends on the head and is useful for *Wei Qi* Deficiency
- LIV-3 is useful to treat *Qi*/Blood Stagnation and support the Liver to prevent Liver Wind
- GV-14 is a distant point on the Governing Vessel that courses over the head to end on the inside of the upper lip as well it is useful to balance the immune system
- LI-11 and ST-36 are useful to balance the immune system
- PC-9 and HT-9 are useful to treat Grade 5-2 Stupor or Grade 1 Coma
- GV-1 is useful to treat seizures
- GB-20 is useful to treat Internal Wind (seizures)
- BL-18 is the Back *Shu* Association point for the Liver
- HT-7 is useful to treat seizures

Herbal Medicine:
- Stasis in Mansion of Mind (JT)[a] 0.5 gm/10-20# orally twice daily to move *Qi* and Blood in the brain

- Combine with Stasis Breaker (JT)[a] 0.5 gm/10-20# twice daily orally to break-up Blood Stasis, soften hardness and clear masses
- If seizures occur also add: *Di Tan Tang* (JT)[a] 0.5 gm/10-20# twice daily orally to clear Internal Wind, stop seizures and eliminate Damp and then reduce the dose of the other two formulas to 0.5 gm/20# twice daily orally
- Administer both herbs for up to 6 months then as needed for maintenance
- A description of all the ingredients of the Chinese herbal medicine listed is beyond the scope of this text, but can be found elsewhere.[8,9]

Food Therapy:

The purpose of the Food therapy is to support the Spleen to transform Phlegm, further promote *Qi*/Blood circulation and tonify *Qi* to support nerve regeneration in the affected region. Foods that are Damp producing or too Cold or Hot are avoided.[16]

- Foods to supplement to support the Spleen and transform Phlegm: Chicken, oats, glutinous rice, brown rice, pumpkin, squash, sweet potato, almond, garlic, ginger, pear, radish, seaweed, thyme
- Foods to supplement to promote *Qi* and Blood circulation include: chicken egg, crab, sweet rice, peaches, carrots, coriander, squash, turnips
- Foods to tonify *Qi*: Beef, chicken, sardines, egg, potato, yam, sweet potato, rice, oats, millet, lentils, carrots, squash, microalgae, dates, figs, molasses, royal jelly
- Damp producing foods to avoid: Pork, eggs, milk, cheese, yoghurt, ghee, bananas, sugar
- Cold foods to avoid: Turkey, duck, duck eggs, conch, clams, mussels, yogurt, millet, barley, spinach, broccoli, celery, egg plant, kelp, alfalfa, cucumbers, pears, bananas, white radishes, watermelon
- Hot foods to avoid: Lamb, shrimp, corn-fed beef, chicken, trout, squash, turnips, sweet rice, basal, caraway, cherries, chilies, cinnamon, ginger, rosemary, sage

Tui-na Procedures:

The purpose of the *Tui-na* therapy is to awaken the brain and reduce Phlegm. The descriptions and actions of each technique are outlined in more detail Chapter 1 Table 8.[15]

- Avoid *Tui-na* of the head
- *Moo-fa* daubing or massaging for 3-5 minutes each at HT-9 and PC-9 to awaken the brain
- Combine *Yi-zhi-chan* single thumb and *Rou-fa* rotary kneading at KID-1 to awaken brain and ST-40 to reduce Phlegm

Daily Life Style Recommendation for Owner Follow-up:

- Avoid massaging the head
- *Moo-fa* daubing or massaging at HT-9, PC-9, GV-26 and KID-1 for 3 minutes each daily to awaken the brain
- Feed nutritious easily digestible food to support the Spleen
- Keep in a low stress environment
- Take for short walks daily
- Report seizure activity

Comments:

The overall prognosis for most brain tumors is poor, but TCVM can be very useful to balance the immune system, support the constitution, relieve pain and generally improve the quality of the life of the animal. More experience is needed using TCVM to treat brain tumors, before an accurate prognosis can be provided. Anecdotal experiences of tumor regression have been shared, but further controlled studies are needed.

2. Blood Stagnation of the Brain

Clinical Signs:
- Chronic progressive dementia, stupor
- May have cranial nerve deficits
- Pain on palpation of the head
- Tongue- purple
- Pulses- wiry

TCVM Diagnosis:
The diagnosis of Blood Stagnation of the Brain is primarily based on knowledge of tumor type and/or tongue and pulse characteristics. The purple tongue and the wiry pulses are typical of Blood Stagnation.

Treatment Principles:
- Resolve the Blood Stagnation to reduce the size of the mass and improve brain function
- Support *Wei Qi* and balance the immune system to reduce further mutation and tumor growth

Acupuncture treatment:
Acupuncture may be combined with corticosteroids to control brain edema secondary to the tumor. A combination of EA, DN and Aqua-AP is usually performed treating both sides to control pain, reduce Blood Stagnation and support the immune system. EA at 20 Hz for 10-15 minutes and 80-120 Hz for 10-15 minutes is recommended. No local acupoints in the area of the tumor are treated, but instead distant acupoints on the Governing Vessel, other Channels that end or begin on the head and acupoints with specific actions can be treated bilaterally. Acupoints that help control pain and balance the immune system are also recommended. Repeat treatments every 1-2 weeks as needed to improve clinical signs and improve the quality of life.

Acupoints recommended
- EA: GB-34/GB-34, BL-17/BL-17, LI-4/LI-4, KID-1/KID-1, LU-7/LU-7
- DN: ST-41, GB-39, TH-5, LIV-3, GV-14, LI-11, ST-36, PC-9, HT-9
- If seizures occur do not use EA and add DN at GV-1, GB-20, BL-18, HT-7
- Aqua-AP: BL-17, GV-14, LI-11

Pertinent acupoint actions
- GB-34 is a distal acupoint of the Gallbladder Channel that begins on the head and is also useful to treat *Qi*/Blood Stagnation
- Bl-17 is the Influential Point for Blood and is useful to treat Blood Stagnation and is also distal acupoint point on the Bladder Channel that begins on the head
- LI-4 is useful to treat pain and balance the immune system
- KID-1 is useful to treat Grade 5-2 Stupor or Grade 1 Coma
- LU-7 is a Master point of the head and neck
- ST-41 is a distal acupoint point on the Stomach Channel that begins on the head and is useful to treat pain of the face and head
- GB-39 is the Influential point for Marrow to support the extraordinary *Fu* organ, the Brain
- TH-5 is an acupoint distal to the head on the Triple Heater Channels that ends on the head and is useful for *Wei Qi* Deficiency
- LIV-3 is useful to treat *Qi*/Blood Stagnation and support the Liver to prevent Liver Wind
- GV-14 is a distant point on the Governing Vessel that courses over the head to end on the inside of the upper lip as well it is useful to balance the immune system
- LI-11 and ST-36 are useful to balance the immune system
- PC-9 and HT-9 are useful to treat Grade 5-2 Stupor or Grade 1 Coma
- GV-1 is useful to treat seizures
- GB-20 is useful to treat Internal Wind (seizures)
- BL-18 is the Back *Shu* Association point for the Liver
- HT-7 is useful to treat seizures

Herbal Medicine:
- Stasis in Mansion of Mind (JT)[a] 0.5 gm/10-20# twice daily orally to move *Qi* and Blood in the brain
- Combine with Stasis Breaker (JT)[a] 0.5 gm/10-20# twice daily orally to break-up Blood Stasis, soften hardness and clear masses.
- Administer both herbs together for up to 6 months, then as needed for maintenance
- If seizures occur also add: *Di Tan Tang* (JT)[a] 0.5 gm/10-20# twice daily orally to clear Internal Wind, stop seizures and eliminate Damp and then reduce the dose of the other two formulas to 0.5 gm/20# twice daily orally
- A description of all the ingredients of the Chinese herbal medicine listed is beyond the scope of this text, but can be found elsewhere.[8,9]

Food Therapy:
The purpose of the Food therapy is to further promote *Qi*/Blood circulation to reduce Blood Stagnation and tonify *Qi* to support nerve regeneration in the affected region. Foods that are Cold or Hot are avoided.[16]
- Foods to supplement to promote *Qi* and Blood circulation include: chicken egg, crab, sweet rice, peaches, carrots, coriander, squash, turnips

- Foods to tonify *Qi*: Beef, chicken, sardines, egg, potato, yam, sweet potato, rice, oats, millet, lentils, carrots, squash, microalgae, dates, figs, molasses, royal jelly
- Cold foods to avoid: Turkey, duck, duck eggs, conch, clams, mussels, yogurt, millet, barley, spinach, broccoli, celery, egg plant, kelp, alfalfa, cucumbers, pears, bananas, white radishes, watermelon
- Hot foods to avoid: Lamb, shrimp, corn-fed beef, chicken, trout, squash, turnips, sweet rice, basal, caraway, cherries, chilies, cinnamon, ginger, rosemary, sage

Tui-na Procedures:
The purpose of the *Tui-na* therapy is to awaken the brain and reduce Blood Stagnation. The descriptions and actions of each technique are outlined in more detail in Chapter 1 Table 8.[15]
- Avoid *Tui-na* of the head
- *Moo-fa* daubing or massaging for 3-5 minutes each at HT-9 and PC-9 to awaken the brain
- Combine *Yi-zhi-chan* single thumb and *Rou-fa* rotary kneading at KID-1 to awaken brain and BL-17 to reduce Blood Stagnation for 3 minutes each

Daily Life Style Recommendation for Owner Follow-up:
- Avoid massaging the head
- *Moo-fa* daubing or massaging at HT-9, PC-9, GV-26 and KID-1 for 3 minutes each daily to awaken the brain
- Feed nutritious easily digestible food to support the Spleen
- Keep in a low stress environment
- Take for short walks daily
- Report seizure activity

Comments:
The overall prognosis for most brain tumors is poor, but TCVM can be very useful to balance the immune system, support the constitution, relieve pain and generally improve the quality of the life of the animal. More experience is needed using TCVM to treat brain tumors, before an accurate prognosis can be provided. Anecdotal experiences of tumor regression have been shared, but further controlled studies are needed.

Footnotes:
[a] (JT) = *Jing Tang* Herbal www.tcvmherbal.com; Reddick, FL

References:
1. De Lahunta A, Glass E. Veterinary Neuroanatomy and Clinical Neurology 3nd Ed. Philadelphia, PA:WB Saunders 2008:95-113,14.
2. Chrisman C, Mariani C, Platt S, Clemmons R. Neurology for the Small Animal Practitioner. Jackson Wy: Teton NewMedia 2003:125-167.
3. Platt S, Olby N (ed). BSAVA Manual of Canine and Feline Neurology 5th Ed. Gloucester, UK:BSAVA Publications 2012:1-500.
4. Platt S, Radaelli ST, McDonnell JJ. The prognostic value of the modified Glasgow Coma Scale in head trauma in dogs. J Vet Intern Med 2001; 15(6):581-584.

5. Xie H, Priest V. Traditional Chinese Veterinary Medicine. Reddick, FL: Jing Tang Publishing 2002:209-293,307-380,409-419.
6. Xie H, Priest V. Xie's Veterinary Acupuncture. Ames, Iowa:Blackwell Publishing 2007:585.
7. Xie H. Personal communications
8. Xie H, Preast V. Xie's Chinese Veterinary Herbology. Ames. IA:Wiley-Blackwell 2010:305-347, 486-510, 387,449-460.
9. Xie H, Preast V. Chinese Veterinary Herbal Handbook 2nd Ed. Reddick, FL: Chi Institute of Chinese Medicine 2008:305-585.
10. Chu NS. Neurology and Traditional Chinese Medicine. In Finger S, Boller F, Tyler KL, (eds). Handbook of Clinical Neurology. Cambridge, MA: Elsevier 2010:755-767.
11. Maciocia G. The Practice of Chinese Medicine. Philadelphia, PA: Churchill Livingstone 2008:1191-1218.
12. http://consensus.nih.gov/1997/1997Acupuncture107html.htm.
13. Kline KL, Caplan ER, Joseph RJ. Acupuncture for neurological disorders. In Schoen AM (ed) Veterinary Acupuncture 2nd Ed. St Louis, Mo: Mosby Publishing 2001:179-192.
14. Still J. Acupuncture in critical care medicine. In Schoen AM (ed) Veterinary Acupuncture 2nd Ed. St Louis, Mo: Mosby Publishing 2001:204-211.
15. Xie H, Ferguson B, Deng X. Application of *Tui-na* in Veterinary Medicine 2nd Ed. Reddick, FL:Chi Institute 2007:1-94,129-132.
16. Leggett D. Helping Ourselves: A Guide to Traditional Chinese Food Energetics. Totnes, England: Meridian Press 2005:21-36.
17. Liu JP, Yang ZL, Wang MS et al. Observation on therapeutic effect of electroacupuncture therapy for promoting consciousness of patients with coma. Zhongguo Zhen Jiu 2010; 30(3):206-8.(in Chinese)
18. Peng F, Chen ZQ, Luo J. Clinical observation on continuous electroacupuncture at Neiguan (PC 6) for arousing consciousness of comatose patients with severe craniocerebral trauma. Zhongguo Zhen Jiu 2010; 30(6):465-8.(in Chinese)
19. Landsberg GM, Denenberg S, Araujo JA. Cognitive dysfunction in cats: a syndrome we used to dismiss as 'old age'. J Feline Med Surg. 2010; 12(11):837-48.
20. Feng BB, Zhang JH, Chen H. Mechanisms of actions of Chinese herbal medicine in the prevention and treatment of cancer. American Journal of Traditional Chinese Veterinary Medicine 2010; 5(1):37-47.
21. Liu LL, Zhao BX, Xie ZH, Fan YP. Changes of electrical property of the twelve source-points in encephaloma patients before and after surgery. Zhen Ci Yan Jiu 2010; 35(1):52-5. (in Chinese)
22. Lu W, Dean-Clower E, Doherty-Gilman A, Rosenthal DS. The value of acupuncture in cancer care. Hematol Oncol Clin North Am 2008; 22(4):631-48.

Seizure Disorders

Cheryl L Chrisman DVM, MS, EdS, DACVIM-Neurology, CVA

The conventional differential diagnosis for seizures in animals includes idiopathic epilepsy, congenital hydrocephalus, meningoencephalitis, hypoglycemia, hepatic encephalopathy, intoxication and brain tumors.[1-3] When an animal is presented with a history of seizures, conventional and TCVM evaluations and a complete blood count, fasting serum biochemistry profile and fasting and post-prandial bile acids can help determine the cause. If a dog has had a history of intermittent seizures for six months or more and has a normal neurological examination and clinicopathological tests, then idiopathic epilepsy is the most likely diagnosis and further invasive tests may not be needed. If other neurological signs such as dementia, behavior changes, stupor, coma, paresis or paralysis develop along with the seizures, idiopathic epilepsy is unlikely and referral to a neurologist for further diagnostic tests may be necessary. A CSF analysis is needed to diagnose meningoencephalitis and MRI or CT is needed to visualize hydrocephalus, meningoencephalitis and brain tumors.[2-4]

From the conventional perspective, seizures are paroxysmal disturbances of the electrical activity of the brain. Generalized seizures involve both sides of the brain and body symmetrically. Generalized seizures may be mild with involuntary tremors and only slightly altered consciousness or severe with loss of consciousness, salivation, tonic, clonic or alternating tono-clonic face, jaw and limb movements, urination and defecation (Grand mal seizures in humans). Symmetrical generalized seizures may be inherited in dogs or associated with toxic, metabolic, nutritional or inflammatory diseases.[1-3]

Focal or partial seizures are associated with an electrical disturbance in one part of the brain and the clinical manifestation varies with the part involved.[2,3] Tremors of one limb or one side of the body, "fly biting" and other episodes of bizarre behavior can be associated with partial seizures an difficult to differentiate from behavioral abnormalities. Behavioral seizures have also been called psychomotor seizures and may involve hysterical running or circling, with or without vocalizations.

A focal seizure that generalizes may initially show a localizing sign at the onset of the seizure, such as lifting one leg then falling on its side unconscious with typical salivating and tono-clonic movements of the face, jaws and limbs.[2,3] Asymmetrical involvement of the face and limbs can be observed, as one side is usually more tono-clonic than the other. Most animals have focal seizures that generalize rather than generalized seizures. These asymmetrical seizures are associated with trauma, meningoencephalitis, brain tumors or an area of damaged neurons from some previous cerebral insult like encephalitis or trauma.

Seizures that are generalized or focal that generalize are brief and last from a few seconds to a few minutes. Seizures can be long and continuous or occur in multiples with brief periods between (status epilepticus).[2,3] Status epilepticus with seizures characterized by loss of consciousness and tono-clonic movements need emergency attention to stop the seizures, as brain damage from hypoxia, hyperthermia, hypoglycemia and lactic acidosis can result. Seizures may also occur in clusters (e.g. multiple seizures a day, but with longer periods between). Status epilepticus and cluster seizures usually require conventional medications to control.

From a TCVM perspective, seizures (*Chou-feng*) are "Wind in the Sea of the Marrow" or Internal Wind. Internal Wind syndromes are related to Phlegm, *Qi*/Blood Stagnation and Deficiencies of *Jing* (Essence), *Yin* and Blood (Table 1).[5,6,9] In TCVM, non-substantial Phlegm is blamed for otherwise unexplainable abnormal behaviors and confusion. Liver *Yang* rising and resultant Fire can lead to non-substantial Phlegm. Substantial Phlegm is usually associated with primary brain tumors like gliomas and meningiomas and some metastatic brain tumors.

Table 1: Common conventional diagnoses and traditional Chinese veterinary medicine (TCVM) patterns and examination findings associated with Internal Wind (seizures) [5,6-9]

Conventional Diagnosis	TCVM Pattern	Clinical Findings	Tongue	Pulses
Idiopathic Epilepsy	Liver *Qi* Stagnation with Internal Profusion of Phlegm-Fire	Wood type personalities Seizures (worse in Spring or when stressed), Irritable, bossy behavior Insomnia Barking and abnormal behavior at night Cool seeking Panting Warm ears, back and feet	Red or purple with a yellow greasy tongue coating	Rapid, slippery, wiry
	Kidney *Jing* Deficiency	Pure breed dogs Familial history of seizures Seizures begin between 6 months and 3 years of age	Pale	Weak, wiry if having cluster seizures
	Liver *Yin* and Kidney *Yin* Deficiencies	Chronic intermittent seizures especially at night or late afternoon Cool seeking Panting Warm ears, back or feet Dry skin and hair Small dandruff flakes	Red, dry, cracked	Deep, weak, worse on left, rapid, thready, wiry if having cluster seizures
	Liver Blood Deficiency	Chronic intermittent seizures Emaciated Severely dry burnt hair Large dandruff flakes Dry cracked pads Cool ears, back or feet	Pale, dry	Deep, weak, worse on left, thready, wiry if having cluster seizures
	Liver Blood, Liver *Yin* and Kidney *Yin* Deficiencies	Chronic intermittent seizures Panting Cool seeking Dry hair Large dandruff flakes Dry cracked pads Warm ears, back or feet	Pale or red, dry	Deep, weak, worse on left, thready, wiry if having cluster seizures

Congenital Hydrocephalus	Kidney *Jing* Deficiency with Spleen *Qi* Deficiency	Intermittent seizures Young toy breed dogs Bilateral deviation of the eyes laterally May or not have an enlarged head Persistent fontanelle	Pale	Deep, weak, wiry if having cluster seizures

As previously described, *Qi*/Blood stagnation with non-substantial Phlegm can occur following head trauma. *Qi*/Blood Stagnation is also associated with lymphoma, hemangiosarcoma and other metastatic blood related tumors. Since Internal Wind comes from the Liver, Liver *Yin* and Blood Deficiencies may manifest as Internal Wind and these are the most common patterns in idiopathic epilepsy. Since the Brain is an organ of the Kidney system, Kidney *Yin* Deficiency may be combined with Liver *Yin* Deficiency to cause seizures. Kidney *Jing* Deficiency can cause seizures as well. Some conventional diagnoses for seizures have more than one TCVM pattern that result in Internal Wind (Table 1). As with other disorders, it is essential to know the correct TCVM pattern diagnosis for seizures to ensure the most effective treatment.[5, 6-9]

There are a variety of local and symptomatic acupoints that may be useful in animals with seizures, but these must be combined with other acupoints that treat the TCVM pattern to ensure the best outcome (Tables 2 and 3).[6] Most animals with chronic intermittent seizures will achieve even better seizure control, if acupuncture is combined with the appropriate Chinese herbal medicine, Food therapy and *Tui-na* (Tables 3 and 4, Chapter 1 Table 8).[7-11] Some simple techniques may be taught to the caretaker to do routinely at home and when seizures occur. The caretaker can be taught to perform *Dian-fa* and apply deep pressure with the thumb and index finger bilaterally at GB-20 and *Nao-shu* to to stop the seizures or control seizures in the car on the way to the emergency clinic (Chapter 1 Table 8, Table 4). The most common conventional diagnoses causing seizures managed with TCVM are: 1) idiopathic epilepsy and 2) congenital hydrocephalus and will be the focus of this section. An overview of the TCVM patterns and treatments for these disorders are listed in Tables 1-3.[6-9]

Table 2: Basic local and symptomatic acupuncture points that can be used to treat seizures associated with most conventional etiologies and Internal Wind TCVM patterns*[6,7]

Clinical Sign	Acupoints	Technique and Acupoint Attributes and Actions
Seizures (Internal Wind)	GV-17	Local acupoint useful to treat seizures and calm *Shen* (*Tien-men* classical acupoint)
	GV-20	Local acupoint useful to treat seizures and calm *Shen*
	GV-1	Distal acupoint on the GV Channel that ends on the head and useful to treat seizures
	Nao-shu	Brain Association acupoint useful to treat seizures; useful to treat during status epilepticus
	Da-feng-men	"Great Wind Gate" useful to treat seizures
	Long-hui	Local acupoint useful to treat seizures
	An-shen	Local acupoint useful to treat seizures and calm *Shen*
	GB-20	Useful to dispel Internal Wind and treat seizures; useful to treat during status epilepticus

		BL-17	Back *Shu* Association point for Blood to support Blood ("Wind suicide") and dispel Internal Wind		
		BL-18	Back *Shu* Association acupoint for Liver to nourish the Liver		
		LIV-3	*Yuan* Source point for Liver to nourish the Liver		
		LU-7	Master point for the head		
		HT-7	Useful point to treat seizures		
		KID-1	"Root" points useful to treat during status epilepticus		

*These acupoints are combined with other acupoints that treat the underlying TCVM pattern (Table 3); Classical acupoint locations: *Nao-shu* (in the temporalis muscle, one third the way along a line from the cranial ear base to the lateral canthus of the eye); *Da-feng-men* (on the dorsal midline at the level of the cranial ear bases); *Long-hui* (on the midline between the temporal fossas); *An-shen* (halfway between GB-20 and TH-17)

Table 3: Treatment strategy, acupuncture points and Chinese herbal medicine used to treat different types of Internal Wind TCVM patterns of dogs resulting in seizures or tremors[6-9]

Conventional Diagnosis	TCVM Pattern	TCVM Treatment Strategy	Acupuncture points	Chinese Herbal Medicine	Comments
Idiopathic Epilepsy	Liver *Qi* Stagnation with Internal Profusion of Phlegm-Fire	Dispel Internal Wind Calm *Shen* Soothe the Liver Clear Fire Expel Phlegm	Table 2 acupoints plus *Er-jian*, GV-14, LI-11, LIV-2, ST-40	*Long Dan Xie Gan* and *Di Tan Tang*	Often require long-term intermittent treatment
	Kidney *Jing* Deficiency	Dispel Internal Wind Support the Liver Nourish Kidney *Jing*	Table 2 acupoints plus BL-23, BL-52, KID-3, SP-6, SP-3	Epimedium Formula and *Di Tan Tang*	Often require long-term intermittent treatment
	Liver *Yin* and Kidney *Yin* Deficiencies	Dispel Internal Wind Support the Liver Tonify Liver *Yin* Tonify Kidney *Yin*	Table 2 acupoints plus BL-23, KID-3, KID-7, KID-6, SP-6, SP-9, LIV-3	*Yang Yin Xi Feng*	May add *Di Tan Tang* if needed; Often require long-term intermittent treatment
	Liver Blood Deficiency	Dispel Internal Wind Support the Liver Tonify Liver Blood	Table 2 acupoints plus SP-10, SP-6	*Bue Xue Xi Feng*	May add *Di Tan Tang* if needed; Often require long-term intermittent treatment
	Liver Blood, Liver *Yin* and Kidney *Yin* Deficiencies	Dispel Internal Wind Support the Liver Tonify Liver Blood and *Yin* Tonify Kidney *Yin*	Table 2 acupoints plus BL-19, SP-10, SP-9, SP-6, LIV-3, BL-23, KID-3, KID-7, KID-6	*Tian Ma* Plus II	May add *Di Tan Tang* if needed; Often require long-term intermittent treatment
Congenital Hydrocephalus	Kidney *Jing* Deficiency	Dispel Internal Wind Support the Liver	GV-1, GB-20, BL-17, BL-18,	Peanut Hydrocephalus	Often require long-term

	with Spleen *Qi* Deficiency	Nourish Kidney *Jing* Tonify Spleen *Qi* Drain Damp	LIV-3, LU-7, HT-7, KID-1 + BL-23, BL-52, KID-3, ST-36, SP-3, SP-6, BL-20, BL-21	Formula *Di Tan Tang* Epimedium Formula	intermittent treatment

The number of acupoints selected and treatment frequency will vary with the animal's condition and response to treatment; Chinese herbal medicine doses are generally 0.5 gm/10-20# orally use 0.5 gm/10 # when signs severe; Do not use electroacupuncture; Use dry needle acupuncture only; All Chinese herbal formulas available from Jing Tang herbal:www.tcvmherbal.com

Table 4: A basic 10-minute *Tui-na* treatment for Internal Wind[10]*

Technique	Description	Duration or Number of Repetitions
An-fa and *Rou-fa*	Combine pressing and rotary kneading using both palms (right hand on top of left hand or vice versa) at *Da-feng-men*, *Nao-shu*	12 times clockwise and 12 times counterclockwise; Caretaker can learn to do to prevent seizures and during a seizure
An-fa and *Tui-fa*	Pressing and pushing from BL-19, BL-18 to BL-17	Repeat 12 times
Yi-zhi-chan and *Rou-fa*	Single thumb and rotary kneading at LIV-3 and GB-34	1 minute at each acupoint
Tui-fa and *Rou-fa*	Pushing and rotary kneading from LU-7 to LU-5	Perform for 1 minute
Anfa and *Rou-fa*	Pressing and rotary kneading at GB-20 and *An-shen*	Perform for 5 minutes; Caretaker can learn to do to prevent seizures and during a seizure

*Other acupoints may be added to treat the underlying pattern

IDIOPATHIC EPILEPSY

A conventional diagnosis of idiopathic epilepsy is suspected in animals with acute onset of seizures for no apparent reason, a normal neurological examination and normal conventional diagnostic tests.[1-3] TCVM practitioners commonly treat idiopathic epilepsy in dogs and cats. From a conventional perspective, idiopathic epilepsy results in recurring seizures with no underlying active disease process like meningoencephalitis or neoplasia. The first seizure is usually manifested between 6 months and 3 years of age. Idiopathic epilepsy may be inherited or due to residual damage from some previous brain insult (e.g. a past head injury or meningoencephalitis).

Most conventional anticonvulsant drugs have adverse side effects (e.g. hepatotoxicity, drowsiness, hyperactivity, ataxia, polyuria, polydipsia and polyphagia).[2,3] The integration of TCVM treatments may result in seizure control with lower doses of anticonvulsant drugs and therefore less adverse side effects.[5,6-9] Depending on the frequency and severity of the seizures, TCVM treatments alone can achieve seizure control. Seizures may be induced by EA in animals and although used in laboratory animal studies of seizures, EA is generally avoided and only DN and Aqua-AP are performed.[4-6,12] In a few cases gold beads or other substances are implanted into acupoints.[13] For intermittent seizures associated with idiopathic epilepsy, acupuncture is performed every 1-4 weeks for 3-5 times, until the seizures are controlled, and then reduced to every 2-4 months. The number of acupuncture treatments for idiopathic epilepsy will be reduced and may eventually discontinued, if the appropriate Chinese herbal medicine, Food therapy and *Tui-na* are also administered.[7-11] If a dog typically has one or more seizures monthly and no seizures have occurred after 3 months of acupuncture and Chinese herbal medicine treatment, the anticonvulsant doses may be reduced by 25% monthly over the next 3-month period and if still seizure-free, the drugs may be discontinued. It is risky to discontinue drugs too rapidly in dogs known to have episodes of status epilepticus or cluster seizures, because the seizure frequency and severity may worsen.

There is only one clinical study of acupoint stimulation for seizure control from idiopathic epilepsy in dogs.[13] Fifty percent or more reduction in the seizure frequency occurred in 9/15 dogs (60%) following gold bead implantation at acupoints. Gold bead implantation of acupoints on the head may create constant low-grade acupoint stimulation and be useful to control frequent seizures. Implanted material in acupoints of the head may result in artifacts that can interfere with interpretation of future brain MRI and CT, so may not be the best choice in young animals.[6] Gold bead implantation should not be performed if a brain tumor is suspected.

There are a few randomized controlled trials in humans and laboratory animals, many case studies and much anecdotal experience that support the treatment of epilepsy with acupuncture.[12,14-16] In two human clinical trials, comparing acupuncture and phenytoin, a 75% or greater reduction in seizure frequency was reported after acupuncture.[14] A reduction of seizure frequency by 75% or more was reported in three other human clinical trials comparing cat gut implantation at acupoints and valproate.[14] Larger and better designed studies are still needed, before specific acupuncture protocols for human and animal epilepsy can be suggested.

Part of the anti-epileptic effects of acupuncture are due increased levels of glycine, taurine and GABA and decreased somatostatin, aspartic acid and glutamine levels in the hippocampus.[12,15] One laboratory animal study that compared EA and vagus nerve stimulation for seizure control, showed both equally inhibited cortical and thalamic epileptiform activities and the authors suggested EA as an alternative to vagus nerve stimulation implants.[16] Further veterinary clinical studies are needed to scientifically verify the strong clinical impressions that acupuncture is an effective therapy for idiopathic epilepsy of animals and to determine the optimum treatment protocol for each TCVM pattern.

Etiology and Pathology

Applying the basic TCVM theories of *Yin/Yang*, Eight Principles, TCVM pathogens, Five Treasures, Five Elements and *Zang Fu* physiology and pathology to make a TCVM diagnosis, idiopathic epilepsy in animals may be associated with one Excess pattern and four Deficiency patterns. The Excess pattern, Liver *Qi* Stagnation, causes Liver Heat that generates Internal Wind (seizures), especially in Wood constitution dogs.[5,6,9] The Heat continues to ascend (Liver *Yang* rising) to affect the Heart since Wood and Fire in Five Element Theory have a "Mother-Child" relationship. When the Heart is affected, a *Shen* disturbance in the form of irritable behavior results. The seizures may be atypical (psychomotor) and the animal may exhibit unusual behavior that in TCVM is often explained by the presence of non-substantial Phlegm. The seizures and *Shen* disturbance may be worse in the Spring, the Wind and Wood season.

Idiopathic epilepsy can also be associated with Internal Wind created by Liver *Yin* and Blood Deficiencies.[5,6] Since the Brain is an Extraordinary *Fu* organ of the Kidney system,

Deficiencies of Kidney *Jing* and *Yin* occur in animals with idiopathic epilepsy. Combinations of Deficiency patterns are common.

1. **Liver *Qi* Stagnation with Internal Profusion of Phlegm-Fire**
   Wood constitution dogs are prone to Liver *Qi* Stagnation, Liver *Yang* rising and Internal profusion of Phlegm-Fire, manifested as irritability, Heat and seizures. The seizures may be characterized by a variety of clinical appearances such as combinations of psychomotor seizures and severe generalized seizures. If Liver *Qi* Stagnation and Heat is chronic, Liver *Yin* can be damaged so TCVM examinations should be performed during each treatment to ensure a Deficiency pattern does not emerge.

2. **Kidney *Jing* Deficiency**
   Idiopathic epilepsy may occur in specific breeds and families as an inherited disorder with an underlying *Jing* Deficiency. The underlying Kidney *Jing* Deficiency affects the Liver ("Sick Mother causes a sick Child", a Five Element theory pathological cycle) and Internal Wind (seizures) result. Seizures usually begin between 6 months and 3 years of age and may have a variety of appearances.

3. **Liver *Yin* and Kidney *Yin* Deficiencies**
   Liver *Yin* Deficiency combined with Kidney *Yin* Deficiency is a common Lower Burner (*Xia Jiao*) pattern.[5] Deficiency of one often leads to Deficiency of the other (the abnormal Five Element Theory cycles of "Sick Mother creates a sick Child" and "Sick Child causes a sick Mother"). Kidney *Yin* can become damaged by chronic poor diet and illness and Kidney *Yin* Deficiency develops. The Kidney fails to nourish the Liver and causes Liver *Yin* Deficiency. The increased Heat associated with the Liver *Yin* Deficiency results in Internal Wind (seizures).

4. **Liver Blood Deficiency**
   Chronic poor nutrition and prolonged illness can stress the Spleen and result in reduced *Gu Qi* needed to make Blood and generalized Blood Deficiency occurs. Since the Liver stores Blood, the Deficiency often manifests as Liver Blood Deficiency. Blood has been known to control Internal Wind, so when Liver Blood become Deficient, Wind increases in the Liver and results in seizures.

5. **Liver Blood, Liver *Yin* and Kidney *Yin* Deficiencies**
   Chronic Liver Blood Deficiency can lead to Liver *Yin* Deficiency, which then causes Kidney *Yin* Deficiency (the abnormal Five Element Theory cycle of "Sick Child creates a sick Mother"). Chronic Liver *Yin* Deficiency can also lead to Liver Blood Deficiency, as *Yin* is needed to nourish Blood. A combination pattern of Liver Blood, Liver *Yin* and Kidney *Yin* Deficiencies is common in animals with chronic idiopathic epilepsy.

Pattern Differentiation and Treatment

1. Liver *Qi* Stagnation with Internal Profusion of Phlegm-Fire

Clinical Signs:

- Seizures
- Bossy, Wood type personality
- Seizures worse in Spring or when stressed
- Barking and abnormal behavior at night
- Cool seeking
- Panting
- Warm ears, back and feet
- Tongue- red or purple with a yellow greasy tongue coat
- Pulses- rapid, slippery, wiry

TCVM Diagnosis:

The diagnosis is based on the history, constitution type and TCVM examination findings including the tongue and pulse characteristics. The bossy, aggressive behavior is typical of Wood constitution animals. Seizures, worse after stress, are typical of this pattern. Increased bossiness and aggression accompanying seizures supports a diagnosis of Liver *Qi* Stagnation with Liver *Yang* rising. Cool seeking, panting, warm ears, back and feet, a red tongue with a yellow coating and rapid pulses reflect the Heat associated with Liver *Yang* rising and Internal Profusion of Fire. A purple tongue and wiry pulses reflect the Liver *Qi* Stagnation. The pulses may be wiry during and shortly after a seizure reflecting the Internal Wind. Abnormal behavior, a greasy tongue coat and slippery pulses are a reflection of Phlegm.

Treatment Principles:
- Dispel Internal Wind
- Calm *Shen*
- Soothe and support the Liver
- Clear Fire
- Expel Phlegm

Acupuncture treatment:

EA is not recommended for animals with Internal Wind. The number of acupoints selected will vary with the age and condition of the animal. Perform DN of local acupoints and those specific to the pattern (Tables 2 and 3). The DN treatment duration is usually 10-30 minutes. Aqua-AP with 0.25-0.5 ml vitamin B12 may be administered to head and other acupoints after the *Tui-na* treatment (Table 4). Treat every 1-3 days for animals with status epilepticus or cluster seizures, otherwise treat every 1-2 weeks for 3-5 times, then every 2-4 months maintenance therapy.

Acupoints recommended
- EA: Not recommended
- DN for seizures and to support the Liver: GV-17, GV-20, GV-1, *Nao-shu, Da-feng-men, Long-hui, An-shen*, GB-20, BL-17, BL-18, LIV-3, LU-7, HT-7, KID-1
- DN to treat underlying pattern: *Er-jian,* GV-14, LI-11, LIV-2, ST-40
- Aqua-AP: *Nao-shu*, GB-20, GV-14, BL-17, BL-18

Pertinent acupoint actions
- See Table 2 for actions of acupoints listed above for seizures and to support the Liver and location of classical acupoints
- *Er-jian* (ear tip) is useful to clear Heat
- GV-14 is useful to clear Heat and treat seizures
- ST-40 is useful to expel Phlegm
- LI-11 and LIV-2 are useful to clear Heat

Herbal Medicine:
- *Long Dan Xie Gan* (JT)[a] 0.5 gm/ 10-20# twice daily orally to clear Liver Heat
- Combine with *Di Tan Tang* (JT)[a] 0.5 gm/ 10-20# twice daily orally to clear Internal Wind, stop seizures and transform Phlegm
- Treat for at least 6 months then as needed
- Do serial TCVM evaluations and if the underlying pattern changes and the herbal medication is no longer effective, then change to treat the underlying pattern.
- A description of all the ingredients of the Chinese herbal medicine listed is beyond the scope of this text, but can be found elsewhere.[8,9]

Food Therapy:
The purpose of Food Therapy is to provide further supportive treatment to soothe the Liver and calm Shen, Clear Fire and Expel Phlegm. Hot foods should be avoided.[11]
- Foods to supplement to soothe Liver *Qi* and calm *Shen*: Crayfish, duck, shrimp, brown rice, oats, spelt, wheat, wheat germ, Belgian endive hearts, celery, cucumbers, kohlrabi, lettuce, legumes, mung beans and sprouts, mushrooms, radishes, rhubarb, seaweed, spinach, sprouts, lemons, apples, mangos, mulberries, schisandra berries, jujube seeds, basil, chamomile, catnip, coriander, dill, ginger in small amount, garlic in small amount, marjoram, skullcap, valerian, vinegar (small amount)
- Foods to supplement to Clear Fire and reduce Phlegm: Grass fed beef, clams, duck, sardines, turkey, deep ocean fish, barley, brown rice, alfalfa sprouts, asparagus, avocado, bok choy, broccoli, celery, Chinese cabbage (Napa cabbage), cucumbers, dandelion greens, mushrooms, potatoes, seaweed, spinach, tofu, tomatoes, bananas, lemons, rhubarb, watermelon
- Hot Foods to avoid: Lamb, shrimp, corn-fed beef, chicken, trout, squash, turnips, sweet rice, basal, caraway, cherries, chilies, cinnamon, ginger, rosemary, sage

Tui-na Procedures:
The purpose of *Tui-na* is to further dispel Internal Wind and nourish the Liver to further control the seizures. A complete description of each technique and their actions can be found in Chapter 1 Table 8.[10]
- *An-fa* pressing and *Rou-fa* rotary kneading at *Da-feng-men* and *Nao-shu* 12 times clockwise and 12 times counterclockwise
- *An-fa* pressing and *Tui-fa* pushing from BL-19 forward to BL-17; repeat 12 times
- *Yi-zhi-chan* single thumb and *Rou-fa* rotary kneading at LIV-3 and GB-34 for 1 minute at each site
- *Tui-fa* pushing and *Rou-fa* rotary kneading from LU-7 the LU-5; repeat for 1 minute

- *Anfa* pressing and *Rou-fa* rotary kneading at GB-20 and *An-shen* for 5 minutes

Daily Life Style Recommendation for Owner Follow-up:
- *Anfa* pressing and *Rou-fa* rotary kneading at GB-20 and *An-shen;* perform for 5 minutes daily to prevent seizures or continuously during a seizure to shorten the duration and severity
- Avoid stress and anxiety which further stress the Liver and give rise to Liver *Qi* Stagnation
- Do aggressive preventative treatment every early Spring

Comments:
TCVM treatment is often very effective for seizure control, but may require long-term maintenance therapy. It is important not to suddenly stop conventional anticonvulsant drugs, but instead taper doses over several months. Chronic episodic Liver *Qi* Stagnation causing Internal Profusion of Phlegm fire can damage *Yin* over time so the TCVM examination should be repeated at each treatment and if Deficiency patterns develop, treated as described below for Liver *Yin* and Kidney *Yin* Deficiencies with or without Liver Blood Deficiency (patterns 3 and 5).

2. Kidney *Jing* Deficiency

Clinical Signs:
- Seizures beginning between 6 months and 3 years
- Seizures common in the breed or specific bloodlines
- Tongue- pale
- Pulses- weak or wiry

TCVM Diagnosis:
The diagnosis of Internal Wind from Kidney *Jing* Deficiency is based on an early onset of seizures for no apparent reason in a breed that is prone to develop epilepsy or has a familial history of epilepsy. The pale tongue and weak pulses reflect the Kidney *Jing* Deficiency. The pulses may be wiry during and shortly after seizures reflecting the Internal Wind.

Treatment Principles:
- Dispel Internal Wind
- Support the Liver
- Nourish Kidney *Jing*

Acupuncture treatment:
EA is not recommended for animals with Internal Wind. The number of acupoints selected will vary with the condition of the animal. Perform DN on local acupoints and those specific to the pattern (Tables 2 and 3). The DN treatment duration is usually 10-30 minutes. Aqua-AP with 0.25-0.5 ml vitamin B12 may be administered to head and other acupoints after the *Tui-na* treatment (Table 4). Treat every 1-3 days for animals with status epilepticus or cluster seizures, otherwise treat every 1-2 weeks for 3-5 times, then every 2-4 months maintenance therapy.

Acupoints recommended
- EA: Not recommended
- DN for seizures and to support the Liver: GV-17, GV-20, GV-1, *Nao-shu, Da-feng-men, Long-hui, An-shen*, GB-20, BL-17, BL-18, LIV-3, LU-7, HT-7, KID-1
- DN for underlying pattern treatment: BL-23, BL-52, KID-3, SP-6, SP-3
- Aqua-AP: *Nao-shu*, GB-20, BL-17, BL-18, BL-23

Pertinent acupoint actions
- See Table 2 for actions of acupoints listed above for seizures and to support the Liver and locations of classical acupoints
- BL-23 is the Back *Shu* Association point for the Kidney to nourish and support the Kidney *Jing*
- BL-52 is 1.5 *cun* lateral to BL-23 and also nourishes and supports the Kidney *Jing*
- KID-3 is the Kidney *Yuan* Source point to support the Kidney *Jing*
- SP-6 is a general *Yin* and Blood tonic useful to support Spleen function and enhance post natal *Jing* to spare pre-natal Kidney *Jing*

Herbal Medicine:
- Epimedium Formula (JT)[a] 0.5 gm/ 10-20# twice daily orally to tonify Kidney *Jing, Yang, Qi* and Blood
- Combine with *Di Tan Tang* (JT)[a] 0.5 gm/ 10-20# twice daily orally to clear Internal Wind, stop seizures and transform Phlegm
- Treat for a least 6 months or longer as needed
- Do serial TCVM evaluations and if the underlying pattern changes and the herbal medication is no longer effective, then change to treat the underlying pattern
- A description of all the ingredients of the Chinese herbal medicine listed is beyond the scope of this text, but can be found elsewhere.[8,9]

Food Therapy:
The purpose of Food Therapy is to provide further support of Kidney *Jing* and support the Liver. Avoid foods that are too Cold or Hot.[11]
- Foods to supplement to tonify *Jing*: Liver, kidneys, fish, bone and bone marrow, millet, quinoa, spelt, wheat, almonds, black sesame, microalgae (e.g. chlorella, spirulina, wild blue-green algae), barley or wheat grass, black soy beans, black beans, kidney beans, seaweed, sea salt, mulberries, raspberries, strawberries, almonds, black sesame, clarified butter (ghee), royal jelly, bee pollen
- Cold foods to avoid: Turkey, duck, duck eggs, conch, clams, mussels, yogurt, millet, barley, spinach, broccoli, celery, egg plant, kelp, alfalfa, cucumbers, pears, bananas, white radishes, watermelon
- Hot foods to avoid: Lamb, shrimp, corn-fed beef, chicken, trout, squash, turnips, sweet rice, basal, caraway, cherries, chilies, cinnamon, ginger, rosemary, sage

Tui-na Procedures:
The purpose of *Tui-na* is to further dispel Internal Wind and nourish the Liver to control the seizures. A complete description of each technique and their actions can be found in Chapter 1 Table 8.[10]
- *An-fa* pressing and *Rou-fa* rotary kneading at *Da-feng-men* and *Nao-shu* 12 times clockwise and 12 times counterclockwise
- *An-fa* pressing and *Tui-fa* pushing from BL-23 forward to BL-17; repeat 12 times
- *Yi-zhi-chan* single thumb and *Rou-fa* rotary kneading at LIV-3 and GB-34 for 1 minute at each site
- *Tui-fa* pushing and *Rou-fa* rotary kneading from LU-7 to LU-5; repeat for 1 minute
- *An-fa* pressing and *Rou-fa* rotary kneading at KID-3, SP-6, GB-20 and *An-shen* 1-3 minutes at each acupoint

Daily Life Style Recommendation for Owner Follow-up:
- *Anfa* pressing and *Rou-fa* rotary kneading at GB-20 and *An-shen*; perform for 5 minutes daily to prevent seizures or continuously during a seizure to shorten the duration and severity
- Good nutrition is important to support Spleen function and create post-natal *Jing* to spare pre-natal Kidney *Jing*.
- Avoid stress as that will increase Liver Heat and the chances of seizures

Comments:
TCVM treatment is often very effective for seizure control, but may require long-term maintenance therapy. It is important not to suddenly stop conventional anticonvulsant drugs, but instead taper doses over several months. The Heat generated during frequent seizures can damage *Yin* over time so the TCVM examination should be repeated at each treatment and if Deficiency patterns develop treat as described below for Liver *Yin* and Kidney *Yin* Deficiencies with or without Liver Blood Deficiency (TCVM patterns 3 and 5).

3. Liver *Yin* and Kidney *Yin* Deficiencies

Clinical Signs:
- Seizures at night or late afternoon
- Cool seeking
- Panting
- Warm ears, back or feet
- Dry skin and hair
- Small dandruff flakes
- Tongue- red, dry, cracked
- Pulses-deep, weak, worse on left and thready in between seizures or wiry shortly after or during a seizure

***TCVM Diagnosis*:**
The diagnosis of Internal Wind from Liver/Kidney *Yin* Deficiency is based on the history, clinical signs and TCVM examination findings, including tongue and pulse characteristics. Seizures that occur at the *Yin* time of day (late afternoon into the night) are common with Liver *Yin* Deficiency. The cool seeking behavior, panting, warm ears, back and feet, dry skin with small dandruff flakes, a red, dry, cracked tongue appearance and weak thready pulses weaker on the left all support Liver/Kidney *Yin* Deficiency.

***Treatment Principles*:**
- Dispel Internal Wind
- Support the Liver
- Tonify Liver *Yin*
- Tonify Kidney *Yin*

***Acupuncture treatment*:**
EA is not recommended for animals with Internal Wind. The number of acupoints selected will vary with the age and condition of the animal. Perform DN on local acupoints and those specific to the pattern (Tables 2 and 3). The DN treatment duration is usually 10-30 minutes. Aqua-AP with 0.25-0.5 ml vitamin B12 may be administered to head and other acupoints after the *Tui-na* treatment (Table 4). Treat every 1-3 days for animals with status epilepticus or cluster seizures, otherwise treat every 1-2 weeks for 3-5 times, then every 2-4 months maintenance therapy.

Acupoints recommended
- EA: Not recommended
- DN for seizures and to support the Liver: GV-17, GV-20, GV-1, *Nao-shu, Da-feng-men, Long-hui, An-shen*, GB-20, BL-17, BL-18, LIV-3, LU-7, HT-7, KID-1
- DN for underlying pattern treatment: BL-23, KID-3, KID-7, KID-6, SP-6, SP-9, LIV-3
- Aqua-AP: *Nao-shu*, GB-20, BL-17, BL-18, BL-23

Pertinent acupoint actions
- See Table 2 for actions of acupoints listed above for seizures and to support the Liver and locations of classical acupoints
- BL-23 is the Back *Shu* Association point for the Kidney
- KID-3 is the Kidney *Yuan* Source point
- KID-7 is the Mother point on the Channel useful to tonify Kidney *Yin*
- KID-6 is the confluent point for the *Yin Qiao* Extraordinary Channel useful to treat *Yin* Deficiencies and epilepsy
- SP-6 is useful to tonify *Yin*
- SP-9 is useful to treat *Yin* Deficiency

Herbal Medicine:
- *Yang Yin Xie Feng* (JT)[a] 0.5 gm/ 10-20# twice daily orally to clear Internal Wind and nourish *Yin* and Blood
- If seizures continue after one month, add *Di Tan Tang* (JT)[a] 0.5 gm/ 10-20# twice daily orally to clear Internal Wind, stop seizures and transform Phlegm
- Treat for a least 6 months or longer as needed
- Do serial TCVM evaluations and if the underlying pattern changes and the herbal medication is no longer effective, then change to treat the underlying pattern
- A description of all the ingredients of the Chinese herbal medicine listed is beyond the scope of this text, but can be found elsewhere.[8,9]

Food Therapy:
The purpose of Food therapy is to clear false Heat and tonify Kidney *Yin*. Cool and Cold foods are supplemented and Hot foods are avoided.[11]
- Foods to Cool and tonify *Yin*: Turkey, pork, duck, clams, crab, eggs, rice, wheat, wheat germ, wheat berries, Belgian endive, string beans, peas, kidney beans, sweet potatoes, yams, tomato, spinach, tofu, kiwi, lemons, rhubarb, pears, bananas, watermelon, sesame, seaweed
- Hot foods to avoid: Lamb, shrimp, corn-fed beef, chicken, trout, squash, turnips, sweet rice, basal, caraway, cherries, chilies, cinnamon, ginger, rosemary, sage

Tui-na Procedures:
The purpose of *Tui-na* is to further dispel Internal Wind and nourish the Liver to treat control the seizures. A complete description of each technique and their actions can be found in Chapter 1 Table 8.[10]
- *An-fa* pressing and *Rou-fa* rotary kneading at *Da-feng-men* and *Nao-shu* 12 times clockwise and 12 times counterclockwise
- *An-fa* pressing and *Tui-fa* pushing from BL-19 forward to BL-17; repeat 12 times
- *Yi-zhi-chan* single thumb and *Rou-fa* rotary kneading at LIV-3 and GB-34 for 1 minute at each site
- *Tui-fa* pushing and *Rou-fa* rotary kneading from LU-7 the LU-5; repeat for 1 minute
- *An-fa* pressing and *Rou-fa* rotary kneading at GB-20 and *An-shen;* perform for 5 minutes

Daily Life Style Recommendation for Owner Follow-up:
- *An-fa* pressing and *Rou-fa* rotary kneading at GB-20 and *An-shen;* perform for 5 minutes daily to prevent seizures or continuously during a seizure to shorten the duration and severity
- Avoid stress as that will stress Liver *Yin* further and increase Liver Heat and the chances of seizures
- Maintain good nutrition to support Liver and Kidney functions

Comments:
TCVM treatment is often very effective for seizure control, but may require long-term maintenance therapy. It is important not to suddenly stop conventional anticonvulsant drugs, but instead taper doses over several months. The TCVM examination should be repeated at each

treatment and as Liver Blood Deficiency could develop from chronic *Yin* Deficiency and the treatment would need to be altered (see pattern 5: Liver Blood, Liver *Yin*, Liver and Kidney *Yin* Deficiencies below)

4. Liver Blood Deficiency

Clinical Signs:
- Chronic intermittent seizures
- May be emaciated
- Severely dry burnt hair
- Large dandruff flakes
- Dry cracked pads
- Cool ears, back or feet
- Tongue- pale, dry
- Pulses-deep, weak, worse on left and thready, wiry

TCVM Diagnosis:

The diagnosis of Internal Wind from Liver Blood Deficiency is based on the history, clinical signs and TCVM examination findings, including tongue and pulse characteristics. The deep, weak pulses are typical of Deficiency patterns. The severely dry burnt hair, large dandruff flakes, dry cracked pads, cool ears, back or feet, pale and dry tongue and thready pulses weaker on the left are associated with Liver Blood Deficiency. The pulses may be wiry during and shortly after seizures.

Treatment Principles:
- Dispel Liver Wind
- Support the Liver
- Tonify Liver Blood

Acupuncture treatment:

EA is not recommended for animals with Internal Wind. The number of acupoints selected will vary with the age and condition of the animal. Perform DN on local acupoints and those specific to the pattern (Tables 2 and 3). The DN treatment duration is usually 10-30 minutes. Aqua-AP with 0.25-0.5 ml vitamin B12 may be administered to head and other acupoints after the *Tui-na* treatment (Table 4). Treat every 1-3 days for animals with status epilepticus or cluster seizures, otherwise treat every 1-2 weeks for 3-5 times, then every 2-4 months maintenance therapy.

Acupoints recommended
- EA: Not recommended
- DN for seizures and to support the Liver: GV-17, GV-20, GV-1, *Nao-shu, Da-feng-men, Long-hui, An-shen*, GB-20, BL-17, BL-18, LIV-3, LU-7, HT-7, KID-1
- DN for underlying pattern treatment: SP-10, SP-6

- Aqua-AP: *Nao-shu*, GB-20, BL-17, BL-18, SP-10

Pertinent acupoint actions
- See Table 2 for actions of acupoints listed above for seizures and to support the Liver and locations of classical acupoints
- SP-10 is useful to nourish Blood
- SP-6 is useful to nourish *Yin*, which will nourish Blood

Herbal Medicine:
- *Bue Xue Xi Feng* (JT)[a] 0.5 gm/ 10-20# twice daily orally to nourish Blood and clear Internal Wind
- If seizures continue after one month, add *Di Tan Tang* (JT)[a] 0.5 gm/ 10-20# twice daily orally to clear Internal Wind, stop seizures and transform Phlegm
- Treat for a least 6 months or longer as needed
- Do serial TCVM evaluations and if the underlying pattern changes and the herbal medication is no longer effective, then change to treat the underlying pattern.
- A description of all the ingredients of the Chinese herbal medicine listed is beyond the scope of this text, but can be found elsewhere.[8,9]

Food Therapy:
The purpose of the Food Therapy is to further tonify Blood. Avoid Hot foods as these foods stress Liver *Yin* needed to support Liver Blood.[11]
- Foods to supplement to tonify Blood: Beef, bone marrow, eggs, liver, heart, pheasant, oysters, salmon, sardines, barley, corn, oats, short grain (glutinous rice), wheat, adzuki, black kidney beans, beet root, carrots, dark leafy greens, kelp, microalgae, cherries, dates, figs, longan, molasses
- Hot Foods to avoid: Lamb, shrimp, corn-fed beef, chicken, trout, squash, turnips, sweet rice, basal, caraway, cherries, chilies, cinnamon, ginger, rosemary, sage

Tui-na Procedures:
The purpose of *Tui-na* is to further control Internal Wind and nourish the Liver to control seizures. A complete description of each technique and their actions can be found in Chapter 1 Table 8.[10]
- *An-fa* pressing and *Rou-fa* rotary kneading at *Da-feng-men* and *Nao-shu* 12 times clockwise and 12 times counterclockwise
- *An-fa* pressing and *Tui-fa* pushing from BL-19 forward to BL-17; repeat 12 times
- *Yi-zhi-chan* single thumb and *Rou-fa* rotary kneading at LIV-3 and GB-34 for 1 minute at each site
- *Tui-fa* pushing and *Rou-fa* rotary kneading from LU-7 the LU-5; repeat for 1 minute
- *An-fa* pressing and *Rou-fa* rotary kneading at GB-20 and *An-shen;* perform for 5 minutes
- *An-fa* pressing and *Rou-fa* rotary kneading at BL-17, Bl-18, SP-10, SP-6 for 1-2 minutes at each site

Daily Life Style Recommendation for Owner Follow-up:
- *An-fa* pressing and *Rou-fa* rotary kneading at GB-20 and *An-shen;* perform for 5 minutes daily to prevent seizures or continuously during a seizure to shorten the duration and severity
- Maintain good nutrition to support Liver Blood
- Avoid stress as that will increase Liver Heat and the chances of seizures

Comments:
TCVM treatment is often very effective for seizure control, but may require long-term maintenance therapy. It is important not to suddenly stop conventional anticonvulsant drugs, but instead taper doses over several months. The Heat generated during frequent seizures can damage *Yin* over time so the TCVM examination should be repeated at each treatment for additional Liver *Yin* and Kidney *Yin* Deficiencies (see pattern 5: Liver Blood, Liver *Yin*, Liver and Kidney *Yin* Deficiencies below).

5. Liver Blood, Liver *Yin* and Kidney *Yin* Deficiencies

Clinical Signs:
- Chronic intermittent seizures
- Panting
- Cool seeking
- Dry burnt hair
- Large dandruff flakes
- Cracked pads
- Warm ears, back or feet
- Tongue- pale or red, dry
- Pulses- deep, weak, worse on left thready or wiry

TCVM Diagnosis:
The diagnosis of Internal Wind from a combination of Liver Blood and Liver and Kidney *Yin* Deficiencies is established by finding clinical signs of both Blood Deficiency and *Yin* Deficiency from the history, clinical and TCVM examination findings, including tongue and pulse characteristics. The weak deep pulses are typical of a Deficiency pattern. The panting, cool seeking behavior, warm ears, back and feet and red, dry tongue are associated with Heat typical of Liver and Kidney *Yin* Deficiencies. The burnt dry hair, cracked pads, large dandruff flakes and pale, dry tongue are typical of Liver Blood Deficiency. Thready pulses reflect the *Yin* Deficiency and pulses weaker on the left are found in *Yin* and Blood Deficiencies. The pulses may be wiry during and shortly after a seizure.

Treatment Principles:
- Dispel Liver Wind
- Support the Liver
- Tonify Liver Blood and *Yin*
- Tonify Kidney *Yin*

Acupuncture treatment:
EA is not recommended for animals with Internal Wind. The number of acupoints selected will vary with the age and condition of the animal. Perform DN on local acupoints and those specific to the pattern (Tables 2 and 3). The DN treatment duration is usually 10-30 minutes. Aqua-AP with 0.25-0.5 ml vitamin B12 may be administered to head and other acupoints after the *Tui-na* treatment (Table 4). Treat every 1-3 days for animals with status epilepticus or cluster seizures, otherwise treat every 1-2 weeks for 3-5 times, then every 2-4 months maintenance therapy.

Acupoints recommended
- EA: Not recommended
- DN for seizures and to support the Liver: GV-17, GV-20, GV-1, *Nao-shu, Da-feng-men, Long-hui, An-shen*, GB-20, BL-17, BL-18, LIV-3, LU-7, HT-7, KID-1
- DN for underlying pattern treatment: BL-19, SP-10, SP-9, SP-6, LIV-3, BL-23, KID-3, KID-7, KID-6
- Aqua-AP: *Nao-shu*, GB-20, BL-17, BL-18, BL-23

Pertinent acupoint actions
- See Table 2 for actions of acupoints listed above for seizures and to support the Liver and locations of classical acupoints
- BL-19 is the Back *Shu* Association point for the Gallbladder to further support the Liver
- SP-10 is useful to tonify Blood
- SP-9 is useful to treat *Yin* Deficiency
- SP-6 is useful to tonify *Yin* which will also nourish Blood
- BL-23 is the Back *Shu* Association point for the Kidney to nourish and support the Kidney
- KID-3 is the Kidney *Yuan* Source point to nourish and support the Kidney
- KID-7 is the mother point on the Kidney Channel useful for tonification of Deficiencies
- KID-6 is the confluent point for the *Yin Qiao* Extraordinary Channel useful to treat *Yin* Deficiencies and epilepsy

Herbal Medicine:
- *Tian Ma* Plus II (JT)[a] 0.5 gm/ 10-20# twice daily orally to clear Internal Wind, tranquilize Liver *Yang*, resolve seizures and nourish *Yin* and Blood
- If seizures continue after one month, add *Di Tan Tang* (JT)[a] 0.5 gm/ 10-20# twice daily orally to clear Internal Wind, stop seizures and transform Phlegm
- Treat for a least 6 months or longer if needed
- Do serial TCVM evaluations and if the underlying pattern changes and the herbal medication is no longer effective, then change to treat the underlying pattern
- A description of all the ingredients of the Chinese herbal medicine listed is beyond the scope of this text, but can be found elsewhere.[8,9]

Food Therapy:

The purpose of the Food Therapy is to further tonify Liver Blood and clear Heat and tonify Liver *Yin*. Hot foods should be avoided.[11]

- Foods to supplement to Tonify Liver Blood: Beef, bone marrow, eggs, liver, heart, pheasant, oysters, salmon, sardines, barley, corn, oats, short grain (glutinous rice), wheat, adzuki, black kidney beans, beet root, carrots, dark leafy greens, kelp, microalgae, cherries, dates, figs, longan, molasses
- Foods to supplement to Tonify Liver *Yin*: Turkey, pork, duck, clams, crab, eggs, rice, wheat, wheat germ, wheat berries, Belgian endive, string beans, peas, kidney beans, sweet potatoes, yams, tomato, spinach, tofu, kiwi, lemons, rhubarb, pears, bananas, watermelon, sesame, seaweed
- Hot foods to avoid: Lamb, shrimp, corn-fed beef, chicken, trout, squash, turnips, sweet rice, basal, caraway, cherries, chilies, cinnamon, ginger, rosemary, sage

Tui-na Procedures:

The purpose of *Tui-na* is to further dispel Internal Wind and nourish the Liver to control the seizures. A complete description of each technique and their actions can be found in Chapter 1 Table 8.[10]

- *An-fa* pressing and *Rou-fa* rotary kneading at *Da-feng-men* and *Nao-shu* 12 times clockwise and 12 times counterclockwise
- *An-fa* pressing and *Tui-fa* pushing from BL-23 forward to BL-17; repeat 12 times
- *Yi-zhi-chan* single thumb and *Rou-fa* rotary kneading at LIV-3 and GB-34 for 1 minute at each site
- *Tui-fa* pushing and *Rou-fa* rotary kneading from LU-7 the LU-5; repeat for 1 minute
- *An-fa* pressing and *Rou-fa* rotary kneading at GB-20 and *An-shen* for 5 minutes
- *An-fa* pressing and *Rou-fa* rotary kneading at KID-3, SP-6, SP-9, SP-10 for 1-2 minutes at each site

Daily Life Style Recommendation for Owner Follow-up:

- *Anfa* pressing and *Rou-fa* rotary kneading at GB-20 and *An-shen;* perform for 5 minutes daily to prevent seizures or continuously during a seizure to shorten the duration and severity
- Avoid stress as that will stress Liver *Yin* further and increase Liver Heat and the chances of seizures
- Maintain good nutrition to support Liver and Kidney functions

Comments:

TCVM treatment is often very effective for seizure control, but may require long-term maintenance therapy. It is important not to suddenly stop conventional anticonvulsant drugs, but instead taper doses over several months.

CONGENITAL HYDROCEPHALUS

Primary hydrocephalus is a congenital brain disorder with a strong breed predisposition for Chihuahuas, Toy Poodles Maltese and brachycephalic dogs, but can occur in other dogs and cats.[1-3] A common clinical sign associated with congenital hydrocephalus is seizures. Seizures usually begin between 3 months and 1 year of age and are often generalized or focal with secondary generalization. Many dogs have no behavior abnormalities and can be normal or have minimal deficits on hopping and conscious proprioception on the neurological examination. Severely affected animals may have enlarged heads and stupor and coma at birth or shortly after and are often euthanized. Surgical shunting of cerebrospinal fluid has been performed in severely affected animals.[3] In animals presented with only seizures, the head may or may not be physically enlarged for the breed, but the skull is often thin, with incomplete closure of the skull sutures. A cranial midline skull opening (persistent cranial fontanelle) can usually be palpated. Enlarged ventricles are often apparent on routine ultrasonography through the open cranial fontanelle, but are most apparent on CT and MRI. The ventricles may be asymmetrically affected. Conventional therapy often involves anticonvulsants alone or with corticosteroids, if behavioral or other neurological deficits are more apparent.

Animals with congenital hydrocephalus are very susceptible to brain injury that can cause acute onset of neurological deficits in a previously stable animal. Even a minor head injury can cause acute stupor or coma from concussion or hemorrhage, because the brain does not have the usual bony protection. If a head injury occurs in an animal with hydrocephalus, the acute phase may be treated as described in the **HEAD INJURY** section above (see **DEMENTIA, STUPOR AND COMA** section). Once recovered, the animal may be treated as described in this section.

There are currently no case reports or clinical studies in english describing acupuncture and Chinese herbal medicine treatment of congenital hydrocephalus, but there are anecdotal reports of efficacy and further investigation is warranted.[7,9] An overview of the TCVM diagnosis and treatment of seizures from congenital hydrocephalus can be found in Tables 1- 3.[6-9]

Etiology and Pathology

From a TCVM perspective, animals with congenital hydrocephalus have an underlying *Jing* Deficiency that results in reduced Spleen *Qi* and increased Damp in the Brain.[6] Damp is usually associated with improper function of the Spleen and because the Brain is an Extraordinary *Fu* organ associated with the Kidney system, in this manifestation of Kidney *Jing* with Spleen *Qi* Deficiency, the Damp collects in the ventricles of the Brain. The underlying Kidney *Jing* Deficiency affects the Liver ("Mother-Child" Five Element Theory pathological cycle) and Spleen *Qi* Deficiency affects the Liver (Grandchild and Grandmother imbalance in Five Element Theory) and Internal Wind (seizures) results.

1. **Kidney *Jing* Deficiency with Spleen *Qi* Deficiency**
   From a TCVM perspective congenital hydrocephalus is associated with Kidney *Jing* Deficiency causing Spleen *Qi* Deficiency and accumulation of Damp in the Brain. Liver Wind develops secondarily from the Kidney *Jing* and Spleen *Qi* Deficiencies.

Pattern Differentiation and Treatment

1. Kidney *Jing* Deficiency with Spleen *Qi* Deficiency

Clinical Signs:
- Intermittent seizures
- Young, toy or brachycephalic breed dog or cat
- May or not have an enlarged head
- Bilateral deviation of eyes
- Persistent cranial fontanelle
- Tongue- pale
- Pulses- deep, weak or wiry

TCVM Diagnosis:
The diagnosis of Internal Wind caused by Kidney *Jing* Deficiency with Spleen *Qi* Deficiency is based on the history, clinical signs and TCVM examination findings, including tongue and pulse characteristics. The onset of seizures in a young animal is typical of Kidney *Jing* Deficiency. Deep, weak pulses and pale tongue in a young animal is also typical of Kidney *Jing* Deficiency, but compatible with Spleen *Qi* Deficiency as well. The accumulation of Damp in the brain reflects the Spleen *Qi* Deficiency and Kidney *Jing* Deficiency. The pulses may be wiry during and shortly after seizures.

Treatment Principles:
- Dispel Internal Wind
- Support the Liver
- Nourish Kidney *Jing*
- Tonify Spleen *Qi*
- Drain Damp

Acupuncture treatment:
EA is not recommended for animals with Internal Wind. Avoid using acupoints directly on the head because of the thinness of the skull and the exposure of the brain. Insertion of acupuncture needles in acupoints of the head could result in a hematoma or brain abscess. The number of acupoints selected will vary with the condition of the animal. A few acupoints may be initially selected and the number increased subsequently, based on the animal's response to treatment. Perform DN on acupoints not located on the head, but known to be useful to control seizures, and those specific to the pattern (Tables 2 and 3). The DN treatment duration is usually 10-30 minutes. Aqua-AP with 0.12-0.25 ml vitamin B12 may be administered in Back *Shu* Association points after the *Tui-na* treatment. Treat every 1-3 days for animals with status epilepticus or cluster seizures, otherwise treat every 1-2 weeks for 3-5 times, then every 2-4 months maintenance therapy.

Acupoints recommended
- EA: Not recommended
- DN for seizures and to support the Liver: GV-1, GB-20, BL-17, BL-18, LIV-3, LU-7, HT-7, KID-1
- DN for underlying pattern: BL-23, BL-52, KID-3, ST-36, SP-3, SP-6, BL-20, BL-21
- Aqua-AP: BL-23, BL-20, BL-21

Pertinent acupoint actions
- See Table 2 for actions of acupoints listed above for seizures and to support the Liver
- BL-23 is the Back *Shu* Association point for the Kidney to nourish Kidney *Jing*
- BL-52 is 1.5 *cun* lateral to BL-23 and also supports the Kidney *Jing*
- KID-3 is the Kidney *Yuan* Source point to nourish Kidney *Jing*
- ST-36 is a general *Qi* tonic useful to tonify Spleen *Qi*
- SP-3 is the *Yuan* Source point of the Spleen to further nourish and support the Spleen
- SP-6 is a general *Yin* and Blood tonic to further nourish and support the Spleen
- SP-9 is a useful acupoint to treat Damp
- BL-20 is the Back *Shu* Association point for the Spleen to further nourish and support the Spleen
- BL-21 is the Back *Shu* Association point for the Stomach to further nourish and support the Stomach and Spleen

Herbal Medicine:
- Peanut Hydrocephalus (JT)[a] 0.5 gm/10-20# twice daily orally is useful to strengthen Spleen *Qi*, regulate water passage, benefit urination and dissipate swelling
- Combine with *Di Tan Tang* (JT)[a] 0.5 gm/10-20# twice daily orally to transform Phlegm, clear Internal Wind and stop the seizures
- Peanut Hydrocephalus may be used for 3 months then discontinue and replaced with Epimedium Formula (JT)[a] 0.5 gm/10-20# twice daily orally to Support Kidney *Jing*, *Yin* and *Yang*
- A description of all the ingredients of the Chinese herbal medicine listed is beyond the scope of this text, but can be found elsewhere.[8,9]

Food Therapy:
The purpose of Food Therapy is to further Drain Damp and support Spleen *Qi* and Kidney *Jing*. Damp producing foods should be avoided.[11]
- Foods to supplement to drain Damp: Eel, mackerel, quail, corn, barley, rye, blueberries, celery, mushrooms
- Foods to tonify Spleen *Qi*: Beef, chicken, sardines, egg, potato, yam, sweet potato, rice, oats, millet, lentils, carrots, squash, microalgae, dates, figs, molasses, royal jelly
- Foods to support Kidney Jing: Liver, kidneys, fish, bone and bone marrow, millet, quinoa, spelt, wheat, almonds, black sesame, microalgae (e.g. chlorella, spirulina, wild blue-green algae), barley, wheat grass, black soy beans, black beans, kidney beans, seaweed, sea salt, mulberries, raspberries, strawberries, almonds, black sesame, clarified butter (ghee), royal jelly, bee pollen
- Damp producing foods to avoid: Pork, eggs, milk, cheese, yoghurt, ghee, bananas, sugar

Tui-na Procedures:

The purpose of *Tui-na* is to nourish the Kidney and Spleen to further Drain Damp. A complete description of each technique and their actions can be found in Chapter 1 Table 8.[10]

- *An-fa* pressing *and Tui-fa* pushing from BL-23 forward to BL-17; repeat 12 times
- *Yi-zhi-chan* single thumb and *Rou-fa* rotary kneading at LIV-3, GB-34, SP-6 for 1 minute at each site
- *Tui-fa* pushing and *Rou-fa* rotary kneading from LU-7 the LU-5; repeat for 1 minute

Daily Life Style Recommendation for Owner Follow-up:

- Because of the persistent cranial fontanelle and fragility of the cervical vertebrae in toy breed dogs, the caretaker should avoid *Tui-na* of the neck and head, but they can do gentle *An-fa* pressing and *Rou-fa* rotary kneading with their finger tips at SP-3, SP-6 and ST-36 of each pelvic limb
- Avoid injury to the head and neck and rough play
- Good nutrition is important to support Spleen function and create post-natal *Jing* to spare pre-natal Kidney *Jing*.

Comments:

Even though many hydrocephalic dogs and cats have virtually no cerebral cortex on CT or MRI, they can still be highly functional pets. It is suspected that the slow loss of neurons or lack of cerebral develop allowed lower centers in the brainstem to take over many of the cerebral functions. Therefore, the seizures may be effectively controlled with TCVM and affected animals can lead a normal life.

Footnotes:

[a] (JT) = *Jing Tang* Herbal www.tcvmherbal.com; Reddick, FL

References:

1. De Lahunta A, Glass E. Veterinary Neuroanatomy and Clinical Neurology 3rd Ed. Philadelphia, PA:WB Saunders 2008:95-113,14.
2. Chrisman C, Mariani C, Platt S, Clemmons R. Neurology for the Small Animal Practitioner. Jackson Wy: Teton NewMedia 2003:125-167.
3. Platt S, Olby N (ed). BSAVA Manual of Canine and Feline Neurology 5th Ed. Gloucester, UK:BSAVA Publications 2011:1-500.
4. Kline KL, Caplan ER, Joseph RJ. Acupuncture for neurological disorders. In Schoen AM (ed) Veterinary Acupuncture 2nd Ed. St Louis, Mo: Mosby Publishing 2001:179-192.
5. Xie H, Priest V. Traditional Chinese Veterinary Medicine. Reddick, FL: Jing Tang Publishing 2002:209-293,307-380,409-419.
6. Xie H, Priest V. Xie's Veterinary Acupuncture. Ames, Iowa:Blackwell Publishing 2007:585.
7. Xie H. Personal communications
8. Xie H, Preast V. Xie's Chinese Veterinary Herbology. Ames. IA:Wiley-Blackwell 2010:305-347, 486-510, 387,449-460.
9. Xie H, Preast V. Chinese Veterinary Herbal Handbook 2nd Ed. Reddick, FL: Chi Institute of Chinese Medicine 2008:305-585.
10. Xie H, Ferguson B, Deng X. Application of *Tui-na* in Veterinary Medicine 2nd Ed. Reddick, FL:Chi Institute 2007:1-94,129-132.

11. Leggett D. Helping Ourselves: A Guide to Traditional Chinese Food Energetics. Totnes, England: Meridian Press 2005:21-36.
12. Li Q, Guo JC, Jin HB et al. Involvement of taurine in penicillin-induced epilepsy and anti-convulsion of acupuncture: a preliminary report. Acupuncture Electrotherapy Research 2005; 30(1-2):1-14.
13. Goiz-Marquez G, Caballero S, Solis H et al. Electroencephalographic evaluation of gold wire implants inserted in acupuncture points in dogs with epileptic seizures. Research in Veterinary Science 2009; 86(1):152-61.
14. Cheuk DK, Wong V. Acupuncture for epilepsy. Cochrane Database Systematic Review 2008; 8(4), CD005062.
15. Shu J, Liu RY, Huang XF. The effects of ear-point stimulation on the contents of somatostatin and amino acid neurotransmitters in brain of rats with experimental seizures. Acupuncture Electrotherapy Research 2004; 29(1-2):43-51.
16. Zhang JL, Zhang SP, Zhang HQ. Antiepileptic effect of electroacupuncture vs. vagus nerve stimulation in the rat thalamus. Neuroscience Letters 2008; 441(2):183-7.

Tremor Disorders

Cheryl L Chrisman DVM, MS, EdS, DACVIM-Neurology, CVA

The conventional differential diagnosis for tremors in dogs includes hypocalcemia, hypoglycemia, toxicity, dysmyelinogenesis, non-suppurative meningoencephalitis (NSME), idiopathic tremors of adult dogs and geriatric pelvic limb tremors.[1-3] Clinicopathological tests are useful to detect low serum calcium or glucose. Dysmyelinogenesis is abnormal myelin development that occurs in Chow Chows and other purebred puppies and improves with age as the myelin matures. Many toxic substances like pyrethrins, pyrethroids, organophosphates, ivermectin, ethylene glycol, chlorinated hydrocarbons, metaldehyde, hexachlorophene, herbicides, poisonous plants, heavy metals and any prescription, over-the-counter or illegal drugs can cause tremors or seizures.[1-3] In TCVM, tremors or seizures associated with toxic substances are Excess patterns described as Heat Toxin or Food Toxin that can generate Liver Heat causing Internal Wind. TCVM treatment can be integrated with conventional treatments for the specific toxic substance and to control tremors or seizures. Hemo-acupuncture at *Er-jian* (ear tip), *Wei-jian* (tail tip) and *Shan-gen* (on the dorsal midline of the nose at the haired, non-haired junction) and DN at LI-4, LI-11, GV-14, LIV-3, GB-34 and ST-36 may be performed for 15-30 minutes. If needed additional acupoints may be added to control seizures (Table 1). Food therapy of fresh ginger and green bean soup (*Lu Dou*) may also be administered.

Tremors from a TCVM perspective are associated with Internal Wind, but differ from seizures, as there is no altered mentation and tremors persist when awake, may worsen when excited and often disappear during sleep. Tremors may be associated with an Excess pattern due to invasion of a TCVM pathogen like Wind-Heat or a Deficiency pattern of the Spleen and Kidney systems that affects the Liver. The most common tremor disorders treated by TCVM practitioners are idiopathic tremors of adult dogs (or NSME) and geriatric pelvic limb tremors.

IDIOPATHIC TREMORS OF ADULT DOGS

Idiopathic tremors of adult dogs and non-suppurative meningoencephalomyelitis (NSME) have the same clinical appearance, treatment and prognosis and may actually be the same disease process. The only difference is the presence of other abnormalities besides tremors on the neurological examination and/or abnormal cerebrospinal fluid in animals with NSME. Animals with idiopathic tremors are normal besides the tremors and the CSF is normal.[2] Both NSME and idiopathic tremors cause acute onset of tremors that last 1-3 months in adult dogs. Often white dogs such as Maltese terriers are affected and the disorder has been referred to as "little white shakers" or "shaky white dog disease".[2,3] Other dogs can also develop idiopathic tremors, so this diagnosis should not be excluded based on coat color or size alone. The tremors may affect only the head and eyes or pelvic limbs, but can be diffuse and affect the whole body. Dogs with NSME may also have a head tilt, ataxia, paraparesis or quadriparesis (see **MENINGOENCEPHALITIS** in the **DEMENTIA, STUPOR AND COMA DISORDERS** section above and **MENINGOMYELITIS** in the **SPINAL CORD DISORDERS** section below for patterns and treatment options, when other signs are present).

If a diagnosis of NSME is made, the conventional treatment is oral prednisone at tapering doses.[2,3] Tremors that are idiopathic or associated with NSME may be conventionally controlled by diazepam. The prognosis for both NSME and idiopathic tremors of adult dogs is excellent and most affected dogs eventually return to normal within 3 months. In the acute stage of tremors, dogs may be referred to TCVM practitioners for evaluation and treatment. From a TCVM perspective, tremors like seizures are a reflection of Internal Wind associated with an imbalance in the Liver. Although there are no descriptions of the TCVM treatment of idiopathic tremors or NSME in dogs, at this time, clinical findings and proposed treatments are outlined in Tables 1 and 2.[4-8] Further studies are needed to determine if TCVM treatments could control the tremors and shorten the course of the disease process.

Table 1: Common conventional diagnoses and traditional Chinese veterinary medicine (TCVM) patterns and examination findings associated with and tremors[2,4-8]

Conventional Diagnosis	TCVM Pattern	Clinical Findings	Tongue	Pulses
Idiopathic tremors of adult dogs	Wind-Heat invasion with Internal Wind	Acute onset of tremors No history of poisoning Often small white dogs	Red, dry, purple	Superficial, forceful, rapid, wiry
Geriatric pelvic limb tremors	Spleen *Qi* and Kidney *Qi* Deficiencies with Internal Wind	Geriatric dogs Pelvic limb tremors when rising and standing Pelvic limb muscle atrophy Pelvic limb weakness	Pale, wet	Deep, weak, worse on right
	Liver Blood, Liver *Yin* and Spleen/Kidney *Qi* Deficiencies	Geriatric animal Pelvic limb tremors when rising and standing Pelvic limb muscle atrophy Pelvic limb weakness Dry burnt hair Large dandruff flakes Cracked pads Panting Cool seeking Warm ears, back or feet	Pale or red, dry	Deep weak, worse on left, thready

Table 2: Treatment strategy, acupuncture points and Chinese herbal medicine used to treat different types of Internal Wind patterns of dogs resulting in tremors[4-7]

Conventional Diagnosis	TCVM Pattern	TCVM Treatment Strategy	Acupuncture points	Chinese Herbal Medicine	Comments
Idiopathic tremors of adult dogs	Wind-Heat invasion with Internal Wind	Dispel Internal Wind Clear Heat Stop tremors	*Tian-men, Long-hui,* GV-20, *Nao-shu, Da-feng-men,* GB-20, GV-1, LU-7, LIV-3, GV-14, LI-4, BL-17, BL-18	*Ding Xian Wan* and *Di Tan Tang*	Treat for 3-4 months

Geriatric pelvic limb tremors	Spleen *Qi* and Kidney *Qi* Deficiency with Internal Wind	Dispel Internal Wind Tonify Spleen *Qi* Tonify Kidney *Qi*	GB-20, LI-10, ST-36, BL-17, BL-18, BL-20, BL-21, BL-23, BL-54, BL-40, BL-39, KID-3, SP-3	*Bu Yang Huan Wu*	Often require long-term intermittent treatment
	Liver Blood, Liver *Yin* and Spleen/Kidney *Qi* Deficiencies	Dispel Internal Wind Tonify Liver Blood Tonify Liver *Yin* Tonify Spleen/Kidney *Qi*	LIV-3, SP-10, BL-17, BL-18, GB-20, LI-10, ST-36, BL-20, BL-21, BL-23, BL-54, BL-40, BL-39, KID-3, KID-6, SP-3	Tendon Ligament Formula	Often require long-term intermittent treatment

Classical acupoint locations: *Nao-shu* (in the temporalis muscle, one third the way along a line from the cranial ear base to the lateral canthus of the eye); *Da-feng-men* (on the dorsal midline at the level of the cranial ear bases); *Long-hui* (on the midline between the temporal fossas); *An-shen* (halfway between GB-20 and TH-17); The number of acupoints selected and treatment frequency will vary with the animal's condition and response to treatment; Chinese herbal medicine doses are generally 0.5 gm/10-20# orally use 0.5 gm/10 # when signs severe; Do not use electroacupuncture; Use dry needle acupuncture only; All Chinese herbal formulas available from Jing Tang herbal:www.tcvmherbal.com

Etiology and Pathology

Applying the basic TCVM theories of *Yin/Yang*, Eight Principles, TCVM pathogens, Five Treasures, Five Elements and *Zang Fu* physiology and pathology to make a TCVM diagnosis, there is currently one pattern associated with idiopathic tremors or NSME. When *Zheng Qi* is weakened from poor nutrition, chronic illness, environmental stress or age, the *Wei Qi* portion of *Zheng Qi* that protects the body's exterior becomes weak and external pathogens such as Wind-Heat or Wind-Cold gain entrance.[2] Although *Yang* animals like Wood and Fire constitutions are more susceptible to Wind-Heat invasion, any animal can have Wind-Heat invasion of the Channels. The Heat reduces Body Fluids and results in Stagnation of non-substantial Phlegm in the brain and the Liver Channels and causes Internal Wind (tremors). The pattern becomes Wind-Heat invasion from *Zheng Qi* Deficiency with Internal Wind. More experience is needed to see if Liver *Qi* Stagnation associated with emotional stress in Wood animals or Wind-Cold invasion in Earth, Metal and Water animals can also produce idiopathic tremors in dogs and cats.

1. **Wind-Heat invasion with *Qi*/Blood Stagnation with Wind**

    When *Wei Qi* becomes weak due to poor nutrition, chronic illness or environmental stress, Wind-Heat invades the Channels and affects the Liver generating Internal Wind in the form of tremors of the head and body.

Pattern Differentiation and Treatment

1. Wind-Heat invasion with Internal Wind

Clinical Signs:
- Acute onset of head, pelvic limb or whole body tremors
- No history of toxic substance exposure
- Often no other neurological deficits
- Cool seeking
- Panting
- Warm ears, back and feet
- Tongue- red, dry, purple
- Pulses- Superficial, forceful, rapid or wiry

TCVM Diagnosis:
The acute onset of tremors is typical of an Excess pattern with invasion of an External pathogen. The diagnosis of Wind-Heat invasion causing Internal Wind is based on the clinical findings. The cool seeking behavior, panting and warmth of the ears, back and feet are typical of a Heat pattern. The tongue is red and dry from the Wind-Heat or purple if Stagnation of Phlegm in the brain is most prominent. The pulses may be superficial, forceful and rapid from the Wind-Heat or wiry from the Stagnation of Phlegm in the brain.

Treatment Principles:
- Dispel Internal Wind
- Clear Wind-Heat and transform Phlegm
- Stop tremors

Acupuncture treatment:
EA is generally not recommended for Internal Wind conditions. Instead DN is recommended in all points for 10-30 minutes. The number of acupoints selected will vary with the condition of the animal. Some acupoints may be initially selected and others may be added subsequently, based on the animal's response to treatment. Aqua-AP is performed after *Tui-na* with 0.25-0.5 ml vitamin B12 at specific acupoints. Acutely acupuncture may be given every 3-5 days for 3 times and then every 1-2 weeks as needed for 3 months or longer if needed.

Acupoints recommended
- DN: *Tian-men, Long-hui,* GV-20, *Nao-shu, Da-feng-men,* GB-20, GV-1, LU-7, LIV-3, GV-14, LI-4, BL-17, BL-18
- Aqua-AP: *Nao-shu,* GB-20, BL-17, BL-18

Pertinent acupoint actions
- *Tian-men* (on the midline level with the caudal ear bases), *Long-hui* (on the midline between the temporal fossae), GV-20 and *Da-feng-men* (on the midline level with the cranial ear bases) are local acupoints to support the Brain
- *Nao-shu* (in the temporalis muscle, a third of the way along a line from the cranial ear base to lateral canthus) is the Brain Association point
- GB-20 and GV-1 are useful to treat Internal Wind
- GV-14 and LI-4 are useful to support the immune system

- BL-17 is an Influential point for Blood that is useful to dispel Internal Wind
- BL-18 is the Back *Shu* Association point for Liver to support the Liver

Herbal Medicine:
- *Ding Xian Wan* (JT)[a] 0.5 gm/10-20# twice daily orally to move *Qi* and Blood in the brain
- Combine with *Di Tan Tang* (JT)[a] 0.5 gm/10-20# twice daily orally to clear Internal Wind and stop tremors
- Treat for 3-4 months
- A description of all the ingredients of the Chinese herbal medicine listed is beyond the scope of this text, but can be found elsewhere.[6,7]

Food Therapy:
The purpose of the Food therapy is to clear Heat so cooling foods are prescribed. Foods to transform Phlegm may also be added. Hot foods and Damp producing foods are avoided.[9]
- Foods to supplement to clear Heat: Turkey, duck, duck eggs, conch, clams, mussels, yogurt, millet, barley, spinach, broccoli, celery, egg plant, kelp, alfalfa, cucumbers, pears, bananas white radishes, peppermint
- Food to supplement to transform Phlegm: sweet potato, almond, garlic, pear, radish, seaweed, thyme
- Hot Foods to avoid: Lamb, shrimp, corn-fed beef, chicken, trout, squash, turnips, sweet rice, basal, caraway, cherries, chilies, cinnamon, ginger, rosemary, sage
- Damp producing foods to avoid: Pork, eggs, milk, cheese, yoghurt, ghee, bananas, sugar

Tui-na Procedures:
The purpose of the *Tui-na* treatment is to further dispel Internal Wind. Because Maltese dogs also have a high incidence of hydrocephalus, do not do this *Tui-na* treatment in toy breed dogs with persistent cranial fontanelle. A description of each technique and their actions can be found in Chapter 1 Table 8.[10]
- *Yi-zhi-chan* single thumb plus *Tui-fa* pushing from *Long-hui* (midline between the temporal fossae) to *Da-feng men* (midline at level of cranial edge of the ear bases) for 3-5 minutes
- *Yi-zhi-chan* single thumb plus *Tui-fa* pushing from *Da-feng men* (midline at level of cranial edge of the ear bases) to TH-23 for 3-5 minutes
- *Yi-zhi-chan* single thumb plus *Tui-fa* pushing from GV-20 to *Nao-shu* (in the temporalis muscle a third of the way along a line from the cranial ear base to lateral canthus) for 3-5 minutes
- *An-fa* pressing and *Rou-fa* rotary kneading using the finger tips at GB-20

Daily Life Style Recommendation for Owner Follow-up:
- *Moo-fa* daubing or massaging at GB-20 for 3 minutes each daily to dispel Internal Wind
- Keep in a quiet restful environment
- Avoid over handling as stimulation makes the tremors worse

Comments:
The purpose of TCVM treatment is to control the tremors to avoid conventional medications that have known adverse effects on the liver of some dogs. Further studies are needed to determine if the TCVM treatment can control signs and shorten the course of the disease process.

GERIATRIC PELVIC LIMB TREMORS

Pelvic limb tremors while standing are commonly seen in geriatric dogs and cats and reduce the quality of life of the animal and distress their caretaker. Many animals also have arthritis and non-steroidal anti-inflammatory drugs may be administered, but often have no effect on the tremors. In conventional veterinary medicine, pelvic limb weakness and tremors are often accepted as part of the aging process and no conventional treatment is suggested.

From a TCVM perspective there may be three causes of geriatric pelvic limb weakness and tremors. *Bi* syndrome results in arthritic changes in the hips, stifles and other joints that cause pain and muscle spasms, when first rising or when standing for long periods of time. An underlying Kidney *Yin* or *Yang* Deficiency often accompanies the *Bi* syndrome of geriatric animals and further description of the TCVM diagnosis and treatment can be found elsewhere in discussions of musculoskeletal disorders.[4-8] In geriatric animals, Liver Blood and/or Liver *Yin* Deficiency can cause Internal Wind (tremors) and with Kidney *Qi* Deficiency, the tremors are manifested in the pelvic limbs. Spleen *Qi* and Kidney *Qi* Deficiencies can affect the Liver in geriatric animals and Internal Wind in the pelvic limbs can result. The last two patterns of geriatric pelvic limb tremors associated with Internal Wind will be discussed in this section. Although there are no case reports or clinical studies of TCVM for geriatric pelvic limb tremors, since TCVM treatments are effective for other Internal Wind disorders, *Wei* syndrome and *Tan-Huan* syndrome, further studies are warranted to improve the quality of life of affected geriatric animals.[4-8]

Etiology and Pathology

Geriatric animals often develop *Wei* syndrome with pelvic limb muscle weakness and atrophy due to Spleen *Qi* Deficiency (weak *Qi* fails to "hold" the limbs) from the aging process, worsened by chronic illness, stress and poor nutrition.[7,8] The Spleen and Kidney have a special relationship, not only as the Grandmother and Grandchild in the Five Element Theory, but also because the Spleen creates post-natal *Jing*, while the Kidney stores the prenatal *Jing*. Post-natal *Jing* replenishes prenatal *Jing*, so when Spleen *Qi* becomes Deficient, the production of post natal *Jing* is reduced and stress is placed on the Kidney *Jing*, resulting in Kidney *Qi* Deficiency and *Tan-Huan* syndrome (paresis).[4,8] According to Five Element Theory a weak Spleen can create imbalance within the Liver, because of their "Grandchild-Grandmother" relationship and a Deficient Kidney *Qi* can also weaken the Liver because of their "Mother-Child" relationship and the pathological cycle of "Sick Mother creates a sick Child". The Liver imbalance can result in Internal Wind. Since the Kidney controls the pelvic limbs, the tremors associated with Kidney *Qi* Deficiency can primarily affect in the pelvic limbs. Spleen *Qi* Deficiency may also result in reduction of Blood production and Kidney *Qi* may fail to nourish the Liver and lead to Liver Blood Deficiency.[2] Because of the close relationship between Blood and *Yin*, chronic Liver Blood Deficiency can lead to Liver *Yin* Deficiency.[8] Tremors can then be associated with Internal Wind from the Liver Blood and *Yin* Deficiencies. As well, since the Liver nourishes the tendons and ligaments, these weaken and further result in weakness and tremors. Although a continuum of a progressive imbalance within the Spleen, Kidney and Liver systems, the TCVM clinical findings and focus of the treatments vary with the stage of the process, so they are dealt with as two separate TCVM patterns.

1. **Spleen *Qi* and Kidney *Qi* Deficiencies:** Aging compounded with long-term poor nutrition, environment and social stress and chronic illness results in both Spleen *Qi* and Kidney *Qi* Deficiencies and *Wei* and *Tan-Huan* syndromes respectively. Imbalance in the Liver results in Internal Wind (tremors) primarily in the pelvic limbs, the area controlled by the Kidney.

2. **Liver Blood, Liver *Yin* and Spleen/Kidney *Qi* Deficiencies:** Spleen *Qi* and Kidney *Qi* Deficiencies cause Deficient Liver Blood and *Yin,* which fail to nourish the tendons and ligaments. Weakness of the tendons and ligaments of the pelvic limbs result in pelvic limb weakness and tremors when standing. As well Liver Blood and *Yin* Deficiencies can result in Internal Wind (tremors) of the pelvic limbs, weakened by Deficient Kidney *Qi*.

Pattern Differentiation and Treatment

1. Spleen *Qi* and Kidney *Qi* Deficiency with Internal Wind

Clinical Signs:
- Geriatric animal
- Pelvic limb tremors when rising and standing
- Pelvic limb muscle atrophy
- Pelvic limb weakness
- Tongue- pale, wet
- Pulses- deep, weak worse on right

TCVM Diagnosis:
Chronic progressive disease and weak pulses are typical of a Deficiency pattern. The diagnosis of Internal Wind is based on the presence of tremors. The pelvic limb weakness and muscle atrophy are associated with Spleen *Qi* Deficiency. Pelvic limb paresis is associated with Kidney *Qi* Deficiency. A pale wet tongue and deep pulses, weaker on the right are typical with Spleen *Qi* ad Kidney *Qi* Deficiency.

Treatment Principles:
- Dispel Internal Wind to reduce tremors
- Tonify Spleen *Qi*
- Tonify Kidney *Qi*

Acupuncture treatment:
EA is generally not recommended in Internal Wind conditions so DN and Aqua-AP are suggested until more experience is gained with this disorder. The number of acupoints selected will vary with the overall condition of the animal and can be increased, once the response to acupuncture has been determined. Aqua-AP is performed after *Tui-na* with 0.25-0.5 ml vitamin

B12 at specific acupoints. Initially acupuncture should be administered every 1-2 weeks for 3-5 times, then every 1-2 months as needed for maintenance.

Acupoints recommended
- EA: Not currently recommended
- DN: GB-20, LI-10, ST-36, BL-17, BL-18, BL-20, BL-21, BL-23, BL-54, BL-40, BL-39, KID-3, SP-3
- Aqua-AP: BL-18, BL-20, BL-23

Pertinent acupoint actions
- GB-20 is a useful acupoint to treat Internal Wind
- LI-10 and ST-36 are general *Qi* tonic acupoints to support Spleen and Kidney *Qi*
- BL-17 is the Back *Shu* Association point for the Blood to reduce Internal Wind ("Blood is Wind suicide")
- BL-18 is the Back *Shu* Association point for the Liver to balance the Liver to reduce Internal Wind
- BL-20 is the Back *Shu* Association point for the Spleen to support Spleen *Qi*
- BL-21 is the Back *Shu* Association point for the Stomach to support Spleen *Qi*
- BL-23 is the Back *Shu* Association point for the Kidney to support Kidney *Qi*
- BL-54 is useful for pelvic limb weakness
- BL-40 is the pelvic limb Master point to strengthen the pelvic limbs
- BL-39 is useful to treat incontinence that can occur in geriatric dogs after treatment of BL-40
- KID-3 is the *Yuan* Source point for the Kidney that supports Kidney *Qi*
- SP-3 is the *Yuan* Source point for the Spleen that supports Spleen *Qi*

Herbal Medicine:
- *Bu Yang Huan Wu* (JT)[a] 0.5gm/10# twice daily orally to tonify Kidney *Qi*
- If the geriatric animal also has pain associated with *Bi* syndrome, add Body Sore (JT)[a] 0.5gm/10# twice daily orally to resolve *Qi*/Blood Stagnation and pain
- Administer Body Sore for 1-2 months or longer if needed
- Administer *Bu Yang Huan Wu* for up to 6 months
- A description of all the ingredients of the Chinese herbal medicine listed is beyond the scope of this text, but can be found elsewhere.[6,7]

Food Therapy:
The purpose of the Food Therapy is to tonify Spleen and Kidney *Qi*. Foods that are too Cold or too Hot are avoided.[9]
- Foods to tonify Spleen and Kidney *Qi*: Beef, chicken, sardines, egg, potato, yam, sweet potato, rice, oats, millet, lentils, carrots, squash, microalgae, dates, figs, molasses, royal jelly

- Cold foods to avoid: Turkey, duck, duck eggs, conch, clams, mussels, yogurt, millet, barley, spinach, broccoli, celery, egg plant, kelp, alfalfa, cucumbers, pears, bananas, white radishes, watermelon
- Hot foods to avoid: Lamb, shrimp, corn-fed beef, chicken, trout, squash, turnips, sweet rice, basal, caraway, cherries, chilies, cinnamon, ginger, rosemary, sage

Tui-na Procedures:

The purpose of *Tui-na* is to further strengthen the pelvic limb and reduce tremors. A description of each technique and their actions can be found in Chapter 1 Table 8.[10]

- *An-fa* pressing and *Tui-fa* pushing from BL-23 forward to BL-17; repeat 12 times
- *Yi-zhi-chan* single thumb and *Rou-fa* rotary kneading at BL-54, BL-40 and BL-39 for 1 minute at each site on each limb
- *Ca-fa* rubbing from the hip to the tarsus on each side for 1 minute
- *Dou-fa* gently shaking for 12 times, *Ba-shen-fa* stretching for 12 times and *Ban-fa* flexing and extending joints for 12 times of each pelvic limb

Daily Life Style Recommendation for Owner Follow-up:

- Gentle *Ca-fa* rubbing from the hip to the tarsus on each side for 1 minute twice daily
- *Dou-fa* gently shaking for 12 times, *Ba-shen-fa* stretching for 12 times and *Ban-fa* flexing and extending joints for 12 times of each pelvic limb twice daily
- Maintain good nutrition to support the Spleen and *Qi*
- Take short walks daily to keep the *Qi* moving
- Keep in a quiet restful low stress environment to support the Liver

Comments:

The purpose of TCVM treatment is to control the tremors and strengthen the pelvic limbs. Further studies are needed to determine if the TCVM treatment can control signs and increase the quality of life for affected geriatric dogs.

2. Liver Blood, Liver *Yin* and Spleen/Kidney *Qi* Deficiencies

Clinical Signs:

- Geriatric animal
- Pelvic limb tremors when rising and standing
- Pelvic limb muscle atrophy
- Pelvic limb weakness
- Dry burnt hair
- Large dandruff flakes
- Cracked pads
- Panting
- Cool seeking
- Warm ears, back or feet
- Tongue- pale or red, dry
- Pulses- deep, weak, worse on left thready

***TCVM Diagnosis*:**
The diagnosis is based on the history, clinical complaint and TCVM examination findings, including tongue and pulse characteristics. The weak deep pulses are typical of a Deficiency pattern. The panting, cool seeking behavior, warm ears, back and feet and red, dry tongue are clinical signs associated with Heat typical of Liver and Kidney *Yin* Deficiencies. The burnt dry hair, cracked pads, large dandruff flakes and pale, dry tongue are typical of Liver Blood Deficiency. Thready pulses reflect the *Yin* Deficiency and pulses weaker on the left are found in *Yin* and Blood Deficiencies.

***Treatment Principles*:**
- Dispel Internal Wind
- Tonify Liver Blood
- Tonify Liver *Yin*
- Tonify Spleen/Kidney *Qi*

***Acupuncture treatment*:**
EA is generally not recommended in Internal Wind conditions so DN and Aqua-AP are suggested until more experience is gained with this disorder. The number of acupoints selected will vary with the overall condition of the animal and can be increased, once the response to acupuncture has been determined. Aqua-AP is performed after *Tui-na* with 0.25-0.5 ml vitamin B12 at specific acupoints. Initially acupuncture should be administered every 1-2 weeks for 3-5 times, then every 1-2 months as needed for maintenance.

Acupoints recommended
- EA: Not currently recommended
- DN: LIV-3, SP-10, BL-17, BL-18, GB-20, LI-10, ST-36, BL-20, BL-21, BL-23, BL-54, BL-40, BL-39, KID-3, KID-6, SP-3
- Aqua-AP: BL-18, BL-20, BL-23

Pertinent acupoint actions
- LIV-3 is the *Yuan* Source point for the Liver that supports Liver *Yin* and Blood
- SP-10 is "the sea of Blood" useful to treat Blood Deficiency
- BL-17 is the Back *Shu* Association point for the Blood to support Liver Blood
- BL-18 is the Back *Shu* Association point for the Liver to support Liver *Yin* and Blood
- GB-20 is a useful acupoint to treat Internal Wind
- LI-10 and ST-36 are general *Qi* tonic acupoints to support Spleen and Kidney *Qi*
- BL-20 is the Back *Shu* Association point for the Spleen to support Spleen *Qi*
- BL-21 is the Back *Shu* Association point for the Stomach to support Spleen *Qi*
- BL-23 is the Back *Shu* Association point for the Kidney to support Kidney *Qi*

- BL-54 is useful for pelvic limb weakness
- BL-40 is the pelvic limb Master point to strengthen the pelvic limbs
- BL-39 is useful to treat incontinence that can occur in geriatric dogs after treatment of BL-40
- KID-3 is the *Yuan* Source point for the Kidney that supports Kidney *Qi*
- KID-6 is the confluent point for the *Yin Qiao* Extraordinary Channel useful to treat *Yin* Deficiencies
- SP-3 is the *Yuan* Source point for the Spleen that supports Spleen *Qi*

Herbal Medicine:
- Tendon Ligament Formula (JT)[a] 0.5gm/10# twice daily orally to tonify Liver Blood and Yin and strengthen the tendons and ligaments
- If the geriatric animal also has pain associated with *Bi* syndrome, add Body Sore (JT)[a] 0.5gm/10# twice daily orally to resolve *Qi*/Blood Stagnation and pain
- Administer Body Sore for 1-2 months or longer if needed
- Administer Tendon Ligament Formula for up to 6 months
- A description of all the ingredients of the Chinese herbal medicine listed is beyond the scope of this text, but can be found elsewhere.[6,7]

Food Therapy:
The purpose of the Food Therapy is to tonify Liver Blood and clear Heat and tonify Liver *Yin*. Hot foods should be avoided.[9]
- Foods to supplement to Tonify Blood: Beef, bone marrow, eggs, liver, heart, pheasant, oysters, salmon, sardines, barley, corn, oats, short grain (glutinous rice), wheat, adzuki, black kidney beans, beet root, carrots, dark leafy greens, kelp, microalgae, cherries, dates, figs, longan, molasses
- Foods to supplement to Cool and tonify *Yin*: Turkey, pork, duck, clams, crab, eggs, rice, wheat, wheat germ, wheat berries, Belgian endive, string beans, peas, kidney beans, sweet potatoes, yams, tomato, spinach, tofu, kiwi, lemons, rhubarb, pears, bananas, watermelon, sesame, seaweed
- Hot foods to avoid: Lamb, shrimp, corn-fed beef, chicken, trout, squash, turnips, sweet rice, basal, caraway, cherries, chilies, cinnamon, ginger, rosemary, sage

Tui-na Procedures:
The purpose of *Tui-na* is to further strengthen the pelvic limb and reduce tremors. A description of each technique and their actions can be found in Chapter 1 Table 8.[10]
- *An-fa* pressing and *Tui-fa* pushing from BL-23 forward to BL-17; repeat 12 times
- *Yi-zhi-chan* single thumb and *Rou-fa* rotary kneading at BL-54, BL-40 and BL-39 for 1 minute at each site on each limb
- *Ca-fa* rubbing from the hip to the tarsus on each side for 1 minute
- *Dou-fa* gently shaking for 12 times, *Ba-shen-fa* stretching for 12 times and *Ban-fa* flexing and extending joints for 12 times of each pelvic limb

Daily Life Style Recommendation for Owner Follow-up:
- Gentle *Ca-fa* rubbing from the hip to the tarsus on each side for 1 minute twice daily

- *Dou-fa* gently shaking for 12 times, *Ba-shen-fa* stretching for 12 times and *Ban-fa* flexing and extending joints for 12 times of each pelvic limb twice daily
- Maintain good nutrition to support the Spleen and *Qi*
- Take short walks daily to keep the *Qi* moving
- Keep in a quiet restful low stress environment to support the Liver

Comments:

The purpose of TCVM treatment is to control the tremors and strengthen the pelvic limbs. Further studies are needed to determine if the TCVM treatment can control signs and increase the quality of life for affected geriatric dogs.

Footnotes:

[a] (JT) = *Jing Tang* Herbal www.tcvmherbal.com; Reddick, FL

References:

1. De Lahunta A, Glass E. Veterinary Neuroanatomy and Clinical Neurology 3rd Ed. Philadelphia, PA:WB Saunders 2008:95-113,14.
2. Chrisman C, Mariani C, Platt S, Clemmons R. Neurology for the Small Animal Practitioner. Jackson Wy: Teton NewMedia 2003:125-167.
3. Platt S, Olby N (ed). BSAVA Manual of Canine and Feline Neurology 5th Ed. Gloucester, UK:BSAVA Publications 2011:1-500.
4. Xie H, Priest V. Xie's Veterinary Acupuncture. Ames, Iowa:Blackwell Publishing 2007:585.
5. Xie H. Personal communications
6. Xie H, Preast V. Xie's Chinese Veterinary Herbology. Ames. IA:Wiley-Blackwell 2010:305-347, 486-510, 387,449-460.
7. Xie H, Preast V. Chinese Veterinary Herbal Handbook 2nd Ed. Reddick, FL: Chi Institute of Chinese Medicine 2008:305-585.
8. Xie H, Priest V. Traditional Chinese Veterinary Medicine. Reddick, FL: Jing Tang Publishing 2002:209-293,307-380,409-419.
9. Leggett D. Helping Ourselves: A Guide to Traditional Chinese Food Energetics. Totnes, England: Meridian Press 2005:21-36.
10. Xie H, Ferguson B, Deng X. Application of *Tui-na* in Veterinary Medicine 2nd Ed. Reddick, FL:Chi Institute 2007:1-94,129-132.

Seizures in a 20 Year Old Quarter Horse Mare

Joan D. Winter, DVM

ABSTRACT:

"Shadow," a fourteen year old Quarter Horse Mare became a patient of mine July 11, 1998, for routine preventive care including vaccines, dental care, and forelimb lameness. On November 13, 2000, based on clinical signs of sore front feet, cresty neck and obese body condition, I drew blood samples in the morning and evening, and mailed the serum to BET Reproductive Laboratories, Inc., for a Thyroxine T4, Insulin, and Cortisol tests:

Thyroxine T4 AM =10.0	Thyroxine T4 PM =15.5	T4 Normal= 12-25ng/ml
Insulin AM=25.2	Insulin PM=54.8	Insulin Normal=2-25 uIU/ml
Cortisol AM=34.2	Cortisol PM=36.0	Cortisol Rhythm Change=5%

Cortisol Rhythm%=(high Value-Low Value)/High Value X 100

Normal Rhythm>30%
Low Rhythm= 20-30%
Poor rhythm=4-20%
No rhythm= <4%

My interpretation included a low morning thyroid value and normal evening thyroid value; normal fasting insulin level in the morning with an elevated insulin level in the evening; Cortisol rhythm change to be poor at 5%.

On November 20, 2000, I started "Shadow" on 0.25mg PerMax tablets from CostCo Human Pharmacy, once daily in the morning. Metaboleeze, a feed additive from Kentucky Performance Products, was included in her feed schedule as of July 24, 2001, to insure adequate chromium intake. Metaboleeze is a supplement source of the micromineral chromium.

Concerning her limbs, I found "Shadow" breaking down in the forelimbs at the level of the pasterns and subject to bruised soles due to flat, rather than concave, soles. I interpreted her pastern lameness due to a possible laxity of the ligaments from excess cortisol secretion. Isoxsuprine (9-30-2002) and Bute (11-29-2001) were added to her daily medication. The isoxsuprine was started to help with her intermittent sore forelimbs soles and navicular syndrome. Previous radiographs of the forelimb feet were taken September 13, 2000, along with nerve blocks of the lame right limb. At that time she responded to a PD nerve block. Nerve blocks were repeated January 3, 2001, of the lame right forelimb and included posterior distal (PD), abaxial, low volar, and high volar with no real improvement. I suspected a high suspensory lesion. On September 18, 2002, I convinced the client to add Rehmannia 14 to the medication regime (2 large scoops twice daily for 30 days). The client discontinued the Herbal Formulation of Rehmannia 14 due to costs and her feelings that the Herbal Formula was not working. On 8-9-2004, "Shadow" became very lame on the right front foot. I injected the right front foot heel points with her blood (aqua acupuncture), applied topical Relief Salve to the coronary band and started *Sang Zhi San* (2 large scoops twice daily for 30 days) for soreness below the carpus and Body Sore (2 large scoops twice daily for 30 days) for compensatory muscle soreness.

Table 1: Ingredients and Actions of Rehmannia 14

Pin Yin Name	English Name	Actions
Bai Shao	Paeonia	Nourish Liver *Yin* and Blood
Fu Ling	Poria	Clear Damp and strengthen Spleen
Fu Zi	Aconite	Warm and tonify Kidney *Yang*
Gui Zhi	Cinnamomum	Warm Kidney *Yang*
Huang Bai	Phellodendron	Clear Heat and nourish *Yin*
Huang Qi	Astragalus	Tonify *Qi*
Mai Men Dong	Ophiopogon	Moisten and nourish Heart and Lung *Yin*
Mu Dan Pi	Moutan	Cool Blood, clear Heat, dissipate stagnation
Shan Yao	Dioscorea	Tonify Qi and *Jing*
Shan Zhu Yu	Cornus	Nourish Liver *Yin*
Sheng Di Huang	Rehmannia	Nourish *Yin* and *Jing*
Wu Wei Zi	Schisandra	Consolidate and nourish Lung *Yin*
Ze Xie	Alisma	Benefit urination and clear deficient Fire
Zhi Mu	Anemarrhena	Clear Heat and promote body fluid and *Yin*

Manufactured and distributed by Jing-tang Herbal, Inc., Reddick, FL

Table 2: Ingredients and Actions of Relief Salve

Pin Yin Name	English Name	Actions
Bai Zhi	Angelica	Clear the surface, relieve pain, promote healing
Bing Pian	Borneol	Open the orifice, dissipate stagnation, clear Heat, relieve pain
Da Huang	Rheum	Break down stasis, dissipate swelling, cool Blood
Dang Gui Wei	Angelica	Invigorates Blood and relieves pain
Feng La	Bees Wax	Carrier
Hai Tong Pi	Erythrina	Dispels Damp, invigorates Channels
Hong Hua	Carthamus	Moves Blood, disperses swelling
Hua Jiao	Zanthoxylum	Warm the middle, dispel Cold, relieve pain, dry up Damp
Mo Yao	Myrrh	Invigorates Blood, relieves pain, repairs tissue
Mu Bie Zi	Momordica	Dissipate swelling and nodules, relieve pain
Ru Xiang	Olibanum	Invigorates Blood, relieves pain, repairs tissue
Xue Jie	Draconis	Dissipate stagnation, relieve pain, promote healing
Yan Hu Suo	Corydalis	Invigorate Blood and relive pain
Zhang Nao	Camphora	Open the orifice, kill parasites, relieve pain
Zhi Wu You	Olive Oil	Carrier
Zhi Zi	Gardenia	Clear Heat, detoxify, cool Blood, dissipate stagnation

Manufactured and distributed by Jing-tang Herbal, Inc., Reddick, FL

Table 3: Ingredients and Actions of *Sang Zhi San*

Pin Yin Name	English Name	Actions
Ba Ji Tian	Morinda	Tonifies Kidney *Yang* and strengthens the bones
Bu Gu Zhi	Psoralea	Tonifies Kidney *Yang*.
Du Huo	Angelica	Dispels Wind, Cold and Dampness; relieves pain

Du Zhong	Eucommia	Tonifies Kidney *Qi* and *Yang*, strengthens back
Fang Feng	Ledebouriella	Clear Wind and open the body surface
Gu Sui Bu	Drynaria	Tonifies Kidney *Yang* and benefits bones
Gui Zhi	Cinnamomum	Warm channel and relieve pain
Niu Xi	Achyranthes	Supports Kidneys, strengthens legs bones.
Qiang Huo	Notopterygium	Clear Wind-Damp and relieve pain
Sang Zhi	Morus	Clear Wind-Cold-Damp in limbs and Channels

Manufactured and distributed by Jing-tang Herbal, Inc., Reddick, FL

On December 31, 2005, "Shadow's" lameness issues seemed to take a back seat. She began that evening to show seizure activity. I observed four partial seizures with muscle fasciculations, vocalization as if squealing, and squirting urine as if in heat. When safe to approach, I gave her 3cc Valium IV and 0.5cc Dormosodan IV. I also used dry acupuncture needles at *Tong-tian* (for Wind pattern and hyperactive behavior), *Er-jian* (for excess heat), and *Da-feng-men* (for Wind pattern and hyperactive behavior). I treated her with more drugs including 2cc Valium IV and 0.75cc Dormosodan IV in order to examine her ears. I needed to rule out an inner ear infection. Her ear drums were unremarkable. She appeared cortically blind on the left side OS. My differential included Brain infection, brain tumor (Cushing's disease) of the pituitary gland putting pressure on the optic chaisma causing seizures, Pergolide overdose, encephalopathy, liver failure, or cholesterol granuloma of the brain. A short telephone consultation with Dr. Tina Kemper, Boarded in Large Animal Internal Medicine, helped me to rule out a cholesterol granuloma based on forced manipulation of the head and the horse's response, or lack of (not collapsing). I ground up *Di Tan Tang* teapills, 50, 2 large scoops of Liver Happy and started "Shadow" on long term course of Stasis in the Mansion of Mind (2 large scoops PO daily BID).

Table 4: Ingredients and Actions of Body Sore

Pin Yin Name	**English Name**	**Actions**
Bu Gu Zhi	Psoralea	Strengthen bone and tonify *Yang*
Chi Shao	Paeonia	Relieve pain and cool Blood
Chuan Xiong	Ligusticum	Relieve pain and activate Blood
Dang Gui	Angelica	Activate Blood, resolve stagnation and relieve pain
Du Huo	Angelica	Relieve pain and eliminate Wind-Damp
Du Zhong	Eucommia	Strengthen back and tonify *Yang*
Hong Hua	Carthamus	Break down Blood stasis, relieve pain
Ji Xue Teng	Millettia	Nourish Blood
Mo Yao	Myrrh	Move Blood, relieve pain
Niu Xi	Achyranthes	Strengthen bones and limbs
Qiang Huo	Notopterygium	Relieve pain and activate Blood
Ru Xiang	Olibanum	Move Blood, relieve pain
Tao Ren	Persica	Break down Blood stasis, relieve pain
Tu Si Zi	Cuscuta	Nourish Kidney and Liver

Yan Hu Suo	Corydalis	Move *Qi*/Blood, resolve stagnation and relieve pain
Yin Yang Huo	Epimedium	Tonify Kidney *Yang* and *Yin*

Manufactured and distributed by Jing-tang Herbal, Inc., Reddick, FL

I ordered and placed "Shadow" on 2 large scoops of *Di Tan Tang* powder PO twice daily. I continued the Stasis in the Mansion of Mind. I allowed the continued use of Bute and Pergalide. I used *Di Tan Tang* for 6 months, then, switched to *Tian Man Bai Zhu* for another 6 months. I followed this protocol until 2007. "Shadow" remained on Stasis in the Mansion of Mind until 2008.

Table 5: Ingredients and Actions of *Di Tan Tang*

Pin Yin Name	English Name	Actions
Chen Pi	Citrus	Move *Qi*, transform phlegm
Dan Nan Xing	Arisaema	Transform phlegm
Fu Ling	Poria	Drain Damp
Gan Cao	Glycyrrhiza	Harmonize
Gan Jiang	Zingiberis	Harmonize
Gou Teng	Uncaria	Extinguish Internal Wind, clear Liver Heat
Hai Zao	Sargassum	Transform phlegm, clear Heat, soften the hardness
Kun Bu	Laminaria	Transform phlegm, soften the hardness, drain water
Ren Shen(Kirin)	Ginseng	Tonify *Qi*
Shi Jue Ming	Haliotis	Clear Liver Heat
Shi Chang Pu	Acorus	Open the orifice, eliminate Damp
Zhi Shi	Aurantium	Move *Qi*
Zhu Ru	Bambusa	Transform phlegm

Manufactured and distributed by Jing-tang Herbal, Inc., Reddick, FL

Table 6: Ingredients and Actions of Liver Happy

Pin Yin Name	English Name	Actions
Bai Shao	Paeonia	Soothe Liver
Bo He	Mentha	Move *Qi*
Chai Hu	Bupleurum	Soothe Liver
Chen Pi	Citrus	Dry up Dampness, move *Qi*
Dang Gui	Angelica	Move Blood
Gan Cao	Glycyrrhiza	Harmonize
Mu Dan Pi	Moutan	Cool Liver
Qing Pi	Citrus	Move *Qi*, Soothe Liver, resolve stagnation
Xiang Fu Zi	Cyperus	Soothe Liver, resolve stagnation
Zhi Zi	Gardenia	Clear Heat

Manufactured and distributed by Jing-tang Herbal, Inc., Reddick, FL

Table 7: Ingredients and Actions of Stasis in Mansion of Mind

Pin Yin Name	English Name	Actions
Bai Zhi	Angelica	Warm the Channel, relieve pain
Ban Xia	Pinellia	Transform phlegm
Chuan Xiong	Ligusticum	Move Blood
Dan Shen	Salvia	Move Blood
Di Long	Lumbricus	Clear Wind, invigorate Channel
Gao Ben	Ligusticum	Relieve pain
Ge Gen	Pueraria	Bring Qi upward
Hong Hua	Carthamus	Break down Blood Stasis
Jiang Can	Bombyx	Transform phlegm, resolve nodule
Quan Xie	Buthus	Break down Blood Stasis
Sheng Ma	Cimicifuga	Ascend Qi
Zhe Bei Mu	Fritillaria	Transform phlegm, resolve nodules

Manufactured and distributed by Jing-tang Herbal, Inc., Reddick, FL

Table 8: Ingredients and Actions of *Tian Ma Bai Zhu*

Pin Yin Name	English Name	Actions
Bai Zhu	Atractylodes	Strengthen Spleen, eliminate Damp
Ban Xia	Pinellia	Transform phlegm, dry up Damp
Chen Pi	Citrus	Move Qi, transform Phlegm
Da Zao	Jujube	Harmonize
Fu Ling	Poria	Drain Damp, strengthen Spleen
Gan Cao	Glycyrrhiza	Harmonize
Gan Jiang	Zingiberis	Harmonize
Tian Ma	Gastrodia Elata	Clear Internal Wind, resolve seizure

Manufactured and distributed by Jing-tang Herbal, Inc., Reddick, FL

On June 28, 2006, I was able to approach "Shadow" as a veterinarian and examine her left eye. Partial vision was assessed with poor blood vessels to the optic disc, in my opinion. Her right eye appeared normal. Since her seizure incident, her next door stable mate, also owned by the same owner, was resistant to leave "Shadow." We later assumed it was because he was her "eyes" when she was cortically blind.

Currently, she is on Pergalide and Bute PO. Her owner finds her well adjusted mentally with no further seizures. After her seizure incident, I was no longer able to go near her safely. Others could, but not me. We have become not friends, but acquaintances - I have haltered her and taken her to the turn out. Her issues today consist of forelimb lameness with broken down pasterns. She is a pet and has been since her seizure activity. Besides, her beloved owner grew into a beautiful woman now in college with little interest in riding.

In my opinion, this is a success story. Horses that have had seizures, unrelated to drug reactions or infectious diseases or organ failure, have been destroyed as there is no long acting medications for seizure activity. In this case, I used an herbal formulation (*Di Tang Tan* and *Tian Man Bai Zhu*) instead of Phenobarbital to control the excess brain activity. I used Stasis in the Mansion of Mind to shrink the pituitary brain tumor (Phlegm caused by underlying Spleen *Qi* deficiency).

References:
1. Tina Kemper, D.V.M. San Louis Rey Equine Hospital, Bonsall, CA, USA
2. BET Reproductive Labs, Lexington, KY, USA

How I Treat Cognitive Dysfunction Syndrome

Huisheng Xie DVM, MS, PhD

Cognitive dysfunction syndrome (CDS) is also known as dementia, which is clinically similar to Alzheimer's disease in humans.[1] With ageing, *beta amyloid* is deposited in the brain. When these proteins have built up over time in the same area of the brain, they form plaque, which impedes the transmission of the brain's electrical signals. Consequently, the CDS patients show disorientation, confusion, memory loss and personality changes.[2]

CDS can affect any breed of dog, but commonly occurs in dogs over eight years old or sooner in large breeds. A large breed such as a Mastiff, may exhibit signs as early as five or six years of age. In one study, 62% of 11-16 year old dogs showed at least one of the clinical sign of CDS listed below.[1,2] CDS can also affect older cats.[3]

TCVM Etiology and Pathology

In Traditional Chinese Veterinary Medicine (TCVM), CDS is due to a loss of *Shen*. The *Shen* is the Spirit or Mind. *Shen* rules mental activities, memory and sleep. *Shen* also refers to the outward appearance of the vital activities of the whole body. It provides an animal with awareness and mental clarity. When *Shen* is healthy, it produces inner peace. The animal with a healthy *Shen* will exhibit normal behaviors and will be alert and responsive to environmental stimuli. When *Shen* is lost, the animal will show poor memory, disorientation, confusion, restlessness, palpitation, anxiety and hyperactivity.

The *Shen* is housed in the Heart. The Heart *Qi* plays an important role in mental activities and brain functions. The plaques formed by *beta amyloid* peptides in the brain are considered Phlegm or local Blood Stagnation. Phlegm is often generated by the abnormal amount of accumulated fluids produced by Spleen *Qi* Deficiency. Phlegm in the brain tends to mist and block the Mind, leading to a loss of *Shen*. The *Shen* also requires nourishment and anchoring from Heart *Yin* and Blood to remain healthy. When Heart *Yin* and Blood are Deficient, the *Shen* lacks anchoring and nourishment, leading to a *Shen* Disturbance and abnormal behavioral changes. Thus, CDS can be divided into two main patterns: Phlegm Misting Mind with Heart/Spleen *Qi* Deficiency and Heart *Yin*-Blood Deficiency with Local Brain Blood Stagnation.

TCVM Pattern Differentiation and Treatment
1) Phlegm Misting the Mind with Heart and Spleen *Qi* Deficiency

Clinical Signs:
- Fire Constitution becomes Metal or Water
    - Stop greeting their family
    - Stop any social interaction or become less responsive
    - Become more aloof or fearful
- Confusion, disorientation, or forgetful
    - Getting lost in corners
    - Not responding to name being called
    - Having indoor accidents
    - Forget how to navigate the stairs

- o Press their heads into corners of walls
- o Wandering through the house
- o Stare blankly at a roof, wall, or door
- o At the end, these animals fail to recognize their owners and friends.
- Sleep more or lack of appetite
- Lethargy or exercise intolerance
- Tongue: pale wet
- Pulse: deep, weaker in the right side

Acupuncture: GV-20, *Da-feng-men, Nao-shu, An-shen*, HT-7, HT-9, BL-14/15/20/21, CV-14/17, ST-40, ST-36

Herbal Medicine: Wen Dan Tang + Stasis in Mansion of Mind.
    Wen Dan Tang strengthens the Spleen to transform Phlegm, and moves *Qi* to resolve Stagnation. Stasis In Mansion of Mind moves Blood to break down Stasis in the brain.

2) Heart *Yin* and Blood Deficiency along with Brain Blood Stagnation

Clinical Signs:
- Listlessness, or anxiety
- Bark, or other abnormal behavior at night or late evening
- Sleep less at night or sleep more during the day
- Forget they ate and want to eat again and again
- Keep their caretakers awake at night pacing
- Become aggressive or develop separation anxiety
- Cats howl at night for no reason, go into closets and can't find their way out
- Stop responding when called or spoken to by the family
- Often forget the family who loves them
- Forget boundary lines or have household accidents
- Tongue: dry, red or pale
- Pulse: deep and thin, weaker on the left side

Acupuncture: GV-20, *Da-feng-men, Nao-shu, An-shen*, HT-7, HT-9, BL-14/15/17/43/44/48, SP-10/6/9, KID-3

Herbal Medicine: Shen Calmer + Stasis in Mansion of Mind
    Shen Calmer tonifies Heart *Yin* and Blood, soothes Liver *Qi*. Stasis In Mansion of Mind moves Blood to break down Stasis in the brain.

Other Considerations:

1) *Jin Gui Shen Qi Wan* (*Ba Wei Di Huang Wan*) benefits in the treatment of dementia in humans. The cognitive function of patients with dementia significantly increased after taking 2 g of this herbal medicine 3 times a day after meals for 8 weeks. [4]
2) Anipryl is a Pfizer drug used in the human treatment of Parkinson's Disease. Anipryl increases the level of the essential neurotransmitter dopamine in the brain. The behavior of approximately 75% of the affected dogs improved within 30 to 60 days.

But 20-25% of the dogs on Anipryl have adverse side effects including vomiting, lethargy, staggering, hyperactivity (restlessness), diarrhea, seizures or anorexia. Anipryl is not recommended for cats because it is very toxic to cats.

3) Antioxidants seem to have some benefit for treatment of CDS. [5]

Case example

"Cinnamon", a Golden Retriever, spayed/female, 11 years old was presented with gradually developed signs of dementia. She showed occasional episodes of disorientation, and unresponsiveness to the owner's when they called her name. Sometimes, her caretaker found her with her head pressed into the corner of the bedroom. Sometimes, she would stand staring blankly at the walls. According to the owner, her appetite, defecation, urination and energy level were good. On the TCVM examination, she had an Earth constitution. Her body temperature and hair coat felt hot. She panted a lot and panting was worse at night. Her *Shen* seemed depressed, and she showed sensitivity on palpation of her head. She had dry skin with lots of dandruff. Her tongue was pale and dry. Her pulse was thin and fast.

The TCVM Pattern was *Yin* and Blood Deficiency with Brain *Qi*-Blood Stagnation.

Acupuncture Treatment
1) Dry needle: GV-20, HT-7, BL-14/15/17, SP-10
2) Electro-acupuncture 10 min 20 Hz and 10 min 80-120 Hz (a total of 20 minutes) at the following pairs of local acupoints:
   Da-feng-men to *Long-hui* (top line)
   Da-feng-men to TH-23 (Line 6, Motor line)
   GV-20 to *Nao-shu* (Line 7, Sensory Line)
3) Aqua-acupuncture (Vitamin B12, 0.5 cc per point): An-*Shen*, HT-7, CV-14, CV-17, ST-40

Herbal Medicine:
1) *Shen* Calmer, 5 grams BID orally for 2 months;
2) Stasis in Mansion of Mind, 5 grams BID for 2 months.

Outcome: She showed a significant improvement (more responsive to the owner's calling her, less time spent staring at the walls) after 2 monthly acupuncture treatments and 2 months of daily herbal medications. She continued to take these two herbal medicines for 1 year and her cognitive function returned to normal. As new problems arose the herbal medication was changed, *Jin Gui Shen Qi* was used for Kidney *Yang* Deficiency renal failure, Hindquarter Weakness Formula was used for Kidney *Yin/Qi* Deficiency (pelvic limb weakness). She had a great life of 4 more years and was euthanized at age of 15 because of diabetes and IVDD.

References:
1. González-Martínez A, Rosado B, Pesini P, Suárez ML, Santamarina G, García-Belenguer S, Villegas A, Monleón I, Sarasa M. Plasma β-amyloid peptides in canine aging and cognitive dysfunction as a model of Alzheimer's disease. Exp Gerontol. 2011 Mar 3. [Epub ahead of print]
2. Ruehl WW, Hart BL: Canine Cognitive Dysfunction. In Psychopharmacology of Animal Behavior Disorders (Dodman NH, Schuster L, eds.). Boston: Blackwell Scientific, 1998; pp. 283-304.

3. Landsberg GM, Denenberg S, Araujo JA. Cognitive dysfunction in cats: a syndrome we used to dismiss as 'old age'. J Feline Med Surg. 2010 Nov;12(11):837-48.
4. Koh Iwasaki, Seiichi Kobayashi, Yuri Chimura, Mayumi Taguchi, Kazumi Inoue, Shigehumi Cho, Tetsuo Akiba, Hiroyuki Arai, Jong-Chol Cyong, and Hidetada Sasaki, A Randomized, Double-Blind, Placebo-Controlled Clinical Trial of the Chinese Herbal Medicine ''Ba Wei Di Huang Wan'' in the Treatment of Dementia. J Am Geriatr Soc 52:1518–1521, 2004.
5. Manteca X. Nutrition and behavior in senior dogs. Top Companion Anim Med. 2011 Feb;26(1):33-6.

How I Treat Hydrocephalus

RM Clemmons, DVM, PhD, CVA, CVFT

Advances in modern medicine have made this an exciting era in the field of veterinary neurology. At no time in the past has the ability to study both the in vivo structure and function of the central nervous system (CNS). New techniques in molecular biology have made it possible to actually diagnose and treat disease at the genetic level or by correcting protein alterations caused by changes at the atomic level. However, in spite these seemingly miraculous enhancements to medicine, we are often left without a practical solution to the patient's problems. The treatment may be beyond the financial or emotional resources of the client so that alternatives to these new treatments need to be available. At the same time, the improved diagnostics that are available are also critical to deciding what constitutes the best approach to treatment whether conventional or not. While owners may have a trouble affording or may not allow processes needed to achieve a diagnosis, they should be encouraged to seek as complete and thorough an answer as possible.

In the case of neurologic conditions, the main things which help are a comprehensive evaluation of the systemic system, including blood tests, urinalysis and radiographic or ultrasound imaging of the body cavities. If these tests are unremarkable or cannot explain the neurologic disease, then specific neurologic tests are indicated. These can include electrodiagnostics such as electromyography (EMG) or electroencephalography (EEG), cerebrospinal fluid (CSF) analysis, and neural imaging such as magnetic resonance imaging (MRI). The latter method (MRI) allows for an anatomic diagnosis and can confirm whether a process is likely to be inflammatory, vascular or neoplastic. This knowledge can direct therapy to be far more specific than without that knowledge. Knowing that the disease is a tumor versus a chronic disk protrusion can make treatments more purposeful and specific.

Hydrocephalus is defined as an abnormal accumulation of cerebrospinal fluid (CSF) within the ventricular system of the brain accompanied by a concomitant loss of cerebral white matter or gray matter.[1-3] This condition is a common neurologic disorder of miniature breed dogs and offers a unique challenge to the clinician for diagnosis and treatment.

Pathophysiology

Hydrocephalus develops as a sequel to excessive formation of CSF, to decreased absorption of CSF, or to a loss of cerebral tissue volume. The pathophysiology of the former two conditions is important because these causes of hydrocephalus are likely to respond to CSF shunting procedures. The third condition is not likely to respond to either surgical or medical management.

As a result of excessive fluid accumulation in the ventricular system from increased formation or decreased absorption of CSF, disequilibrium of forces exists at the ventricular-cerebral interface. Because the ventricular surface is semipermeable, there is a net flux of CSF into the periventricular extracellular fluid compartment. A concomitant decrease must occur in other cranial structures because no "dead space" exists within the cranial cavity. Cerebral vascular structures are most easily compressed, and with increased production of extracellular fluid from the ventricles, the periventricular white matter's reabsorptive capacity is overloaded. The vasculature of the white matter thereby collapses and leads to the development of periventricular white matter ischemia. Because oligodendroglia are sensitive to ischemic insult, demyelination and ventricular enlargement result. Therefore, early treatment must be given for maximal benefit to the patient.

Some authors have not seen elevated intracranial pressure in dogs with hydrocephalus. In human patients likely to benefit from CSF shunting, however, transient or constantly increased ventricular pressure is common. Although the CSF pressure may be within normal levels in most dogs, increased intracranial pressure does occur in hydrocephalus and may play a significant role in the progression of this disorder. Hydrocephalus in the dog is associated with a higher initial resistance to CSF absorption, but an increased absorptive capacity. The mean rate of CSF formation is also found to be reduced. These findings suggest that canine hydrocephalus would be expected to exhibit low or normal ventricular pressures, but that minor changes in CSF volume would result in pressure increases that could not be normally transmitted or dispersed. Fluctuations in intraventricular pressure, as seen in man, would lead to periods of abnormally high pressures.

Diagnosis

The variability of signs of canine hydrocephalus often makes the diagnosis by clinical criteria alone difficult. In young animals in which a dome-shaped calvarium, open fontanelles, and a downcast gaze are also associated with neurologic dysfunction, however, the diagnosis may be easier. Confirmatory laboratory examinations include electroencephalography and radiology.

The electroencephalogram of hydrocephalic dogs is characterized by high-amplitude, slow wave activity. This pattern is accentuated during sleep, but remains abnormal even during the alerting response. Although a correlation does appear to exist between the electroencephalographic changes and the degree of ventricular enlargement, these findings do not correlate with the clinical signs.

Noncontrast radiographs may show some flattening of the gyral impressions upon the calvarium, but such changes are not pathognomonic. Computer-assisted tomography (CAT scan) and MRI have replaced most other methods of brain imaging. Both of these advanced imaging techniques, MRI particularly, can demonstrate the enlarged ventricular system along with changes within the brain's tissues.

Laboratory evaluation of ventricular fluid pressure, volume, and chemical and cellular characteristics may furnish helpful information about the underlying cause of hydrocephalus.

Surgical Correction

The decision to place a ventriculoperitoneal shunt should be based upon the progression of clinical signs. The triad of dementia, gait abnormalities, and incontinence is an accurate predictor of responsiveness to shunting procedures in people and can be used in the dog.

On the other hand, it seems that patients who are less than a year of age seem to do better with shunting than patients over that age. This is probably because of the ability of younger animals to repair and recover from neurologic injuries and from the fact that they may have less overall damage. In older dogs, hydrocephalus may be from loss of neural tissue rather than from increased intracranial pressure as part of normal aging or from canine cognitive dysfunction.

TCVM Diagnosis and Treatment

Hydrocephalus can be the result of Kidney *Jing* deficiency where the Kidney fails to support the development of marrow. The Kidney does not nourish the child (Liver) leading to stagnation of Blood and *Qi*. The grandparent (Kidney) does not control the grandchild (Heart) leading to mania. The grandchild (Kidney) becomes rebellious and insults the grandparent (Spleen) leading to accumulation of Damp. As such, hydrocephalus can be thought of as the result of a Spleen deficient Damp pattern, where the accumulation of Damp affects the Mind and Heart. The treatment principle is to dry the Damp, dissolve the turbidity, eliminate the excess fluid and clear the Mind.

The pattern differentiation of hydrocephalus emphasizes main symptoms in combination with concurrent ones to differentiate whether the disease is deficient or excess in nature. Patients with Kidney deficiency have enlargement of skull, separation of skull sutures, sluggish expression and pale complexion. Spleen deficiency will lead separation of skull sutures without closure and other signs of Spleen *Qi* deficiency such as poor appetite, loose stools and dull expression. On the other hand, stagnation with preponderant Heat will have closed skull sutures, fever, dysphoria, dark urine and constipation. Patients with Blood stasis obstructing Collaterals will have skull enlargement, separation of skull sutures, sluggish expression, and purple lips and tongue.

The treatment principle of hydrocephalus centers upon tonifying the Kidney to promote water metabolism and tonifying the Marrow and the brain. Based on the differences of Wind, water and Dampness, Phlegm and Blood stasis in a given patient, strengthening the Spleen to promote water metabolism, resolving Phlegm and descending *Qi*, calming the Liver to stop endogenous Wind, clearing away Heat and removing toxin, or promoting Blood circulation to remove Blood stasis will need to be adjusted for the specific symptoms of the patient.

Local AP points: BL-10, GV-20, GV-21

Special AP points: GV-26, PC-6, LI-4, SP-6, SP-9, KID-10

TCM herbal: Peanut's Hydrocephalus formula[a]

Table 1: Ingredients and Actions of Peanut's Hydrocephalus formula[a]

Pin Yin Name	English Name	Actions
Bai Zhi	Angelica	Dispel Wind-Cold, Relieve Pain
Bai Zhu	Atractylodes	Strengthen Spleen *Qi*
Ban Xia	Pinellia	Transform Damp and Stops Vomiting
Bo He	Mentha	Dispel Wind-Heat
Cang Zhu	Atractylodes	Dry Up Dampness, Strengthen Spleen *Qi*
Chan Tui	Cicada	Dispel Wind, Move *Qi* to the Head
Dang Shen	Codonopsis	Tonify *Qi*
Deng Xin Cao	Juncus	Clear Heat, Drain Damp-Heat
Fu Ling	Poria	Benefit the Urination
Huang Qi	Astragalus	Tonify Spleen *Qi* and Dissipate Swelling
Jie Geng	Platycodon	Open to the Upper *Jiao*, Transform Phlegm
Jin Yin Hua	Lonicera	Clear Heat, Detoxify

Ju Hua	Chrysanthemum	Clear Heat, Detoxify
Shan Yao	Dioscorea	Tonify Spleen *Qi*
Sheng Ma	Cimcifuga	Clear Wind-Heat, Move *Qi* to the Head
Ze Xie	Alisma	Benefit the Urination
Zhi Ban Xia	Pinellia	Transform Damp and Stops Vomiting
Zhu Ling	Polyporous	Benefit the Urination

References:

1. Clemmons RM: Surgical corrections of hydrocephalus by ventriculoperitoneal shunts. In: MJ Bojrab (ed), Current Techniques in Small Animal Surgery II, Philadelphia, Lea & Febiger, pp. 18-20, 1982.
2. Dewey CW: Encephalopathies: Disorders of the Brain. In: CW Dewey (ed), A Practical Guide to Canine and Feline Neurology, Ames, Wiley-Blackwell, pp. 126-129, 2008.
3. Xie H: Common Disease. In: H Xie (ed), Traditional Chinese Veterinary Medicine, Beijing, Beijing Agricultural University Press, pp. 427-428, 1994.

How I Treat CNS Neoplasia

RM Clemmons, DVM, PhD, CVA, CVFT

Cancer represents a unique state whereby the body's healing system fails to eliminate cells with damaged or altered DNA.[4] This allows these cells to escape the normal regulatory signals leading to uncontrolled cell growth. While most auto-immune diseases represent a failure of the healing system from an over-active immune system, cancer represents the extreme opposite, whereby the immune system is hypoactive (at least in regard to the tumor). On the other hand, both chronic immune diseases and cancer probably represent outcomes from the failure of the healing system brought about by living within a polluted environment, coupled with the genetic make-up of the dog.

While we are beginning to unravel the complex biochemistry of cancer development and have begun to understand how DNA is damaged and repaired, we still have a long way to go before the cure for cancer will be found. Spontaneous healing of cancer has been documented many times in human beings and animals, suggesting that a cure is possible. On the other hand, there is a great deal of information about the potential for preventing many forms of cancer. Most of these techniques involve the use of diet and dietary supplements. We cannot control the air we breathe, unless we do this as a whole. Using alternative means of transportation, car-pooling and clean energy production are good for the environment and for those living in it. It does not pay to fool Mother Nature, she will get even in the end. We can, however, control the food our pets eat and the water they drink; thereby, reducing their pollution load. We can provide our pets with anti-oxidants and bioflavonoids, compounds which help protect DNA and the healing system. We can give them sufficient fiber in their diets to support digestion and protect the GI tract from cellular damage.

Treatment of cancer with traditional Western medicine involves surgery (to remove or de-bulk the tumor mass), ionizing radiation (to expose the tumor to lethal doses radiation, minimizing radiation exposure to surrounding healthy tissue), and chemotherapy (to poison the rapidly growing cancer cells without poisoning the rest of the body). One or all of these methods may be employed in a given patient in an attempt to delay or prevent further cancer growth. On average, the success of Western approaches to cancer provides 1 to 18 months of relief from the cancer. While longer survival times are seen with certain forms of cancer, the long-term prognosis for even the best forms of "systemic" cancer is poor to grave. The best chance for a good prognosis is for localized cancer (particularly benign lesions) that can be removed completely with surgery. When surgical removal of the cancer is not possible, or when the cancer has already spread to other organs (metastasized), control of the tumor may not be possible by conventional means and the owner must make difficult choices about the continued care of their pet. Some of these choices are very expensive. Traditional Western diagnostic methods have advanced dramatically in the last few years and provide the best chance to discover the nature of the tumor and to predict its clinical course. Advanced imaging techniques like diagnostic ultrasound, computer-assisted tomography (CAT scans) and magnetic resonance image (MRI scans) have vastly improve tumor diagnosis. Fine-needle aspirates or "true-cut" biopsies of tumors (sometimes performed in conjunction with an imaging technique) can provide cytological confirmation or histological diagnosis of the tumor type, leading to better therapeutic recommendations.

In isolated cancers where "focused" radioablative surgery can be performed (such as in brain tumors), this can be an excellent treatment option. It is not inexpensive, but can be performed at selective veterinary medical facilities and provides stereotaxic precision to the radiotherapy. In addition, all of the radiotherapy can be done at one time, under a single anesthesia. Stereotaxic radioablation also minimizes damage to surrounding tissues. Moreover, the patient's immune system (and healing system) is not compromised outside the bounds of the tumor, allowing the patient greater potential for healing. While stereotaxic radioablation is currently limited to the brain (and, in some cases, the liver), it offers great potential for good. I am, personally, not enthralled with other forms of radiotherapy or with chemotherapy. Chemotherapy uses compounds thatare toxic to the body and destroys the animal's immune system, hoping that the tumor is killed before the patient. While animals do not suffer all of the side effects as human beings undergoing radiation therapy or chemotherapy, these treatments can still have significant and, in some cases, life threatening side effects in dogs. Owners must weigh the benefits and the risks carefully before making the decision to put their pet through radiation treatments or chemotherapy.

To me, the answer to cancer lies in the immune system. This is the major reason why I have trouble with Western chemotherapy. Spontaneous remission from cancer only occurs when the patient's immune system acts to clear the cancer. Therefore, stimulation of the patient's immune system to selectively attack the cancer seems to be the key to achieving a successful outcome. New methods in immunotherapy and immune-targeted chemotherapy are likely to be the Western methods that lead to the greatest advances in cancer treatment over the next few decades.

Traditional Eastern medicine has also been used successfully in the treatment of cancer for thousands of years, long before we understood the basic pathobiology of tumors. It is not a replacement for Western diagnosis and therapy, but may be used with Western approaches to help heal patients. When the option for Western therapy is lacking, there are Eastern therapies which can be employed to help the patient live a quality life, reducing the rate to cancer expansion or, in some cases, leading to remission of the cancer. Eastern medicine may be best suited to prevention of the development of cancer through healthy living. On the other hand, herbal medications have been shown to lead to spontaneous remissions of cancer. In some cases, these herbal products can be used in conjunction with traditional Western therapies, improving the outcome and reducing the side effects from Western therapy alone. An integrative approach combining the best of both Western and Eastern medicine seems to be the only sensible course of action, providing the best overall care for the patient.

Reducing risk factors for cancer, eating a properly balanced diet (free of pesticides and preservatives), drinking pure water, providing appropriate anti-oxidants, vitamins and minerals, and exercising regularly can help prevent cancer. Once cancer has been found, additional supportive measures are needed. Cancer cells utilize carbohydrates for fuel and compete for the body for amino acids. However, these cancer cells do not metabolize fats. Some data suggests that high fat diets can help the patient overcome the effects of cancer and even reduce cancer expansion. A number of herbal products can stimulate the immune system to attack cancer or block the mediators which the tumor uses to spread to other areas of the body, mediators which the tumor needs to survive. The following is a guide to the integrative treatment of cancer, using those compounds where there is scientific data to support their use in cancer management, helping the patient survive the disease.

Cancer Diet

Although eating healthy is the best too in the fight against cancer, once cancer takes hold certain dietary changes may be help the patient fight against the effects of the cancer. Tumor cells rely heavily upon carbohydrates for their energy and rob the body of amino acids. On the other hand, tumor cells cannot utilize lipids (fats) for energy while the rest of the body can. As such, diets with increased fat content may slow tumor growth, allowing the patient to fight against the tumor. Protein content must be maintained at levels sufficient for tissue repair, but carbohydrates should be held to a minimum. For those who prefer to prepare their dogs food, the following diet contains the ingredients important for cancer patients. In addition, it supplies the important nutrients for cancer protection. For those who cannot cook for their dog, a commercial food should be of good quality, moderate protein (18-22%) content, low carbohydrate (3-13%) content, and high fat (55-60%) content. One of these is Mighty Dog Bacon & Cheese dog food.

Home cooked cancer diet: (for 60-70 pounds body weight)

8 oz	Catfish
8 oz	Tofu
2 tbs	Virgin Olive Oil
2	Whole Carrots
½ cup	Spinach
¼ cup	Green Pepper
½ cup	Broccoli
¼ tsp	Dry Ginger
1	Raw Garlic Cloves
¼ tsp	Dry Mustard
1 tab	Flintstones
1250 mg Calcium	

Prepare by cooking the carrots, green peppers and broccoli in the olive oil in a wok until tender and then add catfish (cubed). Once catfish is beginning to cook, stir in spinach to wilt. When spinach is wilted, turn off heat and crumble tofu into the mixture. Add crushed raw garlic and the additional dry ingredient let cool and serve. Diet contains 1355 Calories with a 27/13/60 percent protein/carbohydrate/fat.

Dietary Supplements:

Vitamins and Antioxidants:

The vitamins and antioxidants for cancer patients are the same for all dogs, including vitamin E, vitamin C, selenium, beta-carotene, ginkgo biloba, green tea and grape seed extract. In addition, the membrane stabilizers omega-3-fatty acids, gammalinolenic acid and coenzyme Q-10 are important for cancer patients. Many of the antioxidants help stabilize DNA and help reduce cancer development or progression. Some data suggests that antioxidants can reduce the effectiveness of radiation and chemotherapy, but this is not well documented. It may be best to stop antioxidants 3 days before radiation therapy or at the start of chemotherapy, reinstituting the antioxidants a few days later. Most of the herbal antioxidants are good for preventing cancer, too.

Immunostimulants:

Echinacea: American Indian medicine gave us a useful native plant that is another immune-system booster: purple coneflower, *Echinacea purpurea* and related species. The root of this ornamental plant is held in high esteem by herbalists, naturopathic doctors and many laypeople, because of its antibiotic and immune-enhancing properties. You can buy echinacea products in any health food store: tinctures, capsules, tablets, and extracts of fresh or dried roots. Although few medical doctors in America are familiar with echinacea, much research on it has been done in Germany, and the plant is in widespread use as a home remedy in Europe and America. Follow the directions for adult dosing.

Astragalus: Another Chinese herbal remedy with similar properties comes from the root of a plant in the pea family, *Astragalus membranaceus*. This plant is a relative of our locoweed, which is toxic to livestock. The Chinese species is nontoxic, the source of a very popular medicine called *Huang Qi* that you can buy in any drugstore in China for use against colds, flu, and other respiratory infections. Recent studies in the West confirm its antiviral and immune-boosting effects, and preparations are now available in most health food stores here. Follow the directions for adult dosing.

Anti-Cancer herbs:

Cat's Claw (una de gato): Cat's claw (name derived from the pattern of thorns found on the vines), *Uncaria tomentosa*, comes from the Peruvian rain forest and was traditionally used by the indigenous people to treat cancer and arthritis. Recent studies indicate that it contains immune-enhancing substances, including several antioxidant compounds. These compounds may account for the antitumor properties reported for cat's claw. Treatments have been reported to lead to remission of brain and other tumors. While published data is lacking, cat's claw should be considered in tumors of the central nervous system. Use ¼ the adult human dose for small dogs, ½ for medium dogs and the equivalent dose in large dogs.

Reishi and Maitake Mushrooms: Like astragalus, mushroom extracts stimulate the patient's immune system by presenting unique macromolecules to the intestinal tract, where they alter the immune regulation by intestinal antigen processing systems. In addition, maitake mushroom extract has been shown to activate NK Killer cells which attack tumor cells and to prevent destruction of T-Helper cells. There is no known toxicity from these mushroom extracts. Use ¼ the adult human dose for small dogs, ½ for medium dogs and the equivalent dose in large dogs.

Pau D'Arco: This herbal extract from the inner bark of trees of the *Tahebuia genus* (found in South American rain forests) contains lapachol which has been reported to induce strong biological activity to cancer. No adverse effects have been reported with the drug. Studies with pure lapachol have not indicated that blood levels are inadequate to provide the anti-cancer and anti-inflammatory actions attributed to Pau D'Arco. On the other hand, its effectiveness may not be related solely to lapachol, but influenced by other phytochemicals in the extract. Use ¼ the adult human dose for small dogs, ½ for medium dogs and the equivalent dose in large dogs.

Other Dietary Supplements:

Milk Thistle: Milk thistle is an herbal product that helps protect the liver from toxic damage. It may be useful in treating chronic active hepatitis or as a prevention of injury from other drugs. It has been used to protect the liver from damage from chemotherapy in human patients. It may help prevent damage from traditional anti-convulsants (phenobarbital). I recommend starting at 1 capsule twice a day.

Shark Cartilage: Mounting evidence suggests that shark cartilage has anti-angiogenic properties, reducing blood vessel development into tumors. While it is not ecologically sound to harvest sharks for their cartilage, it is hard to deny to benefit of reducing tumor blood flow in reducing tumor size and preventing distant metastasis. On the other hand, a recent study using shark cartilage in terminally ill human cancer patients showed no evidence of benefit either in tumor growth or in the quality of life of the patients. If your dog has neoplasia, you can consider using 1000-2000 mg of shark cartilage daily, taking into account that it may do nothing beneficial.

Miscellaneous: You may want to add Essiac tea, Wheatgrass extract, Soybean Concentrate or Chlorella (see www.wheat-grass.com) {these are not proven, only anedoctal}; however, soybean concentrate contains many of the same compounds found in Tofu, in a liquid form. My feeling is that if you use the diet, which is based upon Tofu for much of its protein, you do not need soy concentrates. On the other hand, this might be useful in dogs who remain on commercial dog food.

Basic Cancer Approach:

Cancer remains a unique case. Sadly, in veterinary medicine the goal is to palliate not cure. This is because animals cannot tolerate the protocols used on human beings with cancer. Even so, 1 to 18 month survivals are possible in animals, representing 5-10 year survival times in human beings. My personal belief is that cancer, which can be surgically removed with clean margins, is the only good kind. I am not sure that radiation and chemotherapy are the best option, but owners must decide for themselves what they want to do and put their pets through. There are some things which should be done for all cancer patients regardless of whether they are treated with conventional radiation and chemotherapy. These are outlined here. Other information can be obtained at and http://Dog2Doc.com/chi-files/Acupuncture/TCVM_Diet/TCM_5-E_Diet.ppt about diet and herbal medications. Step in supporting cancer patients:

1. Low-Carbohydrate food (home prepared is best or use Pedigree Weight Loss Formula)
2. Canine basic antioxidant formula (Westlab Pharmacy 800-4WESTLA)
3. Canine arthritis formula (Westlab)
4. Canine cancer formula (Westlab) - use at 2 times prevention dose
5. COX-2 inhibitor (daily- -particularly for carcinomas)
6. Melatonin at night (0.1-0.2 mg/kg, which is now included in the Canine cancer formula)
7. 5-hydroxyurea for meningiomas (50 mg/M2 every 3-4 weeks)
8. Max's formula (0.5 gm/10 lbs BID, Jing Tang) (Table 1)
9. Stasis in the Mansion of the Mind formula (0.5 gm/10 lbs BID, Jing Tang 800-891-1986)

The rationale for each of these products is sound, but more than I wish to explain at the moment. Antioxidants do protect and help stabilize the immune system. Collagen support may help inhibit angiogenesis by the tumor. Mushrooms and astragalus help boost the immune system. COX-2 drugs double life expectancy with carcinomas while melatonin appears to improve survival times in all solid tissue tumors including gliomas. None of these measures will necessarily treat or cure cancer, but they will not do any harm and may provide quality of life. That is probably what is important in cancer that cannot be surgically removed.

TCVM Patterns for Cancer:

Cancer in TCVM represents blood stagnation leading to a mass. It can result from excess conditions that accumulate phlegm and lead to damaged *Qi* and blood flow by the liver. Once the damage is done, generally the pattern of deficiency remains even if there is local stagnation. The underlying deficiencies are: *Qi* and Blood Deficiency and *Qi* and *Yin* Deficiency.

***Qi* and Blood Deficiency:** Patients with the pattern of *Qi* and Blood Deficiency have a lower cell immunity response than normal. Symptoms include: hair loss; dizziness; fatigue; a thin body; shortness of breath; poor appetite; insomnia; palpitations; abdominal pain; a pale complexion; loose stools; scanty urine; a pale tongue with a white tongue coating; and a deep, thin, and weak pulse.

***Qi* and *Yin* Deficiency:** Patients with lung *Qi* deficiency may have a lower lymphocyte transformation rate and lower levels of serum immunoglobulins such as IgM and IgG. Symptoms include: sweating; palpitations; shortness of breath; insomnia; chest congestion; cough without phlegm; lassitude; dry mouth; a thin tongue coating; and a thin pulse.

Local AP points: Surround the Dragon (just don't needle the actual tumor)

Special AP points: GV-14, ST-36, LI-4, TH-5, LIV-3

TCM herbal: While the following two herbs are my main TCVM herbals of choice in treating CNS Neoplasia, they can be redirected by adding additional formulas such as Cervical Formula[a] or Hindquarter Weakness[a] in order to bring the medicines to the affected region of the spinal cord. In addition, Stasis Breaker[a] may be used as a substitute for Stasis in the Mansion of the Mind[a] based upon the preference of the TCVM practitioner.

Table 1: Ingredients and Actions of Max's Formula[a]

Pin Yin Name	English Name	Actions
Bai Zhi	Angelica	Clear Wind-Cold and Relieve Pain
Da Huang	Rheum	Clear Stagnation/Stasis and Clear Heat
Jie Geng	Platycodon	Open the Upper *Jiao* and Transform Phlegm
Mu Li(Shu)	Ostrea	Soften Hardness and Clear Mass
Tian Hua Fen	Trichosanthes	Clear Heat and Promote Body Fluids
Xia Ku Cao	Prunella	Clear Liver Heat and Resolve Nodules
Xuan Shen	Scrophularia	Clear Heat and Cool Blood
Zhe Bei Mu	Fritillaria	Soften Hardness and Resolve Nodules

Table 2: Ingredients and Actions of Stasis in the Mansion of the Mind Formula[a]

Pin Yin Name	English Name	Actions
Bai Zhi	Angelica	Warm the Channel, Relieve Pain
Ban Xia	Pinellia	Transform Phlegm

Chuan Xiong	Ligusticum	Move Blood
Dan Shen	Salvia	Move Blood
Di Long	Lumbricus	Clear Wind, Invigorate Channel
Gao Ben	Ligusticum	Relieve Pain
Ge Gen	Pueraria	Bring *Qi* Upward
Hong Hua	Carthamus	Break Down Blood Stasis
Jiang Can	Bombyx	Transform Phlegm, Resolve Nodules
Quan Xie	Buthus	Break Down Blood Stasis
Sheng Ma	Cimcifuga	Ascend *Qi*
Zhe Bei Mu	Fritillaria	Transform Phlegm, Resolve Nodules

References:
1. Xie H: Common Disease. In: H Xie (ed), Traditional Chinese Veterinary Medicine, Beijing, Beijing Agricultural University Press, pp. 427-428, 1994.
2. Dewey CW: Encephalopathies: Disorders of the Brain. In: CW Dewey (ed), A Practical Guide to Canine and Feline Neurology, Ames, Wiley-Blackwell, pp. 156-172, 2008.

TCVM for Treatment of an Intracranial Lesion in a Dog

Heidi Woog, DVM, CVA, CVCH

Introduction

In recent years there has been a surge in numbers of people seeking Traditional Chinese Veterinary Care for their pets in addition to available Western medicine modalities. The availability of magnetic resonance imaging (MRI) is making it increasingly possible to diagnose brain lesions in the dog. While it is possible to know that a lesion is present with MRI, it is still questionable in Veterinary MRI as to whether these lesions are tumors, inflammatory events, or vascular hemorrhages. Western based treatments for each of these conditions can vary greatly.

Traditional Chinese Veterinary Medicine (TCVM) uses TCVM specific history and physical exam features to elucidate TCVM diagnostic patterns. These patterns can be addressed using acupuncture, Chinese herbal medicine, and dietary changes.

Acute brain injury pathology often includes various combinations of the following diagnostic patterns: Blood Stagnation, Internal Wind, Wind-Stroke, Phlegm, Heat, and Fire, as well as various chronic underlying deficiencies. Tumors, inflammatory events, and non-neoplastic vascular hemorrhages often involve several of these TCVM diagnostic patterns. Blood Stagnation, Wind-Stroke, Wind-Phlegm sequelae with chronic Yin and *Qi* Deficiencies featured prominently in the case discussed below.

Descriptive Case Study

This is a case study involving a 12 year old 48 pound neutered male chow mix, a working avalanche-certified Search and Rescue Canine, that presented with rapid onset of cluster seizures. Phenobarbital and valium were used to control seizure activity. An MRI obtained 4 days after his initial onset of seizure showed a large right-sided intracranial lesion with edema, necrosis, and hemorrhage. It was described as a "strongly enhancing intra-axial lesion in the right rostral piriform lobe of the brain"[a]. This brain mass was initially suspected by the radiologist to be a glioma tumor due to its size, characteristics, and location. A combination of acupuncture and Chinese herbal therapy was instituted with the goal of moving Blood Stagnation and resolving Phlegm in the Mind.

Chronology of Diagnostics and Treatment

Acupuncture was started 3 days after the initial event. Patterns diagnosed and points used for treatments in this case are listed and described in Table 1. Initial MRI was done 4 days post-event. Chinese herbs used to address TCVM patterns diagnosed by both TCVM exam and MRI results are listed in Tables 3 and 5, mushroom extracts in Table 6 EPA/DHA concentrates in Table 7. These herbs and a home prepared diet were all started 10 days post event. Additional Chinese herbal therapy, Table 2, was started 17 days following the initial event (Stasis in the Mansion of Mind to replace Stasis Breaker). A second MRI was completed 27 days (23 days between MRIs) after the initial seizure event. The timing of the second MRI was 24 days post initial acupuncture, herbal, and nutritional intervention and 10 days after the additional Chinese herbal therapy with additional specificity to the brain (Table 2). The second MRI showed a great reduction in the mass, edema, hemorrhage and necrosis. The consulting neurologist stated, "it is almost difficult to see the lesion, because it is greatly reduced in size. Most of the edema is gone, and there is only minimal contrast enhancement."[b] The second MRI included an additional contrast sequence for detecting hemorrhage and showed the area previously considered to be part of the tumor was actually hemorrhage as reflected by the residual iron left behind as the bleed resolved. It is possible that the minimal lesion seen is a small tumor that led to the bleed. The consulting neurologist considered this unlikely and felt that a brain bleed or stroke was the more likely event. "A special MRI sequence that is used for detecting hemorrhage was performed today that was not done on the previous MRI. The area of concern that was previously thought to be a tumor showed up very well on this special sequence, indicating that the lesion is primarily composed of blood, and was likely due to a previous vascular event rather than a tumor. *Based on the fact that the lesion has greatly diminished in size with no treatment and seems to be primarily composed of hemorrhage, a vascular event resulting in hemorrhage is much more likely in this case than a tumor* (emphasis added)."[b] The veterinarians at Colorado State University who contributed to this report did not consider the herbal medicine and acupuncture administered to be "treatment".

Table 1: TCVM for Treatment of Seizure/Wind as Sequelae to Tumor or Stroke/Phlegm and Blood Stagnation[3,4,5,6]

Pattern	Clinical Signs	Acupuncture Points/Herbal Formula
Blood and *Qi* Stagnation/*Bi* Syndrome	Musculoskeletal pain – especially back, hips and knees, lavender tongue	LI-11, GB-29, GB-30, GB-34, GB-39, BL-21, BL-18, BL-40, ST-36, LIV-2, GV-2 EPA/DHA 2 grams
Wind-Stroke/Cerebral Hemorrhage	Seizure as sequelae, dx of Wind-Stroke presumed due to age of onset and confirmed by MRI	ST-40, SP-9, LI-4 Stasis Breaker for first 7 days pending arrival of Stasis in Mansion of Mind
Wind-Phlegm	Seizure, Limb contraction, Wiry Pulse	LIV-2, GB-34, LI-11, GV-14, GV-21, ST-40, SP-9
Liver *Yin* and Blood Deficiency, Hyperactive *Yang*	Dry coarse hair coat, thin hair coat, large skin flakes, behavior moves to arousal/aggression quickly	BL-18, LIV-8, KID-3, LIV-2 *Wei Qi* Booster Dandruff Formula – added for chronic deficiency 4 months post-event Super EPA
Blood Stasis in the Mind	Possible cause of Wind-Phlegm Sequelae due to age of onset and confirmed with MRI, convulsion, lavender tongue, wiry pulse	ST-40, LIV-2, GV-21 *Stasis in Mansion of Mind* *Maitake Mushroom Extract* Super EPA
Spleen *Qi* Deficiency	Muscle atrophy, loss of body weight	SP-9, BL-26 Home Prepared Diet with Sweet Potato
Kidney *Yin* deficiency, Hyperactive *Yang*	Dry skin, cool seeking	KID-3, LIV-8, LIV-2 *Wei Qi* Booster

Wei *Qi* Deficiency	Tumor, general weakness	ST-36, LI-4 *Wei Qi* Booster Maitake Mushroom Extract

Table 2: Ingredients and Actions of *Wei Qi* Booster

Chinese *Pin-Yin*	English Name	Action
Huang Qi	Astragalus	Tonify *Qi* in whole body and *Wei Qi*
Dang Gui	Angelica	Tonify Blood
Dang Shen	Condonopsis	Tonify *Qi* and boost *Wei Qi*
Wu Yao	Lindera	Move *Qi* and clear stagnation
Chen Pi	Citrus	Move *Qi* and transform Phlegm
Ban Zhi Lian	Scutellaria	Inhibit cell mutation, inhibit tumor growth
Bai Hua She She Cao	Oldenlandia	Inhibit cell mutation and tumor growth
Xuan Shen	Scrophularia	Cool Blood and nourish *Yin*

Manufacturer: Jing Tang Herbal[c]

Table 3: Ingredients and Actions of Stasis in Mansion of Mind

Chinese *Pin-Yin*	English Name	Action
Bai Zhi	Angelica	Warm the Channel, relieve pain
Ban Xia	Pinellia	Transform Phlegm
Chuan Xiong	Ligusticum	Move Blood
Dan Shen	Salvia	Move Blood
Di Long	Lumbricus	Clear Wind, invigorate Channel
Gao Ben	Ligusticum	Relieve Pain
Ge Gen	Pueraria	Bring *Qi* upward
Hong Hua	Carthamus	Break down Blood Stasis
Jiang Can	Bombyx	Transform Phlegm, resolve nodule
Sheng Ma	Cimicifuga	Ascend *Qi*
Wu Gong	Scolopendra	Detoxify, resolve nodules
Zhe Bei Mu	Fritillaria	Transform Phlegm, resolve nodules

Manufacturer: Jing Tang Herbal[c]

Table 4: Ingredients and Actions of Dandruff Formula

Chinese *Pin-Yin*	English Name	Action
Dang Gui	Angelica	Nourish Blood
Shu Di Huang	Rehmannia	Nourish *Yin*, Blood and *Jing*
Sheng Di Huang	Rehmannia	Nourish *Yin* and cool Blood
Ji Xue Teng	Millettia	Nourish Blood
He Shou Wu	Polygonum	Nourish Blood
Xuan Shen	Scrophularia	Cool Blood and nourish *Yin*
Dan Shen	Salvia	Cool Blood and activate Blood
Bai Xian Pi	Dictamnus	Clear Wind and relieve itching
Di Fu Zi	Kochia	Clear Heat and relieve itching

Manufacturer: Jing Tang Herbal[c]

Table 5: Ingredients and Actions of Stasis Breaker

Chinese *Pin-Yin*	English Name	Action
Zhe Bei Mu	Fritillaria	Soften hardness and clear nodules
Mu Li	Ostrea	Soften hardness and clear mass
San Leng	Sparaganium	Purge the Interior, break Stasis and clear mass
E Zhu	Zedoaria	Purge the Interior, break Blood Stasis and clear mass
Ban Zhi Lian	Scutellaria	Clear Heat-toxin, inhibit cell mutation, inhibit tumor growth
Bai Hua She She Cao	Oldenlandia	Inhibit cell mutation and tumor growth

Manufacturer: Jing Tang Herbal[3]

Table 6: Ingredients and Actions of Maitake Mushroom Extract

Maitake	Activates immune system, antioxidant, tumor regression[7]

Manufacturer: Kan Herbal[d]

Table 7: Ingredients in Super EPA

EPA/DHA	Anti-inflammatory, *Yin* and Blood tonic

Manufacturer: Thorne Research[e]

Treatment Outcome

Otto has had no additional seizures. He remains on phenobarbital, deramax, herbs, acupuncture and a home prepared diet. He has no neurological deterioration. He returned to a similar quality of life as before the event.

Discussion

Spontaneous Intracerebral Hemorrhage (SICH) in companion animals is still not commonly diagnosed due to lack of MRI in private practice, but many clinicians and owners will often describe "stroke–like" symptoms in pets. The natural history of intracerebral hemorrhage is better understood in human medicine due to a longer history of correlating the use of medical imaging with the clinical course. Whether due to hemorrhagic stroke from an arterio-venous malformation, aneurysm, or due to tumor bulk, the evolution of SICH in humans varies depending on size of hemorrhage and health of the individual. Its pathophysiology includes perihematomal edema and hematoma expansion leading either to death, to severe residual neurologic injury or less often to slow recovery.[1] In one human study, baseline relative edema volume was found to be the strongest predictor of outcome, with a large relative volume being associated with better functional outcome in 3 months than small baseline relative volume.[2] Humans with initially low level edema were more likely to develop additional edema volume during the subsequent 24h than individuals with initially high level edema.[1,2] On average, perihematomal edema increases by approximately 75% during the first 24 hours after ICH.[1] Delayed edema can occur 3 days to 2 weeks after ictus in ICH. Peak edema was found at 5-6 days post ICH onset. In another study this increase in perihematomal edema was strongly related to the volume of underlying hematoma. Significant hematoma expansion was occurring so that the two factors cannot be seen as independent in their effect on ICH outcome. In addition to the parenchymal hematoma, the presence and expansion of intraventricular hemorrhage (IVH) can be a predictor of outcome in ICH. In humans, IVH occurs in 45% of patients with SICH, and is associated with a less favorable outcome.[2]

One great advantage to MRI in diagnosing tumor as a primary cause of Spontaneous Intracerebral Hemorrhage (SICH) vs. non-neoplastic vascular etiology would be to know if primary Blood Stagnation and Phlegm/tumor vs. Wind-Stroke/SICH as the primary TCVM pathology with the Blood Stagnation and Phlegm being the sequelae were the cause. TCVM treatments can be more easily individualized to each pattern, than standard one size fits all allopathic protocols. If animal pathology is similar to published human pathophysiology in spontaneous intracerebral hemorrhage with parenchymal hematoma, cerebral edema, perihematomal edema, and intraventricular hemorrhage, then it is possible that early intervention with acupuncture and Chinese herbs may be helpful in decreasing the hemorrhage and edema, thereby limiting neurological deterioration and preserving brain function.

While the diagnosis is unknown in this case – tumor vs. non-neoplastic vascular SICH and inflammation - the lesion improved significantly in a very short period of time while under a TCVM treatment regimen. The dog has healed with no functional neurological deterioration and has clinical signs that are normal for his age and activity level. While this dog was routinely on deramax, a non-steroidal anti-inflammatory, before, during, and after his event for chronic arthritis post Tibial Plateau Leveling Osteotomy (TPLO), no prednisone or other corticosteroid was administered, and no chemotherapy or radiation were used as treatments. One can presume that if medical intervention was of aid to this dog in reducing his mass/brain bleed both in size and duration that it was due to the intervention of Traditional Chinese Veterinary Medicine and Acupuncture. This case suggests that further research using MRI and biopsy (when possible) is warranted to study the use of Traditional Chinese Veterinary Medicine as a possible primary or adjunctive intervention for brain hemorrhages, edema, and tumors in dogs.

Footnotes
[a.] Pet Rays Veterinary Telemedicine Consultants Record for "Otto" 9.23.10
[b.] Colorado State University Veterinary Teaching Hospital Medical Records for "Otto" 10.14.10
[c.] Xie H. Chinese Veterinary Herbal Handbook. Jing Tang Herbal, Reddick, FL: Chi Institute of Chinese Medicine 2008: 76, 156, 77
[d.] Clinical Guide For Practitioners, Myco Herb, pub 2008 by Kan Herbal Company, Scotts Valley, CA. p 59
[e.] Thorne Veterinary Product List, Veterinarian's Reference Guide, by Thorne Research, Inc., Dover, ID p22

References:
1. Gebel J. etal. Natural History of Perihematomal Edema in Patients With Hyperacute Spontaneous Intracerebral Hemorrhage. Stroke 2002;33;2631-2635
2. Adeoye O. Intracerebral Hemorrhage: Advances in Management. Nat Rev Neurol 2010;6(10)
3. Maciocia G. The Practice of Chinese Medicine: The treatment of Diseases with Acupuncture and Chinese Herbs. Edinburgh, London, Madrid, Melbourne, New York, and Tokyo: Churchill Livingstone 1994: 665-684

4. Maciocia G. The Foundations of Chinese Medicine A comprehensive Text for Acupuncturists and Herbalists. Edinburgh, London, Madrid, Melbourne, New York, and Tokyo: Churchill Livingstone 1989: 187, 195-196
5. Yu C.S., Fei L. A Clinical Guide to Chinese Herbs and Formulae: Edinburgh, London, Madrid, Melbourne, New York, and Tokyo 1993: 220-225
6. Helms J. Acupuncture Point Lists reprinted with permission of Joseph M. Helms, MD and Medical Acupuncture Publishers, editing and addition of veterinary anatomy and indications by Narda G. Robinson, D.O., D.V.M. 1997. A-1-1 – A-14-11
7. Boh B and Berovic M. Grifola frondosa (Dicks.:Fr.) S.F. Gray (Maitake Mushroom): Medicinal Properties, Active Compounds, and Biotechnological Cultivation. International Journal of Medicinal Mushrooms, Volume 9 (2007): 89-108

Right Retrobulbar Squamous Cell Carcinoma in a Dog

Joan D. Winter, DVM, CVA, CVCH, CVTP

ABSTRACT:

I received a telephone request to meet me as a veterinarian integrating Eastern and Western Medicine in November 2006. The gentleman was referred by his closest human friend. The client was a movie producer and of Wood constitution and his best worldly friend was "Chance," a ten year old Golden Retriever.

"Chance" had been seen by Dr. Ayle and treated for brain cancer, squamous cell carcinoma, retrobulbar to the right eye. He had finished his four treatments of radiation and chemotherapy. Chance had done well with radiation/chemotherapy treatments except the last time left him with leucopenia that resolved uneventfully. Dr. Ayle told the owner he could not remove the tumor surgically. His treatment would be palliative. Dr. Ayle hoped to place a perimeter around the tumor. My examination of "Chance" on November 25, 2006, revealed a nice Earth Constitution dog, in good flesh with good *Shen*, *Yang* pulses deficient, somewhat overweight, tongue peachy pink in color to red while panting in the outside hot environment, upper right eyelid drooping with OD entropian and possible corneal ulcer. My Western Veterinary diagnosis was Squamous Cell carcinoma retrobulbar to right eye with corneal ulceration of OD, due to entropian or side effects of treatment leading to dry eye. My TCVM diagnosis was Spleen *Qi* deficiency with *Qi*/Blood stagnation. One must remember that Blood is the mother to *Qi* and *Qi* moves the Blood. Certainly, this older Earth constitution dog could have initially been Blood deficient which led to Spleen *Qi* deficiency and stagnation.

Despite the good report with the client, he declined any Western or Eastern therapy. He was to see Dr. Ayle in three days and would have him evaluate "Chance" and his eye. I sent him a bill and he promptly paid it. It was not until January 2, 2007, that I called the owner to see how "Chance" was. He told me that Dr. Ayle felt that herbal formulas are ok, but rarely hurt. On January 21, 2007, the owner was willing to allow me to order herbal formulas *Wei Qi* Booster and Stasis in the Mansion of Mind, after the tumor had grown into the dogs' oral cavity and had to have surgery to excise it. At this point, the client realized there was no perimeter around the tumor.

The client felt helpless in many ways. He knew Western medicine had failed his best, worldly friend, and that he had to trust me with Eastern medicine, yet, really knew nothing about my art of practice. We had a telephone discussion where we spoke openly and honestly. I had told him of my own dog with metastatic lung cancer and how well he did. The owner accused me of being a failure since I did not cure my dog. I was ready to throw the stone right back at him. I told him I never got to treat my dog when he had a primary abdominal tumor, only as it metastasized to his lungs. He was in a much better place than me, having the opportunity to treat a primary cancerous tumor. I told him I would have loved to be in his boots with my dog! I told him he was not a good friend to his dog if he would forego herbal treatment. He said he would try, but if the dog got diarrhea or any other side effects, I would be at his mercy since the dogs' current quality of life was good. I told the client we would go slowly with the herbal dosage. He wanted me to promise him that if diarrhea occurred I could and would be able to stop it. I made him no such promise. I only reminded him that we are born, pay taxes, and then die!

"Chance" did very well on herbal formulas. I called weekly to encourage him to increase the dose at my recommendation. "Chance" was on the herbal formulas, with no side effects, from

January 21, 2007 until November, 2007. On May 28, 2007, I did add Rehmannia 6 to help "Chance" with his constant panting and Kidney *Yin* deficiency.

This famous movie producer had to leave the country to produce a movie while "Chance" was on herbal formulas. He needed my reassurance that "Chance" was not about to die during his 1 month absence. I gave him my best interpretation based on his clinical description of "Chance" over the telephone.

I heard that "Chance" died in November, 2007. The owner had come home one day and found his rear end paralyzed. He took him to the ER clinic and they put him to rest. A couple of weeks later, I called my client and told him the tumor, being of the brain, most likely spread to the spinal cord as both are controlled by the Water Element. He was amazed that I realized and told him that my treatment, too, did not save his dog. He was thankful that I called as he thought his dog had two separate diseases. He thanked me for giving him and "Chance" quality time together!

In retrospect, "Chance" had a wonderful life and a great human guardian. "Chance's" owner was one of my most difficult clients, questioning everything I did. He explained to me I could be a fraud with all this *Qi*, *Yin* and *Yang* talk, nothing made sense to him. I told him he was luckier than most of my new clients, as his best human friend had referred me. Most people do not have that going for them!

Table 1. Ingredients and Actions of *Wei Qi* Booster

Pin Yin Name	English Name	Actions
Bai Hua She She Cao	Oldenlandia	Inhibit cell mutation and tumor growth
Ban Zhi Lian	Scutellaria	Inhibit cell mutation, inhibit tumor growth
Chen Pi	Citrus	Move *Qi* and transform phlegm
Dang Gui	Angelica	Tonifies Blood
Dang Shen	Codonopsis	Tonify *Qi* and boost *Wei Qi*
Huang Qi	Astragalus	Tonifies *Qi* in whole body and *Wei Qi*
Wu Yao	Lindera	Move *Qi* and clear stagnation
Xuan Shen	Scrophularia	Cool Blood and nourish *Yin*

Manufactured and distributed by Jing-tang Herbal, Inc., Reddick, FL

Table 2. Ingredients and Actions of Stasis in the Mansion of Mind

Pin Yin Name	English Name	Actions
Bai Zhi	Angelica	Warm the Channel, relieve pain
Ban Xia	Pinellia	Transform Phlegm
Chuan Xiong	Ligusticum	Move Blood
Dan Shen	Salvia	Move Blood
Di Long	Lumbricus	Clear Wind, invigorate Channel
Gao Ben	Ligusticum	Relieve pain

Ge Gen	Pueraria	Bring *Qi* upward
Hong Hua	Carthamus	Break down Blood Stasis
Jiang Can	Bombyx	Transform Phlegm, resolve nodule
Quan Xie	Buthus	Break down Blood Stasis
Sheng Ma	Cimcifuga	Ascend *Qi*
Zhe Bei Mu	Fritillaria	Transform phlegm, resolve nodules

Manufactured and distributed by Jing-tang Herbal, Inc., Reddick, FL

Table 3. Ingredients and Actions of Rehmannia 6

Pin Yin Name	**English Name**	**Actions**
Fu Ling	Poria	Drain Damp, strengthen Spleen
Mu Dan Pi	Moutan	Cool Liver
Shan Yao	Dioscorea	Tonify Qi, nourish Kidney *Jing*
Shan Zhu Yu	Cornus	Nourish *Yin*
Shu Di Huang	Rehmannia	Nourish *Yin*, Blood and *Jing*
Ze Xie	Alisma	Drain Damp, clear Kidney false Fire

Manufactured and distributed by Jing-tang Herbal, Inc., Reddick, FL

References:
1. Rodney Ayle, DVM, Specialist in Oncology, Veterinary Medical & Surgical Group, Oxnard, California.

TCVM Pathogenesis of Immune System Excess Diseases

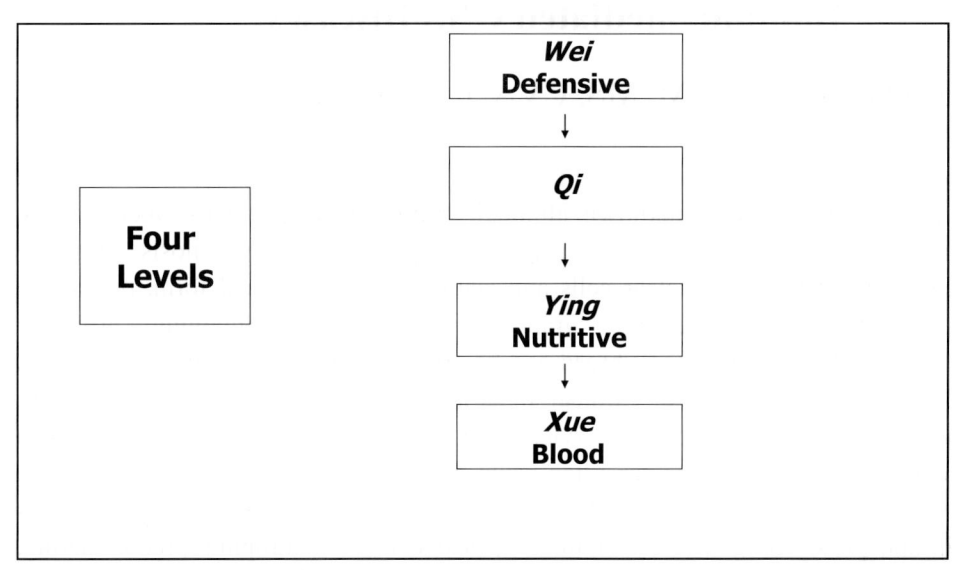

Figure 2. The Four Levels

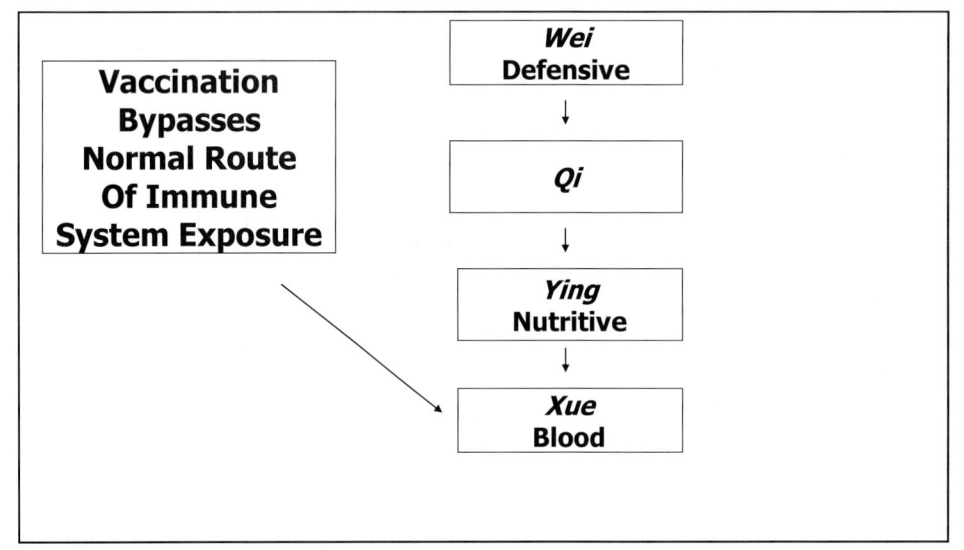

Figure 3. Genesis of Blood Heat by Vaccination

TCVM Pathogenesis
Vaccinations are designed to cause immune system "reactivity" which is Excess and Heat in TCVM. Excess and Heat is introduced directly into the *Xue*/Blood Level by intramuscular or subcutaneous routes of administration. This may then cause Blood Heat either transiently or as a "lingering" or "retained" pathogen.

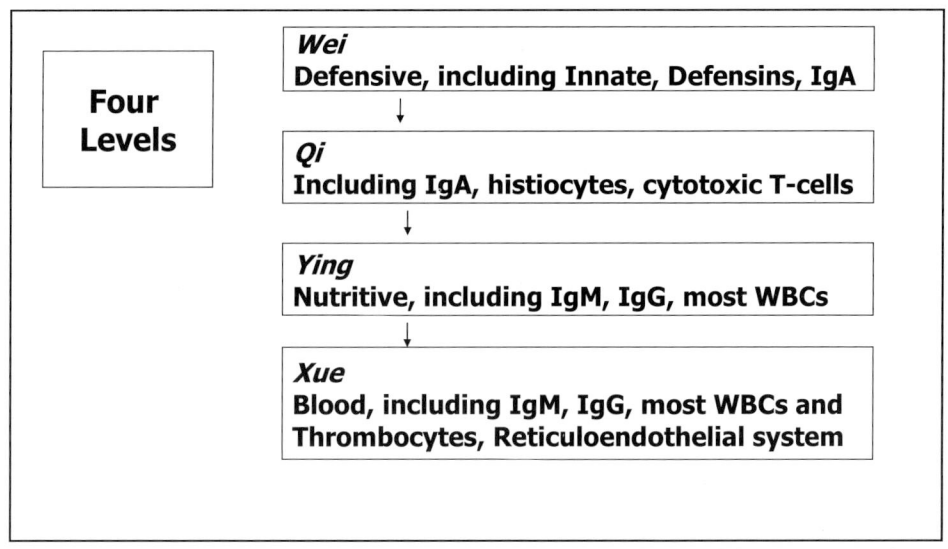

```
┌─────────────────────────────────────────────────────────────┐
│                    ┌──────────────────────────────────────┐ │
│                    │ Wei                                  │ │
│   ┌─────────┐      │ Defensive, including Innate,         │ │
│   │         │      │ Defensins, IgA                       │ │
│   │  Four   │      └──────────────────────────────────────┘ │
│   │ Levels  │                      ↓                        │
│   │         │      ┌──────────────────────────────────────┐ │
│   └─────────┘      │ Qi                                   │ │
│                    │ Including IgA, histiocytes,          │ │
│                    │ cytotoxic T-cells                    │ │
│                    └──────────────────────────────────────┘ │
│                                    ↓                        │
│                    ┌──────────────────────────────────────┐ │
│                    │ Ying                                 │ │
│                    │ Nutritive, including IgM, IgG,       │ │
│                    │ most WBCs                            │ │
│                    └──────────────────────────────────────┘ │
│                                    ↓                        │
│                    ┌──────────────────────────────────────┐ │
│                    │ Xue                                  │ │
│                    │ Blood, including IgM, IgG, most WBCs │ │
│                    │ and Thrombocytes, Reticuloendothelial│ │
│                    │ system                               │ │
│                    └──────────────────────────────────────┘ │
└─────────────────────────────────────────────────────────────┘
```

Figure 4. Proposed Modern Western Biomedical Correlates of the Four Levels

TCVM Treatment Strategies

How does the patient present? Peracute, Acute, Subacute, Chronic, Late Chronic?

Peracute Stage Treatment Strategies

Treating the *Biao* or Branch is usually needed to save the patient from death. 1)TCVM Pattern: Blood Heat. 2)Treatment Strategy: Clear Heat, Cool Blood, Replenish *Yin*. 3)Acupuncture Points: LI-4, LI-10, GV-14, BL-17, SP-10, KID-6. TCVM 4)Herbal Formula: Blood Heat Formula

Table 1: Blood Heat Formula[2]

Pin Yin Name	English Name	Action
Yu Jin	Curcuma	Cool Blood, clear Heat, detoxify
Dan Shen	Salvia	Cool Blood, activate Blood
Chi Shao	Paeonia	Cool Blood, clear Heat
Sheng Di Huang	Rhemannia	Cool Blood, nourish *Yin*
Huang Bai	Phellodendron	Clear Heat, detoxify
Di Fu Zi	Kochia	Clear Heat, detoxify
Xuan Shen	Scrophularia	Cool Blood, clear Heat, resolve nodules
Mai Men Dong	Ophiopogon	Nourish *Yin*
Mu Dan Pi	Moutan	Cool Blood, move Blood, eliminate stagnation

Acute Stage Treatment Strategies

Biao or Branch treatment is still the focus but to begin to address the *Ben* or Root, use assistant herbs. 1)TCVM Patterns: Blood Heat, *Yin* Deficiency, Body Fluid Deficiency. 2)Treatment Strategy: Clear Heat, Cool Blood, Replenish *Yin* and Body Fluids. 3)Acupuncture

Points: LI-4, LI-10, GV-14, BL-17, SP-10, KID-6, CV-12, HT-7, *An Shen*, *Jing*-well point and *Wei Jian* bleeding. 4)TCVM Herbal Formula: Blood Heat Formula or *Qing Ying Tang*.

Table 2: *Qing Ying Tang*[2]

Pin Yin Name	English Name	Action
Mu Dan Pi	Moutan	Cool Blood, resolve stagnation
Sheng Di Huang	Rehmannia	Cool Blood, nourish *Yin*
Xuan Shen	Scrophularia	Cool Blood, clear Heat
Huang Lian	Coptis	Clear Heat, detoxify
Jin Yin Hua	Lonicera	Clear Heat, detoxify
Lian Qiao	Forsythia	Clear Heat, detoxify
Dan Zhu Ye	Bamboo	Clear Heat
Dan Shen	Salvia	Move Blood
Mai Men Dong	Ophiopogon	Nourish *Yin*

Subacute Stage Treatment Strategies

Treat *Biao*/Branch and *Ben*/Root in roughly equal proportions, Using both Emperor and Assistant herbs. 1)TCVM Patterns: Blood Heat, Blood Stagnation, *Yin* Deficiency, Body Fluid Deficiency. 2)Treatment Strategy: Clear Heat, Cool Blood, Move Blood, Replenish *Yin* and Body Fluids. 3)Acupuncture Points: LI-4, LIV-3, LI-10, GV-14, BL-17, SP-10, KID-6, CV-12, *An Shen, Er Jian*. 4)TCVM Herbal Formula: *Mu Dan Pi San* or *Qing Ying Tang*.

Table 3: *Mu Dan Pi San*[2]

Pin Yin Name	English Name	Action
Mu Dan Pi	Moutan	Cool Blood, move Blood, resolve stagnation
Yu Jin	Curcuma	Cool Blood, clear Heat, detoxify
Dan Shen	Salvia	Cool Blood, move Blood
Chi Shao	Paeonia	Cool Blood, clear Heat, resolve stagnation

Chronic Stage Treatment Strategies

Focus on treating the *Ben*/Root and eliminating the lingering pathogen. 1)TCVM Patterns: Blood Heat, Blood Stagnation, Significant *Yin* Deficiency. 2)Treatment Strategy: Clear Heat, Cool Blood, Replenish *Yin*. 3)Acupuncture Points: LI-4, LIV-3, LI-10, GV-14, BL-17, BL-18, SP-10, KID-6, CV-12, BL-23, KID-3, SP-6. 4)TCVM Herbal Formula: *Mu Dan Pi*, Ophiopogon Powder

Table 4: Ophiopogon Powder[2]

Pin Yin Name	English Name	Action
Mai Men Dong	Ophiopogon	Nourish *Yin*
Lu Gen	Phragmites	Clear Heat, promote Body Fluids

Zhi Mu	Anemarrhena	Nourish *Yin*, clear Heat
Tian Hua Fen	Trichosanthes	Clear Heat, promote Body Fluids
Bei Sha Shen	Glehnia	Nourish *Yin*
Zhu Ye	Bambusa	Clear Heat
Ge Gen	Pueraria	Promote Body Fluids
Wu Mei	Mume	Astringently consolidate
Huang Qin	Scutellaria	Clear Heat
Yu Li Ren	Prunus	Move Blood
Shan Zha	Crataegus	Resolve Food Stasis
Shen Qu	Massa Fermentata	Resolve food stasis

Late Chronic Stage Treatment Strategies

Focus on supporting the *Zheng Qi* and eliminating the lingering Pathogen. 1)TCVM Patterns: Blood Deficiency, *Qi* Deficiency. 2)Treatment Strategy: Nourish Blood, Tonify *Qi*. 3)Acupuncture Points: LI-4, LI-10, BL-17, BL-18, BL-20, 21, ST-36, GV-5, CV-6. 4)TCVM Herbal Formula: *Han Lian Cao* and *Gui Pi San*.

Table 5: *Han Lian Cao*[2]

Pin Yin Name	English Name	Action
Han Lian Cao	Eclipta	Cool Blood, stop bleeding
Xian He Cao	Agrimony	Cool Blood, stop bleeding
Hu Zhang	Polygonum	Clear Damp
Tu Fu Ling	Smilax	Clear Damp
Bi Xie	Dioscorea	Clear Damp
Jie Geng	Platycodon	Transform Phlegm
Dang Shen	Codonopsis	Tonify *Qi*
Shan Yao	Dioscorea	Tonify *Qi*
Bai Zhu	Atractylodes	Tonify *Qi*
Suo Yang	Cynomorium	Tonify *Yang*
Yin Yang Huo	Epimedium	Tonify *Yang*

Table 6: *Gui Pi San*[2]

Pin Yin Name	English Name	Action
Ren Shen	Gingseng	Tonify *Qi*
Bai Zhu	Atractylodes	Tonify *Qi* and strengthen Spleen
Huang Qi	Astragalus	Tonify *Qi*
Fu Ling	Poria	Drain Damp, strengthen Spleen
Dang Gui	Angelica	Nourish Blood

Long Yan Rou	Longan	Nourish Blood
Mu Xiang	Saussurea	Move *Qi*
Yuan Zhi	Polygala	Nourish Heart
Suan Zao Ren	Ziziphus	Nourish Heart
Da Zao	Jujube	Harmonize
Zhi Gan Cao	Glychirriza	Harmonize

Conclusion

Immune-system perturbations may lead to neurological diseases such as GME. Correct identification of the TCVM Pattern of Disharmony will suggest treatment strategies. Appropriate use of acupuncture and TCVM herbal medicine may engender healing and give positive results.

References

1. Aiello, S.E., Mays, A. (eds.). The Merck Veterinary Manual. Merck and Company,, Inc. Whitehouse Station, NJ. 1998: 927-928.
2. Xie, H.S. Chinese Veterinary Herbal Handbook. Chi Institute of Chinese Medicine, Reddick, FL. 2004.

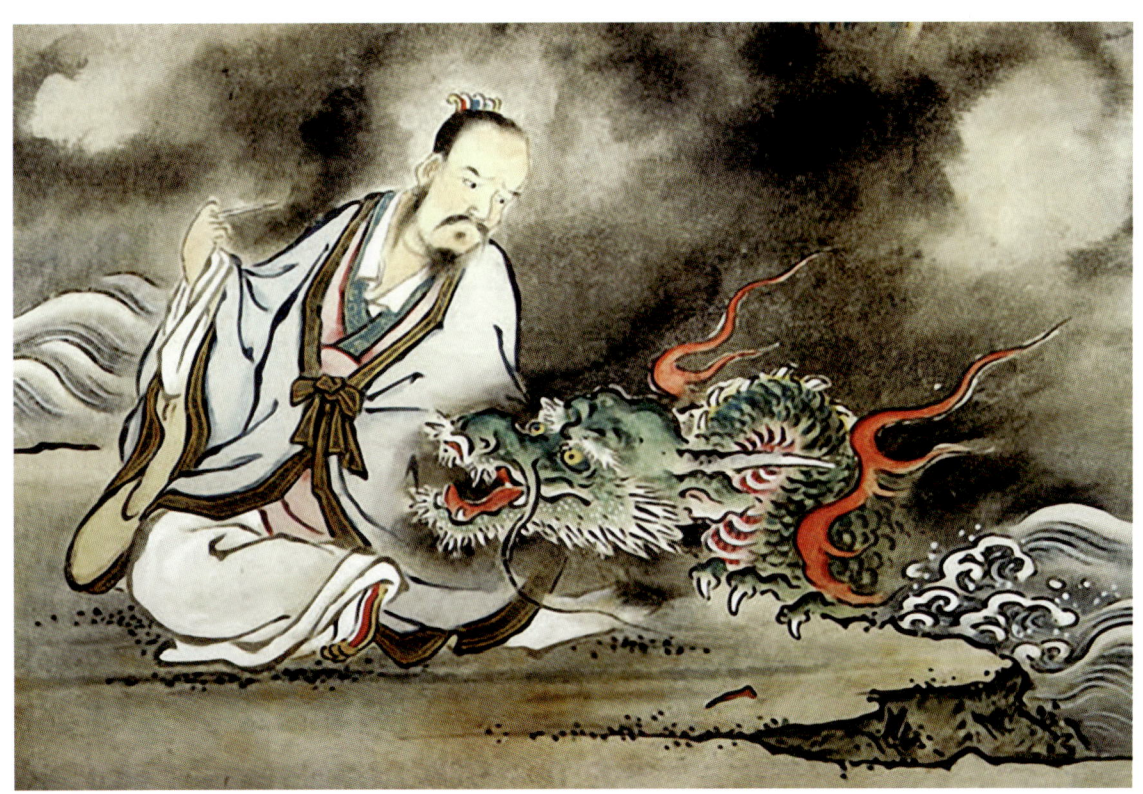

MA SHI HUANG 马师皇

Ma Shi Huang is said to be a famous veterinarian in the Huang Di (Yellow Emperor) Period (2,696 BCE to 2,598 BCE). According to Chinese legend, he is the first man to treat animal diseases with acupuncture and herbal medicines. The book *Lie Xian Zhuan* (Collected Biographies of Immortals) written in the Han Dynasty (206 BCE-220 CE) stated that: "Ma Shi Huang was a veterinarian in the time of the Yellow Emperor. He knew the constitution and vital symptoms of horses. Animal patients would immediately get well after receiving his diagnosis and treatment. Once upon a time, a dragon flew down and approached him with drooping ears and open mouth. Huang said: 'This dragon has illness and knows that I can give recovery.' Then, he needled its upper lip and mouth, and gave it a decoction of *Gan Cao Tang* (Licorice) to swallow, leading to a cure."

CHAPTER 3

Cranial Nerve Disorders

Peripheral Cranial Nerve Disorders

Cheryl L Chrisman DVM, MS, EdS, DACVIM-Neurology, CVA

There are 12 pairs of cranial nerves arranged along the brainstem, each pair associated with a specific brainstem segment.[1-3] Most conventional disease processes that affect the middle to lower brainstem usually affect one or more cranial nerves. Specific tests of cranial nerve function and differentiation of brainstem and peripheral nerve lesions are described in detail elsewhere.[1-3] The brainstem segments, functions, clinical signs and most common conventional diseases of cranial nerves are outlined in Table 1.

When a cranial nerve deficit is found, the challenge is to determine if a peripheral nerve or a brainstem disorder is present. If other neurological deficits are found or more than one cranial nerve is involved, then meningoencephalitis, brainstem neoplasm, polyneuropathy or other neuromuscular disorder are likely and referral to a neurologist is needed for further diagnostic tests. A CSF analysis, CT, MRI, electromyogram (EMG) and further clinicopathological tests may be needed to confirm the diagnosis.[2,3]

Focal peripheral cranial nerve lesions have clinical signs related to the specific cranial nerve and no other abnormal findings on the physical and neurological examinations. Further diagnostic tests may involve only clinicopathological tests for thyroid function and serial neurological examinations. Focal cranial neuropathies may be secondary to trauma, but when clinical signs develop acutely with no known trauma, the cause is often unknown (idiopathic), as all diagnostic tests are normal. Nerve biopsy would only create further damage, so histological evaluation is usually not available to further identify the underlying cause from a conventional perspective. Some of the acute idiopathic cranial neuropathies are suspected to be due to an immune-mediated process causing inflammation (neuritis).[1-3]

The most common cranial neuropathies treated with TCVM are: 1) optic neuritis, 2) trigeminal neuritis 3) facial paralysis, 4) vestibular syndromes, 5) deafness, 6) laryngeal paresis or paralysis and 7) masticatory myositis.[4-10] Since masticatory myositis is treated with TCVM and can be confused with a trigeminal neuropathy, this disorder will be included in the discussion, even though it is due to a primary muscle disease and not direct involvement of the trigeminal nerves. Cranial nerve disorders are treated with TCVM to shorten recovery times and reduce residual neurological deficits.

Peripheral cranial nerves enter and exit specific foramen of the ventral and ventrolateral aspects of the skull.[1,2] Cranial nerves can be traumatized from skull fractures in the area of the foramen or trauma more peripherally. The most common cranial nerves affected by local peripheral trauma are the facial nerves, vestibular nerves and laryngeal nerves (branch of the vagus nerves). From a TCVM perspective, peripheral cranial nerve trauma is due to *Qi*/Blood Stagnation resulting in *Qi* Deficiency (loss of *Qi*/Blood flow) to focal tissues producing peripheral nerve dysfunction.[5,6]

Many cranial nerve disorders and focal myopathies unassociated with trauma are due to an underlying *Zheng Qi* Deficiency.[4-6] The *Zheng Qi* includes all of the processes in the body that protect against the invasion of External Pathogens and their ability to create disease in the body. *Wei Qi* is the part of *Zheng Qi* that protects the body's surface. The *Wei-Qi* can be Deficient due to prenatal *Jing* Deficiency (inherent genetic weaknesses) or postnatal *Jing* Deficiency associated with poor diet or inability to absorb or utilize nutrients to make *Gu Qi*, as in Spleen *Qi*

Deficiency.[4,5] *Wei-Qi* can also become Deficient due to generalized debilitation from stress, over working performance animals or chronic disease.

Table 1: Cranial nerve brainstem locations, functions, signs of dysfunction and most common conventional diagnoses[1-3]

	Cranial nerves	Brain Stem Segments	Functions	Most Common Signs of Disease	Most Common Conventional Diagnoses
1	Olfactory	Diencephalon	Sense of smell	Not eat because can not smell	Olfactory lobe meningioma
2	Optic	Diencephalon	Sense of sight	Blind with dilated pupils, unresponsive to light	Optic neuritis Meningoencephalitis Neoplasia
3	Oculomotor	Midbrain	Motor to extraocular muscles	Ventrolateral strabismus	Meningoencephalitis Neoplasia
4	Trochlear	Midbrain	Motor to extraocular muscles	Rotation of the eyeball (can see in cats as pupils are vertical)	Meningoencephalitis Neoplasia
5	Trigeminal	Pons	Sensation to the head	Face pain	Idiopathic trigeminal neuropathy (rare in animals)
		Pons	Motor to muscles of mastication	Inability to close the mouth	Trigeminal neuritis
6	Abducens	Medulla Oblongata (rostral)	Motor to extraocular muscles	Dorsomedial strabismus	Meningoencephalitis Neoplasia
7	Facial	Medulla Oblongata (rostral)	Motor to muscles of facial expression	Inability to move the ear, eyelids and lips	Idiopathic facial paralysis Middle ear infection Trauma Hypothyroidism
8	Vestibulocochlear	Medulla Oblongata (rostral)	Vestibular portion: equilibrium	Unilateral: head tilt, rolling, circling, nystagmus; Bilateral: falling to both sides and wide swinging head movements	Idiopathic vestibular syndrome Inner ear infection Trauma Hypothyroidism
		Medulla Oblongata	Cochlear portion: Hearing	Deafness	Congenital deafness Middle or inner ear

					infection Geriatric degeneration
		(rostral)			
9	Glossopharyngeal	Medulla Oblongata (caudal)	Pharyngeal sensation and some motor to pharynx, larynx and esophagus	Dysphagia	Usually affected with CN10 vagus nerves May be part of a polyneuropathy or other neuromuscular disease
10	Vagus	Medulla Oblongata (caudal)	Motor to pharynx, larynx and esophagus	Dysphagia, laryngeal paresis or paralysis, megaesophagus	Congenital and idiopathic laryngeal paresis or paralysis; May be part of a polyneuropathy
11	Spinal Accessory	Medulla Oblongata (caudal)	Motor to trapezius muscles	Atrophy of the upper cervical musculature	Rare to have a primary spinal accessory nerve disorder
12	Hypoglossal	Medulla Oblongata (caudal)	Motor to the tongue	Tongue paralysis and atrophy	Trauma Tumor May be part of a polyneuropathy

When *Wei-Qi* is Deficient, Wind enters vulnerable acupoints and causes External disease in the Channels and acute onset of clinical signs (an Excess pattern).[4,5] In a *Yang* animal (Wood and Fire constitutions) the Wind is often accompanied by Heat and a cranial nerve disorder is due to the invasion of Wind-Heat.[4] Damp may also accompany the Wind-Heat and Damp-Heat may enter the Channels, as seen in cases of otitis externa, media and interna caused by Gallbladder Channel Damp Heat.[4] Many *Yin* animals (Earth, Metal and Water constitutions) may be more susceptible to Wind-Cold invasion of the Channels. Wind-Heat, Wind-Damp-Heat and Wind-Cold create local *Qi*/Blood Stagnation in the affected Channels and resultant Deficient *Qi*/Blood flow to surrounding tissues in the area (e.g. peripheral nerves, muscles, tendon and ligaments and connective tissue). The result is acute onset of paresis or paralysis, if motor cranial nerves are affected, or a loss of the sensation normally transmitted by the specific sensory cranial nerve affected.

Although the TCVM etiology and pathology are the same, the clinical manifestations are different because the *Wei Qi* may be weak at different locations in different patients. When Wind-Heat invades the Channels surrounding the eye, blindness due to optic neuritis can result. When Wind-Heat invades the Channels of the face, the result might be inability to close the mouth due to trigeminal neuritis. In another dog, Wind-Heat or Wind-Cold may enter Channels of the face and cause facial paralysis due to blocked *Qi*/Blood failing to nourish the facial nerve. When Wind-Heat, Wind-Damp-Heat or Wind-Cold invades the Channels surrounding the ear and affects the vestibular portion of the vestibulocochlear nerve on one side, the result is a head tilt, nystagmus and loss of equilibrium.[4-6] When Wind-Heat invades Channels near the larynx, the result is laryngeal paresis. When Wind-Heat invades Channels of the head musculature, the resulting *Qi*/Blood Stagnation can cause muscle pain associated with masticatory myositis and eventually muscle atrophy from blocked *Qi*/Blood flow to the muscle tissues.[5,6] Where there is inflammation from a conventional perspective, there is often Heat or Damp-Heat from a TCVM perspective. Therefore, many immune-mediated disorders causing focal cranial nerve or muscle inflammation are due to Wind-Heat.[4]

Congenital disorders like congenital deafness and laryngeal paresis/paralysis are associated with Kidney *Jing* Deficiency and the clinical signs may be present at birth (congenital deafness) or occur at a young age (congenital laryngeal paresis/paralysis). Chronic progressive deafness, associated with aging degeneration, is due to Kidney *Qi* Deficiency. The most common focal peripheral cranial neuropathies and the associated TCVM patterns and clinical findings are listed in Table 2.[2-6]

Table 2: Common conventional diagnoses, TCVM patterns and examination findings of focal peripheral cranial nerve disorders[2,4-7]

Conventional Diagnosis	TCVM Pattern	Clinical Findings	Tongue	Pulses
Optic neuritis	Wind-Heat invasion causing *Qi*/Blood Stagnation and local *Qi* Deficiency	Acute onset Blind, dilated pupils, unresponsive to light	Red, dry or pale	Superficial, forceful, rapid or wiry
	Liver *Qi* Stagnation with Liver *Yang* rising and Liver Heat	Wood constitution Acute onset Blind, dilated pupils, unresponsive to light Irritable Cool seeking Panting Warm ears, feet and back	Red, dry	Superficial, forceful, rapid or wiry
Trigeminal neuritis	Wind-Heat invasion causing *Qi*/Blood Stagnation and local *Qi* Deficiency	Acute onset Inability to close the mouth, prehend or chew food	Red, purple or pale	Superficial, forceful, rapid or wiry
Facial paralysis	Wind-Heat invasion causing *Qi*/Blood Stagnation and local *Qi* Deficiency	Acute onset Inability to close eyelid, move the ear or lips	Red, purple or pale	Superficial, forceful, rapid or wiry
	Wind-Cold invasion causing *Qi*/Blood Stagnation and local *Qi* Deficiency	Acute onset Inability to close eyelid, move the ear or lips	Purple or pale, moist	Superficial, slow or wiry

	Local *Qi*/Blood Stagnation and *Qi* Deficiency	Acute onset History or evidence of trauma Inability to close eyelid, move the ear or lips	Purple	Wiry
	Gallbladder Damp Heat with local *Qi* Deficiency	History or evidence of otitis externa Inability to close eyelid, move the ear or lips	Red, greasy	Forceful, rapid, slippery
Vestibular disorders	Kidney *Jing* Deficiency with Wind-Cold invasion causing *Qi*/Blood Stagnation and local *Qi* Deficiency	Dogs and cats under 1 year of age Acute onset Head tilt, nystagmus, loss of equilibrium	Pale	Wiry then weak
	Wind-Cold invasion causing Damp and Phlegm, *Qi*/Blood Stagnation and local *Qi* Deficiency with underlying Spleen *Qi* Deficiency	Adult or geriatric dogs Acute onset Head tilt, nystagmus, loss of equilibrium	Pale, wet	Wiry, slippery, weak on right side
	Local *Qi*/Blood Stagnation and *Qi* Deficiency	Acute onset History or evidence of trauma Head tilt, nystagmus, loss of equilibrium	Purple	Wiry
	Gallbladder Damp Heat with local *Qi* Deficiency	History or evidence of ear infection Head tilt, nystagmus, loss of equilibrium Seek cool	Red, greasy	Forceful, rapid slippery, wiry
Deafness	Kidney *Jing* Deficiency	Loss of hearing noticed shortly after birth	Pale, swollen	Weak
	Kidney *Qi* Deficiency	Adult onset Chronic progressive hearing loss	Pale, wet	Deep, weak, worse on right
	Gallbladder Damp Heat with local *Qi* Deficiency	Deafness History or evidence of ear infection	Red, greasy	Forceful, rapid slippery

		May have facial paralysis May have a head tilt, Seek cool		
Laryngeal paresis or paralysis	Kidney *Jing* Deficiency with local *Qi* Deficiency	Young purebred dogs or Adult purebred dogs Acute onset Stridor Cyanosis	Pale, swollen, wet, blue	Weak
	Wind-Heat invasion causing *Qi*/Blood Stagnation and local *Qi* Deficiency	Any dog or cat Acute onset Stridor Cyanosis	Red, purple	Superficial, forceful, rapid or wiry
	Local *Qi*/Blood Stagnation and *Qi* Deficiency	Acute onset History or evidence of trauma	Purple, blue	Wiry
Masticatory myopathy	Wind-Heat invasion causing *Qi*/Blood Stagnation and local *Qi* Deficiency	Acute onset Inability to open the mouth due to masticatory muscle pain or atrophy with fibrosis	Acute: Red, dry	Wiry

Acupuncture, Chinese herbal medicine and *Tui-na* can unblock *Qi*/Blood Stagnation, improve *Qi*/Blood flow and treat Kidney *Jing* and *Qi* Deficiencies and are indicated in the treatment of focal cranial neuropathies.[4-10] These TCVM treatments may be combined with conventional medications, when indicated, or used as sole treatments, when no conventional treatment is available. A combination of EA, DN and Aqua-AP is generally recommended. It is important to include EA in the treatment, whenever *Qi*/Blood Stagnation has occurred, because it is more effective to resolve Stagnation than DN alone. One or more acupoint combinations may be selected for EA and for acute onset of signs, 80-120 Hz alternating frequencies for 15-30 minutes once or twice a week, for 3-5 times, are recommended. The frequency can be reduced as the clinical signs improve. If there is associated pain, as with masseter myositis, the EA protocol may be modified for better pain control and 20 Hz for 10-15 minutes is followed by 80-120 hertz frequencies for another 10-15 minutes.[6] Aqua-AP is usually performed by injecting 0.25-0.5 ml vitamin B12 into acupoints.[6] *Tui-na* is useful to treat Kidney *Jing* and *Qi* Deficiencies.[10] Food Therapy can be useful to support Kidney *Jing* and *Qi* and treat other *Zang* organs Deficiencies long-term.[11]

An overview of the TCVM patterns and clinical findings for focal peripheral cranial neuropathies are outlined in Table 2. The acupuncture and Chinese herbal medications for focal cranial neuropathies are listed in Table 3.[5-9] The list is not meant to be exclusive and other TCVM practitioners may have positive clinical outcomes with other acupoints, EA techniques and Chinese herbal medicines. Future clinical studies are needed to determine the optimum treatment protocols.

Table 3: Treatment strategy, acupuncture points and Chinese herbal medicine used to treat different patterns of focal peripheral cranial nerve disorder of dogs and cats[5-9]

Conventional Diagnosis	TCVM Pattern	Acupuncture Points and Technique*[2,3,5,12]	Chinese Herbal Medicine**[13,14,a]	Comments
Optic neuritis	Wind-Heat invasion causing *Qi*/Blood Stagnation and local *Qi* Deficiency	**EA:** GB-20/GB-1, BL-10/B-1, *Tai-yang/Tai-yang* **DN:** GB-14, TH-23, LI-4, TH-5, GV-14, BL-67	*Fang Feng San*	Acutely give AP treatments every 3-5 days for 3 times, then weekly for 3 times, then 1-2 times per month until vision restored; Use herbal formula up to 6 months
	Liver *Qi* Stagnation with Liver *Yang* rising and Liver Heat	**EA:** *Tai-yang/Tai-Yang*, GB-1/GB-1, BL-1/BL-1 **DN:** GV-14, LI-4, BL-18, BL-19, GB-34, LIV-3	*Jue Ming San* (Haliotis Powder)	
Trigeminal neuritis	Wind-Heat invasion causing *Qi*/Blood Stagnation and local *Qi* Deficiency	**EA:** TH-17/TH-17, if not painful ST-6/ST-6, *Nao-shu/Nao-shu* **DN:** *Shang guan*, LI-10, LI-11, LI-4, LU-7, GV-14	*Pu Ji Xiao Du Yin*	AP treatments every 3-5 days for 3 times, then weekly for 3 times; Use herbal formula 2-4 months
Facial paralysis	Wind-Heat invasion causing *Qi*/Blood Stagnation and local *Qi* Deficiency	**EA:** GB-20/GB-14, ST-6/ST-2, TH-17/TH-23 **DN:** GV-14, ST-44, *Tai-yang, An-shen*, SI-19, *Bi-tong*, LI-20, GV-26, CV-24, LI-4, LI-10, ST-36	*Pu Ji Xiao Du Yin*	AP treatments every 1-2 weeks for 6-8 treatments; Use herbal formula 2-4 months
	Wind-Cold invasion causing *Qi*/Blood Stagnation and local	**EA:** GB-20/GB-14, ST-6/ST-2, TH-17/TH-23	Facial P Formula	AP treatments every 1-2 weeks for 6-8 treatments; Use

	Qi Deficiency	**DN:** BL-10, *Tai-yang*, *An-shen*, SI-19, *Bi-tong*, LI-20, GV-26, CV-24, LI-4, LI-10, ST-36		herbal formula for up to 3 months
	Local *Qi*/Blood Stagnation and *Qi* Deficiency	**EA:** GB-20/GB-14, ST-6/ST-2, TH-17/TH-23	Facial P Formula	AP treatments every 1-2 weeks for 6-8 treatments; Use herbal formula for up to 3 months
		DN: *Tai-yang*, *An-shen*, SI-19, *Bi-tong*, LI-20, GV-26, CV-24, LI-4, LI-10, ST-36		
	Gallbladder Damp Heat with local *Qi* Deficiency	**EA:** GB-20/GB-14, ST-6/ST-2, TH-17/TH-23	Ear Damp Heat or *Long Dan Xie Gan* and *Di Er You* topically if otitis externa	AP treatments every 1-2 weeks for 6-8 treatments; Use herbal formula for up to 4 months
		DN: *Er-jian*, GV-14, *Tai-yang*, *An-shen*, SI-19, *Bi-tong*, LI-20, GV-26, CV-24, LI-4, LI-10, ST-36		
Vestibular disorders	Kidney *Jing* Deficiency with Wind-Cold invasion causing *Qi*/Blood Stagnation and local *Qi* Deficiency	**DN only acutely then EA:** PC-6/PC-6, GB-20/GB-2 **DN:** PC-6, GB-20, BL-10, *Da-feng-men*, TH-5, GB-34, LU-7, LI-10, ST-36, SI-19, TH-17, GB-2, TH-21, BL-23, KID-3, BL-20	Stasis in Mansion of Mind and Epimedium Formula	AP treatments every 3-5 days for 3 times, then weekly for 3 times; Use herbal formulas up to 4 months
	Wind-Cold invasion causing Damp and Phlegm, *Qi*/Blood Stagnation and local *Qi* Deficiency with Spleen *Qi* Deficiency	**DN only acutely then EA:** PC-6/PC-6, GB-20/GB-2 **DN:** PC-6, GB-20, BL-10, *Da-feng-men*, TH-5, GB-34, ST-40,	Stasis in Mansion of Mind and Four Gentlemen	AP treatments every 3-5 days for 3 times, then weekly for 3 times; Use herbal formulas up to 4 months

CHAPTER 3   157

		LU-7, LI-10, SI-19, TH-17, GB-2, TH-21, SP-6, SP-9, ST-40		
	Local *Qi*/Blood Stagnation and *Qi* Deficiency	**DN only acutely then EA:** PC-6/PC-6, TH-17/TH-17	Stasis in Mansion of Mind	AP treatments every 3-5 days for 3 times, then weekly for 3 times; Use herbal formula up to 4 months
		DN: PC-6, GB-34, KID-3, BL-23, ST-36, LI-4, LI-10		
	Gallbladder Damp Heat with local *Qi* Deficiency	**DN only acutely then EA:** PC-6/PC-6, TH-17/TH-17	Ear Damp Heat or *Long Dan Xie Gan*; *Di Er You* topically if otitis externa	AP treatments every 1-2 weeks for 6-8 treatments; Use herbal formula for up to 4 months
		DN: GB-20, BL-10, BL-18, LIV-2, SP-6, SP-9, GB-34, BL-40, SP-10, SI-19, GB-2, TH-21, *Er-jian*, *Tai-Yang*		
Deafness	Kidney *Jing* Deficiency	**EA:** SI-16/SI-19, *An-shen/An-shen*, TH-17/TH-17	Epimedium Formula	6-8 AP treatments every 1-2 weeks; Use herbal formula for up to 6 months; Add Food to support *Jing*
		DN: *Shang-guan*, GB-2, TH-21, BL-23, KID-3, TH-3, GB-39, LU-7, LI-10, ST-36, BL-20, BL-21		
	Kidney *Qi* Deficiency	**EA:** SI-16/SI-19, *An-shen/An-shen*, TH-17/TH-17	*Jin Gui Shen Qi Wan*	6-8 AP treatments every 1-2 weeks; Use herbal formula for up to 6 months; Add Food to support *Qi*
		DN: *Shang-guan*, GB-2, TH-21, BL-23, KID-3, TH-3, GB-39, GB-34, LU-7, LI-10, ST-36		
	Gallbladder Damp Heat with local *Qi* Deficiency	**EA:** SI-16/SI-19, *An-shen/An-shen*, TH-17/TH-17	*Long Dan Xie Gan*;	AP treatments every 1-2 weeks for 6-8 treatments; Use

		DN: *Er-jian*, GV-14, SP-6, SP-9, *Shang-guan*, GB-2, TH-21, BL-23, KID-3, TH-3, GB-39, GB-34, LU-7, LI-10, ST-36	*Di Er You* topically if otitis externa	herbal formula for up to 4 months
Laryngeal paresis or paralysis	Kidney *Jing* Deficiency with local *Qi* Deficiency (Young and adult onset)	**EA:** CV-20/CV-24, CV-23a/CV-23b, LI-18/LI-18	Epimedium Formula add *Si Jun Zi* for young dogs or add *Qi* Performance for adult dogs and cats	Repeat acupuncture every 3-5 days for 3-5 times, then every 1-2 weeks until function returns; Use herbal formula for up to 6 months
		DN: CV-1, BL-23, KID-3, GB-39, LU-7, LI-4, LI-10, ST-36, BL-20, BL-21		
		DN: CV-1, BL-23, KID-3, GB-39, LU-7, LI-4, LI-10, ST-36, BL-20, BL-21		
	Wind-Heat invasion causing *Qi*/Blood Stagnation and local *Qi* Deficiency	**EA:** CV-20/CV-24, CV-23a/CV-23b, LI-18/LI-18	*Pu Ji Xiao Du Yin*	Repeat acupuncture every 3-5 days for 3-5 times, then every 1-2 weeks until function returns; Use herbal formula for 2-4 months
		DN: CV-1, GV-14, LI-4, LU-7, LI-10, ST-36		
	Local *Qi*/Blood Stagnation and *Qi* Deficiency	**EA:** GB 21/CV-23a, CV-23/ LI-17, LI-18/LI-18, SI-9/SI-9, SI-17/SI-17	*Bu Yong Yi Qi*	If paresis only, 3-6 AP treatments every 1-2 weeks; Use herbal formula for up to 6 months
		DN: CV-1, BL-23, KID-3, GB-39, LU-7, LI-4, LI-10, ST-36		

Masticatory myopathy	Wind-Heat invasion causing *Qi*/Blood Stagnation and local *Qi* Deficiency	**EA:** Acute pain stage: GB-20/GB-2, TH-17/TH-17 (acupoints on head may be too painful to use); When no longer painful: GB-20/GB-2, TH-17/TH-17, *Da-feng-men/Nao-shu*, ST-6/ST-6	*Pu Ji Xiao Du Yin*	Acute stage: AP treatments every 3-5 days for 3-5 times, then every 1-2 weeks; Chronic stage: AP treatments every 1-2 weeks for 6-8 times then monthly; Use herbal formula for up to 4 months
		DN: *Er-jian* (ear tip), *Tai-Yang*, left LI-4, right LIV-3, LU-7, ST-2, SI-16, TH-21, ST-44, LI-10, ST-36		

The number of acupoints selected and treatment frequency will vary with the animal's condition and response to treatment; Chinese herbal medicine doses are generally 0.5 gm/10-20# orally twice daily, use 0.5 gm/10# signs severe; EA=electro-acupuncture, DN=dry needle acupuncture; All Chinese herbal formulas available from Jing Tang herbal:www.tcvmherbal.com

OPTIC NEURITIS

From a conventional perspective, sudden blindness in dogs and cats with absent pupillary light reflexes and a normal ocular fundus, is usually due to sudden acquired retinal degeneration (SARDS) or optic neuritis.[1-3] Some cases of optic neuritis show swelling of the optic disk, but the optic disk may also appear normal. The electroretinogram (ERG) is abnormal in animals with SARDS, but not in optic neuritis and differentiation of these two diseases is essential, as early diagnosis and treatment of optic neuritis can restore vision.

Optic neuritis may be associated with an infectious agent such as canine distemper virus, feline infectious peritonitis virus, *toxoplasma gondii*, and some fungi, granulomatous meningoencephalitis, a paraneoplastic syndrome, trauma, an immune-mediated disorder or can be idiopathic. Enlarged lymph nodes should be aspirated to detect infection or neoplasia. Evaluation of CSF, serum and CSF organism immunoassays and CT or MRI may be useful to rule out a concurrent meningoencephalitis or neoplasia. Early treatment with corticosteroids (e.g. oral prednisone 1-2mg/kg every 12 hours for 2-3 weeks with subsequent tapering of the dose) often improves vision and is recommended as soon as possible. Integration of TCVM treatments may shorten the recovery time and the degree of vision improvement. Some animals may remain permanently blind, even with early corticosteroid treatment, due to residual optic nerve atrophy, so TCVM may offer hope for these patients.

Although there is little published data using acupuncture and Chinese herbal medicine to treat animals with optic neuritis and resulting optic nerve atrophy, there are a few clinical studies in humans that are encouraging.[12,13] Vision and visual acuity were significantly increased in 85% of patients receiving acupuncture treatment, in one human clinical study of 38 cases (55 affected eyes) of optic nerve atrophy.[12] In another human clinical study of 51 cases (58 affected eyes) of optic nerve atrophy, a combination of the Chinese herbal medicine *Dan Zhi Xiao Yao Yin* and pressing on auricular acupoints resulted in greater improvements in vision compared to patients treated with conventional medications.[13]

Although well-controlled clinical trails are necessary in animals, before specific recommendations can be made, TCVM treatments integrated with conventional medications may be shown to improve the rate and degree of vision recovery in animals with optic neuritis. Treatment of clinical cases is warranted to determine if these therapies will improve the prognosis of optic neuritis in dogs. There are two different TCVM patterns for optic neuritis and the clinical findings are outlined in Table 2. Recommended acupoints, acupuncture techniques and Chinese herbal medicines are listed in Table 3.[6-9] Food therapy and *Tui-na* may further promote recovery.[10,11] Since recovery might occur to some degree without treatment, controlled clinical studies are needed to ensure TCVM treatments are enhancing the recovery process. Based on the positive experiences of practitioners, TCVM treatment of patients with optic neuritis is encouraged to provide the animal with every possible chance for full recovery of vision.[6-9]

Etiology and Pathology

The Bladder, Stomach and Gallbladder Channels, all *Yang* Channels, begin around the eye.[4,6] The Triple Heater Channel also a *Yang* Channel ends near the eye. These Channels may become vulnerable to the entrance of TCVM pathogens. When *Zheng Qi* is weakened and *Wei Qi* allows entrance of Wind-Heat into theses Channels, local *Qi*/Blood Stagnation with resultant local *Qi* Deficiency causes dysfunction of the optic nerves.[4] The eyes are also the opening to the TCVM Liver system and Liver imbalances, especially Liver *Qi* Stagnation, generates Liver *Yang* rising and Heat.[4] The result is ocular disease especially in Wood constitution animals with their susceptibility to Liver *Qi* Stagnation. Applying the basic TCVM theories of *Yin/Yang*, Eight Principles, Five Treasures, Five Elements and *Zang Fu* physiology and pathology to make a TCVM diagnosis, there are 2 basic patterns associated with optic neuritis:

1. **Wind-Heat invasion causing *Qi*/Blood Stagnation and local *Qi* Deficiency**
   When *Wei Qi* becomes weak due to poor nutrition, chronic illness or environmental stress, Wind-Heat invades the Channels surrounding the eye and causes the *Qi*/Blood to Stagnate and optic neuritis and acute blindness result.

2. **Liver *Qi* Stagnation with Liver *Yang* rising and Liver Heat**
   Wood constitution dogs and cats are prone to Liver *Qi* Stagnation and resulting Liver *Yang* Rising. The Liver Heat associated with Liver *Yang* Rising can ascend to the eyes and manifest as optic neuritis.

Pattern Differentiation and Treatment

1. Wind-Heat invasion causing *Qi*/Blood Stagnation and local *Qi* Deficiency

Clinical Signs:
- Acute onset of blindness

- Dilated pupils, unresponsive to light
- May or not have swollen optic disks
- Normal ERG
- Tongue- red, dry or pale
- Pulses- Superficial, forceful, rapid, wiry

TCVM Diagnosis:
The acute onset of blindness is typical of an Excess pattern with invasion of an External pathogen and *Qi*/Blood Stagnation. The diagnosis of Wind-Heat invasion causing *Qi*/Blood Stagnation and local *Qi* Deficiency is based on the clinical signs and TCVM examination findings. The tongue color will vary with the stage of the process. Acutely the tongue is red from the Wind-Heat, purple if *Qi*/Blood Stagnation is most prominent and pale if *Qi* Deficiency is most prominent. The pulses may be forceful and rapid from the Heat or wiry from the Stagnation.

Treatment Principles:
- Clear Wind-Heat
- Resolve *Qi*/Blood Stagnation
- Promote local *Qi* flow and restore optic nerve function

Acupuncture treatment:
For EA use 80-120 Hz alternating frequencies for 15-30 minutes, as EA is more effective to resolve Stagnation than DN alone. Acutely perform AP treatments every 3-5 days for 3 times, then weekly for 3 times, then 1-2 times per month until vision restored. For Aqua-AP inject 0.25-0.5 ml vitamin B12 into the acupoint.

Acupoints recommended
- EA: GB-20/GB-1, BL-10/BL-1, *Tai-yang/Tai-yang*
- DN: GB-14, TH-23, LI-4, TH-5, GV-14, BL-67
- Aqua-AP: GB-20, GV-14, *Tai-yang*

Pertinent acupoint actions
- GB-20 is useful to dispel Wind
- GB-1 and BL-1 are local acupoints around the eye
- BL-10 can connect to BL-1 to bring *Qi* to the area
- *Tai-yang* (one *cun* lateral to the lateral canthus of the eye, above the zygomatic arch) is a local eye acupoint useful to clear Wind-Heat in acute ocular conditions
- GB-14 and TH-23 are local eye acupoints
- LI-4 is the Master point of the face and also balances the immune system
- TH-5 is useful to strengthen *Wei Qi*
- GV-14 is useful to clear Heat and balance the immune system
- BL-67 is a distant acupoint on the Bladder Channel useful for ocular diseases

Herbal Medicine:
- *Fang Feng San* (JT)[a] at 0.5gm/10# twice daily orally to clear Wind and Heat to benefit the eyes
- Administer herbal formula up to 6 months
- A description of all the ingredients of the Chinese herbal medicine listed is beyond the scope of this text, but can be found elsewhere.[8,9]

Food Therapy:
The purpose of the Food therapy is to clear Heat and promote *Qi*/Blood circulation, so cooling foods are prescribed and Hot foods are avoided.[11]
- Foods to supplement to clear Heat: Turkey, duck, duck eggs, conch, clams, mussels, yogurt, millet, barley, spinach, broccoli, celery, egg plant, kelp, alfalfa, cucumbers, pears, bananas, white radishes
- Foods to promote *Qi*/Blood circulation: Chicken egg, crab, sweet rice, peaches, carrots, coriander, turnips
- Hot Foods to avoid: Lamb, shrimp, corn-fed beef, chicken, trout, squash, turnips, sweet rice, basal, caraway, cherries, chilies, cinnamon, ginger, rosemary, sage

Tui-na Procedures:
The purpose of the *Tui-na* is to stimulate *Qi* and Blood flow and promote optic nerve regeneration in the affected region. The descriptions and indications of each technique are outlined in more detail in Chapter 1 Table 8.[10]
- *Rou-fa* rotary kneading of both BL-2 using both thumbs, repeat 20-30 times
- *Anfa* pressing both BL-1 acupoints with the thumb and index finger releasing toward BL-2; repeat 20-30 times
- *Anfa* pressing plus *Rou-fa* rotary kneading of ST-1 with both index fingers; repeat 20-30 times
- *Ca-fa* rubbing upper and lower orbits; repeat 20-30 times
- *Rou-fa* rotary kneading of both Tai-yang acupoints; repeat 20-30 times

Daily Life Style Recommendation for Owner Follow-up:
- *Moo-fa* touching and massaging BL-1, BL-2, ST-1, upper and lower orbits and *Tai Yang* for 3-5 minutes twice daily until vision is restored
- Feed high quality diet to support *Zheng Qi*
- Feed a high quality diet to support *Zheng Qi*
- Keep in a low stress environment to support *Zheng Qi*
- Do not change furniture or other structures in the environment
- Protect the animal from falling down stairs or into the swimming pool

Comments:
Based on clinical studies in humans and anecdotal experiences in animals expect TCVM treatment to shorten the recovery time and improve vision.

2. Liver *Qi* Stagnation with Liver Heat and Liver *Yang* rising

Clinical Signs:
- Wood constitution
- Irritable
- Acute onset of blindness
- Dilated pupils
- May or not have swollen optic disks
- Normal ERG
- Cool seeking
- Panting
- Warm ears, feet and back
- Tongue- red, dry
- Pulses- Superficial, forceful, rapid or wiry

TCVM Diagnosis:
The diagnosis of Liver *Qi* Stagnation with Liver *Yang* rising and Liver Heat is based on the Wood constitution, history and evidence of generalized Heat on the TCVM examination including typical tongue and pulse characteristics.

Treatment Principles:
- Soothe the Liver
- Clear Heat
- Resolve *Qi*/Blood Stagnation to promote local *Qi* flow and restore optic nerve function

Acupuncture treatment:
For EA use 80-120 Hz alternating frequencies for 15-30 minutes, as EA is more effective to resolve Stagnation than DN alone. Acutely perform AP treatments every 3-5 days for 3 times, then weekly for 3 times, then 1-2 times per month until vision restored. For Aqua-AP inject 0.25-0.5 ml vitamin B12 into the acupoint.

Acupoints recommended
- EA: *Tai-yang/Tai-Yang*, GB-1/GB-1, BL-1/BL-1
- DN: GV-14, LI-4, BL-18, BL-19, GB-34, LIV-3, BL-67
- Aqua-AP: GV-14, BL-18

Pertinent acupoint actions
- *Tai-yang* is a local eye acupoint useful to clear Wind-Heat in acute ocular conditions
- BL-1, GB-1 and GB-14 are local acupoints around the eye
- GV-14 is useful to clear Heat
- LI-4 is a Master point of the face
- BL-18 is the Back *Shu* Association point for the Liver
- BL-19 is the Back *Shu* Association point for the Gallbladder
- GB-34 and LIV-3 are useful to treat Liver *Qi* Stagnation

- BL-67 is a distant acupoint on the Bladder Channel useful for ocular disease

Herbal Medicine:
- *Jue Ming San* (Haliotis Powder) (JT)[a] 0.5gm/10# twice daily orally to clear the Liver fire and benefit the eyes
- Administer herbal formula up to 6 months
- A description of all the ingredients of the Chinese herbal medicine listed is beyond the scope of this text, but can be found elsewhere.[8,9]

Food Therapy:
The purpose of the Food therapy is to soothe the Liver, clear Heat and promote *Qi*/Blood circulation, so cooling foods are prescribed and Hot foods are avoided (Table 4).[11]
- Foods to supplement to soothe the Liver: Crayfish, duck, shrimp, brown rice, oats, spelt, wheat, wheat germ, Belgian endive hearts, celery, cucumbers, kohlrabi, lettuce, legumes, mung beans and sprouts, mushrooms, radishes, rhubarb, seaweed, spinach, sprouts, lemons, apples, mangos, mulberries, schisandra berries, jujube seeds, basil, chamomile, catnip, coriander, dill, ginger in small amount, garlic in small amount, marjoram, skullcap, valerian, vinegar (small amount)
- Foods to supplement to clear Heat: Turkey, duck, duck eggs, conch, clams, mussels, yogurt, millet, barley, spinach, broccoli, celery, egg plant, kelp, alfalfa, cucumbers, pears, bananas, white radishes
- Foods to supplement to promote *Qi*/Blood circulation: Chicken egg, crab, sweet rice, peaches, carrots, coriander, squash, turnips
- Foods to avoid: Lamb, shrimp, corn-fed beef, chicken, trout, squash, turnips, sweet rice, basal, caraway, cherries, chilies, cinnamon, ginger, rosemary, sage

Tui-na Procedures:
The purpose of the *Tui-na* is to stimulate *Qi* and Blood flow and promote nerve regeneration in the affected region. The descriptions and indications of each technique are outlined in more detail in Chapter 1 Table 8.[10]
- *Rou-fa* rotary kneading of both BL-2 using both thumbs, repeat 20-30 times
- *Anfa* pressing both BL-1 acupoints with the thumb and index finger releasing toward BL-2; repeat 20-30 times
- *Anfa* pressing plus *Rou-fa* rotary kneading of ST-1 with both index fingers; repeat 20-30 times
- *Ca-fa* rubbing upper and lower orbits; repeat 20-30 times
- *Rou-fa* rotary kneading of both Tai-yang acupoints; repeat 20-30 times

Daily Life Style Recommendation for Owner Follow-up:
- *Moo-fa* touching and massaging BL-1, BL-2, ST-1, upper and lower orbits and *Tai Yang* for 3-5 minutes twice daily until vision is restored
- Feed a high quality diet to support *Zheng Qi*
- Keep in a low stress environment to support *Zheng Qi*
- Keep in a protected environment until vision returns
- Do not change furniture or other structures in the environment

- Protect the animal from falling down stairs or into the swimming pool

Comments:
Based on clinical studies in humans and anecdotal experiences in animals expect TCVM treatment to shorten the recovery time and improve vision.

TRIGEMINAL NEURITIS

Trigeminal neuritis results in acute onset of the inability to close the mouth. The jaw hangs open because the trigeminal nerves (CN5) are not functional and the masticatory muscles are unable to close the temporomandibular joint (TMJ). Swallowing is normal, although saliva often drips from the open mouth. There is no associated pain and sensation of the head is normal. Sometimes unilateral or bilateral Horner's syndrome (ptosis, miosis and enophthalmos) is seen and the third eyelid covers part of the eye. Horner's syndrome can occur because the third order neuron of the sympathetic innervation to the eye traverses for a short distance in the peripheral nerve sheath with the trigeminal motor nerve.[1-3] From a conventional perspective a focal immune-mediated bilateral trigeminal neuritis is suspected.

From a TCVM perspective, trigeminal neuritis is another focal Wind-Heat invasion that results in *Qi*/Blood Stagnation in the distal Triple Heater and Small Intestine Channels and proximal Gallbladder Channels and loss of *Qi*/Blood flow leads to a focal Deficiency that affects the motor portion of the trigeminal nerves bilaterally.[5,7] The TCVM examination findings are listed in Table 2.

There is no conventional therapy for trigeminal neuritis.[1-3] The caretaker must blend dog food into a gruel so the dog can use the tongue to lap food during the recovery period. Most dogs recover the ability to close the jaw and chew soft food in 4-6 weeks, but often have residual weakness in masticatory muscles observed, when chewing hard food and pulling on a toy or rope during play.[2] Acupuncture, Chinese herbal medicine and *Tui-na* may shorten the recovery time, reduce the time the caretaker has to hand-feed the dog and result in less residual muscle weakness. There is one foreign language case report of the acupuncture for a trigeminal neuropathy, but details of the clinical signs and treatment protocol are unknown.[14]

The TCVM examination findings in trigeminal neuritis are listed in Table 2. Recommended acupoints, acupuncture techniques and Chinese herbal medicine are listed in Table 3.[6-9] Since the TCVM etiology and treatment strategy of optic neuritis and trigeminal neuritis are similar, acupuncture techniques should include a combination of EA, DN and Aqua-AP to achieve the best possible results. Again, the TCVM practitioner may administer *Tui-na* treatments after the EA and DN session and before the Aqua-AP and some simple *Tui-na* techniques may also be taught to the caretaker for in-home daily treatments in between TCVM appointments.[10] Cooling foods may also be helpful to clear Heat.[11] Controlled clinical studies are needed to ensure TCVM treatments are enhancing the recovery process, because like optic neuritis, recovery from trigeminal neuritis occurs to some degree without treatment.[1-3,5] Based on the positive experiences of TCVM practitioners, treatment of clinical cases of trigeminal neuritis is encouraged to give the dog every possible chance for a full recovery of normal mastication and jaw strength. Applying the basic TCVM theories of *Yin/Yang*, Eight Principles, Five Treasures, Five Elements and *Zang Fu* physiology and pathology to make a TCVM diagnosis, there is one basic pattern suspected with trigeminal neuritis, but with more TCVM experience other patterns like Wind-Cold invasion or underlying Deficiencies of *Yin* or Blood may also be identified in the future.[5]

Etiology and Pathology

From a TCVM perspective, trigeminal neuritis is another manifestation of a weakened *Zheng Qi* that allows focal Wind-Heat invasion and results in *Qi*/Blood Stagnation in the distal Triple Heater and Small Intestine Channels and proximal Gallbladder Channels. Loss of *Qi*/Blood flow to theses areas causes local *Qi*/Blood Deficiency that affects the motor function of the trigeminal nerves bilaterally.[4,5]

1. **Wind-Heat invasion causing *Qi*/Blood Stagnation and local *Qi* Deficiency**
   When *Zheng Qi* including *Wei Qi* becomes weak due to poor nutrition, chronic illness or environmental stress, Wind-Heat invades the Channels surrounding the eye and causes optic neuritis and acute blindness

Pattern Differentiation and Treatment

1. Wind-Heat invasion causing *Qi*/Blood Stagnation and local *Qi* Deficiency

Clinical Signs:
- Acute onset
- Inability to close the mouth
- Unable to prehend or chew food
- Tongue- red, purple or pale
- Pulses-Superficial, forceful, rapid or wiry

TCVM Diagnosis:
The diagnosis of Wind-Heat invasion causing *Qi*/Blood Stagnation and local *Qi* Deficiency is based on the clinical signs. The tongue color will vary with the stage of the process. Acutely the tongue is red from the Wind-Heat, purple if *Qi*/Blood Stagnation is most prominent and pale if *Qi* Deficiency is most prominent. The pulses may be forceful and rapid from the Heat or wiry from the Stagnation.

Treatment Principles:
- Clear Wind-Heat
- Resolve *Qi*/Blood Stagnation
- Tonify local *Qi* and restore trigeminal nerve function

Acupuncture treatment:
For EA use 80-120 Hz alternating frequencies for 15-30 minutes. EA is more effective to resolve Stagnation than DN alone. Acutely, perform AP treatments every 3-5 days for 3 times, then weekly for 3 times, then 1-2 times per month until jaw strength has returned. For Aqua-AP inject 0.25-0.5 ml vitamin B12 into the acupoint.

Acupoints recommended
- EA: TH-17/TH-17, ST-6/ST-6, *Nao-shu/Nao-shu*

CHAPTER 3

- DN: *Shang guan,* GB-2, SI-19, LI-10, ST-36, LU-7, LI-4, GV-14
- Aqua-AP: ST-6 and *Nao-shu*

Pertinent acupoint actions
- TH-17, GB-2 and SI-19 are local acupoints by the trigeminal nerve
- ST-6 is a local acupoint to move *Qi*/Blood and restore *Qi* to the masseter muscles
- *Nao-shu* (one third of the way along a line form the cranial ear base to the lateral canthus) is a local acupoint to move *Qi*/Blood and restore *Qi* to the temporalis muscles
- *Shang guan* (on the dorsal border of the TMJ) is a local acupoint
- LI-10 and ST-36 are useful to increase *Qi* in Deficiency
- LU-7 is the Master point for the head
- LI-4 is a Master point for the face, clears Heat and balances the immune system
- GV-14 is useful to balance the immune system

Herbal Medicine:
- *Pu Ji Xiao Du Yin* (JT)[a] 0.5gm/10# twice daily orally to clear Heat and disperse Wind-Heat
- Administer herbal formula 2-4 months as needed
- A description of all the ingredients of the Chinese herbal medicine listed is beyond the scope of this text, but can be found elsewhere.[8,9]

Food Therapy:
The purpose of the Food therapy is to clear Heat and promote *Qi*/Blood circulation, so cooling foods are prescribed and Hot foods are avoided.[11]
- Foods to supplement to clear Heat: Turkey, duck, duck eggs, conch, clams, mussels, yogurt, millet, barley, spinach, broccoli, celery, egg plant, kelp, alfalfa, cucumbers, pears, bananas, white radishes
- Foods to promote *Qi*/Blood circulation: Chicken egg, crab, sweet rice, peaches, carrots, coriander, turnips
- Foods to avoid: Lamb, shrimp, corn-fed beef, chicken, trout, squash, turnips, sweet rice, basal, caraway, cherries, chilies, cinnamon, ginger, rosemary, sage

Tui-na Procedures:
The purpose of the *Tui-na* is to stimulate *Qi* and Blood flow and promote nerve regeneration in the affected region. The descriptions and indications of each technique are outlined in more detail in Chapter 1 Table 8.[10]
- *An-fa* pressing and *Ca-fa* rubbing around TH-17, *Xia guan* (upper TMJ) and *Shan guan* (lower TMJ) for 3-5 minutes to relieve *Qi*/Blood Stagnation
- *Ban-fa* wrenching in the form of opening and closing the jaws for TMJ range of motion exercises; repeat 12 times
- *Mo-fa* rubbing the temporal and masseter muscles for 3-5 minutes to improve *Qi*/Blood circulation to the muscles and other tissues

Daily Life Style Recommendation for Owner Follow-up:
- *Moo-fa* massaging under ear base at the TMJ for 3-5 minutes twice daily until function returns
- *Moo-fa* massaging over the masseter muscles for 3-5 minutes twice daily until function returns
- Open and close the jaw 12 times, twice daily until function returns
- Put normal dog food in the blender with water to form a gruel so animals can lap and swallow since they cannot chew
- When function begins to return, allow dog to have toys to chew on and play tug with to provide jaw exercise
- Feed a high quality diet to support *Zheng Qi*
- Keep in a low stress environment to support *Zheng Qi*

Comments:

Based on anecdotal experiences in dogs with trigeminal neuritis, expect TCVM treatment to shorten the recovery time and reduce residual jaw weakness. Further clinical studies are needed.

FACIAL PARALYSIS

Acute facial nerve paralysis may be associated with a middle ear infection, hypothyroidism, trauma or neoplasia, but idiopathic facial nerve paralysis is most common (approximately 75% of cases).[1-3] With idiopathic facial nerve paralysis, there is no history or physical evidence of ear infection or trauma. On neurological examination there is inability to close the eyelid to blink or move the ear or lips on the affected side, but sensation of the face is normal. There may be reduced saliva and tear production on the affected eye and artificial tear administration is essential to prevent corneal ulceration. Facial paralysis is usually unilateral, in some instances both nerves become affected and the signs are bilateral. The remainder of the physical and neurological examinations is normal. Serum thyroxin (T4) and thyroid stimulating hormone (TSH) tests should always be evaluated on every case of acute facial paralysis, as hypothyroidism can cause a focal facial neuropathy with no other findings. Tumors can compress the facial nerve (e.g. nasopharyngeal polyps in the middle ear in cats) or arise from the nerve sheath (e.g. facial nerve schwannoma). The onset of clinical signs with polyps or neoplasia is gradual and progressive, but the caretakers may acutely become aware of the paralysis. Skull radiographs or a CT scan can show bone tumors, but a MRI may be necessary to detect soft tissue or primary nerve sheath tumors.

There is no conventional treatment for idiopathic facial paralysis. Although idiopathic facial nerve paralysis has been treated with EA and Chinese herbal medicine, only two case reports in dogs have been published and well controlled veterinary clinical trials are needed.[5,6,9,15,16] According to a systematic review of human controlled clinical trials, evaluating acupuncture treatment for facial nerve paralysis, significantly positive effects with EA were found and a standardized treatment regime was recommended.[17] Based on the results of another systematic review of several controlled human clinical trials of acupuncture for idiopathic facial nerve paralysis, it was concluded that although preliminary positive results had been reported, higher quality studies with larger numbers of patients were still needed before recommendations regarding acupuncture for idiopathic facial nerve paralysis (Bell's palsy) for humans could be made.[18]

Recommended acupoints, acupuncture techniques and Chinese herbal medicine for facial paralysis associated with different TCVM patterns are listed in Tables 2 and 3.[6-9] Again, a combination of EA, DN and Aqua-AP are recommended acupuncture techniques to ensure optimum recovery of function. The TCVM practitioner also may administer *Tui-na* treatments after the EA and DN session and before the Aqua-AP [10] An example of a *Tui-na* treatment for facial paralysis is outlined in Table 4.[10] Some simple *Tui-na* techniques may be taught to the caretaker for in-home daily treatments in between TCVM appointments. Cooling foods may also be helpful to clear Heat.[11] Controlled clinical studies are needed to ensure TCVM treatments are enhancing the recovery process of idiopathic facial paralysis, because like optic neuritis and trigeminal neuritis, recovery occurs to some degree without treatment.[1-3] Based on the positive experiences of veterinary and human practitioners, TCVM treatment of clinical cases of facial nerve paralysis is encouraged to give the dog every possible chance for full recovery of facial muscle function.[5,6-10]

Etiology and Pathology

The Stomach, Gallbladder, Small Intestine and Large Intestine Channels all traverse the side of the face in the region of the facial nerve. The facial nerve actually crosses the masseter muscle in the same position as the Stomach Channel in that region. From a TCVM perspective, facial paralysis is called *"Wai-zhui-feng"* or oblique facial Wind or deviating mouth Wind.[6,9] Idiopathic facial nerve paralysis may be due to invasion of either Wind-Cold or Wind-Heat into the Channels of the face. The result is local *Qi*/Blood Stagnation and Deficient *Qi*/Blood to the region causing facial nerve dysfunction. Focal *Qi*/Blood Deficiency in the proximal Stomach and Gallbladder Channels causes paralysis of the eyelids. Focal *Qi*/Blood Deficiency in the proximal Stomach Channel also causes paralysis of the lips. Focal *Qi*/Blood Deficiency in the distal Large Intestine Channel results in paralysis of the lips and nose. Focal *Qi*/Blood Deficiency in the distal Small Channel Intestine causes paralysis of the ear.

Facial nerve paralysis from trauma is relatively rare in dogs as compared to horses, but also results in local *Qi*/Blood Stagnation, loss of *Qi*/Blood flow and *Qi*/Blood Deficiency to the region of the affected Channel. Facial nerve paralysis from a middle ear infection is due to middle ear Damp-Heat causing local *Qi*/Blood Stagnation, a loss of *Qi*/Blood flow and *Qi*/Blood Deficiency affecting the facial nerve as it passes through the middle ear. Neoplastic involvement of the facial nerve may be associated with substantial Phlegm (nerve sheath tumors and other non-blood related tumors) or Blood Stagnation (lymphoma and other blood-related tumors). The TCVM examination findings with different disease patterns are listed in Table 2.

Otitis media or middle ear Damp-Heat is usually a bacterial or mycotic infection and is treated with the appropriate conventional medications, but the integration of TCVM treatments may result in a more rapid recovery, less residual damage and prevent recurrences.[19,20] In animals with facial nerve paralysis from hypothyroidism, TCVM treatments integrated with thyroid replacement therapy may resolve clinical signs faster and more completely. There is no conventional therapy for traumatic and idiopathic facial nerve paralysis and some dogs recover function, while others have residual paresis or paralysis. Middle ear Damp-Heat is usually a bacterial infection and is treated with the appropriate antibiotic, but the integration of TCVM treatments may result in a more rapid recovery and less residual damage. Nasopharyngeal polyps are best surgically removed, but TCVM treatments may discourage tumor regrowth.[21] Peripheral nerve neoplasms are not radiosensitive and removal is difficult, so TCVM can be useful to shrink the tumor size and slow or stop tumor growth.[21] In neoplastic processes no local and only distant acupoints are treated. Residual facial nerve damage eventually leads to facial distortion from muscle contracture. Applying the basic TCVM theories of *Yin/Yang*, Eight Principles, Five Treasures, Five Elements and *Zang Fu* physiology and pathology to make a TCVM diagnosis, there are four basic patterns associated with facial paralysis:

1. **Wind-Heat invasion causing *Qi*/Blood Stagnation and local *Qi* Deficiency**
   When *Wei Qi* becomes weak due to poor nutrition, chronic illness or environmental stress, Wind-Heat invades the Channels of the face, especially in *Yang* animals (Wood and Fire constitutions), causing *Qi*/Blood Stagnation, loss of *Qi*/Blood flow and *Qi*/Blood Deficiency to local tissues including the facial nerves. The result is paralysis of facial muscles.

2. **Wind-Cold invasion causing *Qi*/Blood Stagnation and local *Qi* Deficiency**
   When *Wei Qi* becomes weak due to poor nutrition, chronic illness or environmental stress, Wind-Cold invades the Channels of the face especially in *Yin* animals (Earth, Metal and Water constitutions) *Qi*/Blood Stagnation, loss of *Qi*/Blood flow and *Qi*/Blood Deficiency to local tissues including the facial nerves. The result is paralysis of facial muscles.

3. ***Qi*/Blood Stagnation and local *Qi* Deficiency**
   Trauma induces *Qi*/Blood Stagnation, loss of *Qi*/Blood flow and *Qi*/Blood Deficiency to local tissues including facial nerves. The result is paralysis of facial muscles.

4. **Gallbladder Damp Heat with local *Qi* Deficiency (Middle ear)**
   When *Wei Qi* becomes weak due to poor nutrition, chronic illness or environmental stress in any constitution animal, Damp-Heat enters the Gallbladder Channel and causes *Qi*/Blood Stagnation, loss of *Qi*/Blood flow and *Qi*/Blood Deficiency to local tissues causing dysfunction of the facial nerve as it traverses the region of the middle ear.

Pattern Differentiation and Treatment

1. Wind-Heat invasion causing *Qi*/Blood Stagnation and local *Qi* Deficiency

Clinical Signs:
- Acute onset
- Inability to close the eyelids and /or move the nose and lips
- Tongue- red, purple or pale
- Pulses- Superficial, forceful, rapid or wiry

TCVM Diagnosis:
The diagnosis of Wind-Heat invasion causing *Qi*/Blood Stagnation and local *Qi* Deficiency is based on the clinical signs. The tongue color will vary with the stage of the process. Acutely the tongue is red from the Wind-Heat, purple if *Qi*/Blood Stagnation is most prominent and pale if *Qi*/Blood Deficiency is most prominent. The pulses may be forceful and rapid from the Heat or wiry from the Stagnation.

Treatment Principles:
- Clear Wind-Heat
- Resolve *Qi*/Blood Stagnation
- Promote local *Qi*/Blood flow and restore facial nerve function

Acupuncture treatment:

For EA use 80-120 Hz alternating frequencies for 15-30 minutes, as EA is more effective to resolve Stagnation than DN alone. Treat both the normal and abnormal sides. Repeat acupuncture weekly every 1-2 weeks for 6-8 treatments. For Aqua-AP inject 0.25-0.5 ml vitamin B12 into the acupoint.

Acupoints recommended
- EA: GB-20/GB-14, ST-6/ST-2, TH-17/TH-23
- DN: GV-14, ST-44, *Tai-yang*, *An-shen*, SI-19, *Bi-tong*, LI-20, GV-26, CV-24, LI-4, LI-10, ST-36
- Aqua-AP: GB-20

Pertinent acupoint actions
- GB-20 is useful to Dispel Wind
- GV-14 is useful to Clear Heat and balance *Zheng Qi*
- ST-44 is useful to clear Heat in the ST Channel that courses along the side of the face near the facial nerve
- *Tai-yang* (one *cun* lateral to the lateral canthus above the zygomatic arch) is useful to clear Wind-Heat
- GB-14, TH-23 and *Tai-yang* (one *cun* lateral to the lateral canthus above the zygomatic arch) are local acupoints for eyelid paralysis
- *An-shen*, SI-19 and TH-17 are local acupoints for ear paralysis
- ST-2, ST-6, *Bi-tong* (halfway between BL-1 and LI-20), LI-20, GV-26 and CV-24 are local acupoints for paralysis of the lips and nose
- LI-4 is a Master point for the face
- LI-10 and ST-36 tonify *Qi* to encourage *Qi* flow in the Channels

Herbal Medicine:
- *Pu Ji Xiao Du Yin* (JT)[a] 0.5gm/10# twice daily orally to clear Heat and disperse Wind-Heat
- Administer herbal formula 2-4 months as needed
- A description of all the ingredients of the Chinese herbal medicine listed is beyond the scope of this text, but can be found elsewhere.[8,9]

Food Therapy:

The purpose of the Food therapy is to clear Heat and promote *Qi*/Blood circulation, so cooling foods are prescribed and Hot foods are avoided (Table 4).[11]
- Foods to supplement to clear Heat: Turkey, duck, duck eggs, conch, clams, mussels, yogurt, millet, barley, spinach, broccoli, celery, egg plant, kelp, alfalfa, cucumbers, pears, bananas, white radishes

- Foods to promote *Qi*/Blood circulation: Chicken egg, crab, sweet rice, peaches, carrots, coriander, turnips
- Foods to avoid: Lamb, shrimp, corn-fed beef, chicken, trout, squash, turnips, sweet rice, basal, caraway, cherries, chilies, cinnamon, ginger, rosemary, sage

Tui-na Procedures:

The purpose of the *Tui-na* is to stimulate *Qi* and Blood flow and promote nerve regeneration in the affected region. The descriptions and indications of each technique are outlined in more detail in Chapter 1 Table 8.[10]

- A 25-30 minute *Tui-na* treatment for facial paralysis is outlined in Table 4

Table 4: An example of a 25-30 minute *Tui-na* treatment for facial paralysis[10]

Name	Technique	Duration or Number of Repetitions
Moo-fa, then *An-fa* and *Rou-fa*	Massage the face and the top of the neck, then press and perform rotary kneading on the affected side from ST-1, along the obit and upper jaw, cheeks and to the lower jaw	5 minutes
Ban-fa	Open the mouth and stretch	6 times
Yi-zhi-chan and *Tui-fa*	Use the thumb press and perform rotary kneading at GB-14, LI-20, ST-4, ST-6, LU-7 and LI-4	30 seconds/acupoint
Nie-fa	Pinch and lift up on the cheek using both hands from the lower to upper cheek	2 minutes
An-fa and *Na-fa*	Press and pull from GB-20, down the neck to the shoulders	5 minutes
Ca-fa	Rub the cheeks until heat is felt	1-2 minutes

Daily Life Style Recommendation for Owner Follow-up:
- *Moo-fa* rubbing the lips, cheeks and around the ears and eyelids for 10 minutes twice daily until recovers function to improve *Qi*/Blood flow to the facial tissues
- If tear production is reduced, administer artificial tears every 4-6 hours (except during the night), to prevent corneal ulcers
- Feed a high quality diet to support *Zheng Qi*
- Keep in a low stress environment to support *Zheng Qi*

Comments:

Based on clinical studies in humans and anecdotal experiences in animals expect TCVM treatment to shorten the recovery time and improve recovery of facial function.

2. Wind-Cold invasion causing *Qi*/Blood Stagnation and local *Qi* Deficiency

Clinical Signs:
- Acute onset

- Inability to close the eyelids and /or move the nose and lips
- Tongue- purple or pale, moist
- Pulses- Superficial, slow or wiry

TCVM Diagnosis:

The diagnosis of Wind-Cold invasion causing *Qi*/Blood Stagnation and local *Qi*/Blood Deficiency is based on the clinical signs. The tongue color will vary with the stage of the process. Acutely the tongue is purple from the Wind-Cold and *Qi*/Blood Stagnation and then pale if *Qi*/Blood Deficiency is most prominent. The pulses may be slow from the Cold or wiry from the Stagnation.

Treatment Principles:
- Clear Wind-Cold
- Resolve *Qi*/Blood Stagnation
- Promote local *Qi*/Blood flow and restore facial nerve function

Acupuncture treatment:

For EA use 80-120 Hz alternating frequencies for 15-30 minutes, as EA is more effective to resolve Stagnation than DN alone. Treat both the normal and abnormal sides. Repeat acupuncture weekly every 1-2 weeks for 6-8 treatments. For Aqua-AP inject 0.25-0.5 ml vitamin B12 into the acupoint.

Acupoints recommended
- EA: GB-20/GB-14, ST-6/ST-2, TH-17/TH-23
- DN: BL-10, *An-shen, Bi-tong,* CV-24, *Tai-yang*, LI-10, ST-36, LI-4, SI-19, GV-26, LU-7, LI-20, ST-44, GB-14, GB-34
- Aqua-AP: GB-20

Pertinent acupoint actions
- GB-20 is useful to dispel Wind
- BL-10 is useful to dispel Wind-Cold
- GB-14, TH-23 and *Tai-yang* (one *cun* lateral to the lateral canthus above the zygomatic arch) are local acupoints for eyelid paralysis
- *An-shen*, SI-19 and TH-17 are local acupoints for ear paralysis
- ST-2, ST-6, *Bi-tong* (halfway between BL-1 and LI-20), LI-20, GV-26 and CV-24 are local acupoints for paralysis of the lips and nose
- LI-4 is a Master point for the face
- LI-10 and ST-36 tonify *Qi* to encourage *Qi* flow in the Channels

Herbal Medicine:
- Facial P Formula (JT)[a] 0.5gm/10# twice daily orally to clear Wind, invigorate *Qi*/Blood and relieve Stagnation
- Administer herbal formula up to 3 months
- A description of all the ingredients of the Chinese herbal medicine listed is beyond the scope of this text, but can be found elsewhere.[8,9]

Food Therapy:

The purpose of the Food therapy is to clear Cold and promote *Qi*/Blood circulation so warming foods are prescribed and cooling foods are avoided.[11]

- Foods to supplement to clear Cold: Lamb, shrimp, corn-fed beef, chicken, trout, squash, turnips, sweet rice, basal, caraway, cherries, chilies, cinnamon, ginger, rosemary, sage
- Foods to supplement to promote *Qi*/Blood circulation: Chicken egg, crab, sweet rice, peaches, carrots, coriander, squash, turnips
- Foods to avoid: Turkey, duck, clams, white fish, mussels, yogurt, millet, barley, spinach, broccoli, celery, cucumber

Tui-na Procedures:

The purpose of the *Tui-na* is to stimulate *Qi* and Blood flow and promote nerve regeneration in the affected region. The descriptions and indications of each technique are outlined in more detail in Chapter 1 Table 8.[10]

- A 25-30 minute *Tui-na* treatment for facial paralysis is outlined in Table 4

Daily Life Style Recommendation for Owner Follow-up:

- *Moo-fa* rubbing the lips, cheeks and around the ears and eyelids for 10 minutes twice daily until recovers function to improve *Qi*/Blood flow to the facial tissues
- If tear production is reduced, administer artificial tears every 4-6 hours (except during the night), to prevent corneal ulcers
- Feed a high quality diet to support *Zheng Qi*
- Keep in a low stress environment to support *Zheng Qi*

Comments:

Based on clinical studies in humans and anecdotal experiences in animals expect TCVM treatment to shorten the recovery time and improve the recovery of facial function.

3. Local *Qi*/Blood Stagnation and *Qi* Deficiency

Clinical Signs:

- History or evidence of trauma
- Acute onset
- Inability to close the eyelids and /or move the nose and lips
- Tongue- purple
- Pulses- wiry

TCVM Diagnosis:

The diagnosis of *Qi*/Blood Stagnation and local *Qi*/Blood Deficiency is based on a history or physical evidence of trauma. The tongue color is often purple from the *Qi*/Blood Stagnation and the pulses wiry from the Stagnation.

Treatment Principles:

- Resolve *Qi*/Blood Stagnation

- Promote local *Qi*/Blood flow and restore facial nerve function

Acupuncture treatment:

For EA use 80-120 Hz alternating frequencies for 15-30 minutes, as EA is more effective to resolve Stagnation than DN alone. Treat both the normal and abnormal sides. Acutely, perform AP treatments every 3-5 days for 3 times, then weekly for 3 times.

Acupoints recommended
- EA: GB-20/GB-14, ST-6/ST-2, TH-17/TH-23
- DN: *Tai-yang*, *An-shen*, SI-19, *Bi-tong*, LI-20, GV-26, CV-24, LI-4, LI-10, ST-36
- Aqua-AP:

Pertinent acupoint actions
- GB-20 is an acupoint that can be connected to GB-14 during EA to promote *Qi* flow in the Gallbladder Channel
- GB-14, TH-23 and *Tai-yang* (one *cun* lateral to the lateral canthus above the zygomatic arch) are local acupoints for eyelid paralysis
- *An-shen*, SI-19 and TH-17 are local acupoints for ear paralysis
- ST-2, ST-6, *Bi-tong* (halfway between BL-1 and LI-20), LI-20, GV-26 and CV-24 are local acupoints for paralysis of the lips and nose
- LI-4 is a Master point for the face
- LI-10 and ST-36 tonify *Qi* to encourage *Qi* flow in the Channels

Herbal Medicine:
- Facial P Formula (JT)[a] 0.5gm/10# twice daily orally to clear Wind, invigorate *Qi*/Blood and relieve Stagnation
- Administer herbal formula up to 3 months
- A description of all the ingredients of the Chinese herbal medicine listed is beyond the scope of this text, but can be found elsewhere.[8,9]

Food Therapy:

The purpose of the Food therapy is to further promote *Qi*/Blood circulation and tonify *Qi* to support nerve regeneration in the affected region. Foods that are Cold or Hot are avoided.[11]

- Foods to supplement to promote *Qi* and Blood circulation include: chicken egg, crab, sweet rice, peaches, carrots, coriander, squash, turnips
- Foods to tonify *Qi*: Beef, chicken, sardines, egg, potato, yam, sweet potato, rice, oats, millet, lentils, carrots, squash, microalgae, dates, figs, molasses, royal jelly
- Cold foods to avoid: Turkey, duck, duck eggs, conch, clams, mussels, yogurt, millet, barley, spinach, broccoli, celery, egg plant, kelp, alfalfa, cucumbers, pears, bananas, white radishes, watermelon
- Hot foods to avoid: Lamb, shrimp, corn-fed beef, chicken, trout, squash, turnips, sweet rice, basal, caraway, cherries, chilies, cinnamon, ginger, rosemary, sage

Tui-na Procedures:

The purpose of the *Tui-na* is to stimulate *Qi* and Blood flow and promote nerve regeneration in the affected region. The descriptions and indications of each technique are outlined in more detail in Chapter 1 Table 8.[10]
- A 25-30 minute *Tui-na* treatment for facial paralysis is outlined in Table 4

Daily Life Style Recommendation for Owner Follow-up:
- *Moo-fa* rubbing the lips, cheeks and around the ears and eyelids for 10 minutes twice daily until recovers function to improve *Qi*/Blood flow to the facial tissues
- If tear production is reduced, administer artificial tears every 4-6 hours (except during the night), to prevent corneal ulcers
- Feed a high quality diet to support *Zheng Qi*
- Keep in a low stress environment to support *Zheng Qi*

Comments:

Based on clinical studies in humans and anecdotal experiences in animals expect TCVM treatment to shorten the recovery time and improve the recovery of facial function.

4. Gallbladder Damp Heat with local *Qi* Deficiency (Middle Ear)

Clinical Signs:
- Inability to close the eyelids and /or move the nose and lips
- May have otitis externa
- May have Horner's syndrome
- May have a head tilt if inner ear is affected (See Vestibular disorders below)
- Tongue- red, greasy tongue coating
- Pulses- Superficial, forceful, rapid, slippery

TCVM Diagnosis:

The diagnosis of Gallbladder Damp Heat (Middle ear) is based on the history, clinical signs and TCVM examination findings, including tongue and pulse characteristics. The red tongue and superficial, forceful pulses reflect Heat and the greasy tongue coating and slippery pulses reflect the Damp.

Treatment Principles:
- Clear Damp Heat
- Resolve *Qi*/Blood Stagnation to promote local *Qi*/Blood flow and restore facial nerve function

Acupuncture treatment:

For EA use 20 Hz for 10-15 minutes then 80-120 Hz alternating frequencies for 10-15 minutes, to control ear pain and resolve *Qi*/Blood Stagnation. EA is more effective than DN alone to relieve Stagnation. Treat both the normal and abnormal sides. Acutely, perform AP treatments every 3-5 days for 3 times, then weekly for 3 times. For Aqua-AP inject 0.25-0.5 ml vitamin B12 into the acupoint.

Acupoints recommended
- EA: GB-20/GB-14, ST-6/ST-2, TH-17/TH-23
- DN: *Er-jian*, GV-14, *Tai-yang*, *An-shen*, SI-19, *Bi-tong,* LI-20, GV-26, CV-24, LI-4, LI-10, ST-36
- Aqua-AP: BL-10, BL-18

Pertinent acupoint actions
- *Er-jian* (ear tip) is useful to clear Heat
- GV-14 is useful to clear Heat and balance the immune system
- GB-20 is an acupoint that can be connected to GB-14 during EA to promote *Qi* flow in the Gallbladder Channel
- GB-14, TH-23 and *Tai-yang* (one *cun* lateral to the lateral canthus above the zygomatic arch) are local acupoints for eyelid paralysis
- *An-shen*, SI-19 and TH-17 are local acupoints for ear paralysis
- ST-2, ST-6, *Bi-tong* (halfway between BL-1 and LI-20), LI-20, GV-26 and CV-24 are local acupoints for paralysis of the lips and nose
- LI-4 is a Master point for the face and is useful to balance the immune system
- LI-10 and ST-36 tonify *Qi* to encourage *Qi* flow in the Channels

Herbal Medicine:
- Ear Damp Heat (JT)[a] 0.5gm/10# twice daily orally to clear Heat and Damp
- Alternative: *Long Dan Xie Gan* (JT)[a] 0.5gm/10# twice daily orally to clear Heat and Damp
- Administer herbal formulas up to 4 months
- If otitis externa present: also administer *Di Er You* (JT)[a] (Ear drops), 2-7 drops, 5-8 times daily for one month to clear Heat, dry Damp, relieve pruritus and reduce swelling
- A description of all the ingredients of the Chinese herbal medicine listed is beyond the scope of this text, but can be found elsewhere.[8,9]

Food Therapy:
The purpose of the Food therapy is to clear Heat and Damp and promote *Qi*/Blood circulation and nerve regeneration. Cooling foods are prescribed and Damp producing and Hot foods are avoided.[11]
- Foods to supplement to clear Heat: Turkey, duck, duck eggs, conch, clams, mussels, yogurt, millet, barley, spinach, broccoli, celery, egg plant, kelp, alfalfa, cucumbers, pears, bananas, white radishes, watermelon
- Foods to supplement to Drain Damp: Eel, mackerel, quail, corn, barley, rye, blueberries, celery, mushrooms
- Foods to promote *Qi*/Blood circulation: Crab, sweet rice, peaches, carrots, coriander, turnips
- Damp producing foods to avoid: Eggs, milk, cheese, yoghurt, ghee, bananas, sugar

- Hot foods to avoid: Lamb, shrimp, corn-fed beef, chicken, trout, squash, turnips, sweet rice, basal, caraway, cherries, chilies, cinnamon, ginger, rosemary, sage

Tui-na Procedures:

The purpose of the *Tui-na* is to stimulate *Qi* and Blood flow and promote nerve regeneration in the affected region. The descriptions and indications of each technique are outlined in more detail in Chapter 1 Table 8.[10]

- A 25-30 minute *Tui-na* treatment for facial paralysis is outlined in Table 4

Daily Life Style Recommendation for Owner Follow-up:

- *Moo-fa* rubbing the lips, cheeks and around the ears and eyelids for 10 minutes twice daily until recovers function to improve *Qi*/Blood flow to the facial tissues
- If tear production is reduced, administer artificial tears every 4-6 hours (except during the night), to prevent corneal ulcers
- Feed a high quality diet to support *Zheng Qi*
- Keep in a low stress environment to support *Zheng Qi*

Comments:

Based on anecdotal experiences in animals expect TCVM treatment to shorten the recovery time and improve the recovery of facial function.

VESTIBULAR DISORDERS

Acute onset of a head tilt, nystagmus, circling and/or rolling is associated with vestibular disease and is often peripheral (versus brainstem or cerebellar) and idiopathic especially in geriatric dogs and young cats.[1-3] Other causes of acute peripheral vestibular disease are inner ear infection, trauma, hypothyroidism and neoplasia (rare).[1-3] With idiopathic vestibular syndrome, there is no history or physical evidence of ear infection or trauma. On neurological examination, there is always a head tilt (one ear closer to the ground) in unilateral vestibular disease. Acutely there may be horizontal or rotary nystagmus and circling, falling from loss of balance or rolling toward the side of the lesion. The nystagmus and rolling usually last for 1-3 days after the onset of signs, but may have subsided by the time the animal is referred to a TCVM veterinarian for evaluation and treatment. The head tilt, circling and falling may be the only remaining signs and lack of other signs may represent compensation and not true improvement of the underlying problem.[2]

Although idiopathic vestibular syndrome is usually unilateral, in some instances both nerves become affected and the signs are bilateral. If both sides are equally affected there is no head tilt and the animal walks with a drunken, staggering gait, falling to either side due to the generalized disequilibrium. Most bilaterally affected animals are also deaf. There is no hypermetria, so these patients should not be confused with those that have cerebellar disease. With bilateral vestibular disease, the head also has a characteristic side-to-side swinging motion in a horizontal figure eight shape. In cerebellar disease, the head bobs up and down in a "pecking" motion and has intention tremors. Although the balance is affected in animals with peripheral vestibular disease, the limbs are strong, even though animals may lean or crouch to try to keep their balance. Conscious proprioception is always normal in peripheral vestibular nerve disease and is an important test to perform to ensure the lesion is not in the medulla oblongata.

Besides the signs of vestibular dysfunction, the rest of the physical and neurological examinations are normal in idiopathic vestibular syndrome. With middle/inner ear infections, trauma or tumors the facial nerve may also be affected. The sympathetic innervation to the eye in the middle ear can also be affected and a Horner's syndrome (ptosis, miosis and enophthalmos) may be present. If an animal has vestibular signs along with facial nerve paralysis and/or Horner's syndrome, then the diagnosis is not idiopathic vestibular syndrome.

Serum thyroxin (T4) and thyroid stimulating hormone (TSH) tests should always be evaluated on every case of acute vestibular disease since hypothyroidism can cause a focal neuropathy. Vestibular nerve sheath tumors (e.g. vestibular schwannoma or acoustic neuromas) are rare in dogs compared to humans.[2] Neoplasms may also compress the vestibular nerve in the bony labyrinth. There is a gradual and progressive onset of head tilt and usually only a mild loss of balance by the time of presentation. Skull radiographs or CT can show bone tumors, but MRI is necessary to see the details of soft tissue tumors.

There is no conventional treatment for traumatic and idiopathic vestibular syndrome and some animals may appear to effectively recover from the loss of balance, while others retain a head tilt. Some of the clinical improvement is compensation and adaption to the dysfunctional equilibrium, based on normal gravity. If affected animals are placed in water, like a swimming pool or lake, where gravity is changed, they will again lose their equilibrium and begin rolling and drown.[2] Animals, with past vestibular problems, should always be evaluated in the water and if they appear to have dysfunction, they should be protected from contact with any body of water.

Although animals with acute vestibular disease have been treated with acupuncture and Chinese herbal medicines, no case reports or controlled clinical trials in animals have been published.[5-9] Human case reports and controlled clinical trials report successful treatment of acute idiopathic vestibular syndrome (Ménière's disease) with acupuncture.[22] After a recent systematic review of human clinical controlled trials evaluating acupuncture for Ménière's disease, it was concluded that acupuncture was beneficial, but further human clinical studies were needed to clarify questions around the appropriate frequency and number of acupuncture treatments required.[22] Based on the success reported in humans and anecdotally for animals, controlled clinical trials in animals with vestibular dysfunction are warranted.

The TCVM examination findings for the different TCVM patterns associated with acute peripheral vestibular syndromes are listed in Table 2. Recommended acupoints, acupuncture techniques and Chinese herbal medicine for TCVM patterns causing acute vestibular syndromes are listed in Table 3.[5-9] Even though Wind is an important initiating External Pathogen in idiopathic vestibular syndrome, EA of some acupoints is still recommended to treat the *Qi*/Blood Stagnation, after the acute nystagmus phase has passed, as seizures are unlikely with focal vestibular disease. Like the acute loss of function of other cranial nerves, the combination of EA, DN and Aqua-AP techniques is recommended to ensure optimum recovery of equilibrium. As with other cranial neuropathies, the TCVM practitioner may administer *Tui-na* treatments, after the EA and DN session and before the Aqua-AP and Food therapy may be useful to treat the TCVM pattern.[10,11] Simple *Tui-na* techniques may also be taught to the caretaker, for in-home daily treatments in between TCVM appointments. Controlled clinical studies are needed to ensure the TCVM treatments are enhancing the recovery of equilibrium, because recovery from traumatic and idiopathic vestibular syndromes occurs to some degree without treatment.[1-3] Because of the positive experiences of practitioners, TCVM treatment of patients with traumatic and idiopathic vestibular syndrome is encouraged to give the dog every possible chance for full recovery of equilibrium.[5-9] Otitis interna or inner ear Damp-Heat is usually a bacterial or mycotic infection and is treated with the appropriate conventional medications, but the integration of TCVM treatments may result in faster recovery and less residual damage and prevent recurrences.[19,20] In animals with vestibular disease from hypothyroidism, TCVM treatments may be integrated with thyroid replacement therapy to increase the recovery rate and degree of recovery.

Etiology and Pathology

From a TCVM perspective idiopathic vestibular syndrome is mainly due to *Zheng Qi* Deficiency allowing External Wind-Cold invasion in the Triple Heater, Small Intestine and Gallbladder Channels of the region of the inner ear. The result is local *Qi*/Blood Stagnation, loss of *Qi*/Blood flow and *Qi*/Blood Deficiency to the region of the vestibular nerve and the acute loss of equilibrium. In animals under 1 year of age the underlying cause of *Zheng Qi* Deficiency is Kidney *Jing* Deficiency. In adult and geriatric animals the underlying cause of *Zheng Qi* Deficiency is often Spleen *Qi* deficiency which results in the local accumulation of Damp and ultimately Phlegm in the region.[4,7] It is interesting to note that from a conventional perspective, adult onset idiopathic vestibular syndrome in humans is associated with increased fluid within the semicircular canals of the inner ear, which alters the fluid flow and the response of the vestibular sensory receptors in the fluid.

Vestibular nerve dysfunction from trauma and fracture of the petrous temporal bone is less common in dogs, compared to horses that may rear up and strike their poll on the top of a trailer or stall ceiling. As in other cases of peripheral nerve trauma, vestibular nerve trauma results in local *Qi*/Blood Stagnation, reduction of *Qi*/Blood flow and *Qi*/Blood Deficiency to the region of the affected Channels. Like facial paresis, involvement of the vestibular nerve can be due to an inner ear infection. *Zheng Qi* Deficiency allows Damp-Heat invasion of the Gallbladder Channel causing local *Qi*/Blood Stagnation, reduction of *Qi*/Blood flow and local *Qi*/Blood Deficiency affecting the vestibular nerve. Neoplastic involvement of the vestibular nerve may be associated with substantial Phlegm (nerve sheath tumors and other non-blood related tumors) or Blood Stagnation (lymphoma and other blood-related tumors) (See section on **BRAIN TUMORS** above). Applying the basic TCVM theories of *Yin/Yang*, Eight Principles, Five Treasures, Five Elements and *Zang Fu* physiology and pathology to make a TCVM diagnosis, there are four basic patterns associated with vestibular nerve dysfunction, but with more experience other patterns may be identified in the future:

1. **Kidney *Jing* Deficiency with Wind-Cold invasion causing local *Qi*/Blood Stagnation and *Qi* Deficiency**
   An underlying Kidney *Jing* Deficiency results in *Zheng Qi* Deficiency that allows Wind-Cold to enter the Channels around the inner ear and cause *Qi*/Blood Stagnation and local *Qi* Deficiency. The result is acute vestibular dysfunction in a young dog or cat under 1 year of age.

2. **Wind-Cold invasion causing Damp and Phlegm and local *Qi*/Blood Stagnation and *Qi* Deficiency with Spleen *Qi* Deficiency**
   Spleen *Qi* Deficiency makes the animal generally susceptible to the accumulation of Damp and formation of Phlegm. When *Wei-Qi* is also Deficient, Wind-Cold-Damp enters the Channels around the inner ear and causes *Qi*/Blood Stagnation and resulting local *Qi*

Deficiency. Damp and Phlegm also accumulate in the inner ear region, resulting in acute onset of vestibular dysfunction.

3. **Local *Qi*/Blood Stagnation with *Qi* Deficiency**
Trauma induces *Qi*/Blood Stagnation, reduction of *Qi*/Blood flow and *Qi* Deficiency at the site of injury, affecting local tissues including nerves. The result is the acute onset of vestibular signs.

4. **Gallbladder Damp Heat with local *Qi* Deficiency (Inner ear)**
When *Wei-Qi* is Deficient, Damp-Heat enters the Gallbladder Channel and causes local swelling, *Qi*/Blood Stagnation and local *Qi* Deficiency in the inner ear resulting in vestibular signs. The Damp-Heat may extend inward from otitis media and otitis interna.

Pattern Differentiation and Treatment

1. Kidney *Jing* Deficiency with Wind-Cold invasion causing local *Qi*/Blood Stagnation and *Qi* Deficiency

Clinical Signs:
- Young dogs and cats under 1 year of age
- Acute onset
- Head tilt
- Nystagmus
- Loss of equilibrium
- Rolling, circling, falling to one side
- Tongue- pale
- Pulses- wiry acutely, then weak

TCVM Diagnosis:
The diagnosis of an underlying Kidney *Jing* Deficiency is based on acute disequilibrium in a young animal with no history of trauma or infection. The pale tongue is associated with the Kidney *Jing* Deficiency. Wiry pulses reflect the invasion of Wind during the acute phase. Later the pulses may be weak reflecting the Kidney *Jing* Deficiency.

Treatment Principles:
- Tonify Kidney *Jing*
- Clear Wind-Cold
- Promote local *Qi* flow to restore vestibular nerve function

Acupuncture treatment:
Avoid EA for the first 72 hours after the onset of the signs because of the strong Wind component and use only DN in all the recommended acupoints. Treat both the normal and abnormal sides. Once the acute phase has passed, use EA at 80-120 Hz alternating frequencies for 15-20 minutes to stimulate nerve function, as EA is more effective to resolve Stagnation than DN

alone. Discontinue if EA causes nystagmus to return. Repeat acupuncture every 3-5 days for 3 times, then weekly for 3 times; For Aqua-AP inject 0.25-0.5 ml vitamin B12 into the acupoint.

Acupoints recommended
- DN acutely then EA later: PC-6/PC-6, GB-20/GB-2 bilaterally
- DN: PC-6, GB-20, BL-10, *Da-feng-men,* TH-5, GB-34, LU-7, LI-10, ST-36, SI-19, TH-17, GB-2, TH-21, BL-23, KID-3, BL-20
- Aqua-AP: BL-10, BL-23

Pertinent acupoint actions
- PC-6 is useful to treat vertigo and nausea, signs of vestibular dysfunction
- GB-20 is useful to dispel Wind
- BL-10 is useful to dispel Wind-Cold
- *Da-feng-men* (on the midline at the level of the cranial edge of the ear base) is useful to dispel Wind
- TH-5 is useful to strengthen *Zheng Qi*
- GB-34 is useful to break-up Stagnation and is a distant point on the Gallbladder Channel that course around the ear
- LU-7 is the Master point of the head
- LI-10 and ST-36 are useful to tonify *Qi*
- SI-19, TH-17, GB-2 and TH-21 are local acupoints around the ear
- BL-23 is the Back *Shu* Association point for Kidney to tonify Kidney *Jing*
- KID-3 is the *Yuan* Source point for Kidney to support Kidney *Jing*
- BL-20 is the Back *Shu* Association point for Spleen useful to fortify post natal *Jing* to support Kidney *Jing*

Herbal Medicine:
- Stasis in Mansion of Mind (JT)[a] 0.5gm/10# twice daily orally to move Blood and eliminate Blood Stasis
- Epimedium Formula (JT)[a] 0.5gm/10# twice daily orally to tonify Kidney *Jing*
- Administer herbal formula up to 4 months
- A description of all the ingredients of the Chinese herbal medicine listed is beyond the scope of this text, but can be found elsewhere.[8,9]

Food Therapy:
The purpose of the Food therapy is to clear Cold and promote *Qi*/Blood circulation so warming foods are prescribed and Cold foods are avoided.[11]
- Foods to supplement to clear Cold: Lamb, shrimp, corn-fed beef, chicken, trout, squash, turnips, sweet rice, basal, caraway, cherries, chilies, cinnamon, ginger, rosemary, sage
- Foods to supplement to promote *Qi*/Blood circulation: Chicken egg, crab, sweet rice, peaches, carrots, coriander, squash, turnips
- Cold foods to avoid: Turkey, duck, duck eggs, conch, clams, mussels, yogurt, millet, barley, spinach, broccoli, celery, egg plant, kelp, alfalfa, cucumbers, pears, bananas, white radishes, watermelon

Tui-na Procedures:

The purpose of the *Tui-na* is to stimulate *Qi* and Blood flow and promote nerve regeneration in the affected region. The descriptions and indications of each technique are outlined in more detail in Chapter 1 Table 8.[10]

- *An-fa* pressing and *Ca-fa* rubbing with the finger at TH-21, SI-19, GB-2, TH-17, *An-shen* for 2-3 minutes at each site on each ear to invigorate *Qi* Flow
- *Ba-shen-fa* stretching of the ears forward and backward to stimulate *Qi* flow; repeat 12 times on each ear

Daily Life Style Recommendation for Owner Follow-up:

- *Moo-fa* massaging round the ear bases and behind the ears for 5-10 minutes twice daily
- Ensure excellent nutrition to strengthen *Zheng Qi* and Spleen *Qi*, fortify post natal *Jing* to spare Kidney *Jing*
- Keep in a protected environment to prevent falls down stairs, drowning in swimming pools or ponds or attacks by other animals.

Comments:

Based on anecdotal experiences, expect TCVM treatment to shorten the recovery time and improve the degree of vestibular function recovery.

2. Wind-Cold invasion causing Damp and Phlegm, *Qi*/Blood Stagnation and local *Qi* Deficiency with Spleen *Qi* Deficiency

Clinical Signs:

- Acute onset
- Head tilt
- Nystagmus
- Loss of equilibrium
- Rolling, circling, falling to one side
- Tongue- pale, wet
- Pulses- wiry, slippery, weak on right side

TCVM Diagnosis:

The diagnosis of Wind-Cold invasion causing Damp and Phlegm, *Qi*/Blood Stagnation and local *Qi* Deficiency with Spleen *Qi* Deficiency is based on the history, clinical signs and TCVM examination findings, including tongue and pulse characteristics. The acute onset is typical of an Excess pattern. The pale wet tongue and weak pulses, worse on right however reflect the underlying Spleen *Qi* Deficiency. The slippery pulses reflect the Damp and Phlegm. During the acute nystagmus phase the pulses may be wiry reflecting the Wind.

Treatment Principles:

- Clear Wind-Cold
- Expel Damp
- Expel Phlegm

- Tonify Spleen *Qi*

Acupuncture treatment:

Avoid EA for the first 72 hours after the onset of the signs because of the strong Wind component and use only DN in all the recommended acupoints. Treat both the normal and abnormal sides. Once the acute phase has passed, use EA at 80-120 Hz alternating frequencies for 15-20 minutes to stimulate nerve function, as EA is more effective to resolve Stagnation than DN alone. Discontinue if EA causes nystagmus to return. Repeat acupuncture every 3-5 days for 3 times, then weekly for 3 times; For Aqua-AP inject 0.25-0.5 ml vitamin B12 into the acupoint.

Acupoints recommended
- DN acutely then EA later: PC-6/PC-6, GB-20/GB-2
- DN: PC-6, GB-20, BL-10, *Da-feng-men,* TH-5, GB-34, ST-40, LU-9, LI-10, SI-19, TH-17, GB-2, TH-21, SP-6, SP-9, ST-40
- Aqua-AP: GB-20, *Da-feng-men*

Pertinent acupoint actions
- PC-6 is useful to treat vertigo and nausea, signs of vestibular dysfunction
- GB-20 is useful to dispel Wind
- BL-10 is useful to dispel Wind-Cold
- *Da-feng-men* (on the midline at the level of the cranial edge of the ear base) is useful to dispel Wind
- TH-5 is useful to strengthen *Zheng Qi*
- GB-34 is useful to break-up Stagnation and is a distant point on the Gallbladder Channel that course around the ear
- LU-7 is the Master point of the head
- LI-10 and ST-36 are useful to tonify *Qi*
- SI-19, TH-17, GB-2 and TH-21 are local acupoints around the ear
- SP-6 and SP-9 are useful to dispel Damp
- ST-40 is the Influential point for Phlegm to dispel Phlegm

Herbal Medicine:
- Stasis in Mansion of Mind (JT)[a] 0.5gm/10# twice daily orally to move Blood and eliminate Blood Stasis
- *Si Jun Zi* (JT)[a] 0.5gm/10# twice daily orally to tonify *Qi* and strengthen the Spleen
- Administer herbal formulas up to 4 months
- A description of all the ingredients of the Chinese herbal medicines listed is beyond the scope of this text, but can be found elsewhere.[8,9]

Food Therapy:

The purpose of the Food therapy is to clear Cold, promote *Qi*/Blood circulation, strengthen Spleen *Qi* and drain Damp so warming and *Qi* tonifying foods are prescribed and Cold and Damp producing foods and foods are avoided.[11]
- Foods to supplement to clear Cold: Lamb, shrimp, corn-fed beef, chicken, trout, squash, turnips, sweet rice, basal, caraway, cherries, chilies, cinnamon, ginger, rosemary, sage

- Foods to supplement to promote *Qi*/Blood circulation: Chicken egg, crab, sweet rice, peaches, carrots, coriander, squash, turnips
- Foods to tonify *Qi*: Beef, chicken, sardines, egg, potato, yam, sweet potato, rice, oats, millet, lentils, carrots, squash, microalgae, dates, figs, molasses, royal jelly
- Foods to drain Damp: Eel, mackerel, quail, corn, barley, rye, blueberries, celery, mushrooms
- Cold foods to avoid: Turkey, duck, clams, white fish, mussels, yogurt, millet, barley, spinach, broccoli, celery, cucumber
- Damp producing foods to avoid: Pork, eggs, milk, cheese, yoghurt, ghee, bananas, sugar

Tui-na Procedures:

The purpose of the *Tui-na* is to stimulate *Qi* and Blood flow and promote nerve regeneration in the affected region. The descriptions and indications of each technique are outlined in more detail in Chapter 1 Table 8.[10]

- *An-fa* pressing and *Ca-fa* rubbing with the finger at TH-21, SI-19, GB-2, TH-17, *An-shen* for 2-3 minutes at each site on each ear to invigorate *Qi* Flow
- *Ba-shen-fa* stretching of the ears forward and backward to stimulate *Qi* flow; repeat 12 times on each ear

Daily Life Style Recommendation for Owner Follow-up:

- *Moo-fa* massaging round the ear bases and behind the ears for 5-10 minutes twice daily
- Ensure excellent nutrition to strengthen *Zheng Qi* and Spleen *Qi*
- Keep in a protected environment to prevent falls down stairs, drowning in swimming pools or ponds or attacks by other animals.

Comments:

Based on clinical studies in humans and anecdotal experiences in animals expect TCVM treatment to shorten the recovery time and enhance the recovery of vestibular function.

3. *Qi*/Blood Stagnation with local *Qi* Deficiency

Clinical Signs:

- Acute onset
- Head tilt
- Nystagmus
- Loss of equilibrium
- Rolling, circling, falling to one side
- Tongue- purple
- Pulses- wiry

TCVM Diagnosis:

The diagnosis of *Qi*/Blood Stagnation and local *Qi* Deficiency is based on a history or physical evidence of trauma. The tongue color is purple and pulse wiry from the *Qi*/Blood Stagnation.

Treatment Principles:
- Resolve *Qi*/Blood Stagnation
- Tonify local *Qi* and restore vestibular nerve function

Acupuncture treatment:
Avoid EA for the first 72 hours after the onset of the signs because of the strong Wind component and use only DN in all the recommended acupoints. Treat both the normal and abnormal sides. Once the acute phase has passed use EA at 80-120 Hz alternating frequencies for 15-20 minutes to stimulate nerve function, as EA is more effective to resolve Stagnation than DN alone. Repeat acupuncture every 3-5 days for 3 times, then weekly for 3 times; For Aqua-AP inject 0.25-0.5 ml vitamin B12 into the acupoint.

Acupoints recommended
- DN acutely then EA later: PC-6/PC-6, TH-17/TH-17
- DN: PC-6, GB-20, *Da-feng-men,* GB-34, LU-9, LI-10, ST-36, SI-19, TH-17, GB-2, TH-21
- Aqua-AP: GB-20, *Da-feng-men*

Pertinent acupoint actions
- PC-6 is useful to treat vertigo and nausea, signs of vestibular dysfunction
- GB-20 is useful to dispel Wind
- *Da-feng-men* (on the midline at the level of the cranial edge of the ear base) is useful to dispel Wind
- GB-34 is useful to break-up Stagnation and is a distant point on the Gallbladder Channel that course around the ear
- LU-7 is the Master point of the head
- LI-10 and ST-36 are useful to tonify *Qi*
- SI-19, TH-17, GB-2, TH-21 are local acupoints around the ear

Herbal Medicine:
- Stasis in Mansion of Mind (JT)[a] 0.5gm/10# twice daily orally to move Blood and eliminate Blood Stasis
- Administer herbal formula up to 4 months
- A description of all the ingredients of the Chinese herbal medicine listed is beyond the scope of this text, but can be found elsewhere.[8,9]

Food Therapy:
The purpose of the Food therapy is to further promote *Qi*/Blood circulation and tonify *Qi* to support nerve regeneration in the affected region. Foods that are Cold or Hot are avoided.[11]
- Foods to supplement to promote *Qi* and Blood circulation include: chicken egg, crab, sweet rice, peaches, carrots, coriander, squash, turnips
- Foods to tonify *Qi*: Beef, chicken, sardines, egg, potato, yam, sweet potato, rice, oats, millet, lentils, carrots, squash, microalgae, dates, figs, molasses, royal jelly

- Cold foods to avoid: Turkey, duck, duck eggs, conch, clams, mussels, yogurt, millet, barley, spinach, broccoli, celery, egg plant, kelp, alfalfa, cucumbers, pears, bananas, white radishes, watermelon
- Hot foods to avoid: Lamb, shrimp, corn-fed beef, chicken, trout, squash, turnips, sweet rice, basal, caraway, cherries, chilies, cinnamon, ginger, rosemary, sage

Tui-na Procedures:

The purpose of the *Tui-na* is to stimulate *Qi* and Blood flow and promote nerve regeneration in the affected region. The descriptions and indications of each technique are outlined in more detail in Chapter 1 Table 8.[10]

- *An-fa* pressing and *Ca-fa* rubbing with the finger at TH-21, SI-19, GB-2, TH-17, *An-shen* for 2-3 minutes at each site on each ear to invigorate *Qi* Flow
- *Ba-shen-fa* stretching of the ears forward and backward to stimulate *Qi* flow; repeat 12 times on each ear

Daily Life Style Recommendation for Owner Follow-up:

- *Moo-fa* massaging round the ear bases and behind the ears for 5-10 minutes twice daily
- Keep in a protected environment to prevent falls down stairs, drowning in swimming pools or ponds or attacks by other animals.

Comments:

Based on clinical studies in humans and anecdotal experiences in animals expect TCVM treatment to shorten the recovery time and improve the degree of vestibular function recovery.

4. Gallbladder Damp Heat with local *Qi* Deficiency (inner ear)

Clinical Signs:

- Acute onset
- Head tilt
- Nystagmus
- Loss of equilibrium
- Rolling, circling, falling to one side
- May have otitis externa and media
- May have Horner's syndrome (otitis media)
- May have facial paralysis (See FACIAL PARALYSIS above)
- Tongue- red, greasy
- Pulses- forceful, rapid, slippery, wiry

TCVM Diagnosis:

The diagnosis of Gallbladder Damp Heat (Inner ear) is based on the history otitis externa/media if present. The external ear may feel warm and appear red typical of Heat. The red, greasy tongue is typical of Damp-Heat. Forceful and rapid pulses are typical of Excess Heat and slippery pulses are associated with Damp. During the acute phase when nystagmus is present, the pulses may also be wiry.

Treatment Principles:
- Clear Damp Heat
- Resolve local *Qi*/Blood Stagnation and promote local *Qi* flow to restore vestibular nerve function

Acupuncture treatment:
Avoid EA for the first 72 hours after the onset of the signs because of the strong Wind component and use only DN in all the recommended acupoints. Treat both the normal and abnormal sides. For EA use 20 Hz for 10-15 minutes then 80-120 Hz alternating frequencies for 10-15 minutes, to control ear pain and resolve *Qi*/Blood Stagnation. EA is more effective to resolve Stagnation than DN alone. Acutely perform AP treatments every 3-5 days for 3 times, then weekly for 3 times. For Aqua-AP inject 0.25-0.5 ml vitamin B12 into the acupoint.

Acupoints recommended
- DN acutely then EA later: EA: PC-6/PC-6, TH-17/TH-17
- DN: PC-6, GB-20, *Da-feng-men,* GB-34, LU-9, LI-10, ST-36, SI-19, TH-17, GB-2, TH-21, SP-6, SP-9, GV-14, *Er-jian*
- Aqua-AP: GB-20, *Da-feng-men*

Pertinent acupoint actions
- PC-6 is useful to treat vertigo and nausea, signs of vestibular dysfunction
- GB-20 is useful to dispel Wind
- *Da-feng-men* (on the midline at the level of the cranial edge of the ear base) is useful to dispel Wind
- GB-34 is useful to break-up Stagnation and is a distant point on the Gallbladder Channel that course around the ear
- LU-7 is the Master point of the head
- LI-10 and ST-36 are useful to tonify *Qi*
- SI-19, TH-17, GB-2, TH-21 are local acupoints around the ear
- SP-6 and SP-9 are useful to drain Damp
- GV-14 and *Er-jian* (tip of ear) are useful to clear Heat

Herbal Medicine:
- Ear Damp Heat (JT)[a] 0.5gm/10# twice daily orally to drain Damp and clear Heat
- Alternative: *Long Dan Xie Gan* (JT)[a] 0.5gm/10# twice daily orally to drain Damp and clear Heat
- Combine with conventional antibiotic therapy
- Administer herbal formulas up to 4 months
- If otitis externa present: administer *Di Er You* (Ear drops) (JT)[a] 2-7 drops, 5-8 times daily for one month to clear Heat, dry Damp, relieve pruritus and reduce swelling
- A description of all the ingredients of the Chinese herbal medicines listed is beyond the scope of this text, but can be found elsewhere.[8,9]

Food Therapy:

The purpose of the Food therapy is to clear Heat and Damp and promote *Qi*/Blood circulation and nerve regeneration. Cooling foods are prescribed and Damp producing and Hot foods are avoided.[11]

- Foods to supplement to clear Heat: Turkey, duck, duck eggs, conch, clams, mussels, yogurt, millet, barley, spinach, broccoli, celery, egg plant, kelp, alfalfa, cucumbers, pears, bananas, white radishes, watermelon
- Foods to supplement to Drain Damp: Eel, mackerel, quail, corn, barley, rye, blueberries, celery, mushrooms
- Foods to promote *Qi*/Blood circulation: Crab, sweet rice, peaches, carrots, coriander, turnips
- Damp producing foods to avoid: Eggs, milk, cheese, yoghurt, ghee, bananas, sugar
- Hot foods to avoid: Lamb, shrimp, corn-fed beef, chicken, trout, squash, turnips, sweet rice, basal, caraway, cherries, chilies, cinnamon, ginger, rosemary, sage

Tui-na Procedures:

The purpose of the *Tui-na* therapy is to stimulate *Qi* and Blood flow to relieve pain and promote nerve regeneration in the affected region, but *Tui-na* may have to be delayed, until the acupuncture and Chinese herbal medicine control the pain. The techniques descriptions and indications are outlined in more detail in Chapter 1 Table 8.[10]

- *An-fa* pressing and *Ca-fa* rubbing with the finger at TH-21, SI-19, GB-2, TH-17, *An-shen* for 2-3 minutes at each site on each ear to invigorate *Qi* Flow
- *Ba-shen-fa* stretching of the ears forward and backward to stimulate *Qi* flow; repeat 12 times on each ear

Daily Life Style Recommendation for Owner Follow-up:

- *Moo-fa* massaging round the ear bases and behind the ears for 5-10 minutes twice daily
- Keep in a protected environment to prevent falls down stairs, drowning in swimming pools or ponds or attacks by other animals.

Comments:

Based on anecdotal experiences in animals expect TCVM treatment to shorten the recovery time and enhance the recovery of vestibular function.

DEAFNESS

Deafness may be present from birth especially in blue-eyed white cats and certain breeds of dogs (e.g. Dalmatians, Australian shepherds and many others). Brainstem auditory evoked response (BAER) tests may be performed on puppies and kitten at 6-8 weeks of age to detect unilateral and bilateral deafness. There is a genetic lack of development of the sensory receptors associated with the cochlear nerve.

Deafness may also be acquired due to a middle or inner ear infection, ototoxic antibiotics or degeneration associated with aging.[1-3] Deafness may be a feature of young and old animals with bilateral idiopathic vestibular syndrome (see **VESTIBULAR DISORDERS** above), Since unilateral deafness is rarely recognized, most animals have involvement of both cochlear nerves by the time they are presented to a veterinarian.

Previous treatment with ototoxic drugs should be ascertained and a careful examination of the ears performed to detect otitis externa/media in all dogs with acquired deafness.[1-3] Animals with geriatric cochlear receptor and nerve degeneration have chronic progressive loss of hearing with no recent history or physical evidence of an ear infection. The neurological examination is often normal except for the deafness. Deafness associated with debris in the middle ear, as with middle ear infections, is referred to as conduction deafness. Deafness from the lack of sensory receptor development or inflammation and degeneration of the cochlear nerves is referred to as nerve deafness. Electronic otoscopic examination and brain stem auditory response (BAER) tests and skull radiographs, CT or MRI may be needed to determine if conduction or nerve deafness is present.

Congenital deafness may not be responsive to TCVM, because of the anatomic lack of sensory receptors, but might be worth trying to treat the underlying *Jing* Deficiency for 1-2 months to see if there is any response, as there is no conventional treatment. Animals with acquired deafness have been treated with acupuncture and Chinese herbal medicine, but no case reports or clinical controlled trials are available.[5-9] As previous discussed with vestibular diseases, TCVM treatments may be integrated with antibiotic and other conventional treatments for inner ear infections.[19,20]

In a laboratory animal randomized controlled trial of acquired deafness from toxicity, the BAER and the morphology of the sensory endings improved faster and more completely in the group receiving EA.[23] Of sixty clinical reports (1994-2004), regarding the effectiveness of acupuncture for deafness in humans, 71.7% were descriptive studies and 28.3% were clinical trials.[24] Although improved hearing following acupuncture has been reported, after a review of all the studies, it was concluded that higher quality, larger controlled clinical trials were needed, before the efficacy of acupuncture for deafness could be confirmed. Since there are positive effects reported for humans and few other treatment options for dogs and cats with acquired deafness, further studies to explore the potential benefits of acupuncture and Chinese herbal medicine for deaf animals are warranted.

Clinical signs, recommended acupoints, acupuncture techniques and Chinese herbal medicine for deafness associated with the various TCVM patterns are listed in Tables 2 and 3.[6-9] Because of the cochlear nerve dysfunction, EA is recommended along with DN and Aqua-AP. Multiple weekly treatments may be needed before a response is seen. As with the other cranial neuropathies, the TCVM practitioner may administer *Tui-na* treatments, after the EA and DN session and before the Aqua-AP.[10] Simple *Tui-na* techniques may also be taught to the caretaker, for in-home daily treatments in between TCVM appointments. Food therapy may provide long-term support for Kidney *Jing* and *Qi*.[11] Although controlled clinical studies are needed to ensure the TCVM treatments are enhancing the recovery of hearing, TCVM treatment of patients with otitis interna/media and geriatric deafness is encouraged to provide the animal every possible chance for recovery of hearing.

Etiology and Pathology

From a TCVM perspective, congenital deafness is associated with Kidney *Jing* Deficiency and Deficiency of *Qi* flow in the cochlear endings, resulting in lack of development.[5] Idiopathic and geriatric deafness are associated with acquired Kidney *Qi* Deficiency.[4,6] Since the ears are associated with the Kidney, one of the manifestations of Kidney *Qi* Deficiency is local *Qi* Deficiency in the cochlear nerves, reduced nerve function and deafness. As previously discussed otitis media/interna is associated with Gallbladder Damp Heat and Damp Heat can invade the inner ear structures bilaterally and result in deafness.[5,7] Applying the basic TCVM theories of *Yin/Yang*, Eight Principles, Five Treasures, Five Elements and *Zang Fu* physiology and pathology to make a TCVM diagnosis, there are three basic patterns associated with cochlear nerve dysfunction, but with more experience other patterns may be identified in the future:

1. **Kidney *Jing* Deficiency**
   A genetic lack of development of the sensory nerve endings of the cochlear nerves causes deafness from birth associated with Kidney *Jing* Deficiency.

2. **Kidney *Qi* Deficiency**
   Aging, prolonged illness, chronic poor diet and a weak constitution result in reduction of Kidney *Jing* prematurely or as part of the aging process. Since Kidney *Jing* creates Kidney *Qi*, Kidney *Qi* becomes Deficient. Although Kidney *Qi* Deficiency can have many different clinical manifestations, since the ears are the orifices of the Kidney, auditory dysfunction can occur with Kidney *Qi* Deficiency causing local *Qi* Deficiency in the inner ears.

3. **Gallbladder Damp Heat and local *Qi* Deficiency (bilateral middle/inner ears)**
   When *Wei-Qi* is Deficient due to a Deficiency of Kidney *Jing* from genetic disorders, chronic stress, poor diet or aging, Damp-Heat can enter the Gallbladder Channel bilaterally and affect the middle and/or inner ears causing deafness. Damp-Heat causes local swelling, *Qi*/Blood Stagnation and local *Qi* Deficiency resulting in deafness. The Damp-Heat may primarily affect the middle ears and cause conduction deafness from the accumulation of debris or affect the cochlear receptors and nerves in the inner ears and cause nerve deafness.

Pattern Differentiation and Treatment

1. Kidney *Jing* Deficiency

Clinical Signs:
- Loss of hearing noticed shortly after birth
- No response on BAER
- White, blue eyed cats
- Dalmatians and other dog breeds
- Tongue- pale, swollen
- Pulses-weak

TCVM Diagnosis:
The diagnosis of Kidney *Jing* Deficiency is based on the history of neonatal deafness. A pale swollen tongue and weak pulses are associated with Kidney *Jing* Deficiency.

Treatment Principles:
- Tonify Kidney *Jing* and strengthen local *Qi* flow to the cochlear nerve region to attempt to promote nerve regeneration and improve hearing

Acupuncture treatment:

Treat both sides. For EA use 80-120 Hz alternating frequencies for 15-30 minutes to stimulate nerve regeneration. Perform DN to further stimulate *Qi* Flow in the region and support the Kidney. Repeat acupuncture every 1-2 weeks for 6-8 treatments. For Aqua-AP inject 0.25-0.5 ml vitamin B12 into the acupoint.

Acupoints recommended
- EA: SI-16/SI-19, *An-shen/An-shen,* TH-17/TH-17
- DN: *Shang-guan,* GB-2, TH-21, BL-23, KID-3, TH-3, GB-39, LU-7, LI-10, ST-36, BL-20, BL-21
- Aqua-AP: BL-23, BL-20, BL-21

Pertinent acupoint actions
- SI-16 is a point on the Small Intestine Channel useful to bring *Qi* to SI-19 at the ear base during EA
- SI-19, TH-17, *Shang-guan* (caudal end of the temporomandibular joint dorsal to the zygomatic arch), *An-shen* (halfway between GB-20 and TH-17), GB-2 and TH-21 are local acupoints around the ear useful to treat deafness
- BL-23 is the Back *Shu* Association point for Kidney to support Kidney *Jing*
- KID-3 is the *Yuan* Source point of the Kidney to support Kidney *Jing*
- TH-3 is a distant acupoint on the Triple Heater Channel which is useful to treat deafness
- GB-39 is an Influential point for Marrow to support Kidney *Jing*
- LU-7 is the Master point of the head
- LI-10 and ST-36 are useful to tonify *Qi*
- BL-20 is the is the Back *Shu* Association point for Spleen to nourish post natal *Jing* to help support prenatal Kidney *Jing*
- BL-21 is the is the Back *Shu* Association point for Stomach to nourish post natal *Jing* to help support prenatal Kidney *Jing*

Herbal Medicine:
- Epimedium Formula (JT)[a] 0.5gm/10-20# twice daily orally to tonify Kidney *Jing*
- Administer herbal formula up to 6 months
- A description of all the ingredients of the Chinese herbal medicine listed is beyond the scope of this text, but can be found elsewhere.[8,9]

Food Therapy:

The purpose of the Food therapy is to tonify Kidney *Jing* and to promote *Qi*/Blood circulation and nerve regeneration in the affected region. Foods that are Cold or Hot are avoided.[11]

- Foods to tonify *Jing*: Liver, kidneys, fish, bone and bone marrow, millet, quinoa, spelt, wheat, almonds, black sesame, microalgae (e.g. chlorella, spirulina, wild blue-green algae), barley, wheat grass, black soy beans, black beans, kidney beans, seaweed, sea salt, mulberries, raspberries, strawberries, almonds, black sesame, clarified butter (ghee), royal jelly, bee pollen

- Foods to supplement to promote *Qi* and Blood circulation include: chicken egg, crab, sweet rice, peaches, carrots, coriander, squash, turnips
- Cold foods to avoid: Turkey, duck, duck eggs, conch, clams, mussels, yogurt, millet, barley, spinach, broccoli, celery, egg plant, kelp, alfalfa, cucumbers, pears, bananas, white radishes, watermelon
- Hot foods to avoid: Lamb, shrimp, corn-fed beef, chicken, trout, squash, turnips, sweet rice, basal, caraway, cherries, chilies, cinnamon, ginger, rosemary, sage

Tui-na Procedures:

The purpose of the *Tui-na* is to stimulate *Qi* and Blood flow and promote nerve regeneration in the affected region. The descriptions and indications of each technique are outlined in more detail in Chapter 1 Table 8.[10]

- *An-fa* pressing and *Ca-fa* rubbing with the finger at TH-21, SI-19, GB-2, TH-17, *An-shen* for 2-3 minutes at each site on each ear to invigorate *Qi* Flow
- *Ba-shen-fa* stretching of the ears forward and backward to stimulate *Qi* flow; repeat 12 times on each ear

Daily Life Style Recommendation for Owner Follow-up:

- *Moo-fa* massaging round the ear bases and behind the ears for 5-10 minutes twice daily
- Provide high quality nutrition to support production of postnatal *Jing* to spare prenatal Kidney *Jing*
- Keep in a protected environment, as the animal may not be able to hear and avoid automobiles or aggressive animals or people

Comments:

Deafness may not respond to TCVM treatment because some cochlear receptor and nerve function is necessary for a response.

2. Kidney *Qi* Deficiency

Clinical Signs:
- Adult onset of hearing loss
- No response on BAER
- Tongue- pale, wet
- Pulses- deep, weak right side

TCVM Diagnosis:

The diagnosis of Kidney *Qi* Deficiency is based on the history of progressing hearing loss in a geriatric dog. The pale and wet tongue and deep weak pulses, weaker on the right, are associated with Kidney *Qi* Deficiency.

Treatment Principles:
- Tonify Kidney *Qi* to restore auditory nerve function
- Strengthen local *Qi* flow to the cochlear nerve region to promote nerve regeneration and improve hearing

Acupuncture treatment:

Treat both sides. For EA use 80-120 Hz alternating frequencies for 15-30 minutes to stimulate nerve regeneration. Perform DN to further stimulate *Qi* Flow in the region, support the Kidney and resolve deafness. Repeat acupuncture every 1-2 weeks for 6-8 treatments. For Aqua-AP inject 0.25-0.5 ml vitamin B12 into the acupoint.

Acupoints recommended
- EA: SI-16/SI-19, *An-shen* (halfway between GB-20 and TH-17 behind the ear)/*An-shen,* TH-17/TH-17
- DN: *Shang-guan* (caudal end of the temporomandibular joint, dorsal to the zygomatic arch), GB-2, TH-21, BL-23, KID-3, TH-3, GB-39, GB-34, LU-7, LI-10, ST-36
- Aqua-AP: BL-23

Pertinent acupoint actions
- SI-16 is a point on the Small Intestine Channel useful to bring *Qi* to SI-19 at the ear base during EA
- SI-19, TH-17, *Shang-guan, An-shen,* GB-2 and TH-21 are local acupoints around the ear useful to treat deafness
- BL-23 is the Back *Shu* Association point for Kidney to support Kidney *Jing*
- KID-3 is the *Yuan* Source point of the Kidney to support Kidney *Jing*
- TH-3 is a distant acupoint on the Triple Heater Channel which is useful to treat deafness
- GB-39 is an Influential point for Marrow to support Kidney *Jing*
- GB-34 is useful to break-up Stagnation and is a distant point on the Gallbladder Channel that course around the ear
- LU-7 is the Master point of the head
- LI-10 and ST-36 are useful to tonify *Qi*

Herbal Medicine:
- *Jin Gui Shen Qi Wan* (JT)[a] 0.5gm/10-20# twice daily orally to tonify Kidney *Qi* and *Yang*
- Administer herbal formula up to 6 months
- A description of all the ingredients of the Chinese herbal medicine listed is beyond the scope of this text, but can be found elsewhere.[8,9]

Food Therapy:

The purpose of the Food therapy is to tonify Kidney *Qi* to support nerve regeneration in the affected region. Foods that are Cold or Hot are avoided (Table 4).[11]
- Foods to tonify *Qi*: Beef, chicken, sardines, egg, potato, yam, sweet potato, rice, oats, millet, lentils, carrots, squash, microalgae, dates, figs, molasses, royal jelly
- Cold foods to avoid: Turkey, duck, duck eggs, conch, clams, mussels, yogurt, millet, barley, spinach, broccoli, celery, egg plant, kelp, alfalfa, cucumbers, pears, bananas, white radishes, watermelon
- Hot foods to avoid: Lamb, shrimp, corn-fed beef, chicken, trout, squash, turnips, sweet rice, basal, caraway, cherries, chilies, cinnamon, ginger, rosemary, sage

Tui-na Procedures:

The purpose of the *Tui-na* is to stimulate *Qi* and Blood flow and promote nerve regeneration in the affected region. The descriptions and indications of each technique are outlined in more detail in Chapter 1 Table 8.[10]

- *An-fa* pressing and *Ca-fa* rubbing with the finger at TH-21, SI-19, GB-2, TH-17, *An-shen* for 2-3 minutes at each site on each ear to invigorate *Qi* Flow
- *Ba-shen-fa* stretching of the ears forward and backward to stimulate *Qi* flow; repeat 12 times on each ear

Daily Life Style Recommendation for Owner Follow-up:

- *Moo-fa* massaging round the ear bases and behind the ears for 5-10 minutes twice daily
- Provide high quality nutrition to support production of postnatal *Jing* to spare prenatal Kidney *Jing*
- Keep in a protected environment, as the animal may not be able to hear and avoid automobiles or aggressive animals or people

Comments:

Based on clinical studies in humans and anecdotal experiences in animals expect TCVM treatment to improve hearing.

3. Gallbladder Damp Heat with local *Qi* Deficiency

Clinical Signs:

- Deafness
- Usually have chronic otitis externa and media
- May have a Head tilt (otitis interna)
- May have Horner's syndrome (otitis media)
- May facial paralysis (otitis media)
- Tongue- red, greasy
- Pulses- forceful, rapid, slippery

TCVM Diagnosis:

The diagnosis of Gallbladder Damp Heat (Inner ear) is based on a history of otitis externa/media if present. The external ear may feel warm and appear red, typical of Heat. The red, greasy tongue is typical of Damp-Heat. Forceful and rapid pulses are typical of Excess Heat and slippery pulses are typical of Damp.

Treatment Principles:

- Clear Damp Heat
- Resolve local *Qi*/Blood Stagnation and strengthen local *Qi* flow to the cochlear nerve region to promote nerve regeneration and improve hearing

Acupuncture treatment:

For EA use 20 Hz for 10-15 minutes then 80-120 Hz alternating frequencies for 10-15 minutes, to control ear pain and resolve *Qi*/Blood Stagnation. Acutely perform AP treatments every 3-5 days for 3 times, then weekly for 3 times. For Aqua-AP inject 0.25-0.5 ml vitamin B12 into the acupoint.

Acupoints recommended
- EA: SI-16/SI-19, *An-shen/An-shen,* TH-17/TH-17
- DN: *Er-jian* GV-14, SP-6, SP-9, *Shang-guan,* GB-2, TH-21, BL-23, KID-3, TH-3, GB-39, GB-34, LU-7, LI-10, ST-36
- Aqua-AP: BL-23, GV-14

Pertinent acupoint actions
- *Er-jian* (ear tip) and GV-14 are useful to clear Heat
- SP-6 and SP-9 are useful to drain Damp
- SI-16 is a point on the Small Intestine Channel useful to bring *Qi* to SI-19 at the ear during EA
- SI-19, TH-17, *Shang-guan* (caudal end of the temporomandibular joint, dorsal to the zygomatic arch)*, An-shen* (halfway between GB-20 and TH-17 behind the ear)*,* GB-2 and TH-21 are local acupoints around the ear useful to treat deafness
- BL-23 is the Back *Shu* Association point for Kidney to support Kidney *Jing*
- KID-3 is the *Yuan* Source point of the Kidney to support Kidney *Jing*
- TH-3 is a distant acupoint on the Triple Heater Channel which is useful to treat deafness
- GB-39 is an Influential point for Marrow to support Kidney *Jing*
- GB-34 is useful to break-up Stagnation and is a distant point on the Gallbladder Channel that course around the ear
- LU-7 is the Master point of the head
- LI-10 and ST-36 are useful to tonify *Qi*

Herbal Medicine:
- Ear Damp Heat (JT) 0.5gm/10# twice daily orally to drain Damp and clear Heat
- Alternative: *Long Dan Xie Gan* (JT)[a] 0.5gm/10# twice daily orally to drain Damp and clear Heat
- Combine with conventional antibiotic therapy
- Administer herbal formulas up to 4 months
- If otitis externa present: administer *Di Er You* (JT)[a] (Ear drops), 2-7 drops, 5-8 times daily for one month to clear Heat, dry Damp, relieve pruritus and reduce swelling
- A description of all the ingredients of the Chinese herbal medicine listed is beyond the scope of this text, but can be found elsewhere.[8,9]

Food Therapy:
The purpose of the Food therapy is to clear Heat and Damp and promote *Qi*/Blood circulation and nerve regeneration. Cooling foods are prescribed and Damp producing and Hot foods are avoided.[11]
- Foods to supplement to clear Heat: Turkey, duck, duck eggs, conch, clams, mussels, yogurt, millet, barley, spinach, broccoli, celery, egg plant, kelp, alfalfa, cucumbers, pears, bananas, white radishes, watermelon
- Foods to supplement to Drain Damp: Eel, mackerel, quail, corn, barley, rye, blueberries, celery, mushrooms
- Foods to promote *Qi*/Blood circulation: Crab, sweet rice, peaches, carrots, coriander, turnips
- Damp producing foods to avoid: Eggs, milk, cheese, yoghurt, ghee, bananas, sugar
- Hot foods to avoid: Lamb, shrimp, corn-fed beef, chicken, trout, squash, sweet rice, basal, caraway, cherries, chilies, cinnamon, ginger, rosemary, sage

Tui-na Procedures:
The purpose of the *Tui-na* is to stimulate *Qi* and Blood flow and promote nerve regeneration in the affected region. The descriptions and indications of each technique are outlined in more detail in Chapter 1 Table 8.[10]
- The ears may be too painful initially to perform *Tui-na*, but once pain has passed *Tui-na* is recommended to stimulate *Qi* Flow
- *An-fa* pressing and *Ca-fa* rubbing with the finger at TH-21, SI-19, GB-2, TH-17, *An-shen* for 2-3 minutes at each site on each ear to stimulate *Qi* Flow
- *Ba-shen-fa* stretching of the ears forward and backward to stimulate *Qi* flow; repeat 12 times on each ear

Daily Life Style Recommendation for Owner Follow-up:
- When pain has subsided perform *Moo-fa* massaging round the ear bases and behind the ears for 5-10 minutes twice daily
- Provide high quality nutrition to support production of postnatal *Jing* to spare prenatal Kidney *Jing*
- Keep in a protected environment, as the animal may not be able to hear and avoid automobiles or aggressive animals or people

Comments:
Although further clinical studies are needed, based on anecdotal experiences in animals expect TCVM treatment to shorten the recovery time and enhance the recovery of hearing.

LARYNGEAL PARESIS OR PARALYSIS

Acute laryngeal paresis or paralysis is most commonly congenital, associated with hypothyroidism, or idiopathic in dogs and cats, but rarely due to trauma, as in horses.[1-3,6] The presenting complaint of laryngeal paresis is usually stridor, worse with exercise. Reduced movement of one or both vocal folds can be observed during the physical examination and the rest of the neurological examination is normal. Laryngeal paresis may also be part of a polyneuropathy or other neuromuscular disorder, so a thorough neurological examination is important to rule-out these other conditions. Acute paralysis of the laryngeal muscles on both sides is an emergency situation, as the resulting cyanosis can lead to death. Serum thyroxin (T4) and thyroid stimulating hormone (TSH) assays should always be evaluated on every case of acute laryngeal paresis, as hypothyroidism can cause a focal neuropathy with no other findings that responds well to thyroid replacement therapy.

The only conventional treatment for laryngeal paresis or paralysis is surgical, but aspiration pneumonia is a life threatening complication following this surgery, especially if there is a return of some function.[2,3] There is no specific non-surgical conventional treatment and since some dogs and cats spontaneously improve, surgery may not be worth the risk of aspiration pneumonia, if laryngeal paresis is not life threatening. Although EA, DN, Aqua-AP, Chinese herbal medicine and *Tui-na* have been useful to treat laryngeal paresis and hemiplegia, there is only one published case report in a dog and no other reported studies in horses or humans.[5,6-10,25]

The TCVM examination findings associated with each TCVM pattern causing laryngeal paresis or paralysis are listed in Table 2. Recommended acupoints, acupuncture techniques, and Chinese herbal medicine are listed in Table 3.[6-9] Because of the paresis or paralysis, EA with 80-120 Hz alternating frequencies is recommended to most effectively stimulate *Qi* flow. Multiple weekly treatments may be needed in severely affected animals, before a response is seen. As with the other cranial neuropathies, the TCVM practitioner may also administer *Tui-na* treatments, after the EA and DN session and before the Aqua-AP.[10] Simple *Tui-na* techniques may also be taught to the caretaker, for in-home daily treatments in between TCVM appointments. Food therapy may further support recovery.[11] Although controlled clinical studies are needed to ensure that TCVM treatments are enhancing the recovery of laryngeal function, TCVM treatment of patients with laryngeal hemiparesis and bilateral paresis are encouraged prior to surgical intervention to provide the animal the opportunity to recover without the complications that may occur from surgery.

Etiology and Pathology

From a TCVM perspective congenital laryngeal paresis as seen in Siberian Huskies, Bouvier des Flandres and other breeds may be due to an underlying Kidney *Jing* Deficiency and local *Qi* Deficiency. Since some idiopathic adult onset laryngeal paresis also has a breed predisposition (e.g. Labrador Retrievers, Irish Setters and other breeds) there may also be an underlying Kidney *Jing* Deficiency and local *Qi* Deficiency in these cases. *Qi* Deficiency causes reduced *Qi* flow in the Conception Vessel and Stomach and Large Intestine Channels in the area of the laryngeal nerve(s).[4,7] Similar to other focal idiopathic neuropathies, there may be a *Zheng Qi* Deficiency and a weakened *Wei Qi* that allows invasion of Wind-Heat in the Channels around the laryngeal nerves in other cases of idiopathic laryngeal paresis/paralysis in cats and other dogs, With more experience, it may be found that like facial nerve paralysis, Wind-Cold instead of Wind-Heat may invade the Channels in certain animals based on their constitution. Laryngeal hemiplegia from trauma, though relatively rare in dogs, as compared to horses, results in local *Qi*/Blood Stagnation, loss of *Qi*/Blood flow and *Qi*/Blood Deficiency to the laryngeal nerve region. Applying the basic TCVM theories of *Yin/Yang*, Eight Principles, Five Treasures, Five Elements and *Zang Fu* physiology and pathology to make a TCVM diagnosis, there are three basic patterns associated with laryngeal nerve dysfunction, but with more experience other patterns may be identified in the future:

1. **Kidney *Jing* Deficiency with local *Qi* Deficiency**
   Kidney *Jing* Deficiency may result in loss of normal laryngeal nerve development and maturity and cause congenital laryngeal paresis or paralysis in some specific breed dogs. Kidney *Jing* Deficiency may also result in premature degeneration of the laryngeal nerve in other adult dogs of specific breeds. In both of these instances Kidney *Jing* Deficiency is manifested as unilateral or bilateral laryngeal paresis due to a Deficiency in local *Qi* flow to the laryngeal area affecting nerve function.

2. **Wind-Heat invasion causing *Qi*/Blood Stagnation and local *Qi* Deficiency**
   When *Wei Qi* becomes weak due to poor nutrition, chronic illness or environmental stress, Wind-Heat invades the Channels around the larynx causing *Qi*/Blood Stagnation loss of *Qi*/Blood flow and *Qi*/Blood Deficiency to local tissues including nerves. The result is laryngeal paresis or paralysis.

3. ***Qi*/Blood Stagnation and local *Qi* Deficiency**
   Trauma induces *Qi*/Blood Stagnation at the site of injury that results in loss of *Qi*/Blood flow and *Qi*/Blood Deficiency to local tissues including nerves. The result is the acute onset of laryngeal paresis or paralysis.

Pattern Differentiation and Treatment

1. Kidney *Jing* Deficiency with local *Qi* Deficiency

Clinical Signs:
- Acute onset
- Stridor
- Cyanosis
- Young pure breed dog less than 1 year of age
- Adult pure breed dogs
- Tongue- pale, swollen or wet, blue
- Pulses- deep, weak on both sides

TCVM Diagnosis:
   The diagnosis of Kidney *Jing* Deficiency is based on the history of acute onset laryngeal paresis or paralysis in specific breeds of young or adult dogs. The pale, swollen, wet tongue and deep weak pulses bilaterally reflect the Kidney *Jing* Deficiency. The tongue may be blue due to cyanosis.

Treatment Principles:
- Tonify Kidney *Jing*
- Strengthen local *Qi* flow to the laryngeal region to promote nerve regeneration

Acupuncture treatment:
   Treat both sides. For EA use 80-120 Hz alternating frequencies for 15-30 minutes, as EA is more effective to stimulate local *Qi* flow than DN alone. Repeat acupuncture every 1-2 weeks for 6-8 treatments. For Aqua-AP inject 0.25-0.5 ml vitamin B12 into the acupoint.

Acupoints recommended
- EA: CV-20/CV-24, CV-23a/CV-23b, LI-18/LI-18
- DN: CV-1, BL-23, KID-3, GB-39, LU-7, LI-4, LI-10, ST-36, BL-20, BL-21
- Aqua-AP: BL-20, BL-21, BL-23

Pertinent acupoint actions
- CV-20 and CV-24 are points near the larynx that can be connected for EA to stimulate *Qi* flow across the larynx
- CV-23a and CV-23b are on each side of CV-23 at the larynx and are useful to stimulate *Qi* flow at the larynx
- LI-18 is a local acupoint on the neck near the path of the recurrent laryngeal nerve to stimulate *Qi* flow in the region
- CV-1 is a distant point on the Conception Vessel useful to stimulate *Qi* flow along the Channel and across the larynx
- BL-23 is the Back *Shu* Association point for Kidney to support Kidney *Jing*
- KID-3 is the *Yuan* Source point of the Kidney to support Kidney *Jing*
- GB-39 is an Influential point for Marrow to support Kidney *Jing*
- LU-7 is the Master point of the head and neck
- LI-4 is the Master point of the neck and face
- LI-10 and ST-36 are useful to tonify *Qi* to stimulate general *Qi* flow
- BL-20 is the is the Back *Shu* Association point for Spleen to nourish post natal *Jing* to help support prenatal Kidney *Jing*

Herbal Medicine:
- Epimedium Formula (JT)[a] 0.5gm/10-20# twice daily orally to support Kidney *Jing*
- Young dogs: may combine with *Si Jun Zi* (JT)[a] 0.5gm/10-20# twice daily orally to tonify *Qi* and support the Spleen and postnatal *Jing*
- Adult dogs and cats: may combine with *Qi* Performance (JT)[a] 0.5gm/10-20# twice daily orally to support Kidney *Jing*
- Administer herbal formula up to 6 months
- A description of all the ingredients of the Chinese herbal medicine listed is beyond the scope of this text, but can be found elsewhere.[8,9]

Food Therapy:

The purpose of the Food therapy is to tonify Kidney *Jing* and to promote *Qi*/Blood circulation and nerve regeneration in the affected region. Foods that are too Cold or Hot are avoided.[11]

- Foods to tonify *Jing*: Liver, kidneys, fish, bone and bone marrow, millet, quinoa, spelt, wheat, almonds, black sesame, microalgae (e.g. chlorella, spirulina, wild blue-green algae), barley, wheat grass, black soy beans, black beans, kidney beans, seaweed, sea salt, mulberries, raspberries, strawberries, almonds, black sesame, clarified butter (ghee), royal jelly, bee pollen
- Foods to supplement to promote *Qi* and Blood circulation include: chicken egg, crab, sweet rice, peaches, carrots, coriander, squash, turnip

- Cold foods to avoid: Turkey, duck, duck eggs, conch, clams, mussels, yogurt, millet, barley, spinach, broccoli, celery, egg plant, kelp, alfalfa, cucumbers, pears, bananas, white radishes, watermelon
- Hot foods to avoid: Lamb, shrimp, corn-fed beef, chicken, trout, squash, turnips, sweet rice, basal, caraway, cherries, chilies, cinnamon, ginger, rosemary, sage

Tui-na Procedures:

The purpose of the *Tui-na* is to stimulate *Qi* and Blood flow and promote nerve regeneration in the affected region. The descriptions and indications of each technique are outlined in more detail in Chapter 1 Table 8.[10]

- A 25-30 minute *Tui-na* treatment for laryngeal paresis or paralysis is outlined in Table 5

Daily Life Style Recommendation for Owner Follow-up:

- *Moo-fa* massaging along sides of the neck from GB-21 to LI-18 for 3-5 minutes twice daily
- *Moo-fa* massaging along the lower jaw and thoracic inlet region for 3-5 minutes twice daily
- Avoid massage of the affected area, as breathing could be further compromised
- Avoid strenuous activity or overheating while breathing is impaired
- Feed Provide high quality nutrition to support production of postnatal *Jing* to spare prenatal Kidney *Jing*

Comments:

Based on anecdotal experiences in animals expect TCVM treatment to improve laryngeal function. Further clinical studies are needed to ensure that TCVM treatments enhance recovery.

Table 5: An example of a 25-30 minute *Tui-na* treatment for laryngeal paresis or paralysis[10]

Name	Technique	Duration or Number of Repetitions
Moo-fa	Massage the lower jaw and top of neck	3-5 minutes
Ban-fa	Stretch open the mouth	6 times
Yi-zhi-chan and *Rou-fa*	Using the thumb, press and push from GB-21 to LI-18	3 minutes
Ca-fa	Rub from GB-21 to TH-17	2 minutes
Nie-fa and *Na-fa*	Pinch and pull the skin and muscles below and above the larynx; care should be taken not to compromise breathing further	Up to 15 minutes

2. Wind-Heat invasion causing *Qi*/Blood Stagnation and local *Qi* Deficiency

Clinical Signs:
- Acute onset
- Stridor

- Cyanosis
- Adult dogs and cats
- Tongue- red, purple
- Pulses- Superficial, forceful, rapid or wiry

TCVM Diagnosis:

The diagnosis of Wind-Heat invasion causing *Qi*/Blood Stagnation and local *Qi* Deficiency is based on the history of acute onset laryngeal paresis or paralysis in any adult dog or cat. The red and purple tongue reflects the Heat and *Qi*/Blood Stagnation and the superficial, forceful, rapid pulses reflect the Excess pattern associated with the External invasion of Wind-Heat. The wiry pulses reflect the local *Qi*/Blood Stagnation in the area of the larynx.

Treatment Principles:
- Clear Wind-Heat
- Resolve *Qi*/Blood Stagnation
- Promote local *Qi* flow and restore laryngeal nerve function

Acupuncture treatment:

For EA use 80-120 Hz alternating frequencies for 15-30 minutes, as EA is more effective to resolve Stagnation than DN alone. Treat both the normal and abnormal sides. Repeat acupuncture every 3-5 days for 3-5 times, then every 1-2 weeks until function returns; For Aqua-AP inject 0.25-0.5 ml vitamin B12 into the acupoint.

Acupoints recommended
- EA: CV-20/CV-24, CV-23a/CV-23b, LI-18/LI-18
- DN: CV-1, GV-14, LI-4, LU-7, LI-10, ST-36
- Aqua-AP: GV-14

Pertinent acupoint actions
- CV-20 and CV-24 are points near the larynx that can be connected for EA to stimulate *Qi* flow across the larynx
- CV-23a and CV-23b are on each side of CV-23 at the larynx and are useful to stimulate *Qi* flow at the larynx
- LI-18 is a local acupoint on the neck near the path of the recurrent laryngeal nerve to stimulate *Qi* flow in the region
- CV-1 is a distant point on the Conception Vessel useful to stimulate *Qi* flow along the Channel and across the larynx
- GV-1 is useful to clear Wind-Heat
- LI-4 is the Master point of the neck and face
- LU-7 is the Master point of the head and neck
- LI-10 and ST-36 are useful to tonify *Qi* to stimulate general *Qi* flow

Herbal Medicine:
- *Pu Ji Xiao Du Yin* (JT)[a] 0.5gm/10# twice daily orally to clear Heat and disperse Wind-Heat

CHAPTER 3

- Administer herbal formula 2-4 months as needed
- A description of all the ingredients of the Chinese herbal medicine listed is beyond the scope of this text, but can be found elsewhere.[8,9]

Food Therapy:

The purpose of the Food therapy is to clear Heat and promote *Qi*/Blood circulation, so cooling foods are prescribed and Hot foods are avoided.[11]

- Foods to supplement to clear Heat: Turkey, duck, duck eggs, conch, clams, mussels, yogurt, millet, barley, spinach, broccoli, celery, egg plant, kelp, alfalfa, cucumbers, pears, bananas, white radishes, watermelon
- Foods to promote *Qi*/Blood circulation: Chicken egg, crab, sweet rice, peaches, carrots, coriander, turnips
- Foods to avoid: Lamb, shrimp, corn-fed beef, chicken, trout, squash, turnips, sweet rice, basal, caraway, cherries, chilies, cinnamon, ginger, rosemary, sage

Tui-na Procedures:

The purpose of the *Tui-na* is to stimulate *Qi* and Blood flow and promote nerve regeneration in the affected region. The descriptions and indications of each technique are outlined in more detail in Chapter 1 Table 8.[10]

- A 25-30 minute *Tui-na* treatment for laryngeal paresis or paralysis is outlined in Table5

Daily Life Style Recommendation for Owner Follow-up:

- *Moo-fa* massaging along sides of the neck from GB-21 to LI-18 for 3-5 minutes twice daily
- *Moo-fa* massaging along the lower jaw and thoracic inlet region for 3-5 minutes twice daily
- Avoid massage of the affected area, as breathing could be further compromised
- Avoid strenuous activity or overheating while breathing is impaired
- Feed a high quality diet to support *Zheng Qi*
- Keep in a low stress environment to support *Zheng Qi*

Comments:

Based on anecdotal experiences in animals expect TCVM treatment to improve laryngeal function. Further clinical studies are needed to ensure that TCVM treatments enhance recovery.

3. *Qi*/Blood Stagnation and local *Qi* Deficiency

Clinical Signs:

- Acute onset
- Stridor
- Cyanosis
- History or physical evidence of trauma
- Tongue- purple
- Pulses- wiry

TCVM Diagnosis:
The diagnosis of *Qi*/Blood Stagnation and local *Qi* Deficiency is based on a history or physical evidence of trauma and acute onset laryngeal paresis or paralysis. The tongue color is purple from the *Qi*/Blood Stagnation and the pulses wiry from the Stagnation.

Treatment Principles:
- Resolve *Qi*/Blood Stagnation
- Tonify local *Qi* and restore laryngeal nerve function

Acupuncture treatment:
For EA use 80-120 Hz alternating frequencies for 15-30 minutes, as EA is more effective to resolve Stagnation than DN alone. Repeat acupuncture every 3-5 days for 3-5 times, then every 1-2 weeks until function returns.

Acupoints recommended
- EA: GB 21/CV-23a, CV-23/ LI-17, LI-18/LI-18, SI-9/SI-9, SI-17/SI-17
- DN: LI-4, LU-7, LI-10, ST-36, SI-3
- Aqua-AP: B12 injected larynx region may cause further nerve injury

Pertinent acupoint actions
- GB 21/CV-23a, CV-23/ LI-17, LI-18/LI-18, SI-9/SI-9, SI-17/SI-17
- LI-4, LU-7, LI-10, ST-36, SI-3

Herbal Medicine:
- *Bu Yong Yi Qi* (JT)[a] 0.5gm/10-20# twice daily orally to tonify *Qi*
- Administer herbal formula up to 6 months
- A description of all the ingredients of the Chinese herbal medicine listed is beyond the scope of this text, but can be found elsewhere.[8,9]

Food Therapy:
The purpose of the Food therapy is to further promote *Qi*/Blood circulation and tonify *Qi* to support nerve regeneration in the affected region. Foods that are Cold or Hot are avoided.[11]
- Foods to supplement to promote *Qi* and Blood circulation include: chicken egg, crab, sweet rice, peaches, carrots, coriander, squash, turnips
- Foods to tonify *Qi*: Beef, chicken, sardines, egg, potato, yam, sweet potato, rice, oats, millet, lentils, carrots, squash, microalgae, dates, figs, molasses, royal jelly
- Cold foods to avoid: Turkey, duck, duck eggs, conch, clams, mussels, yogurt, millet, barley, spinach, broccoli, celery, egg plant, kelp, alfalfa, cucumbers, pears, bananas, white radishes, watermelon
- Hot foods to avoid: Lamb, shrimp, corn-fed beef, chicken, trout, squash, turnips, sweet rice, basal, caraway, cherries, chilies, cinnamon, ginger, rosemary, sage

Tui-na Procedures:

The purpose of the *Tui-na* is to stimulate *Qi* and Blood flow and promote nerve regeneration in the affected region. The descriptions and indications of each technique are outlined in more detail in Chapter 1 Table 8.[10]
- A 25-30 minute *Tui-na* treatment for laryngeal paresis or paralysis is outlined in Table 5

Daily Life Style Recommendation for Owner Follow-up:
- *Moo-fa* massaging along sides of the neck from GB-21 to LI-18 for 3-5 minutes twice daily
- *Moo-fa* massaging along the lower jaw and thoracic inlet region for 3-5 minutes twice daily
- Avoid massage of the affected area, as breathing could be further compromised
- Avoid strenuous activity, overheating or distress while breathing is impaired
- Provide high quality nutrition to support production of postnatal *Jing* to spare prenatal Kidney *Jing*

Comments:

Based on anecdotal experiences in animals expect TCVM treatment to improve laryngeal function. Further clinical studies are needed to ensure that TCVM treatments enhance recovery.

MASTICATORY MYOSITIS

Atrophy of the temporalis and masseter muscles on one side may be due to unilateral trigeminal neuropathy associated with peripheral nerve or brainstem diseases like trauma, meningoencephalitis or neoplasia.[1-3] Bilateral asymmetrical or symmetrical atrophy of both temporalis and masseter muscles is commonly due to an immune-mediated masticatory myositis in dogs.[1-3,5] There are acute forms where the muscles are primarily painful and atrophy is not as pronounced or chronic forms with progressive non-painful muscle atrophy. The main clinical complaint is an inability to open the mouth completely either due to severe pain (acutely) or restricted movement (chronic muscle fibrosis) resulting in difficulty chewing or eating. The remainder of the physical and neurological examinations is normal, but if pain or atrophy is found in other body or limb muscles, then a polymyositis is the most likely diagnosis (see **POLYMYOSITIS** Chapter 5 **Generalized Neuromuscular Disorders**). An immunoassay detecting antibodies against 2-M type muscle fibers, specific for masticatory muscles, can be useful to confirm the diagnosis. A muscle biopsy usually shows inflammation, muscle fiber degeneration and fibrosis. Conventionally masticatory myositis is treated with immunosuppressive drugs and in chronic cases with muscle fibrosis, the fibrotic material is surgically excised to reduce the restricted chewing movements, so they can lap gruel, but then the jaw often hangs open. Unfortunately, scarring associated with surgery often results in an eventual return of the inability to open the mouth. The overall conventional prognosis for this disease is poor.

The TCVM examination findings in dogs with masticatory myositis are listed in Table 2. Although recommendations for treating masticatory myositis with EA and DN have been suggested, there are no case reports or clinical studies in the human or veterinary literature where any TCVM treatment has been administered for masticatory myositis.[5] Recommended acupoints, acupuncture techniques and Chinese herbal medicine are listed in Table 3.[6-9] Cooling foods may also be helpful to clear Heat.[11] Once pain has subsided *Tui-na* may be helpful to increase range of jaw motion and blood circulation to the masticatory muscles.[10] Because TCVM can balance the immune system and has been successful for pain control and treating other immune-mediated disorders, veterinarians are encouraged to try these treatments in dogs as long-term immunosuppressive drugs usually administered to conventionally treat the disease, have adverse side effects.[21] Further TCVM may be useful to prevent recurrences that are common following conventional treatments.

Etiology and Pathology

From a TCVM perspective masticatory myositis is due to weak *Zheng Qi* with Wind-Heat or Heat-Toxin invasion of the proximal Gallbladder and Stomach Channels with focal *Qi*/Blood Stagnation disrupting normal *Qi*/Blood flow and causing *Qi*/Blood Deficiency.[7] Clinical signs are acute and the muscles feel warm. Muscle biopsies confirm muscle inflammation associated with the Heat. With more experience other TCVM patterns like Wind-Cold invasion may be recognized.[5] Acutely *Qi*/Blood Stagnation of the masticatory muscles cause severe pain. Chronic local *Qi*/Blood Deficiency results in atrophy and fibrosis of the masticatory muscles restricting movement of the temporomandibular joint (TMJ).

1. **Wind-Heat invasion causing *Qi*/Blood Stagnation and local *Qi* Deficiency**
   When *Wei Qi* becomes weak due to poor nutrition, chronic illness or environmental stress, Wind-Heat invades the Channels around the masticatory muscles causing muscle *Qi*/Blood Stagnation, loss of *Qi*/Blood flow and then *Qi*/Blood Deficiency. The result is acute muscle pain or muscle fibrosis.

Pattern Differentiation and Treatment

1. Wind-Heat invasion causing *Qi*/Blood Stagnation and local *Qi* Deficiency

Clinical Signs:
- Inability to open the jaw due to pain or muscle fibrosis of the TMJ
- Acutely temporalis and masseter muscles may be painful and swollen
- Chronically temporalis and masseter muscles are atrophied and fibrotic
- Tongue- acutely red, dry, later may be pale
- Pulses- wiry, forceful and rapid acutely, later may be weak

TCVM Diagnosis:
The diagnosis of Wind-Heat invasion causing *Qi*/Blood Stagnation and local *Qi* Deficiency is based on the clinical signs. The tongue color will vary with the stage of the process. Acutely the tongue is red from the Wind-Heat, and purple if *Qi*/Blood Stagnation is most prominent. Muscles will be painful and swollen at this stage. If chronic progressive with muscle atrophy, the tongue will be pale as Blood/*Qi* Deficiency of the muscles is most prominent. The pulses may be forceful and rapid reflecting the Heat or wiry reflecting the *Qi*/Blood Stagnation, but later may become weak reflecting the *Qi*/Blood Stagnation.

Treatment Principles:
- Clear Wind-Heat
- Resolve *Qi*/Blood Stagnation
- Relieve pain

- Tonify local *Qi* and restore muscle function

Acupuncture treatment:

For EA use 20 Hz for 10-15 minutes then 80-120 Hz alternating frequencies for 10-15 minutes, to control muscle pain and resolve Stagnation. If acute signs, perform AP treatments every 3-5 days for 3 times, then weekly for 3 times, then 1-2 times per month until recovered. May need monthly treatments indefinitely to avoid chronic atrophy. If presented when chronic with muscle atrophy, treat weekly for 5-7 treatments and then see if there is any recovery of function. For Aqua-AP inject 0.25-0.5 ml vitamin B12 into the acupoint.

Acupoints recommended
- EA: Acute pain stage: GB-20/GB-2, TH-17/TH-17 (acupoints on head may be too painful); When no longer painful: GB-20/GB-2, TH-17/TH-17, *Da-feng-men/Nao-shu*, ST-6/ST-6
- DN: *Er-jian*, *Tai-yang*, left LI-4, right LIV-3, LU-7, ST-2, SI-16, TH-21, ST-44, LI-10, ST-36
- Aqua-AP: GB-20

Pertinent acupoint actions
- GB-20 is useful to dispel Wind and is connected to GB-2 during EA to stimulate *Qi* flow in the Gallbladder Channel
- GB-2 is a local acupoint close to masseter muscle and is connected to GB-20 during EA to stimulate *Qi* flow in the Gallbladder Channel
- TH-17 is a local acupoint close to the masseter muscle and can be connected bilaterally during EA to stimulate *Qi* flow to the region of the masseter muscle
- *Da-feng-men* (midline at level of cranial ear bases) is connected *Nao-shu* (in the temporal muscle, one third the way along a line between the cranial ear base and the lateral canthus of the eye) to stimulate *Qi* flow in the area of the temporalis muscles
- ST-6 is local acupoint in the masseter muscles and can be connected bilaterally during EA to promote *Qi* flow in the area
- *Er-jian* (ear tip) and *Tai-yang* (one *cun* lateral to the lateral canthus, above the zygomatic arch) are useful to clear Wind-Heat
- LU-7 is the Master point of the head and is useful to stimulate *Qi* flow and control pain of the head
- LI-4 is the Master point of the face and is useful to stimulate *Qi* flow and control pain of the face
- Left LI-4 and right LIV-3 may be useful to reduce *Qi*/Blood Stagnation and relieve pain
- ST-44 is a distant acupoint to clear Heat in the Stomach Channel
- LI-10 and ST-36 are useful to tonify *Qi* and stimulate *Qi* flow

Herbal Medicine:
- *Pu Ji Xiao Du Yin* (JT)[a] 0.5gm/10# twice daily orally to clear Heat and disperse Wind-Heat
- Administer herbal formula 2-4 months needed
- A description of all the ingredients of each Chinese herbal medicine listed is beyond the scope of this text, but can be found elsewhere.[8,9]

Food Therapy:
The purpose of the Food therapy is to clear Heat and promote *Qi*/Blood circulation, so cooling foods are prescribed and Hot foods are avoided.[11]
- Foods to supplement to clear Heat: Turkey, duck, duck eggs, conch, clams, mussels, yogurt, millet, barley, spinach, broccoli, celery, egg plant, kelp, alfalfa, cucumbers, pears, bananas, white radishes, watermelon
- Foods to promote *Qi*/Blood circulation: Chicken egg, crab, sweet rice, peaches, carrots, coriander, turnips
- Foods to avoid: Lamb, shrimp, corn-fed beef, chicken, trout, squash, turnips, sweet rice, basal, caraway, cherries, chilies, cinnamon, ginger, rosemary, sage

Tui-na Procedures:
The purpose of the *Tui-na* therapy is to stimulate *Qi* and Blood flow and promote muscle regeneration in the affected region. Begin *Tui-na* immediately in dogs that have muscle atrophy and are not painful, but *Tui-na* may have to be delayed in cases with acute pain, until the acupuncture and Chinese herbal medicine control the pain. The techniques descriptions and indications are outlined in more detail in Chapter 1 Table 8.[10]
- *Anfa* pressing and *Ca-fa* rubbing around TH-17, *Xia guan* (upper TMJ) and *Shan guan* (lower TMJ) for 3-5 minutes to relieve *Qi*/Blood Stagnation
- *Ban-fa* wrenching in the form of opening and closing the jaws for TMJ range of motion exercises; repeat 12 times
- *Mo-fa* rubbing the temporal and masseter muscles for 3-5 minutes to improve *Qi*/Blood circulation to the muscles and other tissues

Daily Life Style Recommendation for Owner Follow-up:
- *Moo-fa* massaging under ear base at the TMJ for 3-5 minutes twice daily until function returns
- *Moo-fa* massaging over the temporalis and masseter muscles for 3-5 minutes twice daily until normal function returns
- Open and close the jaw 15-20 times, three times daily stretching the muscles until normal function returns
- Put normal dog food in the blender with water to form a gruel so animals can lap and swallow since they cannot chew
- When function begins to return, allow dog to have toys to chew on and play tug with to provide jaw exercise
- Feed a high quality diet to support *Zheng Qi*
- Keep in a low stress environment to support *Zheng Qi*

Comments:

Based on anecdotal experiences in acute cases with no muscle atrophy, expect TCVM treatment to shorten the recovery time. Since signs tend to recur, intermittent long-term treatment is usually necessary. In chronic cases with inability to open the mouth due to severe muscle atrophy and fibrosis, TCVM may not be helpful, but treatment may be given as a last resort.

Footnotes:

[a] (JT) = *Jing Tang* Herbal www.tcvmherbal.com; Reddick, FL

References:

1. De Lahunta A, Glass E. Veterinary Neuroanatomy and Clinical Neurology 3nd Ed. Philadelphia, PA:WB Saunders 2008:95-113,14.
2. Chrisman C, Mariani C, Platt S, Clemmons R. Neurology for the Small Animal Practitioner. Jackson Wy: Teton NewMedia 2003:125-167.
3. Platt S, Olby N (ed). BSAVA Manual of Canine and Feline Neurology 5th Ed. Gloucester, UK:BSAVA Publications 2012:1-500.
4. Xie H, Priest V. Traditional Chinese Veterinary Medicine. Reddick, FL: Jing Tang Publishing 2002:209-293,307-380,409-419.
5. Kline KL, Caplan ER, Joseph RJ. Acupuncture for neurological disorders. In Schoen AM (ed) Veterinary Acupuncture 2nd Ed. St Louis, Mo: Mosby Publishing 2001:179-192.
6. Xie H, Priest V. Xie's Veterinary Acupuncture. Ames, Iowa:Blackwell Publishing 2007:585.
7. Xie H. Personal communications
8. Xie H, Preast V. Xie's Chinese Veterinary Herbology. Ames. IA:Wiley-Blackwell 2010:305-347, 486-510, 387,449-460.
9. Xie H, Preast V. Chinese Veterinary Herbal Handbook 2nd Ed. Reddick, FL: Chi Institute of Chinese Medicine 2008:305-585.
10. Xie H, Ferguson B, Deng X. Application of *Tui-na* in Veterinary Medicine 2nd Ed. Reddick, FL:Chi Institute 2007:1-94,129-132.
11. Leggett D. Helping Ourselves: A Guide to Traditional Chinese Food Energetics. Totnes, England: Meridian Press 2005:21-36.
12. Liu Y, Yang G, Long YS, Jiao Y. Observation on therapeutic effect of acupuncture for treatment of optic atrophy. Zhongguo Zhen Jiu. 2009; 29(9):714-6. (in Chinese)
13. Yang H. *Dan zhi xiao yao yin* combined with auricular-point-pressing for treatment of optic atrophy-a clinical observation of 51 cases J Tradit Chin Med. 2004; 24(4):259-62.
14. Jeong SM, Yang JW, Jeong ES et al. Electroacupuncture treatment for idiopathic trigeminal nerve paralysis in a dog. Journal of Veterinary Clinics 2001; 18(1): 67-69.
15. Jeong S M, Kim H Y, Lee C H et al. Use of acupuncture for the treatment of idiopathic facial nerve paralysis in a dog. Veterinary Record 2001; 148(20):632-633.
16. Abdel-Rahman HA, Jun HK, Song KH et al. Alternative treatment for facial nerve paralysis in a dog. Journal of Veterinary Clinics 2008; 25(6): 526-528.
17. Zheng H, Li Y, Chen M. Evidence based acupuncture practice recommendations for peripheral facial paralysis. American Journal of Chinese Medicine 2009; 37(1):35-43.
18. Chen N, Zhou M, He L. Acupuncture for Bell's palsy. Cochrane Database Systematic Review 4(8):CD002914.
19. Sánchez-Araujo M, Puchi A. Acupuncture enhances the efficacy of antibiotics treatment for canine otitis crises. Acupunct Electrother Res 1997; 22(3-4):191-206.

20. Sánchez-Araujo M, Puchi A. Acupuncture prevents relapses of recurrent otitis in dogs: a 1-year follow-up of a randomised controlled trial. Acupunct Med 2011; 29(1):21-26.
21. Feng BB, Zhang JH, Chen H. Mechanisms of actions of Chinese herbal medicine in the prevention and treatment of cancer. American Journal of Traditional Chinese Veterinary Medicine 2010; 5(1):37-47.
22. Long AF, Xing M, Morgan K et al. Exploring the evidence base for acupuncture in the treatment of Meniere's syndrome-a systematic review. Evidence Based Complementary and Alternative Medicine 2009:Epub ahead of print.
23. Liu Y, Fang J, Sun D et al. An experimental study of electro-acupuncture on auditory impairment caused by kanamycin in guinea pigs. Journal of Traditional Chinese Medicine 1999; 19(1):59-64.
24. Liu B and Du YH. Evaluation of the literature of clinical studies on acupuncture and moxibustion for the treatment of sensorineural hearing loss. Zhongguo Zhen Jiu 2005; 25(12):893-6.
25. Rosado TW. Acupuncture treatment of laryngeal paralysis in a dog. American Journal of Traditional Chinese Veterinary Medicine 2010; 5 (1):63-6.

Treatment of Head Tilt/Vestibular Disease with Acupuncture and Chinese Herbal Medicine in a Chinese Pug

Daniel King, DVM, CVA, CVCH, CVTP

ABSTRACT

An 11 year old, 6.7 kg male neutered Chinese Pug mix breed dog was presented with severe head tilt of 3 weeks duration. His left side was rotated ventrally, and he would occasionally stumble to the same side. His tongue was pink and tacky. His pulses were superficial and rapid, and somewhat excessive on the left side. His ears were slightly cool to the touch, and his haircoat was very dry. The TCVM pattern diagnosis was Liver *Yin* and Liver Blood Deficiency with Local *Qi*-Blood Stagnation in the vestibular apparatus. The general acupuncture points used to treat this dog were: TH-21/ 20/ 17; GB-2/ 3/ 20; GV-21/ 20/ 17; *An-shen* for *Qi*-Blood Stagnation. Other acupoints used for the underlying deficiencies were GV-14; TH-5; BL-17/ 19/ 23; *Bai-hui*; *Shen-shu*; LIV-3; and CV-12. The Chinese herbal formulas prescribed were *Jia Wei Xiao Yao Wan* tea pills and Stasis in Mansion of Mind. Improvement in the head tilt on occasion and gait stability were noted after the third acupuncture treatment. The head tilt was 95% resolved after four months, with maintenance treatments every 2-3 months for three treatments. The purpose of this case report was to document the use of acupuncture and Chinese herbal medicine to treat vestibular disease with resultant head tilt in the dog.

Initial TCVM Examination and Treatment

An 11 year old, 6.7 kg male neutered Chinese Pug mix breed dog was presented for evaluation and treatment with TCVM for vestibular disease with severe head tilt. Three weeks prior, the dog "Mosey", was diagnosed and treated at a conventional western veterinary medicine clinic for acute onset vestibular disease with head tilt. His clinical history included serum chemistry, CBC, T4, and urinalysis. All results were normal with the following exceptions: The T4 was 1.0 (1.0-4.0) which was borderline low normal with clinical signs. The urinalysis revealed a trace of protein; bilirubin was 1+; sediment showed WBCs 0-3 per HPF, RBCs 0-3 per HPF; and hyaline casts 0-3 per LPF. No bacteria were noted in the sediment. Mosey had been treated with prednisolone 5 mg in a dose decreasing scale: 5mg BID for 5 days; then, 5mg once a day for 5 days; then, 5mg every other day for 5 doses. He was also prescribed Baytril 22.7mg tablets, and he was dosed at one twice a day for ten days.

At the time of initial presentation for TCVM evaluation, Mosey showed severe head tilt with the left side down. His head tilt was approximately 60 degrees relative to a vertical axis. He would occasionally stumble and fall to the left side, particularly when moving faster. He demonstrated horizontal nystagmus with the fast phase to his right. He would regularly circle to his left. Mosey demonstrated good *Shen*. His tongue was pink and tacky. His pulses were superficial, rapid and forceful on the left side. His ears were slightly cool, and his haircoat was very dry, with shedding. Examination of his external ear canals was normal. Mosey was being fed a commercial dry kibble diet with daily commercially prepared treats. The initial TCVM assessment was *Qi*-Blood Stagnation of the vestibular apparatus with Liver *Yin*/ Liver Blood Deficiency.[1]

Mosey was also evaluated and treated for animal chiropractic with the following results:
    1-Decreased R.O.M. at the left occiput-atlas joint

2-Decreased R.O.M. at C4-5 and C5-6 on the left side
3-Left posterior ileum Category I,II, and III
4-Sacrum-left posterior

The goals of TCVM treatment were to resolve the local *Qi*-Blood Stagnation affecting the vestibular apparatus, as well as treating the Liver *Qi*/ Liver Blood deficiency.[2] If the Blood is tonified, the Channels opened, and the Liver is supported, the circulation and innervation to the affected areas is improved restoring homeostasis. To accomplish these goals a combination of acupuncture, Chinese herbal medicine, and Food Therapy were applied. Dry needle acupuncture was performed using ½", 34 gauge *Kingli* needles, some electro-acupuncture was utilized, and aqua- acupuncture was given using Vitamin B12 1000mcg/ mL administered with a syringe and 25 gauge needle.

To resolve the local *Qi*-Blood Stagnation the following local acupoints were selected: TH-21/ 20/ 17 bilaterally; GB-2/ 3/ 20 bilaterally; GV-21/ 20/ 17.(2.) TH-21 is located in a depression just cranial to the supratragic notch dorsal to the condyloid process of the mandible. TH-20 is cranial and dorsal to the ear in a depression at the top of the ear base. TH-17 is located caudoventral to the base of the ear in the depression between the mandible and the mastoid process. TH-17 is the crossing point of the TH and GB Channels. GB-2 is located rostral to the intertragic notch and 1.5 *cun* caudoventral to SI-19 which is at the caudal aspect of the temporomandibular joint. GB-3 is in the depression at the caudal end of the temporomandibular joint, caudal to the masseter muscle, caudodorsal to the zygomatic arch and ST-7. GB-3 is the crossing point of the TH, GB, and ST Channels. GB-20 is on the dorsum of the neck, in the large depression just caudal and lateral to the occipital protuberance, medial to the cranial edge of the wings of the atlas. GB-20 is the crossing point of the GB and *Yang-wei* Channels. GV-21 is located on the dorsal midline at the level of the cranial edge of the ears. GV-20 is on the dorsal midline on a line drawn from the tips of the ears level with the ear canals. GV-20 is the crossing point of the GV and BL Channels. GV-17 is on the dorsal midline at the level of the caudal ear bases. GV-17 is the crossing point between the GV and BL Channels.(3.)

Other acupoints chosen to address deficiency issues were SI-3; LI-4; LU-7; BL-62; KID-6; *Bai-hui*; *Shen-shu*; BL-17; BL-19; BL-23, *Da-feng-men*, CV-12; LIV-3; GV3/ 4. SI-3 is the *Shu-stream* point for Wood, the Mother tonification point for deficiency patterns. It it also the Confluent point of the GV Channel. LI-4 is the Master point for the face and mouth. It is also the *Yuan*-source point. LU-7 is the Master point for the head and neck. It is also the *Luo*-connecting point of the LU Channel, and the Confluent point of the CV Channel. BL-62 is the Confluent point to the *Yang-qiao* Extraordinary Channel. KID-6 is the Confluent point with the *Yin-qiao* Extraordinary Channel. *Bai-hui* is the Classical point of a Hundred Crossings. *Shen-shu* is a tonification point for the Kidney Meridian. BL-17 is the Influential point for Blood. It is also the Back-*shu* Association point for blood deficiency and *Yin* deficiency. BL-19 is the Back-*shu* Association point for Liver and Gallbladder Meridians. BL-23 is the Back-*shu* Association point for the Kidney Meridian. *Da-feng-men* is the Classical point titled the Great Wind Gate which can help vertigo. CV-12 is the Influential point for *Fu* organs, and it is the crossing point of the CV, SI, TH and ST Channels. LIV-3 is the *Shu*-stream point or third level, and it is also the *Yuan*-source point for the Liver Meridian. GV-3 and GV-4 help to tonify the Kidney Meridian.[3]

The Chinese herbal formulas *Jia Wei Xiao Yao Wan* (Free and Easy Wanderer Plus) and Stasis in Mansion of Mind were prescribed. *Jia Wei Xiao Yao Wan* (Free and Easy Wanderer Plus) tea pills were dosed at two teapills twice a day to support the liver.[4] Stasis in

Mansion of Mind was given to treat the local Qi-Blood Stagnation of the vestibular apparatus. The dose was one .5 gram capsule twice a day.[5]

Table 1: Ingredients of the Chinese herbal formula *Jia Wei Xiao Yao Wan* and their actions

English Name	Chinese *Pin Yin*	Action
Paeonia	*Jiu chao bai*	Sooth liver
Poria	*Fu ling*	Strengthen Spleen; Drain the Damp
Atractylodes	*Bai zhu*	Dry up Damp; Strengthen Spleen
Moutan	*Mu dan pi*	Cool Liver
Gardenia	*Zhi zi*	Clear Heat
Bupleurum	*Chai hu*	Soothe Liver
Angelica	*Dang gui*	Move Blood
Zingiberis	*Sheng jiang*	Warm the middle
Glycyrrhiza	*Gan cao*	Harmonize
Mentha	*Bo he*	Dispel Wind-Heat

Manufacturer - Mayway Corp, Oakland, CA

Table 2: Ingredients of the Chinese herbal formula Stasis in Mansion of Mind and their actions

English Name	Chinese *Pin Yin*	Actions
Angelica	*Bai zhi*	Warm the Channel, relieve pain
Pinellia	*Ban xia*	Transform Phlegm
Ligusticum	*Chuan xiong*	Move Blood
Salvia	*Dan shen*	Move Blood
Lumbricus	*Di long*	Clear Wind, invigorate Channel
Ligusticum	*Gao ben*	Relieve pain
Pueraria	*Ge gen*	Bring *Qi* upward
Carthamus	*Hong hua*	Break down Blood Stasis
Bombyx	*Jiang can*	Transform phlegm, resolve nodule
Buthus	*Quan xie*	Break down Blood Stasis
Cimicifuga	*Sheng ma*	Ascend *Qi*
Scolopendra	*Wu gong*	Detoxify, resolve nodule
Fritillaria	*Zhe bei mu*	Transform Phlegm, resolve nodule

Manufacturer Jing Tang Herbal, Inc., Reddick, FL

Food Therapy to promote better homeostasis and nutrition was also implemented. Initially, for one month he was fed 1/3 cup of his dry kibble in the morning only. His afternoon meal consisted of lightly steamed ground turkey, so as to leave it rare, mixed with green veggies i.e. chopped green beans, chopped spinach, chopped kale, broccoli, or asparagus. These were combined in a 50:50 ratio of meat to veggies. Bio-Preparation, a complete nutritional supplement, was given once a day to provide vitamins, minerals, essential amino acids, and essential fatty acids. He was also supplemented with Iosol Drops at 1-2 drops once a day in his afternoon meal. Blood tonics were fed every other day in small amounts like treats. A raw egg was mixed with his afternoon meal twice a week. Sardines packed in water were fed once a week. After one month, the morning dry kibble meal was eliminated. Wet canned food was fed avoiding Lamb, Chicken, or Venison. The Lamb and Venison were too hot energetically in this case, and the Chicken which goes into the pet food industry is too contaminated with antibiotics, causing further Liver *Qi* Stagnation.[6]

Followup Treatments

Treatments were performed at two week intervals for the first six treatments utilizing all the points prescribed. In order to treat the patient with the local points selected, he was sedated using 0.1 mL by intramuscular injection of a combination of Xylazine and Ketamine mixed 1 part to 2 parts respectively. Dry needle acupuncture was performed for the first two treatments. Electro-acupuncture was introduced at the third treatment session. The electrodes were paired between GB-2 and GB-20 bilaterally; BL-17 bilaterally; and *Shen-shu* bilaterally. The settings were pulsed at 20 Hz for 10 minutes; then, changed to 80/ 120 Hz for 10 minutes. The Chinese herbals and Food Therapy were continued as prescribed. Two weeks later, the fourth acupuncture session, electro-acupuncture was again performed along with the dry needle acupuncture. The electrodes were paired at GV-20 and GV-17; between GB-2 and GB-20 bilaterally; and at BL-23. The owner reported that Mosey was more energetic, had a good appetite, and he was tracking straight when walking (no more circling), and at times his head tilt was better. Two weeks later at the fifth acupuncture session, electro-acupuncture was performed along with the dry needle acupuncture. The leads were paired at GB-2, and between TH-17 and TH-21 bilaterally. The owner's report was similar to the previous treatment session, with the added comment that the head tilt was better for longer periods of time. Two weeks later at the sixth treatment session, electro-acupuncture was performed along with dry needle acupuncture. The leads were paired between TH-17 and TH-21 on the left side only, and between GB-2 and GB-3 on the left side only. The owner reported that the patient's head tilt was resolved approximately 50% of the time. He also noted that his head tilt was always better on his walks. The next two acupuncture sessions were performed at one month intervals. Electro-acupuncture was again performed along with dry needle acupuncture. The leads were paired at GB-2; between TH-17 and TH-21 bilaterally; and between GV-20 and GV-17. One month later no electro-acupuncture was performed. Aqua-acupuncture was performed along with the dry needle acupuncture. Vitamin B-12 (1000 mcg per mL) was injected using a 25 gauge needle at GV-20, GV-22, GV-14, and TH-21 bilaterally; GB-2 bilaterally; and BL-62 bilaterally. The owner reported that the patient's head tilt was 95% resolved the majority of the time. Two months later the patient was again treated in similar manner to the previous session. Four months later, Mosey was treated with dry needle acupuncture at GV-21/ 20/ 17; TH-21/ 20/ 17; GB-2/ 8; *An-shen*; and LI-11 bilaterally. He continued to take the Chinese herbals for three more months at which time they were discontinued. Mosey continues to do well with only his Food Therapy.

References:
1. Xie H. TCVM Clinical Approach/ Herbology: Liver and Endocrinology Module. Liver Physiology and Pathology. Reddick, FL:Chi Institute of Chinese Medicine. 2006:17-19.
2. Xie H. E-mail [AATCVM] Vestibular Disease. December 23, 2009.
3. Xie H, Preast V. Xie's Veterinary Acupuncture. Ames, IA: Blackwell Publishing 2007: 129-204.

4. Wrinkle A, Stropes L & Potts T. A Practitioner's Formula Guide. Oakland, CA: Elemental Essentials Press 2008:42.
5. Xie H Chinese Veterinary Herbal Handbook 2nd edition. Reddick, FL:Chi Institute of Chinese Medicine. 2008:156.
6. Xie H. Veterinary Food Therapy Training Program. Reddick, FL:Chi Institute of Chinese Medicine. 2007.

TCVM Treatment of Severe Canine Geriatric Vestibular Disease

Margaret Fowler, DVM, CVA, CVCH, CVTP, CVFT

Canine Geriatric Vestibular Disease is an acute nonprogressive disturbance of the peripheral vestibular system in dogs typically 8 years of age or older. The specific cause is unknown but is suspected to be an abnormal flow of fluid in the semicircular canals of the inner ear or an inflammation of the vestibulocochlear nerve (cranial nerve VIII). It is marked by a sudden onset of imbalance, disorientation, reluctance to stand, and possibly nausea. Clinical signs include a head tilt toward the side of the lesion, nystagmus, and ataxia with a tendency to lean or fall in the direction of the head tilt. Although dogs tend to return to normal with little treatment within 2-3 weeks, severe cases may require hospitalization, fluid support, physical rehabilitative therapy, and some may be left with a residual head tilt. [1]

Background:

A blind 11.5 year old male Boston Terrier was seen at an emergency clinic for an acute onset of a severe head tilt to the right, marked disorientation, severe ataxia and inability to stand or walk. Bloodwork was within normal limits except for an elevated alkaline phosphatase and no abnormalities were noted in the outer ears or tympanic membranes. A presumptive diagnosis of geriatric vestibular disease was made and conservative treatment was initiated with anti-histamines and antibiotics. After 2 weeks of no improvement, the owner sought treatment at the University of Florida Acupuncture Department where the dog was treated with TCVM including dry needle and electro-acupuncture, aquapuncture, and the TCVM herbal formulas Stasis in the Mansion of Mind and *Yi Lin Gai Cuo* (*Bu Yang Huan Wu*), both manufactured by Jing Tang Herbal. The dog showed some improvement after the treatment and was instructed to follow-up with additional acupuncture sessions. After returning home, the owner sought treatment with another TCVM veterinarian one week later. The treatment was limited to aquapuncture which was not well received by the dog. The owner then sought another session with Acupuncture and Holistic Veterinary Services of NW Florida.

TCVM Evaluation:

On presentation one week later (4 weeks after the onset), the Boston Terrier still could not stand or walk without assistance and had a severe head tilt to the right. A TCVM evaluation revealed a Wood personality, a purple tongue, normal temperature, mildly decreased *Shen*, weak rear leg pulses, and muscle atrophy in the rear legs.

TCVM Patterns:

Two TCVM patterns were identified. The first was local *Qi* Stagnation of the head as evidenced by the purple tongue, severe head tilt and vestibular dysfunction, and decrease in *Shen*. The second pattern was one of Kidney and Spleen *Qi* Deficiency as evidenced by the inability to stand or walk, weak pulses, rear leg weakness and muscle atrophy. In TCVM, the Kidney controls the rear legs, opens in the ears and dominates the marrow including the brain; the Spleen controls the muscles. [2]

Treatment Strategies:

The treatment strategies were to resolve the *Qi* Stagnation of the head thereby decreasing vestibular disease signs and to tonify the Kidney and Spleen *Qi* Deficiency thereby improving ear and brain function, movement ability and muscle tone.

Treatment:

To accomplish these goals, the dog was continued on Stasis in the Mansion of Mind for an additional for 6 months which is designed to break down stagnation in the head area, and *Yi Lin Gai Cuo* (*Bu Yang Huan Wu*) for 3 months which is designed to tonify *Qi* and rear weakness especially in cases of ataxia. As the weather warmed into the Florida spring, the *Qi* deficiency improved, the dog's tongue changed to a dark pink reddish color, his pulses became fast and thin, and he started panting excessively. His Kidney *Qi* Deficiency had shifted to a Kidney *Qi* and *Yin* Deficiency, so *Yi Lin Gai* Cuo (*Bu Yang Huan Wu*) was replaced with *Bu Qi Zi Yin Tang* (Hindquarter Weakness) manufactured by Jing Tang Herbal for 3 months which is better designed for the Kidney *Yin* Deficiency and rear end weakness. [3]

Aquapuncture was avoided due to the objection of the dog, so dry needle and electro-acupuncture were used in 4 sessions over 2 months. Points were chosen from the following list: KID-1 (powerful rear Root point for rear weakness), KID-3 and BL-23 (Kidney Source point and Kidney Association point to tonify Kidney *Qi*), LIV-3 (Liver Source point to support Wood constitution and one of Four Gate points to move stagnated *Qi*), LI-4 (Four Gate Point to move stagnated *Qi*), SI-3 and BL-62 (ataxia, confluent points of GV Meridian), BL-20 and SP-3 (Spleen Association point and Source point to tonify Spleen *Qi*), *Tian-Men* (dizziness, relaxation effect), GV-20 (relaxation effect, *Shen* disturbance), *Nao-Shu* (Brain Association point, Spleen Deficiency, Shen disturbance), GB-20 and TH-17 (proximity to inner ear), ST-36 (general and Earth element *Qi* tonification) [4], and scalp points along the motor function line . Generally points were paired in the following combinations for electro-acupuncture: ST-36 + KID-1, SI-3 + BL-62, GB-20 +TH-17, scalp points + scalp points, and BL-20 + BL-23, stimulating 10 minutes at 20 hertz and 10 minutes at 80 + 120 hertz. Points were rotated in different sessions to avoid point exhaustion.

Tui-na was prescribed for the owner to do for 15 minutes on a daily basis at home at the following areas: stroking on the facial midline from *Da-feng-men* to *Tian-men* (for relaxation and shen issues), and along the scalp motor lines, and *Ca-fa* (rubbing) at KID-1 and GB-20.

Table 1. Ingredients and Actions of Stasis in the Mansion of Mind

English Name	Chinese *Pin-Yin*	Actions
Angelica	*Bai Zhi*	Warm the Channel, relieve pain
Pinellia	*Ban Xia*	Transform Phlegm
Ligusticum	*Chuan Xiong*	Move Blood
Salvia	*Dan Shen*	Move Blood
Lumbricus	*Di Long*	Clear Wind, invigorate Channel
Ligusticum	*Gao Ben*	Relieve pain
Pueraria	*Ge Gen*	Bring *Qi* upward
Carthamus	*Hong Hua*	Break down Blood Stasis
Bombyx	*Jiang Can*	Transform Phlegm, resolve nodules
Scorpion	*Quan Xie*	Break down Blood Stasis
Cimicifuga	*Sheng Ma*	Ascend *Qi*

| Scolopendra | *Wu Gong* | Detoxify, resolve nodules |
| Fritillary | *Zhe Bei Mu* | Transform Phlegm, resolve nodules |

Manufactured by Jing Tang Herbal

Table 2. Ingredients and Actions of *Yi Lin Gai Cuo* (*Bu Yang Huan Wu*)

English Name	Chinese *Pin-Yin*	Actions
Astragalus	*Huang Qi*	Warm and tonify *Qi*
Angelica	*Dang Gui*	Nourish Blood
Paoenia	*Bai Shao*	Nourish Blood and *Yin*, soothe Liver *Yang*
Earthworm	*Di Long*	Beak Blood stagnation
Ligusticum	*Chuan Xiong*	Activate Blood and relieve pain
Carthamus	*Hong Hua*	Break Blood Stasis and relieve pain
Persica	*Tao Ren*	Break Stasis and relieve pain

Manufactured by Jing Tang Herbal

Table 3. Ingredients and Actions of *Bu Qi Zi Yin Tang* (Hindquarter Weakness)

English Name	Chinese *Pin-Yin*	Actions
Eucommia	*Du Zhong*	Tonify Kidney and strengthen back
Achyranthes	*Niu Xi*	Tonify Kidney and strengthen the hind limbs
Lindera	*Wu Yao*	Move *Qi* and relieve pain
Astragalus	*Huang Qi*	Tonify *Qi*
Apis	*Feng Hua Fen*	Tonify *Qi* and *Yin*
Morinda	*Ba Ji Tian*	Warm and strengthen the back
Angelica	*Dang Gui*	Nourish Blood
Rehmannia	*Shu Di Huang*	Nourish *Yin* and *Jing*
Cinnamon	*Gui Zhi*	Warm the Channels and benefit the limbs

Manufactured by Jing Tang Herbal

Outcome:

The dog was cooperative at the first session and his coordination improved significantly by the time of the next session 10 days later. At this time he was able to stand and walk with difficulty but without assistance. His Shen improved also and unfortunately this meant a stronger, less cooperative and somewhat aggressive Wood personality, necessitating a muzzle. Over the remaining 3 sessions, the dog's ataxia, head tilt, muscle atrophy and walking continued to improve and his owners' were very pleased with the outcome. After the 4th and final session, he was walking nearly normal and only had a mild residual head tilt. A follow up phone call 9 months later, revealed the Boston Terrier was still doing well and ambulating well on his own but was left with a permanent mild head tilt.

Conclusion:

Although most cases of Geriatric Vestibular Disease typically recover within a few days to 3 weeks with no treatment, this dog's severe case showed no indication of improving until TCVM therapy was aggressively pursued. It is unlikely this old dog would have recovered as well as he did without acupuncture, *Tui-na* and TCVM herbal therapy, despite his difficult personality.

References:
1. Tilley, Larry, DVM and Smith, Francis, DVM. The Five Minute Veterinary Consult, Canine and Feline, 3rd Edition. Lippincott Williams and Wilkins, 2004, pg 1350-1351.
2. Xie, Huisheng, DVM. The North American Veterinary Conference Post Graduate Institute, Acupuncture Class Notes. Chi Institute of Chinese Medicine, 2005, pg 154-162.
3. Xie, Huisheng, DVM and Preast, Vanessa, DVM, and Liu, Wen, PhD. Chinese Veterinary Herbal Handbook, 2nd Edition. Chi Institute of Chinese Medicine, 2008, pg 156, 85, 86.
4. Xie, Huisheng, DVM. The North American Veterinary Conference Post Graduate Institute, Acupuncture Class Notes. Chi Institute of Chinese Medicine, 2008, pg 135-142.

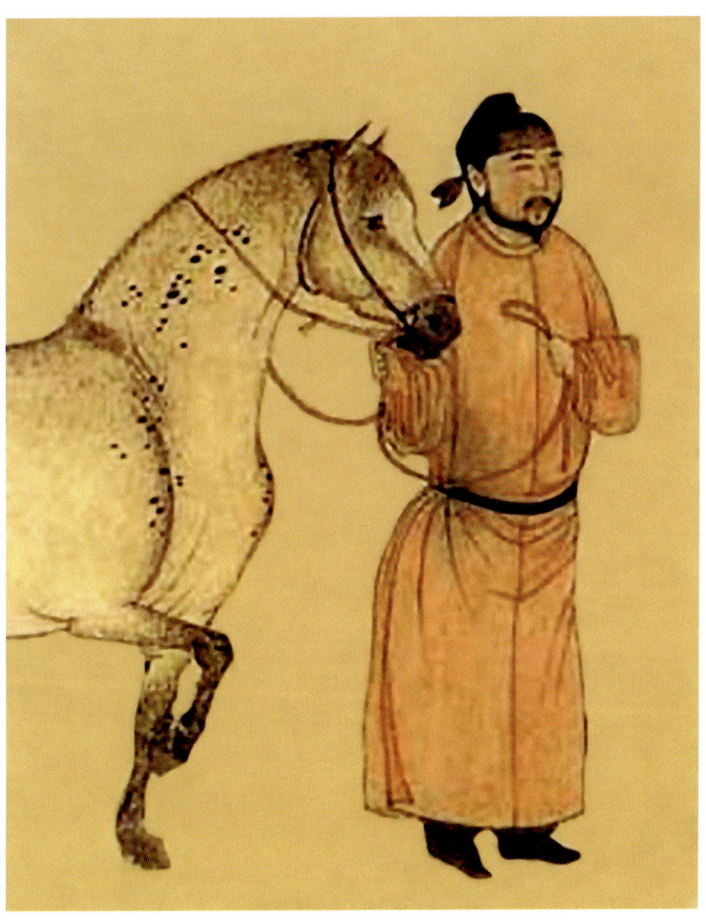

ZHAO FU 造父

Zhao Fu started veterinary acupuncture during the *Zhou-mu-gong* period (947 to 848 BCE.). For example, historical books indicated that he used hemo-acupuncture at *Jing-mai* to treat diseases in horses. He was the chief personnel and veterinarian who took care of the Emperor's and Royal horses. *Shi Ji* (The *Records of the Grand Historian*), the first systematic Chinese historical text written by Sima Qian from 109 BCE to 91 BCE, states that "Zhao Fu is an expert of horses…..Once upon a time, the King Zhou-mu-gong went to the west to hunt and forgot to return to the palace. Prince Xu tried to assassinate the King. Zhao Fu rescued the King with a cart with fast horses. After running 1,000 Chinese miles (approximately 312 American miles) in one day, Zhao Fu was able to bring the King back to the palace. Thereafter, the King built a city and named it Zhao to award his successful assassination rescue." Other ancient texts including *Si Mu An Ji Ji* (Simu's Collection of Equine Medicine) written during the *Tang* dynasty (618-907 CE) recorded the medical care of horses conducted by Zhao Fu.

Professor Yu Chuan (1924-2005), the most important figure in modern TCVM history, believed that there is enough historical evidence and written documents to verify Zhao Fu as the first veterinarian of China. Even though Ma Shi Huang in the Huang Di Period (2,696 BCE to 2,598 BCE) appeared to be the earliest veterinarian according to the mythological texts, these stories are too shrouded by legend to be validated with historical evidence.

CHAPTER 4

Spinal Cord Disorders

Spinal Cord Disorders

Cheryl L Chrisman DVM, MS, EdS, DACVIM-Neurology, CVA

The most common conventional spinal cord disorders that a TCVM practitioner will be asked to treat are: 1) intervertebral disc disease, 2) spinal cord trauma from external causes, 3) cervical spondylomyelopathy ("wobbler" syndrome) 4) fibrocartilaginous embolism (spinal cord infarction), 5) pain from diskospondylitis and 6) degenerative myelopathy.[1-6] Other less common spinal cord disorders that might be treated with TCVM are 1) atlantoaxial malformation 2) meningomyelitis and 3) neoplasia. Dogs with focal spinal cord lesions have normal mentation, head coordination and posture and cranial nerves. On occasion, with cervical fibrocartilaginous embolism and spinal cord tumors, ptosis, miosis and enophthalmos (Horner's syndrome) will be present on the side of the lesion.

Evaluation of the gait and the hemiwalking, wheelbarrowing, hopping and conscious proprioception tests help to localize a spinal cord lesion to the cervical or thoracolumbar area and determine the severity of the signs. The severity of neurological deficits may be graded from 1-5 (1= mildest and 5= most severe) based on the neurological examination findings as follows:

1. Grade 1= Neck or back pain and no other deficits
2. Grade 2= Ataxia in all four limbs or pelvic limbs with or without conscious proprioceptive deficits and hemiparesis, quadriparesis or paraparesis with ambulation spared
3. Grade 3= Non-ambulatory hemiparesis, quadriparesis or paraparesis with or without urinary or fecal incontinence; may or not have a reduced or absent cutaneous trunci responses
4. Grade 4= Quadriplegia and paraplegia (no voluntary movement) with preserved deep pain sensation and typically have fecal and urinary incontinence and reduced or absent cutaneous trunci responses
5. Grade 5= Quadriplegia with no deep pain (rare as they usually die from respiratory paralysis) and paraplegia with no deep pain sensation

Paresis is defined as varying degrees of weakness with preservation of some voluntary movements. Voluntary movements should not be confused with the movements observed during reflex testing, as these movements are involuntary and may still be present even when the spinal cord is severed.[1-3] The term "plegia" means paralysis or total loss of voluntary movement (Grade 4 or 5), but depending on the lesion location, the spinal reflexes may still be spared. Squeezing the digital bones with hemostatic forceps, until the animal cries, growls or provides some behavioral response, tests the deep pain response. Withdrawal of the limb is only a reflex and does not indicate that the animal has deep pain. It is best to pinch the digit strongly with hemostatic forceps and test all toes and then if no response is elicited, deep pain is truly absent. Pinching digits or webbing with the fingers is not enough stimuli to test deep pain. Insertion of an acupuncture needle at KID-1 or *Liu-feng* (three acupoints on each foot, between the digits through the webbing just dorsal to each metatarsophalangeal or metacarpophalangeal joint) is not enough stimulation to effectively test deep pain to differentiate between a Grade 4 and 5 spinal cord lesion. The periosteum of the digits has a much higher concentration of small unmyelinated C-fibers that carry the sensation of deep pain, compared to the skin and subdermal structures of the digital webbing, so the periosteum must be stimulated to accurately test deep pain.[1,2] Loss of deep pain means the spinal cord lesion is severe, but is not hopeless and over 50% of these dogs recover, if treated appropriately.[2,3]

Focal pain, spinal cord reflexes and the cutaneous trunci muscle responses are the evaluations useful to localize spinal cord lesions. Neck and back pain localize the lesion to the painful site. Spinal reflexes of the cervical region involve five large spinal cord segments and most mild compressive lesions from intervertebral disk disease or "wobbler" syndrome are not long enough to affect all the segments to cause loss of the thoracic limb flexor (withdrawal) reflex. The flexor reflex is the most reliable reflex in the cervical region. A cervical fibrocartilaginous embolism may cause hemiplegia and loss of the thoracic limb flexor reflex on the affected side, because the lesion can involve all the segments associated with the reflex (Table 1). Usually there will be Horner's syndrome of the eye on that side as well, especially in C6-T2 lesions, where both 1st order and 2nd order sympathetic neurons can be affected. Spinal cord lesions between T3-L3 will have normal to hyperactive pelvic limb reflexes, even though they may have Grade 3-5 severity of deficits (Table 1). Focal lesions at L4-5 will have a depressed or absent patellar reflex, but the other reflexes will be normal. Focal lesions from L6-S2 will have a normal or slightly exaggerated patellar reflex (from loss of opposing muscle tone) (Table 1). The flexor, cranial tibial muscle and sciatic nerve reflexes will be depressed or absent with L6-S2 lesions. If the S1-S3 spinal cord segments or nerve roots are affected, then the anal reflex will be depressed or absent and there will be no tone on rectal palpation.

Table 1: Neurological signs, gait, tests of subtle dysfunction and spinal cord reflex and sensation changes with lesions of the spinal cord and cauda equina nerve roots[1-3]

Lesion Location	Neurological Signs	Gait Coordination and Strength	Tests of Subtle Limb Dysfunction*	Spinal Cord Reflexes and Sensation
Spinal Cord C1- C5 Vertebrae C1- C4 -dog	+/- Horner's syndrome Normal brain and cranial nerves, fecal and/or urinary incontinence, +/- neck pain	Ataxia, hemiparesis, paraparesis, quadriparesis, quadriplegia (respiratory paralysis)	Normal, decreased or absent in one or more limbs	Normal or increased reflexes in all four limbs
Spinal Cord C6-T2 Vertebrae C5-T2 dog	+/- Horner's syndrome Normal brain and cranial nerves, fecal and/or urinary incontinence, +/- neck pain, atrophy of scapular muscles,	Ataxia, hemiparesis, paraparesis, quadriparesis, quadriplegia (respiratory paralysis)	Normal, decreased or absent in one or more limbs	Normal, decreased or absent reflexes in thoracic limbs, normal or increased reflexes in pelvic limbs

Spinal Cord T3-L3 Vertebrae T3-L2 dog	Normal brain and cranial nerves and thoracic limbs, fecal and urinary incontinence, +/- back pain	Pelvic limb ataxia, paraparesis/ paraplegia	Normal thoracic limbs, decreased or absent in one or both pelvic limbs	Normal reflexes in thoracic limbs, normal or increased reflexes in pelvic limbs, depressed or absent cutaneous trunci response from lesion site caudally, +/- deep pain
Spinal Cord and cauda equina nerve roots L4-S2 Vertebrae L3- L7 dog	Normal brain and cranial nerves and thoracic limbs, fecal and urinary incontinence, pelvic limb muscle atrophy, +/- back pain	Pelvic limb ataxia, paraparesis/ paraplegia	Normal thoracic limbs, decreased or absent in one or both pelvic limbs	Normal reflexes in thoracic limbs
				Decreased or absent patellar reflex with lesions at L4-5 (vertebrae L3-5)
				Decreased or absent flexor, gastrocnemius, and cranial tibial reflexes with lesions at L6-S2 (vertebrae L5-7)
				Decreased or absent anal reflex with lesions at S1-3 (vertebrae L5-S3)
				+/- deep pain
Cauda Equina nerve roots S1-Cd5 Vertebrae L5-S3 dog	Normal brain and cranial nerves and thoracic and pelvic limbs, mild pelvic limb ataxia and mild paraparesis, tail paralysis, fecal and urinary incontinence +/- sacrocaudal pain	Normal or may have mild pelvic limb ataxia or paresis	Normal thoracic and pelvic limbs or slightly decreased in one or both pelvic limbs	Normal reflexes in thoracic and pelvic limbs, decreased/absent anal reflex with S1-3 (vertebrae L5-S3) lesions, decreased or absent tail reflex with lesions at Cd1-5 (vertebrae L6-Cd)

*Tests of subtle dysfunction = hemistanding, hemiwalking, wheelbarrowing, hopping and conscious proprioception; May have one or more clinical signs; Clinical signs are always on the same side as the lesion; Horner's syndrome= ptosis, miosis, enophthalmos due to loss of sympathetic innervation to the eye

From a TCVM perspective, most spinal cord disorders cause focal *Qi* Stagnation with or without Blood Stagnation and if weakness is present there is *Qi* Deficiency in the spinal cord causing paresis or paralysis caudal to the lesion. In other disorders there is also an underlying Kidney Deficiency. An overview of the TCVM patterns and diagnosis of the most common spinal cord disorders is outlined in Table 2.[4-8] Acute spinal cord lesions causing Grade 3-5 deficits (non-ambulatory) always have some Blood Stagnation and often have edema as well. When the neurological deficits are Grades 2-5 (paresis or paralysis), *Qi* Deficiency is present as well.

Table 2: Conventional diagnoses of spinal cord disorders and the associated TCVM patterns and examination findings[4-8]

Conventional Diagnosis	TCVM Patterns	Clinical Findings Grade of Deficits**	Tongue	Pulse
Degenerative Intervertebral Disk Disease	Wind-Cold-Damp Invasion with External *Qi*/Blood Stagnation	Grade 1 Acute neck or back pain No paresis or paralysis	Purple	Superficial, strong, slow, wiry
	Kidney *Yin* Deficiency with External *Qi*/Blood Stagnation	Grade 1 Acute neck or back pain No paresis or paralysis Panting Cool seeking Warm ears, back, feet Dry skin	Reddish purple, dry	Deep, weak, worse on left, rapid, thready or wiry
	Kidney *Yang* Deficiency with External *Qi*/Blood Stagnation	Grade 1 Acute neck or back pain No paresis or paralysis Heat seeking Cold ears, back, feet	Purple	Deep, weak, worse on right or wiry
	Spinal cord *Qi*/Blood Stagnation with Kidney *Qi* Deficiency	Grades 2-5 deficits Acute or chronic Paresis or paralysis +/- Neck or back pain	Pale purple, wet	Deep, weak worse on right or wiry
	Spinal cord *Qi*/Blood Stagnation with Kidney *Yang* Deficiency	Grades 2-5 deficits Acute or chronic Paresis or paralysis +/- Neck or back pain Heat seeking Cold ears, back, feet	Pale purple, wet	Deep, weak (weaker on right), slow, may be wiry
	Spinal cord *Qi*/Blood Stagnation with Kidney *Yin* and *Qi* Deficiencies	Grades 2-5 deficits Acute or chronic Paresis or paralysis +/- Neck or back pain Panting	Pale or red, purple, wet or dry, cracked (chronic)	Deep, weak, may be on both sides, rapid, thready, may be wiry

		Cool seeking Warm ears, back, feet Dry skin		
	Spinal cord *Qi*/Blood Stagnation with Kidney *Yin* and *Yang* Deficiencies	Grades 2-5 deficits Acute or chronic Paresis or paralysis +/- Neck or back pain back pain Seeks Heat or Cold May or nor pant Warm or Cold ears, back, feet May be Warm in front and Cold in back	Pale, red or purple, wet or dry	Deep, weak pulses on both sides, may be rapid or slow or wiry
Spinal Cord Trauma (accidents and falls)	Spinal cord *Qi*/Blood Stagnation and Kidney *Qi* Deficiency	History or evidence of trauma Acute non-progressive paresis or paralysis Grades 2-5 deficits	Pale, purple	Wiry or weak
Cervical Spondylomyelopathy (Wobbler syndrome)	Spinal cord *Qi*/Blood Stagnation and Kidney *Jing* and *Qi* Deficiencies	Great Danes and other large breed dogs Young dogs < 5 years old Chronic progressive ataxia, quadriparesis or quadriplegia (Grades 2-4) May or not have neck pain	Pale, purple wet, swollen	Deep, weak bilaterally or wiry
	Spinal cord *Qi*/Blood Stagnation and Kidney *Qi* Deficiency	Doberman Pinschers and other large breed dogs Older dogs > 5years Chronic progressive ataxia, quadriparesis or quadriplegia (Grades 2-5) May or not have neck pain	Pale, purple wet	Deep, weak worse on right or wiry

	Spinal cord *Qi*/Blood Stagnation and Kidney *Yang* Deficiency	Doberman Pinschers and other large breed dogs Older dogs > 5years Chronic progressive ataxia, quadriparesis or quadriplegia (Grades 2-5) May or not have neck pain Heat seeking Cold ears, back and toes	Pale, purple, wet or swollen	Deep, slow, weak worse on right or wiry
	Spinal cord *Qi*/Blood Stagnation and Kidney *Yin* and *Qi* Deficiencies	Doberman Pinschers and other large breed dogs Older dogs > 5years Chronic progressive ataxia, quadriparesis or quadriplegia (Grades 2-5) May or not have neck pain Panting Cool seeking Warm ears, back, feet Dry skin	Pale or red, purple, wet or dry, cracked (chronic)	Deep, weak both sides, rapid, thready, may be wiry
	Spinal cord *Qi*/Blood Stagnation and Kidney *Yin* and *Yang* Deficiencies	Doberman Pinschers and other large breed dogs Older dogs > 5years Chronic progressive ataxia, quadriparesis or quadriplegia (Grades 2-5) May or not have neck pain Seeks Heat or Cold May or nor pant Warm or Cold ears, back, feet May be Warm in front and Cold in back	Pale purple and wet or reddish purple, dry and cracked or a combination of these	Deep, weak on both sides or wiry
Fibrocartilaginous Embolism	Spinal cord *Qi*/Blood Stagnation and	Grades 3-5 deficits Acute non-progressive	Purple, pale, purple, wet	Wiry (acute), deep, weak (later) worse on

	Kidney *Qi* Deficiency	hemiparesis, asymmetrical paraparesis or paraplegia		the right
Diskospondylitis	Damp Heat in the vertebrae and disks (Heat Toxin)	Grades 1-4 deficits Severe neck or back pain May have fever Panting Cool seeking Warm ears, back and feet Anorexia	Red, yellow coating, dry	Superficial, strong, forceful, rapid and wiry
Degenerative Myelopathy	Kidney *Jing*, Spleen *Qi* and Kidney *Qi* Deficiencies	German shepherds Boxers, Welsh Corgis 5 years of age or older Grades 2-4 deficits Chronic progressive paraparesis	Pale, wet	Deep, weak, weaker on right
	Kidney *Jing*, Spleen *Qi* and Kidney *Yang* Deficiencies	German shepherds Boxers, Welsh Corgis 5 years of age or older Grades 2-4 deficits Chronic progressive paraparesis Heat Seeking Cold ears, back and feet	Pale or purple, wet or swollen	Deep, slow, weak, weaker on right
	Kidney *Jing*, Spleen *Qi*, Kidney *Qi* and Kidney/Liver *Yin* Deficiencies	German shepherds Boxers, Welsh Corgis 5 years of age or older Grades 2-4 deficits Chronic progressive Cool Seeking Panting Warm ears, back, feet	Pale or red, dry, cracked	Deep, rapid, thready, weak on both sides or weaker on the left

	Kidney *Jing*, Spleen *Qi*, Kidney *Yang* and Kidney/Liver *Yin* Deficiencies	German shepherds Boxers, Welsh Corgis 5 years of age or older Grades 2-4 deficits Chronic progressive paraparesis Seeks Heat or Cold May or not pant Warm or Cold ears, back, feet May be Warm in front and Cold in back	Red, dry, cracked or pale purple and wet	Deep, weak both sides
Atlantoaxial malformation	Spinal cord *Qi*/Blood Stagnation and Kidney *Jing* and *Qi* Deficiencies	Acute neck pain (Grade 1) May or not have Grade 2-5 neurological deficits Acute, chronic progressive Toy breed dogs	Pale, purple	Deep, weak or wiry
Meningitis Meningomyelitis	Damp-Heat of the Spinal Cord with *Qi*/Blood Stagnation and Kidney *Qi* Deficiency	Acute neck pain (Grade 1) May or not have Grade 2-5 neurological deficits May or not have fever Panting Warm ears, back, feet	Red, dry	Strong, forceful, rapid, wiry if painful
Spinal cord tumor	Spinal cord Phlegm	Acute neck pain (Grade 1) May or not have Grade 2-5 neurological deficits Types: Primary spinal cord tumors and non-blood related metastatic tumors	Pale with white greasy coating, purple if painful	Slippery, wiry if painful
	Spinal cord Blood Stagnation	Acute neck pain (Grade 1) May or not have	Purple	Wiry

| | | Grade 1-5 neurological deficits Types: Lymphoma, hemangiosarcoma and other blood related metastatic tumors | | |

The conventional diagnosis is often known or strongly suspected; Severity of neurological deficits: Grade 1= Neck or back pain and no other deficits, Grade 2= Ataxia in all four limbs with or without mild hemiparesis, quadriparesis or paraparesis; Grade 3= Non-ambulatory hemiparesis, quadriparesis or paraparesis; Grade 4= Quadriplegia and paraplegia with preserved deep pain sensation, Grade 5= Quadriplegia or paraplegia with no deep pain sensation

INTEGRATED TREATMENT OF ACUTE PARALYSIS

There are several interesting clinical and experimental studies supporting the use of EA for the treatment of acute paralysis from intervertebral disk herniation or external trauma.[9-16] A secondary progressive neurodegenerative process occurs within the first 72 hours, following acute spinal cord trauma.[10,11] Inhibition of this secondary process improves the chances of recovery and has been the focus of research attention for many decades. The benefits and mechanisms of EA to reduce neuronal and glial cell death and axonal loss and improve functional recovery have been demonstrated in many laboratory animal studies.[10,12]

Acute Grades 4 and 5 neurological deficits are considered an emergency and the animal should be evaluated and treated conventionally within 3 hours. If the animal is presented within 3 hours of the onset of signs, the current standard of care, based on human trials, is to administer methylprednisone sodium succinate (MPSS) intravenously in a bolus of 30 mg/kg followed by a constant rate infusion (CRI) of MPSS at 5.4 mg/kg/hr for 24 hours.[2,3] If the animal is presented between 3-8 hours of the onset of signs, the current standard of care, based on human trials, is to administer MPSS intravenously in a bolus of 30 mg/kg followed by a CRI of MPSS at 5.4 mg/kg/hr for 48 hours. High dose MPSS therapy is contraindicated, if it has been more than 8 hours after the onset of paresis or paralysis and for dogs with Grades 1-3 neurological deficits.

If MPSS is not indicated, because of the delay in treatment following injury or the grade of the neurological deficits, then a decreasing dose of oral prednisone is given (e.g. 0.5 mg/kg twice daily for 3 days, followed by 0.5 mg/kg once daily for 5 days and then 0.5 mg/kg every other day for 5 days).[2,13] To protect against adverse gastrointestinal side effects from the prednisone, oral famotidine (0.5-1 mg/kg every 12-24 hours) or ranitidine (2 mg/kg every 12 hours) for 5-7 days is also recommended.[2] Tramadol (2 mg/kg every 8 hours for 7 days) is usually administered for pain control.[13] Acupuncture and Chinese herbal medicine may be integrated with all these drugs. Surgery to decompress the spinal cord should be performed as soon as possible and ideally within 24 hours of onset.[2,3]

OVERVIEW OF TCVM TREATMENT FOR SPINAL CORD DISORDERS

There has been hesitancy by some TCVM practitioners to administer acupuncture, while an animal is receiving steroids, as it was feared that the steroids would reduce the acupuncture effects. Also some TCVM practitioners have thought acupuncture should not be administered to a patient with acute injury. Based on the results of the clinical studies on intervertebral disk disease in dogs, acupuncture can be combined with steroids and other medications and surgery and should be begun as soon as possible.[13-15] Experimental and clinical studies have shown that a combination of EA and DN enhances recovery.[10,12-16] The current clinical recommendation for EA is 10-15 minutes at 20 Hz constant frequency rate followed by 10-15 minutes at alternating frequencies between 80 and 120 Hz since most dogs have a combination of pain and paresis or paralysis.[5] Dry needles are left in position un-manipulated for 20-30 minutes. To perform Aqua-AP, 0.25-1 ml vitamin B12 is injected into the acupoint.

Acupoints on the Governing Vessel in the area of the incision for a dorsal decompression surgery and *Hua-tuo-jia-ji* and inner Bladder Channel acupoints on the side of a hemilaminectomy are avoided to reduce the possibility of wound contamination. The paravertebral musculature on the side of the hemilaminectomy, where the *Hua-tuo jia-ji* and inner Bladder Channel acupoints are located, is elevated and retracted to expose the bone and it is unknown whether these acupoints need time to recover after being physically traumatized during surgery. As well acupoints on the Conception Vessel in the area of the incision for ventral decompression in the cervical region are also avoided for the same reasons.

The acupuncture session can begin by inserting dry needles into GV-20 and *Bai-hui* to calm the animal and open the GV Channel that traverses directly above the spinal cord. The GV Channel along with the other Extraordinary Channels (Vessels) control, store and regulate the flow of *Qi* and Blood in the twelve regular Channels.[17] Because of its close proximity to the spinal cord and powerful effect on *Qi* and Blood flow, the GV Channel acupoints are very effective to treat the spinal cord *Qi*/Blood Stagnation associated with most spinal cord disorders. For EA of lesions between vertebrae C7-L5, at least one acupoint on the Governing Vessel above the lesion (e.g. GV-14) should be connected to one acupoint below the lesion (e.g. GV-4 or GV-3), based on the results of experimental spinal cord injuries studies in rats.[10,16] In one study in rats with a T10 lesion, EA at GV-6 and GV-9 was compared to EA at *Hua-tuo-jia-ji* lateral to the lesion at T10 and parameters of neuroprotection were measured.[16] The results indicated that EA of GV acupoints may result in greater neuroprotection than EA of *Hua-tuo-jia-ji* acupoints. There is also some research evidence that EA treatments should be bilateral and not just unilateral in paired Channels.[18] The acupoints, commonly selected to treat neck and back pain and spinal cord injuries from intervertebral disk herniation, external trauma and other spinal cord lesions with *Qi*/Blood Stagnation, are outlined in Table 3.[5] These acupoints are combined with acupoints to treat the underlying TCVM pattern outlined in Table 4.[5]

The number of acupoints selected and the frequency of treatment will vary with the condition and severity of neurological deficits in each patient. For Grade 4 and 5 neurological deficits, EA and DN should be administered every 1-3 days for 3-5 times, depending on the patient's response, then reduced to once every 1-2 weeks until ambulatory. For Grades 2 and 3, the acupuncture treatments may be weekly or every other week. The addition of Chinese herbal medicine may reduce the number and frequency of acupuncture treatments needed and will relieve pain and improve function even faster (Table 4).[7,8]

Table 3: The location, attributes, indications and actions of acupuncture points suggested to treat *Qi*/Blood Stagnation associated with spinal cord disorders[5]

\multicolumn{3}{c}{**Cervical Spinal Cord Lesions**}
Acupoint*	**Technique**	**Indications and Actions**
GB-20	EA connected to GB-21 on same side Treat both sides Aqua-AP	Cervical spinal cord lesions between C1-C7 *Qi*/Blood Stagnation Crossing point of the Gallbladder Channel and *Yang Wei* Extraordinary Channel
GB-21	EA connected to GB-20 on same side Treat both sides Aqua-AP	Cervical spinal cord lesions between C1-C7 *Qi*/Blood Stagnation
SI-16	EA connected to SI-9 on same side treat both sides Aqua-AP	Cervical spinal cord lesions between C1-C7 *Qi*/Blood Stagnation
SI-9	EA connected to SI-16 on same side; Treat both sides Aqua-AP	Cervical spinal cord lesions between C1-C7 *Qi*/Blood Stagnation
Jing-jia-ji	EA connected bilaterally or on one side	Cervical spinal cord lesions between C1-C7 *Qi*/Blood Stagnation
LU-7	Dry needle	Master point of the head and neck
\multicolumn{3}{c}{**Thoracolumbar Spinal Cord Lesions**}
Acupoint*	**Technique**	**Indications and Actions**
GV-14	EA connected to GV-4, GV-3 or *Bai-hui* Aqua-AP	Thoracolumbar spinal cord lesions between C7-L3 *Qi*/Blood Stagnation
GV-4	EA connected to GV-14	Thoracolumbar spinal cord lesions between C7-L3 *Qi*/Blood Stagnation
GV-3	EA connected to GV-14	Thoracolumbar spinal cord lesions between C7-L3 *Qi*/Blood Stagnation
Bai-hui	EA connected to GV-14	Thoracolumbar spinal cord lesions between C7-S-1 *Qi*/Blood Stagnation

KID-1	EA connected to a Back-*Shu* Association point (BL Channel) cranial to the spinal lesion	Thoracolumbar spinal cord lesions between C7-S1 *Qi*/Blood Stagnation
Hua-tuo-jia-ji	EA connected bilaterally or longitudinally above and below the lesion if surgery, can be in area of the lesion, if no surgery performed Aqua-AP	Thoracolumbar spinal cord lesions between C7-L3 *Qi*/Blood Stagnation
BL 11 through BL-28 (use as local acupoints)	EA connected bilaterally or longitudinally above and below the lesion if surgery, can be in area of the lesion if no surgery performed Aqua-AP	Thoracolumbar spinal cord lesions and nerve root lesions between T1-S1 *Qi*/Blood Stagnation
Liu-feng	EA connected bilaterally	Thoracolumbar spinal cord lesions between C7-S1 *Qi*/Blood Stagnation

Acupoints Added to Treat External Channel and Spinal Cord *Qi*/Blood Stagnation and other General Signs

Acupoint*	Technique	Indications and Actions
LIV-3	DN	*Qi*/Blood Stagnation, pelvic limb paresis or paralysis
LI-4	DN	Pair with LIV-3 contralaterally for generalized pain control
BL-60	DN	Generalized pain control; Can simultaneously treat KID-3 and support the Kidney and Marrow
BL-62	DN	Confluent point of the *Yang-Qiao* Extraordinary Channel for ataxia and weakness of all 4 limbs or only the pelvic limbs
BL-17	DN or EA (if not at an incision) For EA connect to the other BL-17 or another BL Channel acupoint Aqua-AP	Influential point for Blood Move *Qi* and Blood
LI-10	DN	Generalized or hind limb weakness, lameness or paresis or paralysis of thoracic limb
ST-36	DN	General *Qi* tonic, generalized weakness, hind limb weakness

BL-40	EA connected bilaterally or to BL-54 Treat both sides Aqua-AP	Paraparesis or paraplegia, Master point of the caudal back, urinary incontinence and pelvic limb paresis or paralysis
BL-54	EA connected to BL-40	Paraparesis or paraplegia
BL-39	DN, Aqua-AP	Urinary incontinence
CV-3	DN	Urinary incontinence
KID-10	DN	Dysuria
GV-1	DN	*Luo*-connecting point of the Governing Vessel, crossing point for GV, GB and KID Channels
PC-8	DN	Thoracic limb "root" acupoints; if non-ambulatory quadriparesis or quadriplegia; treat both sides
KID-1	DN	Pelvic limb "root" acupoints; if non-ambulatory quadriparesis/paraparesis or quadriplegia/paraplegia; treat both sides
GB-39	DN	Influential point for marrow to promote recovery of the spinal cord

*Combine with other acupoints for other TCVM patterns present (Table 3); The number of acupoints selected will vary with the patient and response to treatment; EA= electro-acupuncture; DN= dry needle acupuncture; Aqua-AP= aqua-acupuncture; Location of Classical acupoints: *Jing-jia-ji* (from C1-C7, above and below the lateral processes of the cervical vertebrae), *Bai-hui* (midline between L7-S1), *Hua-tuo-jia-ji* (between T1-L7, 0.5 *cun* lateral to dorsal spinous process of each vertebra), *Liu-feng* (through the webbing between the digits to metacarpal or metatarsal joint- 3 on each side)

Table 4: Conventional diagnosis, TCVM pattern and suggested acupuncture points to use in combination with acupoints from Table 3 and Chinese herbal medicine for spinal cord disorders[4-8]

Conventional Diagnosis	TCVM Patterns	Acupuncture Points and Technique	Chinese Herbal Medicine	Comments
Degenerative Intervertebral Disk Disease	Wind-Cold-Damp Invasion with External *Qi*/Blood Stagnation	Acupoints for EA and DN from Table 3 plus DN of BL-10 and moxibustion at GV-3 and GV-4	Double P II If neck pain, add Cervical formula	Use herbal formulae as needed up to 4 months
	Kidney *Yin* Deficiency with External *Qi*/Blood Stagnation	Acupoints for EA and DN from Table 3 plus BL-23, KID-3/BL-60, SI-3, Left LI-4 and right LIV-3, KID-6, SP-6	Double P II and *Di Gu Pi*; If neck pain, add Cervical formula (reduce dose to 0.5 g/20#)	Double P II until pain resolves; Use *Di Gu Pi* (with Cervical formula if needed) up to 6 months

	Pattern	Acupuncture	Herbal Medicine	Duration
	Kidney *Yang* Deficiency with External *Qi*/Blood Stagnation	Acupoints for EA and DN from Table 3 plus DN of BL-23, KID-3 and moxibustion of GV-3, GV-4, *Bai-hui, Shen-shu, Shen-peng, Shen-jiao*	Double P II and *Bu Yang Huan Wu* with Cervical Formula of needed	Double P II until pain resolves; Use *Bu Yang Huan Huan* (with Cervical formula if needed) up to 6 months
	Spinal cord *Qi*/Blood Stagnation with Kidney *Qi* Deficiency	Acupoints for EA and DN from Table 3 plus BL-23, KID-3, KID-7, *Bai-hui, Shen-shu, Shen-peng, Shen-jiao*	Body Sore (Grade 2) or Double P II (Grades 3-5) and *Bu Yang Huan Wu* or Cervical Formula	Body Sore until pain resolves or Double P II for 1-2 months, then continue *Bu Yang Huan Wu* or Cervical Formula alone until recovered up to 6 months; If chronic may have to treat on and off long-term
	Spinal cord *Qi*/Blood Stagnation with Kidney *Yang* Deficiency	Acupoints for EA and DN from Table 3 plus BL-23, KID-3 and moxibustion of GV-3, GV-4, *Bai-hui, Shen-shu, Shen-peng, Shen-jiao*	Body Sore (Grade 2) or Double P II (Grades 3-5) and *Bu Yang Huan Wu* or Cervical Formula	Body Sore until pain resolves or Double P II for 1-2 months, then continue *Bu Yang Huan Wu* or Cervical Formula alone until recovered; If chronic may have to treat on and off long-term
	Spinal cord *Qi*/Blood Stagnation with Kidney *Yin* and *Qi* Deficiencies	Acupoints for EA and DN from Table 3 plus BL-23, KID-3, KID-6, SP-6	Body Sore (Grade 2) or Double P II (Grades 3-5) and *Di Gu Pi;* If neck pain, may combine with Cervical formula (0.5 g/20#)	Body sore until pain resolves or Double P II for 1-2 months, then *Di Gu Pi* alone or with Cervical Formula for up to 6 months; If chronic may treat on and off long-term

	Spinal cord *Qi*/Blood Stagnation with Kidney *Yin* and *Yang* Deficiencies	Acupoints for EA and DN from Table 3 plus BL-23, KID-3, KID-6, SP-6, GV-3, GV-4, *Shen-shu, Shen-peng, Shen-jiao*	Body Sore (Grade 2) or Double P II (Grades 3-5) and Hind Quarter Weakness; If neck pain, may combine with Cervical formula (0.5 g/20#)	Body sore until pain resolves or Double P II for 1-2 months, then *Di Gu Pi* alone or with Cervical Formula for up to 6 months; If chronic may treat on and off long-term
Spinal cord Trauma (accidents and falls)	Spinal cord *Qi*/Blood Stagnation with Kidney *Qi* Deficiency	Acupoints for EA and DN from Table 3 plus BL-23, KID-7, KID-3	Double P II and *Bu Yang Huan Wu* or Cervical Formula	Double P II for 1-2 months then *Bu Yang Huan Wu* alone until recovered
Cervical spondylomyelopathy	Spinal cord *Qi*/Blood Stagnation and Kidney *Jing* and *Qi* Deficiencies	Acupoints for EA and DN from Table 3 plus BL-20, BL-21, BL-23, BL-26, BL-62, KID-3, SI-3	Cervical Formula and Double P II then add Epimedium Formula	Double P II for 1-5 months then continue Cervical Formula and add Epimedium Formula
	Spinal cord *Qi*/Blood Stagnation with Kidney *Qi* Deficiency	Acupoints for EA and DN from Table 3 plus BL-23, KID-3, SI-3, BL-62	Cervical Formula and *Bu Yang Huan Wu* alone with mild deficits or with Double P II (moderate to severe deficits); Reduce dose of Cervical Formula and *Bu Yang Huan Wu* while on Double P II	Cervical Formula and *Bu Yang Huan Wu* for 6 or more months; Double P II for 1-5 months
	Spinal cord *Qi*/Blood Stagnation and Kidney *Yang* Deficiency	Acupoints for EA and DN from Table 3 plus BL-23, SI-3, BL-62 and moxibustion GV-3, GV-4, *Bai-hui, Shen-shu, Shen-peng, Shen-jiao*	Cervical Formula and *Bu Yang Huan Wu* alone with mild deficits or with Double P II (moderate to severe deficits); Reduce dose of Cervical Formula and *Bu Yang Huan Wu* while on Double P II	Cervical Formula and *Bu Yang Huan Wu* for 6 or more months; Double P II for 1-5 months

	Spinal cord *Qi*/Blood Stagnation with Kidney *Yin* and *Qi* Deficiencies (Grade 2-5)	Acupoints for EA and DN from Table 3 plus BL-23, KID-3, KID-6, SP-6, SI-3	Cervical Formula and *Hu Qian Wan* (or Hindquarter Weakness) alone with mild deficits or with Double P II (moderate to severe deficits); Reduce dose of Cervical Formula and *Hu Qian Wan* while on Double P II	Cervical Formula and *Hu Qian Wan* (or Hind Quarter Formula) for 6 or more months; Double P II for 1-5 months
	Spinal cord *Qi*/Blood Stagnation and Kidney *Yin* and *Yang* Deficiencies	Acupoints for EA and DN from Table 3 plus BL-23, KID-3, KID-6, SP-6, GV-3, GV-4, *Shen-shu, Shen-peng, Shen-jiao,* BL-62, SI-3	Cervical Formula and *Di Huang Yi Zi* (or Hindquarter Weakness) alone with mild deficits or with Double P II (moderate to severe deficits); Reduce dose of Cervical Formula and *Di Huang Yi Zi* (or Hindquarter Weakness) while on Double P II	Cervical Formula and *Di Huang Yi Zi* (or Hind Quarter Formula) for 6 or more months; Double P II for 1-5 months
Fibrocartilaginous embolism	Spinal cord *Qi*/Blood Stagnation With Kidney *Qi* Deficiency	Acupoints for EA and DN from Table 3 plus BL-23, KID-3	Double P II and Cervical Formula (if cervical) or *Bu Yang Huan Wu* (if thoracolumbar)	Double P II for 1-2 months then continue Cervical Formula or *Bu Yang Huan Wu* until recovered
Diskospondylitis	Heat Toxin Damp Heat in the vertebrae and disks	Acupoints for EA and DN from Table 3 plus GV-14, LI-11, *Er-jian, Wei-jian,* BL-11	*Qing Ying Tang* and *Pu Ju Xiao Du* (if high fever)	*Qing Ying Tang* for 2-3 months, but monitor for signs of Spleen *Qi* Deficiency; *Pu Ju Xiao Du* for 1-2 weeks; Use antibiotics and conventional pain medication also

Degenerative myelopathy	Kidney *Jing*, Spleen *Qi* and Kidney *Qi* Deficiencies	Acupoints for EA and DN from Table 3 plus BL-20, BL-21, BL-23, KID-3	Epimedium Formula and *Bu Yang Huan Wu*	Long-term treatment to prolong life quality
	Kidney *Jing*, Spleen *Qi* and Kidney *Yang* Deficiencies	Acupoints for EA and DN from Table 3 plus BL-20, BL-21, BL-23, KID-3 and moxibustion at GV-3, GV-4, *Bai-hui, Shen-shu, Shen-peng, Shen-jiao*	*You Gui Wan, Jin Gui Shen Qi Wan* or *Ba Ji San*	Long-term treatment to prolong life quality
	Kidney *Jing*, Spleen *Qi*, Kidney *Qi* and Kidney/Liver *Yin* Deficiencies	Acupoints for EA and DN from Table 3 plus BL-18, BL-20, BL-21, BL-23, KID-3, KID-6, SP-6	*Hu Qian Wan* or Hindquarter Weakness	Long-term treatment to prolong life quality
	Kidney *Jing*, Spleen *Qi*, Kidney *Yang* and Kidney/Liver *Yin* Deficiencies	Acupoints for EA and DN from Table 3 plus BL-20, BL-21, BL-23, KID-3, KID-6, SP-6, GV-3, GV-4, *Shen-shu, Shen-peng, Shen-jiao*, BL-62 (no moxibustion)	*Di Huang Yin Zi*	Long-term treatment to prolong life quality
Atlantoaxial malformation	Kidney *Jing* Deficiency resulting in Spinal cord *Qi*/Blood Stagnation with Kidney *Qi* Deficiency	Acupoints for EA and DN from Table 3 (see text if a brace is present) plus BL-20, BL-21, BL-23, LI-10, KID-7, KID-3,	Double P II and Cervical formula	Double P II for 1-2 months then Cervical formula and Epimedium Formula
Meningitis Meningomyelitis	Damp-Heat of the Spinal Cord with *Qi*/Blood Stagnation and Kidney *Qi* Deficiency	Acupoints for EA and DN from Table 3 plus GV-14, LI-11*Er-jian, Wei-jian*	*Wu Wei Xiao Du Yin* and then *Zhi Bai Di Huang*	*Wu Wei Xiao Du* for 1 month then *Zhi Bai Di Huang* until recovered May initially need corticosteroids as well
Spinal cord tumors	Spinal Cord Phlegm and Kidney *Qi* Deficiency with or without	Cervical tumors: GV-20, GV-1, TH-5, LI-4, LI-11, LIV-3, ST-36, LI-10, LIV-3, LU-7, ST-40, SP-6,	Max's Formula or Stasis Breaker *Wei Qi* Booster May combine with Body Sore or	Max's Formula or Stasis Breaker for 3 months or longer as needed then continue

	Qi/Blood Stagnation	SP-9, BL-23, KID-3	Double PII if pain is severe	Wei Qi Booster indefinitely
		Thoracolumbar tumors: GV-20, GV-1, TH-5, LI-4, LI-11, LIV-3, ST-36, LI-10, ST-40, SP-6, SP-9, BL-40, KID-3		
	Spinal Cord Blood Stagnation	Cervical tumors: GV-20, GV-1, LI-4, LI-11, ST-36, LI-10, LIV-3, LU-7, BL-23, KID-3, BL-17, SP-10	Stasis Breaker Wei Qi Booster May combine with Body Sore or Double P II if pain is severe	Max's Formula or Stasis Breaker for 3 months or longer as needed then continue Wei Qi Booster indefinitely
		Thoracolumbar tumors: GV-20, GV-1, LI-4, LI-11, LIV-3, ST-36, LI-10, BL-40, KID-3, SP-10		

The number of acupoints selected and treatment frequency will vary with the animal's condition and response to treatment; Location of classical acupoints: *Bai-hui* (on the midline at L7-S1); *Shen-shu* (one *cun* lateral to *Bai-hui*), *Shen-peng* (one *cun* cranial to *Shen-shu*) and *Shen-jiao* (one *cun* caudal to *Shen-shu*); Chinese herbal medicine doses are generally 0.5 gm/10-20# orally twice daily, reduced doses are 0.5 gm/20#; EA=electro-acupuncture, DN=dry needle acupuncture; All Chinese herbal formulas available from Jing Tang herbal:www.tcvmherbal.com

There are also many experimental and clinical studies that support the use of EA for *Qi/Blood Stagnation* causing only neck and back pain (Grade 1 severity).[18,19] If the pain is acute and severe, EA every 1-3 days, combined with conventional pain medication may be needed. As the pain subsides, the conventional medication may be decreased and discontinued and the EA frequency reduced. If the pain is due to intervertebral disk disease or vertebral degeneration known to cause recurrent painful episodes, the underlying TCVM pattern should also be treated with acupuncture every 1-3 months along with herbal medicine and *Tui-na* to prevent recurrences.[5-8,20]

Spinal cord injuries often result in acute and chronic bladder dysfunction in animals.[1-3] In a spinal cord injury laboratory animal study, EA reduced detrusor hyper-reflexia compared to controls.[21] In two human clinical trials, EA had positive effects on the functional recovery of bladder function.[22] Improvement of fecal incontinence with EA has also been reported in humans.[23] The use of EA to manage bladder and bowel dysfunction of animals, following spinal cord injury, should be further evaluated, as EA could be an effective complement to enhance recovery.

The effects of Chinese herbal medicines on spinal cord regeneration and functional recovery following injury have also been studied.[24-27] The Chinese herbal medicine *Bu Yang Huan Wu* has been used for hundreds of years in China to treat human paralysis and for approximately the past 25 years in dogs.[7,8] *Bu Yang Huan Wu* has recently been shown to enhance spinal cord regeneration and reduce damage from ischemia and reperfusion in rat spinal cord trauma models.[24,25] The Chinese herbal medicine *Sheng Mai San* and *Sui Fu Kang* have been reported to reduce the size of spinal cord lesions and increase many biological parameters that indicate spinal cord regeneration and axonal regrowth in laboratory animal spinal cord injury studies.[26,27]

Double P II (JT)[a], is a commonly prescribed powerful formula for spinal cord injuries (*Qi*/Blood Stagnation causing paresis or paralysis).[8] The usual dose of most Chinese herbal formulas is 0.5 grams/10-20# of body weight twice daily orally. Double P II may cause diarrhea, especially in patients with Spleen *Qi* Deficiency. If a concurrent Spleen *Qi* Deficiency is suspected, the lower dose is initially recommended to determine how well the dog tolerates the herbal medicine. Double P II should be administered for no more than 5 months.[8] Patients should be evaluated every 1-2 months to determine if the TCVM pattern has changed or if further treatment is needed. In chronic degenerative or neoplastic vertebral or spinal cord disorders, periodic acupuncture and constant or intermittent Chinese herbal medicine treatment may be needed long-term.

Since *Tui-na* is especially useful to treat disorders of *Qi* and Blood Stagnation, it is ideal to reduce painful muscle spasms, nerve root pain and paresis or paralysis associated with vertebral and spinal cord disorders.[20] Fractured or bruised sites, areas of extreme pain or tumors should be avoided and only mild techniques should be applied to traumatized, weak or debilitated animals. The TCVM practitioner can do *Tui-na* treatments periodically and the frequency of treatments will vary with the severity of the signs, the TCVM patterns, the condition of the animal and the response to therapy. Sample 20-30 minute *Tui-na* sessions for cervical and thoracolumbar *Qi*/Blood Stagnation for intervertebral disk disease, cervical spondylomyelopathy, fibrocartilaginous embolism and degenerative myelopathy are outlined in Tables 5 and 6.[20]

Table 5: A 15-30 minute *Tui-na* session for neck pain and Grades 2-5 neurological deficits of all 4 limbs from intervertebral disk disease, cervical spondylomyelopathy and cervical fibrocartilaginous embolism[20]

Name	Technique	Duration or Number of Repetitions
Mo-fa and *Rou-fa*	First, touch and palpate the skin (*Mo-fa*) to detect *Ah-shi* points and areas of muscle tension, and then perform rotary kneading (*Rou-fa*) to release the tension and Stagnation.	Repeat for 2 to 5 minutes.
Gun-fa	Rolling technique of the *Ah-shi* points and areas of tension	For 1-3 minutes
An-fa	Pressing on SI-3 and LU-7	For 5-10 seconds per acupoint
Dian-fa	Knocking on SI-19, B-21, SI-16, BL-10, GB-20	For 2-5 second per acupoint
Nie-fa	Pinching all along the Governing Vessel from the tail to the neck	Repeat 12 times
Tui-fa	Pushing forward along *Jing-jia-ji*	Repeat 12 times
Yao-fa	Flexing, extending and rocking each front limb	Repeat 12 times
Ba-shen-fa and *An-fa*	Stretching each limb while pressing on LI-10, and TH-5, then LI-11 and LI-4 for 1 minute each	Repeat for 2-3 minutes
Dou-fa	Shake each limb	Repeat 12 times
Nian-fa	Holding and kneading each of the digits and	Repeat 12 times

	distal extremities	
Rou-fa	Rotary kneading of the neck and shoulders	Up to 10 minutes
Ca-fa	Rubbing cranial to caudal to end the *Tui-na* treatment	Until the neck feels warm and relaxed

Table 6: A 15-30 minute *Tui-na* session for back pain and Grades 2-5 neurological deficits of the pelvic from intervertebral disk disease, thoracolumbar fibrocartilaginous embolism and degenerative myelopathy[20]

Name	Technique	Duration or Number of Repetitions
Moo-fa	Massaging using the palms at *Da-feng-men* (dorsal midline at cranial edge of ear bases), GV-14, *Bai-hui* (L7-S1), then from BL-13 to BL-35 and from BL-42- to BL-52	Repeat 10-20 times
An-fa and *Rou-fa*	Perform pressing and rotary kneading from *Bai-hui* to GV-14 with both palms or finger tips in a clockwise direction 12 times then counterclockwise for 12 time	Repeat 12 times
An-fa and *Tui-fa*	Pressing and pushing from BL-26 to BL-13	Repeat 12 times
Ca-fa	Rub the back from caudal to cranial until the tissues are warm	For 1-3 minutes
Yi-zhi-chan and *Rou-fa*	Single thumb and rotary kneading at BL-40, KID-1 and LIV-3	Repeat 12 times
Nie-fa	Holding and pinching the skin form *Bai-hui* to GV-14	Repeat 12 times
Na-fa	Pull the tail	Repeat 12 times
Dou-fa	Gently shake each pelvic limb	
Ba-shen-fa	Stretch the pelvic limbs	Repeat 12 times
Ban-fa	Flex and extend all the limb joints	Repeat 12 times
Rou-fa	Finish with rotary kneading from *Bai-hui* to GV-14	For 5-10 minutes

Some simple *Tui-na* techniques may be taught to caretakers for daily treatment at home. *Tui-na* can also be integrated with conventional physical rehabilitation techniques like swimming and underwater treadmill therapy. Dogs with Kidney *Qi, Yin, Yang* or *Jing* Deficiencies can benefit long-term from Food therapy.[28] The addition of Food therapy may reduce the number of acupuncture treatments and the length of time Chinese herbal medicine is needed especially in dogs with chronic disorders.

Many neurological disorders of the spinal cord respond well to TCVM treatments, which may be combined with conventional treatments for acute spinal injury and bacterial infections or used alone for chronic progressive disorders, to delay or reduce progression of the neurological signs and increase the length and quality of life.

INTERVERTEBRAL DISK DISEASE

Intervertebral disk herniation (extrusion) is the most common cause of acute neck or back pain (Grade 1) and ataxia, quadriparesis, quadriplegia, paraparesis and paraplegia (Grades 2-5) of dogs.[1-3] An intervertebral disk rarely extrudes into the spinal canal between vertebrae T2-T10. In this region the conjugal (intercapital) ligament, which traverses the space between the rib heads immediately dorsal to the disk, adds a protective barrier between the disk and the spinal cord. The mobility of the thoracolumbar junction region results in a high incidence of intervertebral disk extrusions between vertebrae T11-L2. Jumping off the couch or any other sudden impact or twisting of the vertebral column can cause the intervertebral disk to extrude with a force that can render the dog paralyzed for life. Dachshunds, Pekingese, Lhasa Apsos, Beagles, Cocker Spaniels, Shih Tzus and many other small breed dogs and some large breed dogs like German Shepherds and Doberman Pinschers develop degenerative intervertebral disk disease, but the incidence in Dachshunds exceeds other dogs. The onset of signs can occur any time after 1 year of age. Extrusion of a degenerated intervertebral disk occurs occasionally in elderly cats. Herniation of a non-degenerated intervertebral disk can occur secondary to trauma in any dog or cat at any age (see section entitled **SPINAL CORD TRAUMA** below). Acute paralysis is always an emergency and should be conventionally treated as described above in the section entitled **INTEGRATED TREATMENT OF ACUTE PARALYSIS**.

One of the most exciting areas for the integration of TCVM treatments with conventional treatment is for animals with spinal cord injuries.[10-16] For many years, TCVM practitioners have found that animals with neurological deficits from intervertebral disk disease and other traumatic spinal cord injuries had shorter recovery times, more complete recovery and reduced recurrence of problems, when treated with acupuncture, Chinese herbal medicine, *Tui-na* and Food therapy and now there are experimental and clinical studies to support these clinical impressions.[4-17,24-27,29]

In a pilot experimental spinal cord compression study, 20 paraplegic dogs with preserved deep pain were divided into four treatment groups and recovery time was monitored, using daily neurological examinations and somatosensory evoked potentials.[12] Five dogs received corticosteroids alone, another five EA alone, five others a combination of corticosteroids and EA and the final five dogs received no treatment. Dogs receiving corticosteroids or EA alone recovered significantly faster than the dogs receiving no treatment, but were not significantly different from each other. The dogs receiving a combination of corticosteroids and EA recovered significantly faster than all other dogs, supporting the clinical impression that integration of acupuncture with conventional treatments improves patient outcomes.

There have been three recent clinical studies involving a total of 170 dogs, with spinal cord injuries from intervertebral disk disease.[13-15] The effect of EA on recovery was evaluated in one clinical study of 50 dogs with neurological deficits from confirmed intervertebral disk disease.[13] All dogs were treated with tapering doses of prednisone and one group also received EA weekly or bi-weekly for paraplegic dogs with no deep pain (Grade 5 neurological deficits). The time to recover ambulation, in 7 non-ambulatory dogs (Grade 3 and 4 neurological deficits) treated with EA, was significantly less than 9 similarly affected dogs not receiving EA. Deep pain perception and ambulation was regained in 50% (3/6) of dogs, with Grade 5 dysfunction, treated with EA and 12.5% (1/8) of dogs in the control group, but the difference was not statistically significant.

In another study of 40 non-ambulatory paraplegic dogs with Grades 4 and 5 neurological deficits from intervertebral disk disease, all dogs received conventional treatment with tapering doses of prednisone, but some were also treated with surgery, some with surgery plus EA and other with EA alone.[14] Recovery rate (Grade 4 or 5 becoming Grade 1-2 within 6 months) was significantly higher for dogs treated with EA alone (15/19) and EA plus surgery (8/11), than for dogs that only had surgery (4/10). The investigators concluded that if early surgical intervention (within 24 hours) was not possible, dogs with Grade 4 or 5 neurological deficits might benefit from tapering doses of prednisone and EA. Larger veterinary clinical studies of the effects of EA, integrated with conventional medications and rehabilitation, on recovery from spinal cord injuries are needed, but these results are encouraging.

The effects of a combination of EA and DN were compared in a retrospective study of 80 paraplegic dogs with intact deep pain associated with intervertebral disk disease.[15] Back pain relief and recovery (ambulation) times and recovery and relapse rates were compared for a group receiving prednisone alone (n=37) and a group receiving prednisone plus EA/DN (n=43). Dogs receiving prednisone plus EA/DN had a significantly shorter time for pain relief and recovery, a better overall rate of recovery and fewer relapses than dogs treated with prednisone alone.

Etiology and Pathology

Intervertebral disk disease and vertebral degeneration are considered forms of Bony *Bi* syndrome.[5,29] *Bi* syndromes that cause neck and back pain are most commonly associated with Wind-Cold-Damp invasion and Deficiencies of Kidney *Yin,* Kidney *Yang* or a combination of both causing Bony *Bi*. Applying the basic TCVM theories of *Yin/Yang*, Eight Principles, Five Treasures, Five Elements and *Zang Fu* physiology and pathology to make a TCVM diagnosis, there are seven patterns associated with the clinical signs of intervertebral disk disease and each requires a different treatment (Tables 2-4).

Three TCVM patterns cause *Qi*/Blood Stagnation in External Channels that results in neck or back pain originating from intervertebral disks, vertebrae, vertebral joints and ligaments, peripheral nerve roots and paravertebral muscles, tendons and connective tissue.[29] The immediate focus of treatment in these External patterns is to resolve the *Qi*/Blood Stagnation in the Channels to relieve the pain, which is often severe. Underlying Deficiencies of *Yin* or *Yang* must also be treated to prevent recurrence of pain or Internal involvement of the Spinal Cord (capitalized as it is an Extraordinary *Fu* organ associated with the Kidney system). The other four TCVM patterns are associated with ataxia, paresis or paralysis due to *Qi*/Blood Stagnation in the Spinal Cord. Although *Qi*/Blood Stagnation in External Channels may still be present in animals that have neck or back pain, once neurological deficits are present and the Spinal Cord is affected, the disease has become Internal. With neurological deficits, the primary TCVM pattern is Spinal Cord *Qi*/Blood Stagnation with Kidney *Qi, Yang* and/or *Yin* Deficiencies. Resolving pain associated with *Qi*/Blood Stagnation in the External Channels is important, but when *Tan-Huan* syndrome (Grades 2-5 paresis or paralysis) is present, aggressive treatment of the Spinal Cord *Qi*/Blood Stagnation becomes of utmost importance to reduce further neuronal damage and promote nerve function and regeneration to ensure recovery of function. Treatment of Kidney *Yin* or *Yang* Deficient Bony *Bi* is important to prevent further intervertebral disk degeneration and recurrence of Spinal Cord *Qi*/Blood Stagnation. The seven TCVM patterns are as follows:

1. **Wind-Cold-Damp Invasion with External *Qi*/Blood Stagnation**
   Acute onset of neck or back pain (Grade 1 neurological deficits) with no trauma may be due to the External invasion of Wind-Cold-Damp in the Governing Vessel and Bladder Channels of the neck and back. When *Wei Qi* becomes weak due to chronic poor nutrition, illness, environmental stress and possibly genetic factors (breed

predisposition for IVDD), Wind-Cold-Damp invades the Channels and causes *Qi*/Blood Stagnation. Because the pattern is External the Spinal Cord is not involved and there is no ataxia, paresis or paralysis (Grades 2-5 neurological deficits), but the pain can be extreme. With multiple episodes of invasion as in chronic cases, damage to the Kidney can lead to *Yin* or *Yang* Deficient Bony *Bi*.

2. **Kidney *Yin* Deficiency with External *Qi*/Blood Stagnation**
   Acute onset of neck or back pain (Grade 1 neurological deficits) with no trauma, but with evidence of Heat and weak pulses, especially on the left is typical of Kidney *Yin* Deficiency. Kidney *Yin* becomes damaged by chronic poor nutrition, illness, environmental stress and possibly genetic factors (breed predisposition for IVDD) and results in intervertebral disk degeneration, especially in *Yang* animals (Wood and Fire constitutions). Dogs with Kidney *Yin* Deficiency often have Bony *Bi* and difficulty rising due to pain from *Qi*/Blood Stagnation in the External Channels that affect the surrounding vertebral and paravertebral structures. If ataxia, paresis or paralysis develops, the Spinal Cord has become affected and the disease is now also Internal and must be treated as Spinal Cord *Qi*/Blood Stagnation with Kidney *Qi* and *Yin* Deficiency (see below).

3. **Kidney *Yang* Deficiency with External *Qi*/Blood Stagnation**
   Acute onset of neck or back pain (Grade 1 neurological deficits) with no trauma, but evidence of Cold and weak pulses, especially on the right, on the TCVM examination is typical of the presence of Kidney *Yang* Deficiency. Kidney *Yang* become damaged by chronic poor nutrition, illness and environmental stress and possibly genetic factors (breed predisposition for IVDD) and results in intervertebral disk degeneration, especially in *Yin* animals (Earth, Metal and Water constitutions). Dogs with Kidney *Yang* Deficiency often have Bony *Bi* and difficulty rising due to pain from *Qi*/Blood Stagnation in the External Channels that affect the surrounding vertebral and paravertebral structures. If ataxia, paresis or paralysis develops, the Spinal Cord has become affected and the disease is now also Internal and must be treated as Spinal Cord *Qi*/Blood Stagnation with Kidney *Yang* Deficiency (see below).

4. **Spinal Cord *Qi*/Blood Stagnation with Kidney *Qi* Deficiency**
   Protrusion or extrusion of intervertebral disk material can compress or contuse the spinal cord and result in acute ataxia, paresis or paralysis, with or without pain (Grades 2-5 neurological deficits). From a TCVM perspective Spinal Cord *Qi*/Blood Stagnation with focal *Qi*/Blood Deficiency has occurred. Local Spinal Cord *Qi*/Blood Deficiency reduces the normal function and results in neurological deficits caudal to the lesion. Ataxia, paresis or paralysis (*Tan-Huan* syndrome) with no evidence of Cold or Heat on the TCVM examination is typical of an Internal TCVM pattern of Spinal Cord *Qi*/Blood Stagnation with Kidney *Qi* Deficiency. Serial neurological and TCVM examinations are important, as worsening of the signs and evidence of one of the other TCVM patterns (e.g. *Yin* or *Yang* Deficiency or both) may become evident and alters the treatment.

5. **Spinal Cord *Qi*/Blood Stagnation with Kidney *Yang* Deficiency**
   Kidney *Yang* Deficiency is associated with chronic poor nutrition, illness, and environmental stress and possibly genetic factors (breed predisposition for IVDD) and results in Bony *Bi* with intervertebral disk degeneration, especially in *Yin* animals (Earth, Metal and Water constitutions). Protrusion or extrusion of intervertebral disk material can compress or contuse the spinal cord and result in ataxia, paresis or paralysis, with or without pain (Grades 2-5 neurological deficits). From a TCVM perspective, Spinal Cord *Qi*/Blood Stagnation causes local *Qi*/Blood Deficiency that reduces normal spinal cord functions and results in neurological deficits caudal to the lesion. Ataxia, paresis or paralysis (*Tan-Huan* syndrome), with evidence of Cold on the TCVM examination, is typical of an Internal TCVM pattern of Spinal Cord *Qi*/Blood Stagnation with Kidney *Yang* Deficiency (*Qi* Deficiency plus Cold = *Yang* Deficiency). Serial neurological and TCVM examinations are important, as worsening of the signs and evidence of Heat may also be found indicating the pattern has now changed to Spinal Cord *Qi*/Blood Stagnation with Kidney *Yin* and *Yang* Deficiencies, which alters the treatment (see below).

6. **Spinal Cord *Qi*/Blood Stagnation with Kidney *Qi* and *Yin* Deficiencies**
   Kidney *Yin* Deficiency is associated with chronic poor nutrition, illness, and environmental stress and possibly genetic factors (breed predisposition for IVDD) and results in Bony *Bi* with intervertebral disk degeneration, especially in *Yang* animals (Wood and Fire constitutions). Protrusion or extrusion of intervertebral disk material can compress or contuse the spinal cord and result in ataxia, paresis or paralysis, with or without pain (Grades 2-5 neurological deficits). From a TCVM perspective, Spinal Cord *Qi*/Blood Stagnation causes local *Qi*/Blood Deficiency that reduces normal spinal cord functions and results in neurological deficits caudal to the lesion. Ataxia, paresis or paralysis (*Tan-Huan* syndrome) is associated with Kidney *Qi* Deficiency. Evidence of Heat on the TCVM examination is typical of a concurrent Kidney *Yin* Deficiency. The two Deficiencies combine as the Internal TCVM pattern of Spinal Cord *Qi*/Blood Stagnation with Kidney *Qi* and Kidney *Yin* Deficiencies. Serial neurological and TCVM examinations are important, as worsening of the signs and evidence of Cold may also be found that indicate the pattern has now changed to Spinal Cord *Qi*/Blood Stagnation with Kidney *Yin* and *Yang* Deficiencies, which alters the treatment (see below).

7. **Spinal Cord *Qi*/Blood Stagnation with Kidney *Yin* and *Yang* Deficiencies**
   Chronic poor nutrition, illness, environmental stress and possibly genetic factors (breed predisposition for IVDD) can damage both Kidney *Yang* and *Yin* and result in Bony *Bi* with intervertebral disk degeneration. Protrusion or extrusion of intervertebral disk material can compress or contuse the spinal cord and result in ataxia, paresis or paralysis with or without pain (Grades 2-5 neurological deficits). From a TCVM perspective, Spinal Cord *Qi*/Blood Stagnation causes local *Qi*/Blood Deficiency that reduces normal spinal cord functions and results in neurological deficits caudal to the lesion. When clinical evidence of Heat and Cold are found on the TCVM examination, the pattern then becomes Spinal Cord *Qi*/Blood Stagnation with Kidney *Yin* and *Yang* Deficiencies.

Pattern Differentiation and Treatment

1. Wind-Cold-Damp Invasion with External *Qi*/Blood Stagnation

Clinical Signs:
- Acute neck or back pain only (Grade 1 on neurological deficit scale)
- No paresis or paralysis
- Tongue- purple
- Pulses- superficial, strong, slow, wiry

TCVM Diagnosis:
The acute onset of neck or back pain with no neurological deficits and superficial, strong pulses are typical of an Exterior and Excess pattern. The superficial, strong slow pulses and purple tongue are typical of an Exterior Cold pattern. The purple tongue and wiry pulses reflect the *Qi*/Blood Stagnation in the Exterior Channels.

Treatment Principles:
- Clear Wind-Cold-Damp
- Warm the Channels to dispel Cold, resolve *Qi*/Blood Stagnation and relieve pain

Acupuncture treatment:
EA is more effective than DN to control pain. For EA use 20 Hz for 10-15 minutes then 80-120 Hz alternating frequencies for 10-15 minutes. EA is combined with DN and Aqua-AP. For Aqua-AP inject 0.25-0.5 ml vitamin B12 into the acupoint after *Tui-na*. For severe pain administer conventional pain medications and perform EA and DN every 1-3 days for 3-5 times, depending on the patient's response, then reduced to once every 1-2 weeks until the pain is gone, when the conventional medications are discontinued.

Acupoints recommended
- EA: Select appropriate acupoints in Table 3 depending on the lesion location
- DN: Select acupoints in Table 3 plus BL-10,
- Moxibustion at: GV-3 and GV-4
- Aqua-AP: BL-10

Pertinent acupoint actions
- See Table 3 for indications and actions of acupoints recommended for EA and DN and locations of classical acupoints
- Bl-10 is useful to clear Wind-Cold and resolve *Qi*/Blood Stagnation of the Bladder Channels
- GV-3 and GV-4 moxibustion is useful to clear Cold from the Governing Vessel Channel that traverses the vertebral column

Herbal Medicine:
- Double P II (JT)[a] 0.5gm/10# twice daily orally to move *Qi*, activate Blood and resolve Stagnation and pain (may reduce the dose if needed to 0.5gm/20# after the pain is controlled)
- For cervical pain, combine with Cervical Formula (JT)[a] 0.5gm/10-20# twice daily orally to move *Qi*, activate Blood and resolve Stagnation and pain especially in the cervical region
- Administer the herbal formulas for 4 months, then as needed if signs recur
- A description of all the ingredients of the Chinese herbal medicine listed is beyond the scope of this text, but can be found elsewhere.[7,8]

Food Therapy:
The purpose of the Food therapy is to Clear Cold from the Channels and to promote *Qi*/Blood circulation and relieve pain in the affected region. Foods that are Cold are avoided.[28]
- Foods to supplement to Clear Wind-Cold: Lamb, shrimp, corn-fed beef, chicken, trout, squash, turnips, sweet rice, basal, caraway, cherries, chilies, cinnamon, ginger, rosemary, sage
- Foods to supplement to promote *Qi* and Blood circulation include: chicken egg, crab, sweet rice, peaches, carrots, coriander, squash, turnips
- Foods to tonify *Qi*: Beef, chicken, sardines, egg, potato, yam, sweet potato, rice, oats, millet, lentils, carrots, squash, microalgae, dates, figs, molasses, royal jelly
- Cold foods to avoid: Turkey, duck, duck eggs, conch, clams, mussels, yogurt, millet, barley, spinach, broccoli, celery, egg plant, kelp, alfalfa, cucumbers, pears, bananas, white radishes, watermelon

Tui-na Procedures:
The purpose of the *Tui-na* is to stimulate *Qi* and Blood flow to relieve pain and promote nerve regeneration in the affected region. If pain is severe, avoid *Tui-na* in the painful region until acupuncture and Chinese herbal medicine have relieved the pain. The descriptions and indications of each technique are outlined in more detail in Chapter 1 Table 8.[20]
- A *Tui-na* protocol for cervical disk disease is outlined in Table 5
- A *Tui-na* protocol for thoracolumbar disk disease is outlined in Table 6

Daily Life Style Recommendation for Owner Follow-up:
- Gentle *Moo-fa* (Daubing or massaging) of the neck or back for 3 minutes
- Gentle *Ca-fa* (Rubbing) of neck or back for a few minutes until it feels warm, once or twice daily for 14-21 days
- Can put warm pads on neck and back (not too Hot or heavy)
- Keep warm
- Avoid prolong periods outdoors when weather is Cold and Damp
- Avoid collars and walk with a harness, as even if the problem is in the thoracolumbar region, cervical intervertebral disks may cause problems in the future
- Avoid jumping on and off furniture and rough play

Comments:
Based on clinical experiences and current research, the TCVM treatments should relieve the pain and reduce recurrences.

2. Kidney *Yin* Deficiency with External *Qi*/Blood Stagnation

Clinical Signs:
- Acute or recurrent neck or back pain only (Grade 1 on neurological deficit scale)
- No ataxia, paresis or paralysis
- History of cool seeking
- Panting episodes
- Warm ears, back and/or feet
- Dry skin
- Tongue- reddish purple and dry
- Pulses- deep, weak worse on the left, rapid and thready or wiry

TCVM Diagnosis:
The Cool seeking behavior, panting episodes and warm ears, back and feet with deep, rapid, thready pulses weaker on the left and red, dry tongue are typical of Kidney *Yin* Deficiency. The neck and back pain with no neurological deficits, purple tongue and wiry pulses are typical of External Channel *Qi*/Blood Stagnation. A combination of a Deficiency and Excess pattern is present.

Treatment Principles:
- Resolve *Qi*/Blood Stagnation to return proper *Qi*/Blood flow in the External Channels to relieve pain
- Tonify Kidney *Yin* to prevent recurrence of pain

Acupuncture treatment:
EA is more effective than DN to resolve *Qi*/Blood Stagnation and control pain. For EA use 20 Hz for 10-15 minutes then 80-120 Hz alternating frequencies for 10-15 minutes. EA is combined with DN and Aqua-AP. For Aqua-AP inject 0.25-0.5 ml vitamin B12 into the acupoint after *Tui-na*. For severe pain, integrate acupuncture with conventional medications. Then EA and DN should be administered every 1-3 days for 3-5 times, depending on the patient's response, then reduced to once every 1-2 weeks until the pain resolves. If the pain is controlled initially, acupuncture treatments may be weekly or every other week and conventional medication doses decreased and then discontinued once the acupuncture controls the pain.

Acupoints recommended
- EA: Select appropriate acupoints in Table 3 depending on the lesion location
- DN: Select suggested acupoints in Table 3 plus BL-23, KID-3/BL-60, SI-3, Left LI-4 and right LIV-3, KID-6, SP-6
- Aqua-AP: BL-23, SP-6, GB-21, SI-9

Pertinent acupoint actions
- See Table 3 for indications and actions of acupoints recommended for EA and DN and locations of classical acupoints
- BL-23 is the Back *Shu* Association point for the Kidney which nourishes the intervertebral disks
- KID-3 is the *Yuan* Source point for the Kidney which nourishes the intervertebral disks
- BL-60 is useful for pain control
- SI-3 is useful for pain control
- Left LI-4 and right LIV-3 are useful for pain control
- KID-6 is the confluent point with the *Yin Qiao* Extraordinary Channel useful to treat *Yin* Deficiencies
- SP-6 tonifies *Yin* and Blood

Herbal Medicine:
- Double P II (JT)[a] 0.5gm/10-20# twice daily orally to move *Qi*, activate Blood and eliminate Stagnation and pain
- Combine with *Di Gu Pi* (JT)[a] to nourish *Yin* and clear Deficient Heat
- For cervical pain, add Cervical Formula (JT)[a] 0.5gm/10-20# twice daily orally to move *Qi*, activate Blood and resolve Stagnation and pain in the cervical region.
- In elderly dogs administer 0.5gm/20# doses of *Di Gu Pi* and Cervical Formula if combine all three herbal formulas together
- Administer Double P II for 1-2 months until the pain resolves; Administer *Di Gu Pi* (with Cervical formula if needed) up to 6 months
- If recurrent signs, may treat on and off long-term
- A description of all the ingredients of the Chinese herbal medicine listed is beyond the scope of this text, but can be found elsewhere.[7,8]

Food Therapy:
The purpose of Food therapy is to promote *Qi*/Blood circulation, clear false Heat and tonify Kidney *Yin* to support nerve regeneration. Foods that are Hot are avoided.[28]
- Foods to supplement to promote *Qi* and Blood circulation include: chicken egg, crab, sweet rice, peaches, carrots, coriander, squash, turnips
- Foods to Cool and tonify *Yin*: Turkey, pork, duck, clams, crab, eggs, rice, wheat, wheat germ, wheat berries, Belgian endive, string beans, peas, kidney beans, sweet potatoes, yams, tomato, spinach, tofu, kiwi, lemons, rhubarb, pears, bananas, watermelon, sesame, seaweed
- Hot foods to avoid: Lamb, shrimp, corn-fed beef, chicken, trout, squash, turnips, sweet rice, basal, caraway, cherries, chilies, cinnamon, ginger, rosemary, sage

Tui-na Procedures:
The purpose of the *Tui-na* is to stimulate *Qi* and Blood flow to relieve pain and promote nerve regeneration in the affected region. If pain is severe, avoid *Tui-na* in the region of the pain until acupuncture and Chinese herbal medicine have relieved the pain. The descriptions and indications of each technique are outlined in more detail in Chapter 1 Table 8.[20]

- A *Tui-na* protocol for cervical disk disease is outlined in Table 5
- A *Tui-na* protocol for thoracolumbar disk disease is outlined in Table 6

Daily Life Style Recommendation for Owner Follow-up:
- Gentle *Moo-fa* (Daubing or massaging) of the neck or back for 3 minutes
- Gentle *Ca-fa* (Rubbing) of neck or back for a few minutes until it feels warm, once daily for 14-21 days
- Keep cool
- Avoid prolong periods outdoors when weather is Hot
- Avoid collars and walk with a harness, as even if the problem is in the thoracolumbar region, cervical intervertebral disks may cause problems in the future
- Avoid jumping on and off furniture and rough play

Comments:
Based on clinical experiences and current research, the TCVM treatments should relieve the pain and reduce recurrences.

3. Kidney *Yang* Deficiency with External *Qi*/Blood Stagnation

Clinical Signs:
- Acute or recurrent neck or back pain only (Grade 1 on neurological deficit scale)
- No ataxia, paresis or paralysis
- Seeks Heat
- Cold ears, back, feet
- Tongue- purple
- Pulses- deep, weak, slow, worse on right or wiry

TCVM Diagnosis:
The Heat seeking behavior and cold ears, back and feet with deep, slow pulses weaker on the right and purple tongue are typical of Kidney *Yang* Deficiency. The neck and back pain with no neurological deficits, purple tongue and wiry pulses are typical of External Channel *Qi*/Blood Stagnation. A combination of a Deficiency and Excess pattern is present.

Treatment Principles:
- Resolve *Qi*/Blood Stagnation to return proper *Qi*/Blood flow in the External Channels to relieve pain
- Tonify Kidney *Yang* to prevent recurrence of pain

Acupuncture treatment:
EA is more effective than DN to resolve *Qi*/Blood Stagnation and control pain. For EA use 20 Hz for 10-15 minutes then 80-120 Hz alternating frequencies for 10-15 minutes. EA is combined with DN, moxibustion and Aqua-AP. For Aqua-AP inject 0.25-0.5 ml vitamin B12 into the acupoint after *Tui-na*. For severe pain, integrate acupuncture with conventional medications. Then EA and DN should be administered every 1-3 days for 3-5 times, depending on the patient's response, then reduced to once every 1-2 weeks until the pain resolves. If the pain is controlled

initially, acupuncture treatments may be weekly or every other week and conventional medication doses decreased and then discontinued once the acupuncture controls the pain.

Acupoints recommended
- EA: Select appropriate acupoints in Table 3 depending on the lesion location
- DN: Select acupoints in Table 3 plus BL-23, KID-3
- Moxibustion: GV-3, GV-4, *Bai-hui, Shen-shu, Shen-peng, Shen-jiao*
- Aqua-AP: BL-23, *Jing-jia-ji* or *Hua-tuo-jia-ji*

Pertinent acupoint actions
- See Table 3 for indications and actions of acupoints recommended for EA and DN and locations of classical acupoints
- BL-23 is the Back *Shu* Association point for the Kidney to support the Kidney and nourish the intervertebral disks
- KID-3 is the *Yuan* Source point for the Kidney to support the Kidney and nourish the intervertebral disks
- GV-3, GV-4 *Bai-hui* (on the midline between L7-S1) are useful to treat Kidney *Yang* Deficiency with back pain
- *Shen-shu* (one *cun* lateral to *Bai-hui*), *Shen-peng* (one *cun* cranial to *Shen-shu*) and *Shen-jiao* (one *cun* caudal to *Shen-shu*) are useful to treat Kidney *Yang* Deficiency and back pain

Herbal Medicine:
- Double P II (JT)[a] 0.5gm/10-20# twice daily orally to move *Qi* and Blood and eliminate Stagnation and pain
- *Bu Yang Huan Wu* (JT)[a] 0.5gm/10-20# twice daily orally to move and nourish Blood and tonify *Qi* and *Yang*
- If neck may combine with Cervical Formula (JT)[a] 0.5gm/20# twice daily orally to activate Blood, move *Qi*, eliminate Stagnation and pain in the cervical region
- Administer Double P II for 1-2 months then continue *Bu Yang Huan Wu* with or without Cervical Formula until recovered up to 6 months
- A description of all the ingredients of the Chinese herbal medicine listed is beyond the scope of this text, but can be found elsewhere.[7,8]

Food Therapy:
The purpose of Food therapy is to promote *Qi*/Blood circulation, clear false Cold and tonify Kidney *Yang*. Foods that are Cold are avoided.[28]
- Foods to supplement to promote *Qi* and Blood circulation include: chicken egg, crab, sweet rice, peaches, carrots, coriander, squash, turnips
- Foods to clear false Cold and tonify *Yang*: Chicken, lamb, corn fed beef, corn, millet, oats, brown rice, microalgae, pumpkin, squash, rutabaga, shiitake mushrooms, yams, sweet potatoes, winter squash, cherries, dates, figs, hawthorn fruit, lychees, molasses, royal jelly

- Cold foods to avoid: Turkey, duck, duck eggs, conch, clams, mussels, yogurt, millet, barley, spinach, broccoli, celery, egg plant, kelp, alfalfa, cucumbers, pears, bananas, white radishes, watermelon

Tui-na Procedures:

The purpose of the *Tui-na* is to stimulate *Qi* and Blood flow to relieve pain and promote nerve regeneration in the affected region. If pain is severe, avoid *Tui-na* in the painful region until acupuncture and Chinese herbal medicine have relieved the pain. The descriptions and indications of each technique are outlined in more detail in Chapter 1 Table 8.[20]
- A *Tui-na* protocol for cervical disk disease is outlined in Table 5
- A *Tui-na* protocol for thoracolumbar disk disease is outlined in Table 6

Daily Life Style Recommendation for Owner Follow-up:
- Gentle *Moo-fa* (Daubing or massaging) of the neck or back for 3 minutes
- Gentle *Ca-fa* (Rubbing) of neck or back for a few minutes until it feels warm, once daily for 14-21 days
- Can put warm pads on neck and back (not too hot or heavy)
- Keep warm
- Avoid prolong periods outdoors when weather is cold
- Avoid collars and walk with a harness, as even if the problem is in the thoracolumbar region, cervical intervertebral disks may cause problems in the future
- Once recovered avoid jumping on and off furniture and rough play

Comments:

Based on clinical experiences and current research, the TCVM treatments should shorten the recovery time, improve the degree of functional recovery and reduce recurrences.

4. Spinal cord *Qi*/Blood Stagnation and Kidney *Qi* Deficiency

Clinical Signs:
- Acute or chronic paresis or paralysis (Grades 2-5 neurological deficits)
- With or without neck or back pain
- Tongue- pale, purple, wet
- Pulses- deep, weak worse on right or wiry

TCVM Diagnosis:

The diagnosis is made based on the presence of paresis or paralysis (Grades 2-5 neurological deficits) of all four limbs or the pelvic limbs alone with no evidence of a concurrent Deficient Heat and/or Deficient Cold pattern. The purple of the tongue is typical of *Qi*/Blood Stagnation and the pale wet tongue is associated with *Qi* Deficiency. The pulses can vary and may be wiry reflecting acute *Qi*/Blood Stagnation or deep and weak worse on the right reflecting the *Qi* Deficiency.

Treatment Principles:
- Resolve *Qi*/Blood Stagnation to return proper *Qi*/Blood flow, relieve pain and resolve paresis and paralysis
- Tonify Kidney *Qi* to resolve paresis or paralysis

Acupuncture treatment:

EA is more effective than DN to control pain, resolve *Qi*/Blood Stagnation and promote nerve regeneration. For EA use 20 Hz for 10-15 minutes then 80-120 Hz alternating frequencies for 10-15 minutes. EA is combined with DN and Aqua-AP. For Aqua-AP inject 0.25-0.5 ml vitamin B12 into the acupoint after *Tui-na*. For acute Grades 3-5 paresis or paralysis, EA and DN should be administered every 1-3 days for 3-5 times, depending on the patient's response, then reduced to once every 1-2 weeks until ambulatory. For Grade 2 ataxia or paresis, the acupuncture treatments may be weekly or every other week.

Acupoints recommended
- EA: Select appropriate acupoints in Table 3 depending on the lesion location
- DN: Select acupoints in Table 3 plus BL-23, KID-3, KID-7, *Bai-hui, Shen-shu, Shen-peng, Shen-jiao*
- Aqua-AP: BL-23, *Jing-jia-ji* or *Hua-tuo-jia-ji*

Pertinent acupoint actions
- See Table 3 for indications and actions of acupoints recommended for EA and DN and locations of classical acupoints
- BL-23 is the Back *Shu* Association point for the Kidney to tonify Kidney *Qi* and resolve paresis and paralysis and nourish the spinal cord and intervertebral disks
- KID-3 is the *Yuan* Source point for the Kidney to treat *Qi* Deficiency and resolve paresis of paralysis and nourish the intervertebral disks
- KID-7 is the mother (Metal) point on the Channel to treat *Qi* Deficiency and resolve paresis of paralysis
- *Shen-shu* (one *cun* lateral to *Bai-hui*), *Shen-peng* (one *cun* cranial to *Shen-shu*) and *Shen-jiao* (one *cun* caudal to *Shen-shu*) are useful to treat Kidney *Qi* and *Yang* Deficiency and pelvic limb paresis or paralysis

Herbal Medicine:
- For Grade 2 paresis administer Body Sore (JT)[a] 0.5gm/10-20# twice daily orally to move *Qi* and Blood and eliminate Stagnation and pain
- For Grades 3-5 paresis or paralysis administer Double P II (JT)[a] 0.5gm/10-20# twice daily orally to move *Qi* and Blood and eliminate Stagnation and pain
- If pelvic limb paresis or paralysis is present, combine with *Bu Yang Huan Wu* (JT)[a] 0.5gm/10-20# twice daily orally to move and nourish Blood and tonify *Qi*
- If all four limbs are affected, instead combine with Cervical Formula (JT)[a] 0.5gm/10-20# twice daily orally to activate Blood, move *Qi*, eliminate Stagnation and pain
- Administer Body Sore until pain resolves or Double P II for 1-2 months, then continue *Bu Yang Huan Wu* or Cervical Formula until recovered up to 6 months

- A description of all the ingredients of the Chinese herbal medicine listed is beyond the scope of this text, but can be found elsewhere.[7,8]

Food Therapy:
The purpose of the Food therapy is to promote *Qi*/Blood circulation and tonify Kidney *Qi* to support nerve regeneration in the affected region. Foods that are Cold or Hot are avoided.[28]
- Foods to supplement to promote *Qi* and Blood circulation include: chicken egg, crab, sweet rice, peaches, carrots, coriander, squash, turnips
- Foods to tonify *Qi*: beef, chicken, sardines, egg, potato, yam, sweet potato, rice, oats, millet, lentils, carrots, squash, microalgae, dates, figs, molasses, royal jelly
- Cold foods to avoid: turkey, duck, duck eggs, conch, clams, mussels, yogurt, millet, barley, spinach, broccoli, celery, egg plant, kelp, alfalfa, cucumbers, pears, bananas, white radishes, watermelon
- Hot foods to avoid: lamb, shrimp, corn-fed beef, chicken, trout, squash, turnips, sweet rice, basal, caraway, cherries, chilies, cinnamon, ginger, rosemary, sage

Tui-na Procedures:
The purpose of the *Tui-na* is to stimulate *Qi* and Blood flow to relieve pain and promote nerve regeneration in the affected region. If pain is severe, avoid *Tui-na* in the region of the pain until acupuncture and Chinese herbal medicine have relieved the pain. The descriptions and indications of each technique are outlined in more detail in Chapter 1 Table 8.[20]
- A *Tui-na* protocol for cervical disk disease is outlined in Table 5
- A *Tui-na* protocol for thoracolumbar disk disease is outlined in Table 6

Daily Life Style Recommendation for Owner Follow-up:
- If Grades 3-5 paresis or paralysis, turn (if in lateral recumbency) or move every 4-6 hours to prevent lung atelectasis and decubitus ulcers
- Keep on padding to avoid decubitus ulcers on shoulders, hips or tuber ischii
- Keep dry and clean of feces and urine
- Gentle *Moo-fa* (Daubing or massaging) of the neck or back for 3 minutes
- Gentle *Ca-fa* (Rubbing) of neck or back for a few minutes until it feels warm, once daily for 14-21 days
- *Ba-shen-fa* (Stretching) and range of motion exercises of all the limbs for 12 times twice daily until can walk
- Assist to walk with a sling if needed
- Swim with support and supervision
- Avoid collars and walk with a harness, as even if the problem is in the thoracolumbar region, cervical intervertebral disks may cause problems in the future
- Once recovered avoid jumping on and off furniture and rough play

Comments:
Based on clinical experiences and current research, the TCVM treatments should shorten the recovery time, improve the degree of functional recovery and reduce recurrences. On serial TCVM evaluations if *Yin* or *Yang* Deficiency develops, see the treatment of Kidney *Qi* and *Yin*

Deficiencies, Kidney *Yang* Deficiency and Kidney *Yin* and *Yang* Deficiency described below in this section.

5. Spinal cord *Qi*/Blood Stagnation and Kidney *Yang* Deficiency

Clinical Signs:
- Acute or chronic paresis or paralysis (Grades 2-5 neurological deficits)
- With or without neck or back pain
- Seeks Heat
- Cold ears, back, feet
- Tongue- pale purple and wet
- Pulses- deep, weak, slow, worse on right or may be wiry

TCVM Diagnosis:
The diagnosis is made based on the presence of paresis or paralysis (Grades 2-5 neurological deficits) of all four limbs or the pelvic limbs alone with evidence of a Deficient Cold pattern. Along with the paresis or paralysis, the animal will also seek Heat and have cold ears, back and feet, typical of a Kidney *Yang* Deficiency. The pale purple of the tongue is typical of *Qi*/Blood Stagnation and *Yang* Deficiency. The tongue is usually wet since the disorder is often chronic. The pulses can vary and may be deep and weak worse on the right reflecting the *Yang* Deficiency, but may also be wiry reflecting the *Qi*/Blood Stagnation if in the acute stage.

Treatment Principles:
- Resolve *Qi*/Blood Stagnation to return proper *Qi*/Blood flow, relieve pain and resolve paresis and paralysis
- Tonify Kidney *Yang* and resolve paresis or paralysis

Acupuncture treatment:
EA is more effective than DN to control pain, resolve *Qi*/Blood Stagnation and promote nerve regeneration. For EA use 20 Hz for 10-15 minutes then 80-120 Hz alternating frequencies for 10-15 minutes. EA is combined with DN and Aqua-AP. For Aqua-AP inject 0.25-0.5 ml vitamin B12 into the acupoint after *Tui-na*. For acute Grades 3-5 paresis or paralysis, EA and DN should be administered every 1-3 days for 3-5 times, depending on the patient's response, then reduced to once every 1-2 weeks until ambulatory. For Grade 2 ataxia or paresis, the acupuncture treatments may be weekly or every other week.

Acupoints recommended
- EA: Select appropriate acupoints in Table 3 depending on the lesion location
- DN: Select acupoints in Table 3 plus BL-23, KID-3
- Moxibustion: GV-3, GV-4, *Bai-hui, Shen-shu, Shen-peng, Shen-jiao*
- Aqua-AP: GV-4, BL-23, *Jing-jia-ji* or *Hua-tuo-jia-ji*

Pertinent acupoint actions
- See Table 3 for indications and actions of acupoints recommended for EA and DN and locations of classical acupoints
- BL-23 is the Back *Shu* Association point for the Kidney to tonify Kidney *Qi*, resolve paresis and paralysis and nourish the spinal cord and intervertebral disks
- KID-3 is the *Yuan* Source point for the Kidney to treat *Qi* Deficiency resolve paresis and paralysis and nourish intervertebral disks
- GV-3, GV-4 *Bai-hui* are useful to treat Kidney *Yang* and *Qi* Deficiency with back pain and pelvic limb paresis or paralysis
- *Shen-shu* (one *cun* lateral to *Bai-hui*), *Shen-peng* (one *cun* cranial to *Shen-shu*) and *Shen-jiao* (one *cun* caudal to *Shen-shu*) are useful to treat Kidney *Qi* and *Yang* Deficiency and pelvic limb paresis or paralysis

Herbal Medicine:
- For Grade 2 paresis administer Body Sore (JT)[a] 0.5gm/10-20# twice daily orally to move *Qi* and Blood and eliminate Stagnation and pain
- For Grades 3-5 paresis or paralysis administer Double P II (JT)[a] 0.5gm/10-20# twice daily orally to move *Qi* and Blood and eliminate Stagnation and pain
- If pelvic limb paresis or paralysis, combine with *Bu Yang Huan Wu* (JT)[a] 0.5gm/10-20# twice daily orally to move and nourish Blood and tonify *Qi*
- If all four limbs are affected, instead combine with Cervical Formula (JT)[a] 0.5gm/10-20# twice daily orally to activate Blood, move *Qi*, eliminate Stagnation and pain
- Administer Body Sore until pain is resolved or Double P II for 1-2 months then continue *Bu Yang Huan Wu* or Cervical Formula until recovered up to 6 months
- A description of all the ingredients of the Chinese herbal medicine listed is beyond the scope of this text, but can be found elsewhere.[7,8]

Food Therapy:
The purpose of Food therapy is to promote *Qi*/Blood circulation, clear false Cold and tonify Kidney *Yang* to support nerve regeneration. Foods that are Cold are avoided.[28]
- Foods to supplement to promote *Qi* and Blood circulation include: chicken egg, crab, sweet rice, peaches, carrots, coriander, squash, turnips
- Foods to clear false Cold and tonify *Yang*: Chicken, lamb, corn fed beef, corn, millet, oats, brown rice, microalgae, pumpkin, squash, rutabaga, shiitake mushrooms, yams, sweet potatoes, winter squash, cherries, dates, figs, hawthorn fruit, lychees, molasses, royal jelly
- Cold foods to avoid: Turkey, duck, duck eggs, conch, clams, mussels, yogurt, millet, barley, spinach, broccoli, celery, egg plant, kelp, alfalfa, cucumbers, pears, bananas, white radishes, watermelon

Tui-na Procedures:
The purpose of the *Tui-na* is to stimulate *Qi* and Blood flow to relieve pain and promote nerve regeneration in the affected region. If pain is severe, avoid *Tui-na* in the region of the pain

until acupuncture and Chinese herbal medicine have relieved the pain. The descriptions and indications of each technique are outlined in more detail in Chapter 1 Table 8.[20]

- A *Tui-na* protocol for cervical disk disease is outlined in Table 5
- A *Tui-na* protocol for thoracolumbar disk disease is outlined in Table 6

Daily Life Style Recommendation for Owner Follow-up:
- If Grades 3-5 paresis or paralysis, turn (if in lateral recumbency) or move every 4-6 hours to prevent lung atelectasis and decubitus ulcers
- Keep on padding to avoid decubitus ulcers on shoulders, hips or tuber ischii
- Keep dry and clean of feces and urine
- Gentle *Moo-fa* (Daubing or massaging) of the neck or back for 3 minutes
- Gentle *Ca-fa* (Rubbing) of neck or back for a few minutes until it feels warm, once daily for 14-21 days
- *Ba-shen-fa* (Stretching) and range of motion exercises of all the limbs for 12 times twice daily until can walk
- Assist to walk with a sling if needed
- Do not swim as the body may become chilled further and put unneeded stress on the body's *Yang*
- For severely *Yang* Deficient dogs, select clients may be taught to administer moxibustion at GV-3, GV-4, *Bai-hui, Shen-shu, Shen-peng, Shen-jiao* in-between veterinary visits
- Avoid prolong periods outdoors when weather is Cold
- Avoid collars and walk with a harness, as even if the problem is in the thoracolumbar region, cervical intervertebral disks may cause problems in the future
- Once recovered avoid jumping on and off furniture and rough play

Comments:
Based on clinical experiences and current research, the TCVM treatments should shorten the recovery time, improve the degree of functional recovery and reduce recurrences.

6. Spinal cord *Qi*/Blood Stagnation and Kidney *Yin* and *Qi* Deficiency

Clinical Signs:
- Acute or chronic paresis or paralysis (Grades 2-5 neurological deficits)
- With or without neck or back pain
- Panting
- Cool seeking
- Warm ears, back, feet
- Dry skin
- Tongue- pale or red, purple, wet or dry, may be cracked if chronic *Yin* Deficiency
- Pulses- deep, weak, may be weak on both sides or worse on left, rapid, thready, may be wiry

***TCVM Diagnosis*:**
The diagnosis is made based on the presence of paresis or paralysis (Grades 2-5 neurological deficits) of all four limbs or the pelvic limbs alone with evidence of a Deficient Heat pattern on the TCVM examination. The paresis or paralysis is typical of Spinal Cord *Qi*/Blood Stagnation with Kidney *Qi* Deficiency. The animal will also be cool seeking, have panting episodes, warm ears, back and feet and dry skin, typical of a Kidney *Yin* Deficiency. The tongue characteristics can vary depending on which pattern is primarily reflected. A pale purple and wet tongue reflects the *Qi*/Blood Stagnation and Kidney *Qi* Deficiency. The reddish purple and dry tongue reflects the *Qi*/Blood Stagnation and Kidney *Yin* Deficiency. The tongue may be cracked, if the *Yin* Deficiency is chronic. The pulses can vary and may be wiry reflecting acute *Qi*/Blood Stagnation or be deep and weak on both sides reflecting the combination of *Yin* and *Qi* Deficiency.

***Treatment Principles*:**
- Resolve *Qi*/Blood Stagnation to return proper *Qi*/Blood flow, relieve pain and resolve paresis and paralysis
- Tonify Kidney *Yin* to nourish intervertebral disks
- Tonify Kidney *Qi* to resolve paresis or paralysis

***Acupuncture treatment*:**
EA is more effective than DN to control pain, resolve *Qi*/Blood Stagnation and promote nerve regeneration. For EA use 20 Hz for 10-15 minutes then 80-120 Hz alternating frequencies for 10-15 minutes. EA is combined with DN and Aqua-AP. For Aqua-AP inject 0.25-0.5 ml vitamin B12 into the acupoint after *Tui-na*. For acute Grades 3-5 paresis or paralysis, EA and DN should be administered every 1-3 days for 3-5 times, depending on the patient's response, then reduced to once every 1-2 weeks until ambulatory. For Grade 2 ataxia or paresis, the acupuncture treatments may be weekly or every other week.

Acupoints recommended
- EA: Select appropriate acupoints in Table 3 depending on the lesion location
- DN: Select acupoints in Table 3 plus BL-23, KID-3, KID-6, SP-6
- Aqua-AP: BL-23, *Jing-jia-ji* or *Hua-tuo-jia-ji*

Pertinent acupoint actions
- See Table 3 for indications and actions of acupoints recommended for EA and DN and locations of classical acupoints
- BL-23 is the Back *Shu* Association point for the Kidney which tonifies the Kidney *Qi* to resolve paresis and paralysis and nourish the spinal cord and intervertebral disks
- KID-3 is the *Yuan* Source point for the Kidney which tonifies the Kidney *Qi* to resolve paresis and paralysis and nourish intervertebral disks
- KID-6 is the confluent point with the *Yin Qiao* Extraordinary Channel useful to treat *Yin* Deficiencies
- SP-6 tonifies *Yin* and Blood

Herbal Medicine:

- For Grade 2 paresis administer Body Sore (JT)[a] 0.5gm/10-20# twice daily orally to move *Qi* and Blood and eliminate Stagnation and pain
- For Grades 3-5 paresis and paralysis administer Double P II (JT)[a] 0.5gm/10-20# twice daily orally to move *Qi* and Blood and eliminate Stagnation and pain
- Combine with *Di Gu Pi* (JT)[a] 0.5gm/10-20# twice daily orally to nourish *Yin* and clear Deficient Heat and tonify Kidney *Qi*
- If all four limbs are affected, also add Cervical Formula (JT)[a] 0.5gm/10-20# twice daily orally to move *Qi*, activate Blood and resolve Stagnation and pain especially in the cervical region.
- In elderly dogs administer 0.5gm/20# doses of *Di Gu Pi* and Cervical Formula if combine all three herbal formulas together
- Administer the Double P II for 1-2 months; Administer *Di Gu Pi* (with Cervical formula if needed) up to 6 months
- If recurrent signs may treat on and off long-term
- A description of all the ingredients of each Chinese herbal medicine listed is beyond the scope of this text, but can be found elsewhere.[7,8]

Food Therapy:

The purpose of Food therapy is to promote *Qi*/Blood circulation, tonify Kidney *Qi*, clear false Heat and tonify Kidney *Yin* to support nerve regeneration. Foods that are Hot are avoided.[28]

- Foods to supplement to promote *Qi* and Blood circulation include: chicken egg, crab, sweet rice, peaches, carrots, coriander, squash, turnips
- Foods to tonify *Qi*: Beef, chicken, sardines, egg, potato, yam, sweet potato, rice, oats, millet, lentils, carrots, squash, microalgae, dates, figs, molasses, royal jelly
- Foods to Cool and tonify *Yin*: Turkey, pork, duck, clams, crab, eggs, rice, wheat, wheat germ, wheat berries, Belgian endive, string beans, peas, kidney beans, sweet potatoes, yams, tomato, spinach, tofu, kiwi, lemons, rhubarb, pears, bananas, watermelon, sesame, seaweed
- Hot foods to avoid: Lamb, shrimp, corn-fed beef, chicken, trout, squash, turnips, sweet rice, basal, caraway, cherries, chilies, cinnamon, ginger, rosemary, sage

Tui-na Procedures:

The purpose of the *Tui-na* is to stimulate *Qi* and Blood flow to relieve pain and promote nerve regeneration in the affected region. If pain is severe, avoid *Tui-na* in the region of the pain until acupuncture and Chinese herbal medicine have relieved the pain. The descriptions and indications of each technique are outlined in more detail in Chapter 1 Table 8.[20]

- A *Tui-na* protocol for cervical disk disease is outlined in Table 5
- A *Tui-na* protocol for thoracolumbar disk disease is outlined in Table 6

Daily Life Style Recommendation for Owner Follow-up:

- If Grades 3-5 paresis or paralysis, turn (if in lateral recumbency) or move every 4-6 hours to prevent lung atelectasis and decubitus ulcers
- Keep on padding to avoid decubitus ulcers on shoulders, hips or tuber ischii
- Keep dry and clean of feces and urine

- Gentle *Moo-fa* (Daubing or massaging) of the neck or back for 3 minutes
- Gentle *Ca-fa* (Rubbing) of neck or back for a few minutes until it feels warm, once daily for 14-21 days
- *Ba-shen-fa* (Stretching) and range of motion exercises of all the limbs for 12 times twice daily until can walk
- Assist to walk with a sling if needed
- Swim with support and supervision
- Avoid prolong periods outdoors when weather is Hot
- Avoid collars and walk with a harness, as even if the problem is in the thoracolumbar region, cervical intervertebral disks may cause problems in the future
- Once recovered avoid jumping on and off furniture and rough play

Comments:
Based on clinical experiences and current research, the TCVM treatments should shorten the recovery time, improve the degree of functional recovery and reduce recurrences.

7. Spinal cord *Qi*/Blood Stagnation and Kidney *Yin* and *Yang* Deficiencies

Clinical Signs:
- Acute or chronic paresis or paralysis (Grades 2-5 neurological deficits)
- With or without neck or back pain
- May have panting, warm ears, back or feet and seek cool
- May have cold ears, back or feet and seek heat
- Tongue- may vary and be pale purple and wet or reddish purple, dry and cracked or a combination
- Pulses- deep, weak both sides; may be rapid, thready, slow or wiry

TCVM Diagnosis:
The diagnosis is made based on the presence of paresis or paralysis (Grades 2-5 neurological deficits) of all four limbs or the pelvic limbs alone with clinical evidence of a combination of Heat and Cold on the TCVM examination. The paresis or paralysis with cold ears, back or feet is typical of Spinal Cord *Qi*/Blood Stagnation with Kidney *Yang* Deficiency. The animal may at times have panting episodes, warm ears, back and feet and dry skin, typical of a Kidney *Yin* Deficiency. The tongue characteristics can vary, depending on which pattern is primarily reflected. A pale purple and wet tongue reflects the *Qi*/Blood Stagnation and Kidney *Yang* Deficiency. A reddish purple and dry tongue reflects the *Qi*/Blood Stagnation and Kidney *Yin* Deficiency. The tongue may be cracked, if *Yin* Deficiency is chronic. The pulses can vary and may be wiry reflecting an acute *Qi*/Blood Stagnation or be deep and weak on both sides reflecting the combination of *Yin* and *Qi* Deficiency. A combination of warm ears and front feet and cold back and hind feet is one example of the mixed TCVM examination findings typical of Cold and Heat in an animal with concurrent *Yang* and *Yin* Deficiency patterns.

- Assist to walk with a sling if needed
- Do not swim as the body may become chilled further and put unneeded stress on the body's *Yang*
- Avoid collars and walk with a harness, as even if the problem is in the thoracolumbar region, cervical intervertebral disks may cause problems in the future
- Once recovered avoid jumping on and off furniture and rough play

Comments:

Based on clinical experiences and current research, the TCVM treatments should shorten the recovery time, improve the degree of functional recovery and reduce recurrences.

SPINAL CORD TRAUMA

Spinal cord injury from automobile accidents, gun shot wounds, falls and other sources of trauma are common in dogs and cats.[1-4,10] Clinical signs of acute paresis or paralysis of all four limbs or the pelvic limbs alone may be associated with a traumatic intervertebral disk herniation, fractured vertebrae with or without luxation or vertebral column ligament tears. Spinal cord contusion (hemorrhage and edema) usually results. Acute paralysis is always an emergency and should be treated as described above in the section entitled **INTEGRATED TREATMENT OF ACUTE PARALYSIS**. Referral for TCVM treatment is common after 72 hours, as conventional treatments have less effect and other treatment options are sought.[2,3,5] As discussed above, studies have supported the use of EA and DN to promote neuronal regeneration and recovery from spinal trauma.[10] In five human clinical trials, patients receiving EA integrated with conventional drugs and rehabilitation had significantly increased recovery rates compared to those receiving only conventional drugs and rehabilitation for spinal cord injury.[22] As discussed for intervertebral disk related spinal cord injuries, Chinese herbal medicine can promote neural regeneration in experimental spinal cord injury studies.[24-27]

Stem cell transplantation research has been increasing to promote spinal cord regeneration following injury.[30] Stem cell differentiation may be effected by EA and the combination of EA and stem cell transplantation may prove to be superior to stem cell transplantation alone. In a recent spinal cord injury study in laboratory animals, the group that had mesenchymal stem cell (MSC) implantation plus EA had significantly higher numbers of neuron-like cells, oligodendrocyte-like cells and 5-hydroxytryptophan positive nerve fibers than groups receiving only MSC implantation, EA alone or no treatment.[31]

Etiology and Pathology

From a TCVM perspective, spinal cord trauma results in Stagnation of *Qi*/Blood flow with *Qi* Deficiency locally that affects spinal cord function.[4,5] The Deficiency and Stagnation of *Qi* and bleeding, associated with the spinal cord contusion, depletes Blood and *Gu Qi* that nourish the neurons and other cells of the region and degeneration and demyelination occurs. Kidney *Qi* Deficiency is also present, if the animal has pelvic limb or generalized limb paresis or paralysis (*Tan-Huan* syndrome). Applying the basic TCVM theories of *Yin/Yang*, Eight Principles, Five Treasures, Five Elements and *Zang Fu* physiology and pathology to make a TCVM diagnosis, there is one main TCVM pattern associated with spinal cord trauma (Table 2):

1. **Spinal cord *Qi*/Blood Stagnation and Kidney *Qi* Deficiency**
    External trauma to the spinal cord causes spinal cord *Qi*/Blood Stagnation, local bleeding and *Qi* Deficiency and Kidney *Qi* Deficiency causing paresis or paralysis.

Pattern Differentiation and Treatment

1. Spinal cord *Qi*/Blood Stagnation and Kidney *Qi* Deficiency

Clinical Signs:
- Acute Grades 2-5 paresis or paralysis
- May or not have pain
- Tongue- pale, purple
- Pulses- wiry or weak

TCVM Diagnosis:
There is usually a history or physical evidence of a traumatic event. Conventional medical treatment with MPSS is important within the first 8 hours of onset of Grades 4-5 paralysis. Spinal radiographs are obtained prior to manipulation to detect vertebral fractures that might worsen with handling or need to be surgically repaired. Neck or back pain is usually present in animals with vertebral fractures. Spinal cord *Qi*/Blood Stagnation with Kidney *Qi* Deficiency is the primary TCVM pattern commonly associated with spinal trauma causing Grades 2-5 paresis or paralysis. The tongue may be purple reflecting the *Qi*/Blood Stagnation, but can also be pale associated with shock or Kidney *Qi* Deficiency. The pulses are wiry reflecting the *Qi*/Blood Stagnation or weak reflecting shock or Kidney *Qi* Deficiency.

Treatment Principles:
- Resolve *Qi*/Blood Stagnation to return proper *Qi*/Blood flow, relieve pain and resolve paresis and paralysis
- Tonify Kidney *Qi* and resolve paresis or paralysis

Acupuncture treatment:
EA is more effective than DN to control pain, resolve *Qi*/Blood Stagnation and promote nerve regeneration. For EA use 20 Hz for 10-15 minutes then 80-120 Hz alternating frequencies for 10-15 minutes. EA is combined with DN and Aqua-AP. For Aqua-AP inject 0.25-0.5 ml vitamin B12 into the acupoint after *Tui-na*. For Grade 4-5 neurological deficits, EA and DN should be administered every 1-3 days for 3-5 times, depending on the patient's response, then reduced to once every 1-2 weeks until ambulatory. For Grades 2 and 3, the acupuncture treatments may be weekly or every other week.

Acupoints recommended
- EA: Select appropriate acupoints in Table 3 depending on the lesion location
- DN: Select acupoints in Table 3 plus BL-23, KID-7, KID-3
- Aqua-AP: BL-23

Pertinent acupoint actions
- See Table 3 for indications and actions of acupoints recommended for EA and DN
- BL-23 is the Back *Shu* Association point for the Kidney to support Kidney *Qi* and resolve paresis or paralysis and nourish the spinal cord
- KID-7 is the Mother point on the Channel useful to treat Kidney Deficiencies
- KID-3 is the *Yuan* Source point useful to treat Kidney *Qi* Deficiency and resolve paresis and paralysis

Herbal Medicine:
- For Grades 2-5 paresis or paralysis administer Double P II (JT)[a] 0.5gm/10-20# twice daily orally to move *Qi* and Blood and eliminate Stagnation and pain
- If pelvic limb paresis or paralysis, add *Bu Yang Huan Wu* (JT)[a] 0.5gm/10-20# twice daily orally to move and nourish Blood and tonify *Qi*
- If all four limbs are affected, administer Cervical Formula (JT)[a] 0.5gm/10-20# twice daily orally to activate Blood, move *Qi*, eliminate Stagnation and pain
- Administer Double P II for 1-2 months then continue *Bu Yang Huan Wu* or Cervical Formula until recovered up to 6 months
- A description of all the ingredients of the Chinese herbal medicine listed is beyond the scope of this text, but can be found elsewhere.[7,8]

Food Therapy:
The purpose of the Food therapy is to promote *Qi*/Blood circulation and tonify Kidney *Qi* to support nerve regeneration in the affected region. Foods that are Cold or Hot are avoided.[28]
- Foods to supplement to promote *Qi* and Blood circulation include: chicken egg, crab, sweet rice, peaches, carrots, coriander, squash, turnips
- Foods to tonify *Qi*: Beef, chicken, sardines, egg, potato, yam, sweet potato, rice, oats, millet, lentils, carrots, squash, microalgae, dates, figs, molasses, royal jelly
- Cold foods to avoid: Turkey, duck, duck eggs, conch, clams, mussels, yogurt, millet, barley, spinach, broccoli, celery, egg plant, kelp, alfalfa, cucumbers, pears, bananas, white radishes, watermelon
- Hot foods to avoid: Lamb, shrimp, corn-fed beef, chicken, trout, squash, turnips, sweet rice, basal, caraway, cherries, chilies, cinnamon, ginger, rosemary, sage

Tui-na Procedures:
The purpose of the *Tui-na* is to stimulate *Qi* and Blood flow to relieve pain and promote nerve regeneration in the affected region. The descriptions and indications of each technique are outlined in more detail in Chapter 1 Table 8.[20]
- If fractured vertebrae are present avoid manipulation of the neck and back
- *An-fa* pressing of SI-3, LI-4, TH-5 and LU-7 for 5-10 seconds per acupoint
- *Nian-fa* holding and kneading each of the digits and distal extremities repeat 12 times
- Once pain and has been controlled and fractured vertebrae have been stabilized further *Tui-na* can be performed
- *Ca-fa* rubbing from the scapula to the carpus and/or from the hip to the tarsus on each side for 1 minute on each limb

- *Dou-fa* gently shaking for 12 times, *Ba-shen-fa* stretching for 12 times and *Ban-fa* flexing and extending joints for 12 times; perform on each limb

Daily Life Style Recommendation for Owner Follow-up:
- If Grades 3-5 paresis or paralysis, turn (if in lateral recumbency) or move every 4-6 hours to prevent lung atelectasis and decubitus ulcers
- *Nian-fa* holding and kneading each of the digits and distal extremities repeat 12 times twice daily
- Keep on padding to avoid decubitus ulcers on shoulders, hips or tuber ischii
- Keep dry and clean of feces and urine
- Assist to walk with a sling if needed
- Swim with support and supervision
- Once recovered avoid jumping on and off furniture and rough play

Comments:
Based on clinical experiences and current research, the TCVM treatments should shorten the recovery time and improve the degree of functional recovery. On serial TCVM evaluations if *Yin* or *Yang* Deficiency develops, see the treatment of Kidney *Qi* and *Yin* Deficiencies, Kidney *Yang* Deficiency and Kidney *Yin* and *Yang* Deficiency described above in the section on **INTERVERTEBRAL DISK DISEASE**.

CERVICAL SPONDYLOMYELOPATHY (WOBBLER SYNDROME)

"Wobbler" syndrome (cervical spondylomyelopathy) occurs in both young and old large breed dogs. A potentially inherited malformation and malarticulation of the cervical vertebrae that might be accentuated by a high protein diet, produces a stenosis of the vertebral canal and spinal cord compression in young dogs.[2,3] In older dogs vertebral canal stenosis and spinal cord compression are associated with ligamentous degeneration and hypertrophy, cervical vertebral joint laxity with vertebral degeneration and remodeling with or without intervertebral disk disease degeneration and protrusion.[2,3] Although many different large breed dogs can be affected, 1-2 year old Great Danes and 5-10 year old Doberman Pinchers are most common. Wobbler syndrome is therefore a specific cervical spondylomyelopathy and the term should not be used to simply describe an ataxic dog. Most ataxic small breed dogs have intervertebral disk disease or some other spinal cord disorder. Large breed dogs can also have intervertebral disk disease and not all the other vertebral and ligamentous changes associated with Wobbler syndrome as well as many other spinal cord disorders.

The onset of clinical signs is most often slow and insidious, but can be acute, if associated with a minimal traumatic event. Ataxia is present in all four limbs, although the pelvic limbs often appear more affected. The limbs circumduct during ambulation and the hips wobble from side to side and it was this characteristic gait that resulted in the syndrome name "wobbler". The thoracic limb deficits are often misconstrued as compensation for the pelvic limb ataxia and a lesion below T2 may be initially suspected, but on closer examination and utilizing the tests of subtle dysfunction on the neurological examination a stiff, stilted short-strided gait, conscious proprioceptive deficits and paresis of the thoracic limbs can often be found. There may be atrophy or fasciculation of the deltoid, biceps, infraspinatus and supraspinatus muscles. A "root signature" (slight lifting of one thoracic limb) may be apparent. Conscious proprioceptive deficits may be seen in the pelvic limbs alone or both the thoracic and pelvic limbs. One side may be more affected than the other. There may be some degree of neck pain on palpation and manipulation, although this is often subtle. Rarely dogs are presented for acute non-ambulatory quadriparesis (Grades 3 or 4 neurological deficits) associated with a minor neck injury. Other dogs are presented to the TCVM practitioner with non-ambulatory quadriparesis (Grade 3 or 4 neurological deficits) post-operatively or as a natural progression of the disease.

An MRI with the neck extended then flexed is essential to appreciate the location and extent of the spinal cord compression prior to surgical intervention. Conventional treatments involve the chronic administration of corticosteroids and/or ventral decompression and distraction/fusion surgery. All conventional treatments carry a risk for long-term adverse side effects and affected animals may benefit first from TCVM treatments that have no adverse side effects.

In one clinical study of 40 dogs with "wobbler" syndrome (cervical spondylomyelopathy), dogs were graded based on the severity of their neurological deficits and then randomly assigned to one of two groups to ensure equal overall severity between groups.[32] Group 1 consisted of 20 dogs that received surgery and conventional medicine and Group 2 consisted of 20 dogs that received EA with or without surgery and conventional medicine. The authors reported an overall success rate of 85% for dogs that received EA and 20% for dogs that received surgery and conventional medication alone. The surgical success rate in this study was lower than other reports, but the benefit of EA warrants further investigation.[2,3] In a retrospective study of "wobbler" syndrome in 13 large breed dogs, 6 dogs were diagnosed with caudal cervical IVDD and 7 with "wobbler" syndrome.[33] All dogs were graded using the standard 1-5 scale of neurological deficits described above and ranged from 2-4. All dogs, except two, received prednisone or non-steroidal anti-inflammatory drugs. A combination of EA, DN and Aqua-AP was performed from 3-16 times with an average of 7.6 treatments. Seven dogs returned to normal (1 dog with Grade 3 and 6 dogs with Grade 2). Four dogs improved to Grade 1 (3 dogs with Grade 3 and 1 dog with Grade 2). One dog with Grade 4 improved to Grade 2 and one dog with Grade 5 did not improve after 3 acupuncture treatments. Although further clinical studies are needed, there is enough evidence to warrant further investigation and treatment of wobblers with TCVM. An overview of the TCVM patterns associated with "wobbler" syndrome and suggested TCVM treatments are outlined in Tables 2-4.[5-8] Food therapy may be useful to treat underlying TCVM patterns and *Tui-na* can be integrated into the treatment (Table 5).[20,28]

Etiology and Pathology

Since "wobbler" syndrome results in chronic repeated mild spinal cord injury from cervical vertebral instability and spinal cord compression, the signs of *Tan-Huan* syndrome (paresis or paralysis) may be more chronic progressive than with other forms of spinal cord injury. However the result is still spinal cord *Qi*/Blood Stagnation with resulting Kidney *Qi* Deficiency.[5] As with other types of trauma and compression, in "wobbler" syndrome, local Stagnation and Deficiency of *Qi*/Blood depletes Blood and *Gu Qi* necessary to nourish the neurons and other cells of the spinal cord and degeneration and demyelination occurs. Kidney *Qi* Deficiency is also present, if the animal develops pelvic limb or generalized limb paresis or paralysis. Either *Jing* Deficiency (pre-natal) or *Bi* syndrome is the primary basic disorder that accounts for the vertebral and intervertebral disk degeneration associated with wobbler's syndrome. Pre-natal *Jing* Deficiency usually takes three forms: 1) Malformations (birth defects), 2) Genetic disorders and 3) Premature degeneration (aging). *Jing* Deficient "wobbler" syndrome may result in malformation and premature aging (in the form of vertebral and ligamentous degeneration) and although there is a breed predisposition the genetic basis is still unclear and currently under investigation. Kidney *Yin* or *Yang* Bony *Bi* may produce the disease in older dogs. Applying the basic TCVM theories of *Yin/Yang*, Eight Principles, Five Treasures, Five Elements and *Zang Fu* physiology and pathology to make a TCVM diagnosis, there are five basic patterns associated with wobbler syndrome in dogs:

1. **Spinal cord *Qi*/Blood Stagnation and Kidney *Jing* and *Qi* Deficiencies**
   In these young Great Danes and other large breed dogs an underlying Kidney *Jing* Deficiency causes the abnormalities in vertebral and ligamentous development that lead to cervical vertebral malformation and instability. The result is repeated focal spinal cord trauma and compression causing *Qi*/Blood Stagnation, local spinal cord *Qi*/Blood Deficiency and ataxia, paresis or paralysis (usually Grades 2-4 neurological deficits). Since the spinal cord is associated with the Kidney and the pelvic limbs are often most prominently affected, the paresis or paralysis is associated with Kidney *Qi* Deficiency.

2. **Spinal cord *Qi*/Blood Stagnation and Kidney *Qi* Deficiency**
   In these adult Doberman Pinschers and other large breed dogs, *Bi* syndrome is present and vertebral and intervertebral disk degeneration is associated with this form of "wobbler" syndrome. Progressive spinal cord trauma and compression cause focal spinal cord *Qi*/Blood Stagnation and *Qi*/Blood Deficiency with clinical signs of ataxia, quadriparesis or quadriplegia (Grades 2-5 neurological deficits). Since the spinal cord is associated with the Kidney and the pelvic limbs are often most prominently affected, the paresis or paralysis is due to Kidney *Qi* Deficiency. Serial neurological and TCVM examinations are important, as evidence of one of the other underlying TCVM patterns (e.g. Kidney *Yin* or *Yang* Deficiency) may become evident and also need to be treated.

3. **Spinal cord *Qi*/Blood Stagnation and Kidney *Yang* Deficiency**
   Kidney *Yang* Deficiency *Bi* Syndrome develops due to chronic stress, illness or poor nutrition and results in vertebral and intervertebral disk degeneration especially in *Yin* animals (Earth, Metal and Water constitutions). When animals with Kidney *Qi* Deficiency develop clinical signs of Cold, the pattern becomes Kidney *Yang* Deficiency (*Qi* Deficiency plus Cold = *Yang* Deficiency). In these adult Doberman Pinschers and other large breed dogs, *Bi* syndrome is present and vertebral and intervertebral disk degeneration is associated with this form of "wobbler" syndrome. Progressive spinal cord trauma and compression cause focal spinal cord *Qi*/Blood Stagnation and *Qi*/Blood Deficiency with clinical signs of ataxia, quadriparesis or quadriplegia (Grades 2-5 neurological deficits). Since the spinal cord is associated with the Kidney and the pelvic limbs are often affected most prominently, the paresis or paralysis is due to Kidney *Qi* Deficiency. Evidence of Cold is found on the TCVM history and examination.

4. **Spinal cord *Qi*/Blood Stagnation and Kidney *Qi* and *Yin* Deficiency**
   Kidney *Yin* Deficiency *Bi* Syndrome occurs from chronic stress, illness or poor nutrition and results in vertebral and intervertebral disk degeneration especially in *Yang* animals (Wood and Fire constitutions). In these adult Doberman Pinschers and other large breed dogs, *Bi* syndrome is present and vertebral and intervertebral disk degeneration is associated with this form of "wobbler" syndrome. Progressive spinal cord trauma and compression cause focal spinal cord *Qi*/Blood Stagnation and *Qi*/Blood Deficiency with clinical signs of ataxia, quadriparesis or quadriplegia (Grades 2-5 neurological deficits). Since the spinal cord is associated with the Kidney and the pelvic limbs are often affected most prominently, the paresis or paralysis is due to Kidney *Qi* Deficiency. Clinical evidence of Heat on the TCVM examination is typical of a concurrent *Yin* Deficiency. The pattern then becomes Spinal cord *Qi*/Blood Stagnation with Kidney *Qi* and *Yin* Deficiency.

5. **Spinal cord *Qi*/Blood Stagnation and Kidney *Yin* and *Yang* Deficiencies**
   In these adult Doberman Pinschers and other large breed dogs, *Bi* syndrome is present and vertebral and intervertebral disk degeneration is associated with this form of "wobbler" syndrome. Progressive spinal cord trauma and compression cause focal spinal cord *Qi*/Blood Stagnation and *Qi*/Blood Deficiency with clinical signs of ataxia, quadriparesis or quadriplegia (Grades 2-5 neurological deficits). Since the spinal cord is associated with the Kidney and the pelvic limbs are often affected most prominently, the paresis or paralysis is associated with Kidney *Qi* Deficiency. Kidney *Qi* Deficiency and clinical signs of Cold are typical of Kidney *Yang* Deficiency. Clinical evidence of Heat is associated with a concurrent Kidney *Yin* Deficiency. The TCVM pattern then becomes Spinal cord *Qi*/Blood Stagnation with underlying Kidney *Yin* and *Yang* Deficiencies. Both Kidney *Yin* and *Yang* Deficiency *Bi* Syndrome occur from chronic stress, illness or poor nutrition and results in vertebral and intervertebral disk degeneration.

Pattern Differentiation and Treatment

1. Spinal cord *Qi*/Blood Stagnation and Kidney *Jing* and *Qi* Deficiencies

<u>Clinical Signs:</u>
- Great Danes and other large breed dogs usually less than 5 years of age
- Chronic progressive ataxia, quadriparesis or quadriplegia (Grades 2-4 neurological deficits)
- May or not have neck pain
- Tongue- pale, purple, wet and may be swollen
- Pulses- deep, weak bilaterally or wiry

<u>TCVM Diagnosis</u>:
The diagnosis is made based on the presence of ataxia, paresis or paralysis (Grades 2-5 neurological deficits) of all four limbs usually worse in the pelvic limbs in a young large breed dog, commonly Great Danes. The onset of clinical signs when the dog is less than 5 years of age suggests a Kidney *Jing* Deficiency. The ataxia, paresis or paralysis (Grades 2-5 neurological

deficits) of all four limbs is associated with a Kidney *Qi* Deficiency. The purple of the tongue is typical of *Qi*/Blood Stagnation and the paleness reflects the Kidney *Jing* and *Qi* Deficiencies. The tongue is usually wet with Kidney *Jing* and *Qi* Deficiencies. The pulses can vary and may be wiry, reflecting the *Qi*/Blood Stagnation, or be deep and weak on both sides reflecting the Kidney *Jing* and *Qi* Deficiencies.

Treatment Principles:
- Resolve *Qi*/Blood Stagnation to return proper *Qi*/Blood flow, relieve pain and resolve ataxia, quadriparesis and quadriplegia
- Tonify Kidney *Jing*
- Tonify Kidney *Qi* to resolve ataxia, quadriparesis and quadriplegia

Acupuncture treatment:
EA is more effective than DN to control pain, resolve *Qi*/Blood Stagnation and promote nerve regeneration. For EA use 20 Hz for 10-15 minutes then 80-120 Hz alternating frequencies for 10-15 minutes. EA is combined with DN and Aqua-AP. For Aqua-AP inject 0.25-0.5 ml vitamin B12 into the acupoint after *Tui-na*. For non-ambulatory quadriparesis or quadriplegia (Grades 3-5 neurological deficits), EA and DN should be administered every 3-5 days for 3-5 times, depending on the patient's response, then reduced to once every 1-2 weeks until ambulatory. For ataxia and mild paresis (Grade 2), the acupuncture treatments may be weekly or every other week for 5-7 times and then every 4-6 weeks for maintenance, as needed.

Acupoints recommended
- EA: Select appropriate acupoints in Table 3 for cervical spinal cord lesions
- DN: Select acupoints in Table 3 plus BL-20, BL-21, BL-23, BL-26, BL-62, KID-3, SI-3
- Aqua-AP: BL-23, *Jing-jia-ji*

Pertinent acupoint actions
- See Table 3 for indications and actions of acupoints recommended for EA and DN and classical point locations
- BL-20 is the Back *Shu* Association point for the Spleen to support the production of post-natal *Jing* to reduce the use of pre-natal Kidney *Jing*
- BL-21 is the Back *Shu* Association point for the Stomach to support the production of post-natal *Jing* to reduce the use of pre-natal Kidney *Jing*
- BL-23 is the Back *Shu* Association point for the Kidney to tonify Kidney *Qi* and resolve quadriparesis and quadriplegia and nourish the spinal cord, vertebrae and intervertebral disks
- BL-26 is the Gate of *Yuan* Source *Qi* and is useful to treat Kidney *Yang* and *Qi* Deficiency and resolve quadriparesis and quadriplegia
- BL-62 is the confluent point with the *Yang Qiao* Extraordinary Channel useful to treat ataxia and weakness of all four limbs
- KID-3 is the *Yuan* Source point for the Kidney to treat *Qi* Deficiency and resolve quadriparesis and quadriplegia and nourish the Kidney
- SI-3 is useful to treat cervical *Qi*/Blood Stagnation

Herbal Medicine:
- For ataxia and mild quadriparesis (mild Grade 2 neurological deficits) administer Cervical Formula (JT)[a] 0.5gm/10-20# twice daily orally to move *Qi* and Blood and eliminate Stagnation and pain, ataxia and paresis
- If the quadriparesis is moderate (moderate Grade 2 neurological deficits) or the dog has non-ambulatory quadriparesis or quadriplegia (Grades 3-5 neurological deficits) combine Cervical Formula (JT)[a] with Double P II (JT)[a] 0.5gm/10-20# twice daily orally for 1-5 months as needed to further move *Qi* and Blood and eliminate Stagnation and pain, ataxia, paresis or paralysis
- When Double P II is no longer needed, discontinue and add Epimedium Formula (JT)[a] 0.5gm/10-20# twice daily orally to support Kidney *Jing*
- Epimedium Formula and Cervical Formula are often administered for 6-9 months or longer if needed
- If signs are recurrent, may treat on and off long-term
- A description of all the ingredients of the Chinese herbal medicine listed is beyond the scope of this text, but can be found elsewhere.[7,8]

Food Therapy:
The purpose of the Food therapy is to resolve *Qi*/Blood Stagnation and tonify Kidney *Jing* and Kidney *Qi* to promote nerve regeneration in the affected region and strengthen limbs. Foods that are Cold or Hot are avoided.[28]
- Foods to supplement to promote *Qi* and Blood circulation include: chicken egg, crab, sweet rice, peaches, carrots, coriander, squash, turnips
- Foods to tonify *Jing*: Liver, kidneys, fish, bone and bone marrow, millet, quinoa, spelt, wheat, almonds, black sesame, microalgae (e.g. chlorella, spirulina, wild blue-green algae), barley, wheat grass, black soy beans, black beans, kidney beans, seaweed, sea salt, mulberries, raspberries, strawberries, almonds, black sesame, clarified butter (ghee), royal jelly, bee pollen
- Foods to tonify Kidney *Qi*: Beef, chicken, sardines, egg, potato, yam, sweet potato, rice, oats, millet, lentils, carrots, squash, microalgae, dates, figs, molasses, royal jelly
- Cold foods to avoid: Turkey, duck, duck eggs, conch, clams, mussels, yogurt, millet, barley, spinach, broccoli, celery, egg plant, kelp, alfalfa, cucumbers, pears, bananas, white radishes, watermelon
- Hot foods to avoid: Lamb, shrimp, corn-fed beef, chicken, trout, squash, turnips, sweet rice, basal, caraway, cherries, chilies, cinnamon, ginger, rosemary, sage

Tui-na Procedures:
The purpose of the *Tui-na* is to stimulate *Qi* and Blood flow to relieve pain and promote nerve regeneration in the affected region. The descriptions and indications of each technique are outlined in more detail in Chapter 1 Table 8.[20]
- A *Tui-na* protocol for cervical spondylomyelopathy (wobbler syndrome) is outlined in Table 5.

Daily Life Style Recommendation for Owner Follow-up:
- *Moo-fa* (Daubing or massaging) of the neck for 3 minutes

- *Ca-fa* (Rubbing) of neck for a few minutes until it feels warm, once daily for 14-21 days
- *Ba-shen-fa* and stretch the neck and front limbs for 12 times once a day for 7 days
- Remove all collars and walk with a harness
- No rough play involving the neck

Comments:

With acupuncture, Chinese herbal therapy, *Tui-na* and Food therapy corticosteroids and surgery may be avoided and a high quality of life maintained.

2. Spinal cord *Qi*/Blood Stagnation and Kidney *Qi* Deficiency

Clinical Signs:
- Doberman Pinschers and other large breed dogs greater than 5 years of age
- Chronic progressive ataxia, quadriparesis or quadriplegia (Grades 2-5 neurological deficits)
- May or not have neck pain
- Tongue- pale, purple, wet
- Pulses- deep, weak worse on right or wiry

TCVM Diagnosis:

The diagnosis is made based on the presence of ataxia, paresis or paralysis (Grades 2-5 neurological deficits) of all four limbs with no evidence of concurrent Deficient Heat and/or Cold patterns. The purple tongue is typical of *Qi*/Blood Stagnation and the pale, wet tongue reflects the Kidney *Qi* Deficiency. The pulses can vary and may be wiry reflecting the *Qi*/Blood Stagnation or be deep and weak worse on the right reflecting the Kidney *Qi* Deficiency.

Treatment Principles:
- Resolve *Qi*/Blood Stagnation to return proper *Qi*/Blood flow, relieve pain and resolve ataxia, quadriparesis and quadriplegia
- Tonify Kidney *Qi* to resolve quadriparesis and quadriplegia

Acupuncture treatment:

EA is more effective than DN to control pain, resolve *Qi*/Blood Stagnation and promote nerve regeneration. For EA use 20 Hz for 10-15 minutes then 80-120 Hz alternating frequencies for 10-15 minutes. EA is combined with DN and Aqua-AP. For Aqua-AP inject 0.25-0.5 ml vitamin B12 into the acupoint after *Tui-na*. For non-ambulatory quadriparesis or quadriplegia (Grades 3-5 neurological deficits), EA and DN should be administered every 3-5 days for 3-5 times, depending on the patient's response, then reduced to once every 1-2 weeks until ambulatory. For ataxia and mild paresis (Grade 2 neurological deficits), the acupuncture treatments may be weekly or every other week for 5-7 times and then every 4-6 weeks for maintenance, as needed.

Acupoints recommended
- EA: Select appropriate acupoints in Table 3 for cervical spinal cord lesions

- DN: Select acupoints in Table 3 plus BL-23, KID-3, SI-3, BL-62
- Aqua-AP: BL-23, *Jing-jia-ji*

Pertinent acupoint actions
- See Table 3 for indications and actions of acupoints recommended for EA and DN and classical point locations
- BL-23 is the Back *Shu* Association point for the Kidney to tonify Kidney *Qi* and resolve ataxia, quadriparesis and quadriplegia and nourish the spinal cord, vertebrae and intervertebral disks
- KID-3 is the *Yuan* Source point for the Kidney to treat *Qi* Deficiency and resolve quadriparesis and quadriplegia and nourish the Kidney
- SI-3 is useful to treat cervical *Qi*/Blood Stagnation
- BL-62 is the confluent point with the *Yang Qiao* Extraordinary Channel useful to treat ataxia, quadriparesis and quadriplegia

Herbal Medicine:
- For ataxia and mild quadriparesis (mild Grade 2 neurological deficits) administer Cervical Formula (JT)[a] 0.5gm/10-20# twice daily orally to move *Qi* and Blood and eliminate Stagnation and pain, ataxia and paresis
- Combine with *Bu Yang Huan Wu* (JT)[a] 0.5gm/10-20# twice daily orally to further move *Qi*/Blood, nourish Blood and tonify *Qi* and *Yang*
- If the quadriparesis is moderate (moderate Grade 2) or the dog has non-ambulatory quadriparesis or quadriplegia (Grades 3-5 neurological deficits) also add Double P II (JT)[a] 0.5gm/10-20# twice daily orally for 1-5 months as needed to further move *Qi* and Blood and eliminate Stagnation and pain, ataxia, paresis or paralysis
- If Cervical Formula, Double P II and *Bu Yang Huan Wu* are combined, then reduce the dose of Cervical Formula and *Bu Yang Huan Wu* to 0.5gm/20# twice daily orally especially in geriatric dogs
- Administer Double P II for 1-5 months, then continue Cervical Formula and *Bu Yang Huan Wu*, increasing the doses to 0.5gm/10# twice daily orally for 6 months or longer if needed
- If signs are recurrent, may treat on and off long-term
- A description of all the ingredients of the Chinese herbal medicine listed is beyond the scope of this text, but can be found elsewhere.[7,8]

Food Therapy:

The purpose of the Food therapy is to promote *Qi*/Blood circulation and tonify Kidney *Qi* to support nerve regeneration in the affected region. Foods that are Cold or Hot are avoided.[28]
- Foods to supplement to promote *Qi* and Blood circulation include: chicken egg, crab, sweet rice, peaches, carrots, coriander, squash, turnips
- Foods to tonify *Qi*: Beef, chicken, sardines, egg, potato, yam, sweet potato, rice, oats, millet, lentils, carrots, squash, microalgae, dates, figs, molasses, royal jelly
- Cold foods to avoid: Turkey, duck, duck eggs, conch, clams, mussels, yogurt, millet, barley, spinach, broccoli, celery, egg plant, kelp, alfalfa, cucumbers, pears, bananas, white radishes, watermelon

- Hot foods to avoid: Lamb, shrimp, corn-fed beef, chicken, trout, squash, turnips, sweet rice, basal, caraway, cherries, chilies, cinnamon, ginger, rosemary, sage

Tui-na Procedures:

The purpose of the *Tui-na* is to stimulate *Qi* and Blood flow to relieve pain and promote nerve regeneration in the affected region. The descriptions and indications of each technique are outlined in more detail in Chapter 1 Table 8.[20]

- A *Tui-na* protocol for cervical spondylomyelopathy (wobbler syndrome) is outlined in Table 5.

Daily Life Style Recommendation for Owner Follow-up:

- If Grades 3-5 paresis or paralysis, turn every 4-6 hours to prevent lung atelectasis and decubitus ulcers
- Keep on padding to avoid decubitus ulcers on shoulders, hips or tuber ischii
- Keep dry and clean of feces and urine
- Gentle *Moo-fa* (Daubing or massaging) of the neck or back for 3 minutes
- Gentle *Ca-fa* (Rubbing) of neck or back for a few minutes until it feels warm, once daily for 14-21 days
- *Ba-shen-fa* (Stretching) and range of motion exercises of all the limbs for 12 times twice daily for 7 days if ambulatory or until can walk if non-ambulatory
- Assist to walk with a sling if needed
- Swim with support and supervision if needed
- Remove all collars and walk with a harness
- No rough play involving the neck

Comments:

With acupuncture, Chinese herbal therapy, *Tui-na* and Food therapy corticosteroids and surgery may be avoided and a high quality of life maintained. On serial TCVM evaluations if *Yin* or *Yang* Deficiency develops, treat as described for those patterns below.

3. Spinal cord *Qi*/Blood Stagnation and Kidney *Yang* Deficiency

Clinical Signs:

- Doberman Pinschers and other large breed dogs greater than 5 years of age
- Chronic progressive ataxia, quadriparesis or quadriplegia (Grades 2-5 neurological deficits)
- May or not have neck pain
- Seeks Heat
- Cold ears, back, feet
- Tongue- pale purple, wet and may be swollen
- Pulses- deep, weak, slow, worse on right or may be wiry

TCVM Diagnosis:

The diagnosis is made based on the presence of ataxia, paresis or paralysis (Grades 2-5 neurological deficits) of all four limbs with evidence of a Cold pattern indicated by Heat seeking behavior and cold ears, back and feet. The purple tongue is typical of *Qi*/Blood Stagnation and *Yang* Deficiency and the tongue paleness is typical of Kidney *Qi* Deficiency. The tongue is often also wet and swollen from the Kidney *Yang/Qi* Deficiency. The deep, slow weak pulses, worse on the right, also reflect the Kidney *Yang* Deficiency. The pulses may also be wiry reflecting the *Qi*/Blood Stagnation.

Treatment Principles:
- Resolve *Qi*/Blood Stagnation to return proper *Qi*/Blood flow, relieve pain and resolve ataxia, quadriparesis and quadriplegia
- Tonify Kidney *Yang* and resolve quadriparesis and quadriplegia

Acupuncture treatment:

EA is more effective than DN to control pain, resolve *Qi*/Blood Stagnation and promote nerve regeneration. For EA use 20 Hz for 10-15 minutes then 80-120 Hz alternating frequencies for 10-15 minutes. EA is combined with DN and Aqua-AP. For Aqua-AP inject 0.25-0.5 ml vitamin B12 into the acupoint after *Tui-na*. For non-ambulatory quadriparesis or quadriplegia (Grades 3-5 neurological deficits), EA and DN should be administered every 3-5 days for 3-5 times, depending on the patient's response, then reduced to once every 1-2 weeks until ambulatory. For ataxia and mild paresis (Grade 2 neurological deficits), the acupuncture treatments may be weekly or every other week for 5-7 times and then every 4-6 weeks for maintenance, as needed.

Acupoints recommended
- EA: Select appropriate acupoints in Table 3 for cervical spinal cord lesions
- DN: Select acupoints in Table 3 plus BL-23, SI-3, BL-62
- Moxibustion: GV-3, GV-4, *Bai-hui*, *Shen-shu*, *Shen-peng*, *Shen-jiao*
- Aqua-AP: GV-4, BL-23, *Jing-jia-ji* or *Hua-tuo-jia-ji*

Pertinent acupoint actions
- See Table 3 for indications and actions of acupoints recommended for EA and DN and classical point locations
- BL-23 is the Back *Shu* Association point for the Kidney to tonify Kidney *Qi*, resolve paresis and paralysis and nourish the spinal cord, vertebrae and intervertebral disks
- *Shen-shu* (one *cun* lateral to *Bai-hui*), *Shen-peng* (one *cun* cranial to *Shen-shu*), *Shen-jiao* (one *cun* caudal to *Shen-shu*) are useful to treat Kidney *Qi* and *Yang* Deficiency and resolve quadriparesis and quadriplegia
- GV-3, GV-4 and *Bai-hui* are useful to treat Kidney *Yang* and *Qi* Deficiency and resolve quadriparesis and quadriplegia
- LI-10 and ST-36 are *Qi* Tonic acupoints useful to treat Kidney *Qi* Deficiency and resolve quadriparesis and quadriplegia

- KID-1 and PC-8 are pelvic and thoracic limb "root" acupoints useful to treat Grades 3-5 quadriparesis or quadriplegia
- SI-3 is useful to treat cervical *Qi*/Blood Stagnation
- BL-62 is the confluent point with the *Yang Qiao* Extraordinary Channel useful to treat *Yang* Deficiency and ataxia, quadriparesis and quadriplegia

Herbal Medicine:
- For ataxia and mild quadriparesis (mild Grade 2 neurological deficits) administer Cervical Formula (JT)[a] 0.5gm/10-20# twice daily orally to move *Qi* and Blood and eliminate Stagnation and pain, ataxia and paresis
- Combine with *Bu Yang Huan Wu* (JT)[a] 0.5gm/10-20# twice daily orally to further move *Qi*/Blood, nourish Blood and tonify *Qi* and *Yang*
- If the quadriparesis is moderate (moderate Grade 2 neurological deficits) or the dog has non-ambulatory quadriparesis or quadriplegia (Grades 3-5 neurological deficits) also add Double P II (JT)[a] 0.5gm/10-20# twice daily orally for 1-5 months as needed to further move *Qi* and Blood and eliminate Stagnation and pain, ataxia, paresis or paralysis
- If Cervical Formula, Double P II and *Bu Yang Huan Wu* are combined, then reduce the dose of Cervical Formula and *Bu Yang Huan Wu* to 0.5gm/20# twice daily orally especially in geriatric dogs
- Administer Double P II for 1-5 months, then continue Cervical Formula and *Bu Yang Huan Wu*, increasing the doses to 0.5gm/10# twice daily orally for 6 months or longer if needed
- If signs are recurrent, may treat on and off long-term
- A description of all the ingredients of the Chinese herbal medicine listed is beyond the scope of this text, but can be found elsewhere.[7,8]

Food Therapy:
The purpose of Food therapy is to promote *Qi*/Blood circulation, clear false Cold and tonify Kidney *Yang* to support nerve regeneration. Foods that are Cold are avoided.[28]
- Foods to supplement to promote *Qi* and Blood circulation include: chicken egg, crab, sweet rice, peaches, carrots, coriander, squash, turnips
- Foods to clear false Cold and tonify *Yang*: Chicken, lamb, corn fed beef, corn, millet, oats, brown rice, microalgae, pumpkin, squash, rutabaga, shiitake mushrooms, yams, sweet potatoes, winter squash, cherries, dates, figs, hawthorn fruit, lychees, molasses, royal jelly
- Cold foods to avoid: Turkey, duck, duck eggs, conch, clams, mussels, yogurt, millet, barley, spinach, broccoli, celery, egg plant, kelp, alfalfa, cucumbers, pears, bananas, white radishes, watermelon

Tui-na Procedures:
The purpose of the *Tui-na* is to stimulate *Qi* and Blood flow to relieve pain and promote nerve regeneration in the affected region. The descriptions and indications of each technique are outlined in more detail in Chapter 1 Table 8.[20]
- A *Tui-na* protocol for cervical spondylomyelopathy (wobbler syndrome) is outlined in Table 5

Daily Life Style Recommendation for Owner Follow-up:
- If Grades 3-5 paresis or paralysis, turn every 4-6 hours to prevent lung atelectasis and decubitus ulcers
- Keep on padding to avoid decubitus ulcers on shoulders, hips or tuber ischii
- Keep dry and clean of feces and urine
- Gentle *Moo-fa* (Daubing or massaging) of the neck or back for 3 minutes
- Gentle *Ca-fa* (Rubbing) of neck or back for a few minutes until it feels warm, once daily for 14-21 days
- *Ba-shen-fa* (Stretching) and range of motion exercises of all the limbs for 12 times twice daily for 7 days if ambulatory or until can walk if non-ambulatory
- Assist to walk with a sling if needed
- Do not swim as the body may become chilled further and put unneeded stress on the body's *Yang*
- Remove all collars and walk with a harness
- No rough play involving the neck
- For severely *Yang* Deficient dogs, select clients may be taught to administer moxibustion at GV-3, GV-4, *Bai-hui, Shen-shu, Shen-peng, Shen-jiao* in-between veterinary visits

Comments:
With acupuncture, Chinese herbal therapy, *Tui-na* and Food therapy corticosteroids and surgery may be avoided and a high quality of life maintained.

4. Spinal cord *Qi/*Blood Stagnation and Kidney *Yin* and *Qi* Deficiencies

Clinical Signs:
- Doberman Pinschers and other large breed dogs greater than 5 years of age
- Chronic progressive ataxia, quadriparesis or quadriplegia (Grades 2-5 neurological deficits)
- With or without neck or back pain
- Panting
- Cool seeking
- Warm ears, back, feet
- Dry skin
- Tongue- pale or red, purple, wet or dry, may be cracked (chronic)
- Pulses- deep, weak on both sides, rapid thready or wiry

TCVM Diagnosis:
The diagnosis is made based on the presence of paresis or paralysis (Grades 2-5 neurological deficits) of all four limbs with evidence of a Deficient Heat pattern. The paresis or paralysis is associated with Spinal Cord *Qi*/Blood Stagnation with Kidney *Qi* Deficiency. The animal will also be cool seeking, have panting episodes, warm ears, back and feet and dry skin, typical of a Kidney *Yin* Deficiency. The tongue characteristics can vary depending on which pattern is primarily reflected. A pale purple and wet tongue reflects the *Qi*/Blood Stagnation and Kidney *Qi* Deficiency. The reddish purple and dry tongue reflects the *Qi*/Blood Stagnation and

Kidney *Yin* Deficiency. The tongue may be cracked, if the *Yin* Deficiency is chronic. The pulses can vary and may be deep and weak on both sides reflecting the combination of *Yin* and *Qi* Deficiency or be wiry reflecting the *Qi*/Blood Stagnation.

Treatment Principles:
- Resolve *Qi*/Blood Stagnation to return proper *Qi*/Blood flow, relieve pain and resolve ataxia, quadriparesis and quadriplegia
- Tonify Kidney *Yin* to nourish the vertebrae and intervertebral disks
- Tonify Kidney *Qi* to resolve quadriparesis and quadriplegia

Acupuncture treatment:
EA is more effective than DN to control pain, resolve *Qi*/Blood Stagnation and promote nerve regeneration. For EA use 20 Hz for 10-15 minutes then 80-120 Hz alternating frequencies for 10-15 minutes. EA is combined with DN and Aqua-AP. For Aqua-AP inject 0.25-0.5 ml vitamin B12 into the acupoint after *Tui-na*. For non-ambulatory quadriparesis or quadriplegia (Grades 3-5 neurological deficits), EA and DN should be administered every 3-5 days for 3-5 times, depending on the patient's response, then reduced to once every 1-2 weeks until ambulatory. For ataxia and mild quadriparesis (Grade 2 neurological deficits), the acupuncture treatments may be weekly or every other week for 5-7 times and then every 4-6 weeks for maintenance, as needed.

Acupoints recommended
- EA: Select appropriate acupoints in Table 3 for cervical spinal cord lesions
- DN: Select acupoints in Table 3 plus BL-23, KID-3, KID-6, SP-6, SI-3
- Aqua-AP: BL-23, *Jing-jia-ji*

Pertinent acupoint actions
- See Table 3 for indications and actions of acupoints recommended for EA and DN and classical point locations
- BL-23 is the Back *Shu* Association point for the Kidney which tonifies the Kidney *Qi* to resolve quadriparesis and quadriplegia and nourish the spinal cord, vertebrae and intervertebral disks
- KID-3 is the *Yuan* Source point for the Kidney which tonifies the Kidney *Qi* to resolve quadriparesis and quadriplegia and nourish the vertebrae and intervertebral disks
- KID-6 is the confluent point with the *Yin Qiao* Extraordinary Channel useful to treat *Yin* Deficiency
- SP-6 tonifies *Yin* and Blood
- SI-3 is useful to treat cervical *Qi*/Blood Stagnation

Herbal Medicine:
- For ataxia and mild quadriparesis (mild Grade 2 neurological deficits) administer Cervical Formula (JT)[a] 0.5gm/10-20# twice daily orally to move *Qi* and Blood and eliminate Stagnation and resolve pain, ataxia and paresis

- Combine with *Hu Qian Wan* (JT)[a] 0.5gm/10-20# twice daily orally to further move nourish *Yin* and clear Deficient Heat
- Hind Quarter Weakness (JT)[a] 0.5gm/10-20# twice daily orally to tonify Kidney *Yin* and *Qi* and treat generalized weakness can be administered instead of *Hu Qian Wan*
- If the quadriparesis is moderate (moderate Grade 2) or the dog has non-ambulatory quadriparesis or quadriplegia (Grades 3-5), also add Double P (JT)[a] 0.5gm/10-20# twice daily orally for 1-5 months as needed to further move *Qi* and Blood and eliminate Stagnation and pain, ataxia, paresis or paralysis
- If Cervical Formula, Double P II and *Hu Qian Wan* (or Hind Quarter Weakness) are combined, then reduce the dose of Cervical Formula and *Hu Qian Wan* (or Hind Quarter Weakness) to 0.5gm/20# twice daily orally especially in geriatric dogs
- Administer Double P II for 1-5 months, then continue Cervical Formula and *Hu Qian Wan* (or Hind Quarter Weakness) alone at doses of 0.5gm/10-20# twice daily orally for 6 months or longer if needed
- If signs are recurrent, may treat on and off long-term
- A description of all the ingredients of the Chinese herbal medicine listed is beyond the scope of this text, but can be found elsewhere.[7,8]

Food Therapy:

The purpose of Food therapy is to promote *Qi*/Blood circulation, clear false Heat and tonify Kidney *Yin* and tonify Kidney *Qi* to support nerve regeneration. Foods that are Hot are avoided.[28]

- Foods to supplement to promote *Qi* and Blood circulation include: chicken egg, crab, sweet rice, peaches, carrots, coriander, squash, turnips
- Foods to Cool and tonify *Yin*: Turkey, pork, duck, clams, crab, eggs, rice, wheat, wheat germ, wheat berries, Belgian endive, string beans, peas, kidney beans, sweet potatoes, yams, tomato, spinach, tofu, kiwi, lemons, rhubarb, pears, bananas, watermelon, sesame, seaweed
- Foods to tonify *Qi*: Beef, chicken, sardines, egg, potato, yam, sweet potato, rice, oats, millet, lentils, carrots, squash, microalgae, dates, figs, molasses, royal jelly
- Hot foods to avoid: Lamb, shrimp, corn-fed beef, chicken, trout, squash, turnips, sweet rice, basal, caraway, cherries, chilies, cinnamon, ginger, rosemary, sage

Tui-na Procedures:

The purpose of the *Tui-na* is to stimulate *Qi* and Blood flow to relieve pain and promote nerve regeneration in the affected region. The descriptions and indications of each technique are outlined in more detail in Chapter 1 Table 8.[20]

- A *Tui-na* protocol for cervical spondylomyelopathy (wobbler syndrome) is outlined in Table 5

Daily Life Style Recommendation for Owner Follow-up:

- If Grades 3-5 paresis or paralysis, turn every 4-6 hours to prevent lung atelectasis and decubitus ulcers
- Keep on padding to avoid decubitus ulcers on shoulders, hips or tuber ischii
- Keep dry and clean of feces and urine

- Gentle *Moo-fa* (Daubing or massaging) of the neck or back for 3 minutes
- Gentle *Ca-fa* (Rubbing) of neck or back for a few minutes until it feels warm, once daily for 14-21 days
- *Ba-shen-fa* (Stretching) and range of motion exercises of all the limbs for 12 times twice daily for 7 days if ambulatory or until can walk if non-ambulatory
- Assist to walk with a sling if needed
- Swim with support and supervision if needed
- Remove all collars and walk with a harness
- No rough play involving the neck
- Avoid collars and walk with a harness, as even if the problem is in the thoracolumbar region, cervical intervertebral disks may cause problems in the future
- Once recovered avoid jumping on and off furniture and rough play

Comments:

With acupuncture, Chinese herbal therapy, *Tui-na* and Food therapy corticosteroids and surgery may be avoided and a high quality of life maintained.

5. Spinal cord *Qi*/Blood Stagnation and Kidney *Yin* and *Yang* Deficiencies

Clinical Signs:
- Doberman Pinschers and other large breed dogs greater than 5 years of age
- Chronic progressive ataxia, quadriparesis or quadriplegia (Grades 2-5 neurological deficits)
- With or without neck or back pain
- May have panting, warm ears, back or feet and seek cool
- May have cold ears, back or feet and seek heat
- Tongue- may vary and be pale purple and wet or reddish purple, dry and cracked or a combination of these
- Pulses- deep, weak both sides; may be rapid, thready, slow or wiry

TCVM Diagnosis:

The diagnosis is made based on the presence of paresis or paralysis (Grades 2-5 neurological deficits) of all four limbs with evidence of a combination of Deficient Heat and Deficient Cold patterns. The paresis or paralysis with cold ears, back or feet is typical of Spinal Cord *Qi*/Blood Stagnation with Kidney *Yang* Deficiency. The animal may at times have panting episodes, warm ears, back and feet and dry skin, typical of a Kidney *Yin* Deficiency. Warm ears and front feet and cold back and hind feet may be present and reflect the combination of *Yin* and *Yang* Deficiency patterns. The tongue characteristics can vary depending on which pattern is primarily reflected. A pale purple and wet tongue reflects the *Qi*/Blood Stagnation and Kidney *Yang* Deficiency. The reddish purple and dry tongue reflects the *Qi*/Blood Stagnation and Kidney *Yin* Deficiency. The tongue may be cracked, if *Yin* Deficiency is chronic. The pulses can vary and may be wiry reflecting an acute *Qi*/Blood Stagnation or be deep and weak on both sides reflecting the combination of *Yin* and *Qi* Deficiency.

Treatment Principles:
- Resolve *Qi*/Blood Stagnation to return proper *Qi*/Blood flow, relieve pain and resolve ataxia, quadriparesis and quadriplegia
- Tonify Kidney *Yin* to nourish the vertebrae and intervertebral disks
- Tonify Kidney *Yang* to resolve quadriparesis and quadriplegia

Acupuncture treatment:

EA is more effective than DN to control pain, resolve *Qi*/Blood Stagnation and promote nerve regeneration. For EA use 20 Hz for 10-15 minutes then 80-120 Hz alternating frequencies for 10-15 minutes. EA is combined with DN and Aqua-AP. For Aqua-AP inject 0.25-0.5 ml vitamin B12 into the acupoint after *Tui-na*. For non-ambulatory quadriparesis or quadriplegia (Grades 3-5 neurological deficits), EA and DN should be administered every 3-5 days for 3-5 times, depending on the patient's response, then reduced to once every 1-2 weeks until ambulatory. For ataxia and mild paresis (Grade 2), the acupuncture treatments may be weekly or every other week for 5-7 times and then every 4-6 weeks for maintenance, as needed.

Acupoints recommended
- EA: Select appropriate acupoints in Table 3 for cervical spinal cord lesions
- DN: Select acupoints in Table 3 plus a combination of points to support both Kidney *Yin* and *Yang* such as BL-23, KID-3, KID-6, SP-6, GV-3, GV-4, *Shen-shu, Shen-peng, Shen-jiao,* BL-62, SI-3
- Moxibustion: Do not administer moxibustion because of the *Yin* Deficiency
- Aqua-AP: BL-23, GV-3 or GV-4, *Jing-jia-ji*

Pertinent acupoint actions
- See Table 3 for indications and actions of acupoints recommended for EA and DN and classical point locations
- BL-23 is the Back *Shu* Association point for the Kidney which tonifies the Kidney *Qi* to resolve quadriparesis and quadriplegia and nourish the spinal cord, vertebrae and intervertebral disks
- KID-3 is the *Yuan* Source point for the Kidney which tonifies the Kidney *Qi* to resolve quadriparesis and quadriplegia and nourish the vertebrae and intervertebral disks
- KID-6 is the confluent point with the *Yin Qiao* Extraordinary Vessel useful to treat *Yin* Deficiencies
- SP-6 tonifies *Yin* and Blood
- GV-3 and GV-4 are useful to treat Kidney *Yang* and *Qi* Deficiency and resolve quadriparesis and quadriplegia
- *Shen-shu* (one *cun* lateral to *Bai-hui*), *Shen-peng* (one *cun* cranial to *Shen-shu*) and *Shen-jiao* (one *cun* caudal to *Shen-shu*) are useful to treat Kidney *Qi* and *Yang* Deficiency and resolve quadriparesis and quadriplegia
- BL-62 is the confluent point with the *Yang Qiao* Extraordinary Channel useful to treat *Yang* Deficiency and resolve ataxia, quadriparesis and quadriplegia
- SI-3 is useful to treat cervical *Qi*/Blood Stagnation

Herbal Medicine:

- For ataxia and mild quadriparesis (mild Grade 2 neurological deficits) administer Cervical Formula (JT)[a] 0.5gm/10-20# twice daily orally to move *Qi* and Blood and eliminate Stagnation and resolve pain, ataxia and paresis
- Combine with *Di Huang Yin Zi* (JT)[a] 0.5gm/10-20# twice daily orally to tonify Kidney *Yin* and *Yang*
- Alternative: Hind Quarter Weakness (JT)[a] 0.5gm/10-20# twice daily orally may be administered instead of *Di Huang Yin Zi* to tonify Kidney *Yin* and *Qi* and treat generalized weakness
- If the quadriparesis is moderate (moderate Grade 2 neurological deficits) or the dog has non-ambulatory quadriparesis or quadriplegia (Grades 3-5 neurological deficits), also add Double P II (JT)[a] 0.5gm/10-20# twice daily orally for 1-5 months as needed to further move *Qi* and Blood and eliminate Stagnation and pain, ataxia, paresis or paralysis
- If Cervical Formula, Double P II and *Di Huang Yi Zi* (or Hind Quarter Weakness) are combined, then reduce the dose of Cervical Formula and *Di Huang Yi Zi* (or Hind Quarter Weakness) to 0.5gm/20# twice daily orally especially in geriatric dogs
- Administer Double P II for 1-5 months, then continue Cervical Formula and *Di Huang Yi Zi* (or Hind Quarter Weakness) alone at doses of 0.5gm/10-20# twice daily orally for 6 months or longer if needed
- If signs are recurrent, may treat on and off long-term
- A description of all the ingredients of the Chinese herbal medicine listed is beyond the scope of this text, but can be found elsewhere.[7,8]

Food Therapy:

The purpose of the Food therapy is to promote *Qi*/Blood circulation and tonify Kidney *Qi* to support nerve regeneration in the affected region. Since both Kidney *Yin* and Kidney *Yang* are Deficient, foods that are Cold or Hot are avoided.[28]

- Foods to supplement to promote *Qi* and Blood circulation include: chicken egg, crab, sweet rice, peaches, carrots, coriander, squash, turnips
- Foods to tonify *Qi*: Beef, chicken, sardines, egg, potato, yam, sweet potato, rice, oats, millet, lentils, carrots, squash, microalgae, dates, figs, molasses, royal jelly
- Cold foods to avoid: Turkey, duck, duck eggs, conch, clams, mussels, yogurt, millet, barley, spinach, broccoli, celery, egg plant, kelp, alfalfa, cucumbers, pears, bananas, white radishes, watermelon
- Hot foods to avoid: Lamb, shrimp, corn-fed beef, chicken, trout, squash, turnips, sweet rice, basal, caraway, cherries, chilies, cinnamon, ginger, rosemary, sage

Tui-na Procedures:

The purpose of the *Tui-na* is to stimulate *Qi* and Blood flow to relieve pain and promote nerve regeneration in the affected region. The descriptions and indications of each technique are outlined in more detail in Chapter 1 Table 8.[20]

- A *Tui-na* protocol for cervical spondylomyelopathy (wobbler syndrome) is outlined in Table 5

Daily Life Style Recommendation for Owner Follow-up:
- If Grades 3-5 paresis or paralysis, turn every 4-6 hours to prevent lung atelectasis and decubitus ulcers
- Keep on padding to avoid decubitus ulcers on shoulders, hips or tuber ischii
- Keep dry and clean of feces and urine
- Gentle *Moo-fa* (Daubing or massaging) of the neck or back for 3 minutes
- Gentle *Ca-fa* (Rubbing) of neck or back for a few minutes until it feels warm, once daily for 14-21 days
- *Ba-shen-fa* (Stretching) and range of motion exercises of all the limbs for 12 times twice daily for 7 days if ambulatory or until can walk if non-ambulatory
- Assist to walk with a sling if needed
- Do not swim as the body may become chilled further and put unneeded stress on the body's *Yang*
- Remove all collars and walk with a harness
- No rough play involving the neck

Comments:

With acupuncture, Chinese herbal therapy, *Tui-na* and Food therapy corticosteroids and surgery may be avoided and a high quality of life maintained.

FIBROCARTILAGINOUS EMBOLISM

Fibrocartilaginous embolism and infarction of the spinal cord is the most common nervous system vascular disorder of dogs.[2,3] Young, large breed dogs, Miniature Schnauzers and very rarely cats are presented with acute asymmetrical quadriparesis, hemiparesis or hemiplegia for no apparent reason. Asymmetrical paraparesis with paralysis of one pelvic limb is also common with fibrocartilaginous embolism of the thoracic and lumbar spinal cord. Infarction of the spinal cord is due to the occlusion of either arteries or veins with fibrocartilage. The origin of the fibrocartilage is unknown, although most theories suggest that it arises from degenerating intervertebral disk material that gains entrance to the spinal cord vasculature. The route of entrance is still speculative. A history of acute collapse with or without vigorous exercise is common. The clinical signs may worsen within the first few hours, but are usually non-progressive by the time veterinary help is obtained. Initially the animal may be painful, but this usually passes in a few hours and pain is usually not evident on palpation of the neck or back. If the lesion involves the caudal cervical region, hyporeflexia or areflexia of one or both thoracic limbs with Horner's syndrome and/or symmetrical loss of the cutaneous trunci reflex may be observed. With severe cervical infarctions, respiratory compromise may be evident. The diagnosis is typically one of exclusion, although an acute, non-progressive, non-painful, asymmetric paresis or paralysis in a young, large breed dog is highly suggestive of fibrocartilaginous embolism. Dogs may be referred to TCVM practitioners to shorten recovery time and improve the recovery outcome.[4] There is currently one case report of the integration of TCVM with conventional rehabilitation techniques for the treatment of a fibrocartilaginous embolism strongly suspected from MRI findings.[34]

Etiology and Pathology

From a TCVM perspective, spinal cord ischemia results in Stagnation of *Qi*/Blood flow with *Qi* Deficiency locally that affects spinal cord function.[4,34] The Deficiency and Stagnation of *Qi*/Blood, depletes *Gu Qi* that nourishes the neurons and other cells of the region and degeneration and demyelination occurs. Kidney *Qi* Deficiency is also present, if the animal has pelvic limb or generalized limb paresis or paralysis (*Tan-Huan* syndrome). Applying the basic TCVM theories of *Yin/Yang*, Eight Principles, Five Treasures, Five Elements and *Zang Fu* physiology and pathology to make a TCVM diagnosis, there is one basic TCVM pattern (Table X):

1. **Spinal cord *Qi*/Blood Stagnation and Kidney *Qi* Deficiency**
   Focal spinal cord ischemia causes *Qi*/Blood Stagnation and *Qi* Deficiency with loss of function and acute paresis or paralysis caudal to the lesion. Since the spinal cord is associated with the Kidney, paresis or paralysis is a sign of Kidney *Qi* Deficiency. Serial neurological and TCVM examinations are important, as evidence of one of the other underlying TCVM patterns (e.g. *Yin* or *Yang* Deficiencies) may become evident and also need to be treated.

Pattern Differentiation and Treatment

1. Spinal cord *Qi*/Blood Stagnation and Kidney *Qi* Deficiency

Clinical Signs:
- Any adult dog (large breed dogs most common)
- Acute non-progressive hemiparesis or symmetrical paraparesis or paraplegia (Grade 3-5 neurological deficits)
- Tongue- purple, pale purple, wet
- Pulses- wiry (acute), deep, weak (later) worse on the right

TCVM Diagnosis:
The diagnosis is made based on the presence of acute asymmetrical quadriparesis or paraparesis or paraplegia (Grades 2-5 neurological deficits) with no evidence of concurrent Deficient Heat and/or Cold patterns. The purple tongue is typical of *Qi*/Blood Stagnation and the tongue paleness is typical of *Qi* Deficiency. The tongue may be wet. The pulses can vary and may be wiry reflecting the *Qi*/Blood Stagnation or be deep and weak worse on the right reflecting the Kidney *Qi* Deficiency.

Treatment Principles:
- Resolve *Qi*/Blood Stagnation to return proper *Qi*/Blood flow and resolve hemiparesis, quadriparesis, paraparesis or paraplegia
- Tonify Kidney *Qi* to resolve hemiparesis, quadriparesis, paraparesis or paraplegia

Acupuncture treatment:
EA is more effective than DN to resolve *Qi*/Blood Stagnation and promote nerve regeneration. For EA use 80-120 Hz alternating frequencies for 15-30 minutes since pain is usually not present. EA is combined with DN and Aqua-AP. For Aqua-AP inject 0.25-0.5 ml

vitamin B12 into the acupoint after *Tui-na*. For Grade 4-5 neurological deficits, EA and DN should be administered every 1-3 days for 3-5 times, depending on the patient's response, then reduced to once every 1-2 weeks until ambulatory. For Grades 2 and 3 neurological deficits, the acupuncture treatments may be weekly or every other week.

Acupoints recommended
- EA: Select appropriate acupoints in Table 3 depending on the lesion location
- DN: Select acupoints in Table 3 plus BL-23, KID-3
- Aqua-AP: BL-23

Pertinent acupoint actions
- See Table 3 for indications and actions of acupoints recommended for EA and DN
- BL-23 is the Back *Shu* Association point for the Kidney which tonifies the Kidney *Qi* to resolve quadriparesis and quadriplegia and nourish the spinal cord
- KID-3 is the *Yuan* Source point for the Kidney which tonifies the Kidney *Qi* to resolve quadriparesis and quadriplegia and nourish the spinal cord

Herbal Medicine:
- For Grades 3-5 paresis or paralysis administer Double P II (JT)[a] 0.5gm/10-20# twice daily orally to move *Qi* and Blood and eliminate Stagnation and pain
- If pelvic limb paresis or paralysis is present, combine with *Bu Yang Huan Wu* (JT)[a] 0.5gm/10-20# twice daily orally to move and nourish Blood and tonify *Qi*
- If all four limbs are affected, instead combine with Cervical Formula (JT)[a] 0.5gm/10-20# twice daily orally to activate Blood, move *Qi*, eliminate Stagnation and pain
- Administer Double P II for 1-2 months, then continue *Bu Yang Huan Wu* or Cervical Formula alone until recovered up to 6 months
- A description of all the ingredients of the Chinese herbal medicine listed is beyond the scope of this text, but can be found elsewhere.[7,8]

Food Therapy:
The purpose of the Food therapy is to promote *Qi*/Blood circulation and tonify Kidney *Qi* to support nerve regeneration in the affected region. Foods that are Cold or Hot are avoided.[28]
- Foods to supplement to promote *Qi* and Blood circulation include: chicken egg, crab, sweet rice, peaches, carrots, coriander, squash, turnips
- Foods to tonify Kidney *Qi*: Beef, chicken, sardines, egg, potato, yam, sweet potato, rice, oats, millet, lentils, carrots, squash, microalgae, dates, figs, molasses, royal jelly
- Cold foods to avoid: Turkey, duck, duck eggs, conch, clams, mussels, yogurt, millet, barley, spinach, broccoli, celery, egg plant, kelp, alfalfa, cucumbers, pears, bananas, white radishes, watermelon
- Hot foods to avoid: Lamb, shrimp, corn-fed beef, chicken, trout, squash, turnips, sweet rice, basal, caraway, cherries, chilies, cinnamon, ginger, rosemary, sage

Tui-na Procedures:
The purpose of the *Tui-na* is to stimulate *Qi* and Blood flow to relieve pain and promote nerve regeneration in the affected region. The descriptions and indications of each technique are outlined in more detail in Chapter 1 Table 8.[20]
- A *Tui-na* protocol for cervical fibrocartilaginous embolism in outlined in Table 5
- A *Tui-na* protocol for thoracolumbar fibrocartilaginous embolism in outlined in Table 6

Daily Life Style Recommendation for Owner Follow-up:
- If Grades 3-5 paresis or paralysis, turn (if in lateral recumbency) or move every 4-6 hours to prevent lung atelectasis and decubitus ulcers
- Keep on padding to avoid decubitus ulcers on shoulders, hips or tuber ischii
- Keep dry and clean of feces and urine
- Gentle *Moo-fa* (Daubing or massaging) of the neck or back for 3 minutes
- Gentle *Ca-fa* (Rubbing) of neck or back for a few minutes until it feels warm, once daily for 14-21 days
- *Ba-shen-fa* (Stretching) and range of motion exercises of all the limbs for 12 times twice daily until can walk
- Assist to walk with a sling if needed
- Swim with support and supervision
- Avoid collars and walk with a harness
- Once recovered avoid jumping on and off furniture and rough play

Comments:
Based on clinical experiences, the TCVM treatments should shorten the recovery time and improve the degree of functional recovery. On serial TCVM evaluations if *Yin* or *Yang* Deficiency develops, see the treatment of Kidney *Qi* and *Yin* Deficiencies, Kidney *Yang* Deficiency and Kidney *Yin* and *Yang* Deficiency described above in the section on **INTERVERTEBRAL DISK DISEASE**.

DISKOSPONDYLITIS AND SPONDYLITIS
Diskospondylitis is a very painful infection of the intervertebral disk and vertebral endplates.[1-3] Spondylitis (vertebral osteomyelitis) is a very painful infection of the vertebral body. Diskospondylitis is more common than spondylitis and both are usually caused by a bacterial infection. Fungal infections such as aspergillosis, foreign body migrations such as grass awns and aberrant parasites are infrequent. *Staphylococcus aureus* and *intermedius* that arrive via a hematogenous route are the most frequent bacteria isolated, although *Streptococcus canis*, *Escherichia coli, Brucella canis* and others have also been cultured. Pre-existing or concurrent skin, urinary tract or cardiopulmonary infections are often present. Focal lesions at the lumbosacral, thoracolumbar and cervicothoracic junctions and the mid-thoracic regions are common, but multiple lesions can also occur. Paresis and paralysis (Grades 2-5 neurological deficits) can occur, if left untreated, due to compression and infection involving the spinal cord (see MENINGOMYELITIS section below).

Pyrexia may or may not be present. Sites of systemic infection should be investigated by performing a thorough physical examination accompanied by a complete blood count, serum chemistry profile, urinalysis and urine culture. The complete blood count may be normal or show a neutrophilic leukocytosis, but the fibrinogen is usually elevated. Cystitis is common and the bacterial organism isolated from the urine is often also infecting the disk and vertebrae. Fungal hyphae associated with *Aspergillus sp.* may occasionally be seen on examination of the urine sediment. Several bacterial cultures of the blood taken at different intervals may also help identify the causal organism, but cultures are negative more than half of the time. Serology for *Brucella canis* is often performed due to the public health significance of this infection. Radiographs can be useful to confirm the diagnosis of diskospondylitis and spondylitis. Characteristic routine radiographic changes may take 1-2 weeks to after the onset of signs to become obvious and repeat radiographs may be necessary to demonstrate the lesions in some cases. Radiographic abnormalities include lysis of adjacent vertebral endplates with collapsed intervertebral disk spaces or vertebrae. Imaging with CT or MRI may show lesions earlier and detail the changes better than routine radiographs. Treatment requires intensive appropriate antibiotic or anti-fungal therapy. Bacterial infections usually clear in 4 weeks, but recurrence are seen if antibiotic therapy is inappropriate or not administered for long enough. From a TCVM perspective vertebral and intervertebral disk infections are associated with Damp-Heat or Heat Toxins invading the Channels affecting the spinal column causing Qi/Blood Stagnation in the Exterior Channels.

The primary problem is pain, but if left untreated the infection can move to the Interior and produce Spinal Cord *Qi*/Blood Stagnation. TCVM treatments may be integrated with conventional pain medications and antibiotic and anti-fungal therapy to further control pain and support the immune system.[19,35] Further investigations are needed to determine if acupuncture can enhance the effectiveness of antibiotics as suggested in Gallbladder Damp-Heat.[36,37]

Etiology and Pathology
  1. **Heat Toxin, Damp Heat in the vertebrae and disks**
     Chronic poor nutrition, illness and environmental stress can cause *Zheng Qi* to become Deficient and Deficient *Wei Qi* allows the invasion of Exterior pathogens, Heat Toxins (bacteria and fungi), to enter the Governing Vessel and Bladder Channels and invade the vertebral column causing Damp Heat in the intervertebral disks and vertebrae as well as local *Qi*/Blood Stagnation of vertebral and paravertebral structures causing pain.[8] Although the disease is usually Exterior (involving skeletal structures), it can be challenging to treat because of the presence of Heat Toxins (organisms). Serial neurological examinations are important because paresis or paralysis occurs if the Heat Toxin moves into the Interior and affects the Spinal Cord.

Pattern Differentiation and Treatment

1. Heat Toxin, Damp Heat in the vertebrae and disks

Clinical Signs:
- Any age, breed sex of dog or cat
- Acute severe pain of the neck, back or both locations
- Anorexia
- May have a low grade or high fever
- Ears, back and feet feel warm

- Animal may pant
- Tongue- red, yellow coating, dry
- Pulses- Superficial, forceful, rapid and wiry

TCVM Diagnosis:
The diagnosis of Heat Toxin is based on the evidence of a bacterial or fungal infection and Heat on the TCVM examination with a possible fever and warm ears, back and feet and panting. A red tongue with a yellow coating also reflects Heat in the body. Superficial, forceful and rapid pulses are typical of Excess Heat and the wiry pulses reflect the *Qi*/Blood Stagnation causing the clinical sign of pain.

Treatment Principles:
- Resolve *Qi*/Blood Stagnation to control pain
- Clear Heat
- Clear Damp

Acupuncture treatment:
Combine acupuncture with antimicrobial therapy and pain medications. EA is more effective than DN to control pain, resolve *Qi*/Blood Stagnation and promote regeneration. For EA use 20 Hz for 10-15 minutes then 80-120 Hz alternating frequencies for 10-15 minutes. EA is combined with DN and Aqua-AP. For Aqua-AP inject 0.25-0.5 ml vitamin B12 into acupoints distant to the area of pain. Acutely for severe pain, may have to treat every 3 days for 3-5 times, then reduce to ever 1-2 weeks until clinical signs resolve.

Acupoints recommended
- EA: Select appropriate acupoints in Table 3 depending on the lesion location; avoid acupoints in the immediate area of the lesion as it may be too painful
- DN: Select acupoints in Table 3 plus GV-14, *Er-jian*, *Wei-jian*, BL-11,
- Aqua-AP: GV-14

Pertinent acupoint actions
- See Table 3 for indications and actions of acupoints recommended for EA and DN
- GV-14, LI-11, *Er-jian* (ear tip) and *Wei-jian* (tail tip) are useful to clear Heat
- GV-14 and LI-11 can also support the immune system
- BL-11 is the Influential point for bones and is useful to promote bone healing

Herbal Medicine:
- *Qing Ying Tang* (JT)[a] 0.5gm/10-20# twice daily orally to clear Heat Toxins combined with conventional pain medications and antibiotics.
- If a high fever add *Pu Ju Xiao Du* (P)[b] 0.5gm/10-20# twice daily orally for 1-2 weeks to clear Heat and detoxify
- Administer *Qing Ying Tang* for 2-3 months, but monitor for signs of Spleen *Qi* Deficiency

- Administer *Qing Ying Tang* with caution in animals with a history or signs of Spleen *Qi* Deficiency
- A description of all the ingredients of the Chinese herbal medicine listed is beyond the scope of this text, but can be found elsewhere.[7,8]

Food Therapy:

The purpose of the Food therapy is to clear Heat and Damp and promote *Qi*/Blood circulation and nerve regeneration. Cooling foods are prescribed and Damp producing and Hot foods are avoided.[28]

- Foods to supplement to clear Heat: Turkey, duck, duck eggs, conch, clams, mussels, yogurt, millet, barley, spinach, broccoli, celery, egg plant, kelp, alfalfa, cucumbers, pears, bananas, white radishes, watermelon
- Foods to supplement to Drain Damp: Eel, mackerel, quail, corn, barley, rye, blueberries, celery, mushrooms
- Foods to promote *Qi*/Blood circulation: Crab, sweet rice, peaches, carrots, coriander, turnips
- Damp producing foods to avoid: Eggs, milk, cheese, yoghurt, ghee, bananas, sugar
- Hot foods to avoid: Lamb, shrimp, corn-fed beef, chicken, trout, squash, turnips, sweet rice, basal, caraway, cherries, chilies, cinnamon, ginger, rosemary, sage

Tui-na Procedures:

The purpose of the *Tui-na* is to stimulate *Qi* and Blood flow to relieve pain and promote nerve regeneration in the affected region. The descriptions and indications of each technique are outlined in more detail in Chapter 1 Table 8.[20]

- Initially pain is usually severe and manipulation of the neck and back are avoided
- *An-fa* pressing of SI-3, LI-4, TH-5 and LU-7 for 5-10 seconds per acupoint
- *Nian-fa* holding and kneading each of the digits and distal extremities repeat 12 times
- Later can select techniques outlined in Tables 5 and 6 useful to treat cervical or thoracolumbar *Qi*/Blood Stagnation.

Daily Life Style Recommendation for Owner Follow-up:

- Usually too painful for *Tui-na*
- Keep quiet and resting during recovery
- Once the pain is controlled begin short walks with assistance if needed

Comments:

Heat toxins may require intensive and prolong treatment to ensure recovery. Combine TCVM and conventional treatments for 1-2 months and then continue TCVM treatment for 6-9 months.

DEGENERATIVE MYELOPATHY

Degenerative myelopathy occurs in German Shepherds, Boxers, Welsh/Pembroke Corgis and a few other large breed dogs. Clinical signs usually begin between 5-14 years of age.[1-3] The etiology is unknown, but a type of breed specific immune-mediated disease process is suspected to be the cause of spinal cord degeneration.[2] A non-painful pelvic limb ataxia and paresis develops over the course of several months and clinical signs may wax and wan, but ultimately the disorder is progressive. Weakness evident on rising may be the first sign of problems. As many large breed dogs may concurrently develop osteoarthritis of the hips and stifles and spondylosis deformans, difficulty rising might be initially attributed to discomfort associated with these disorders. If reduced or absent conscious proprioception is found in one or both pelvic limbs, then a neurological problem is present.

As degenerative myelopathy progresses over the following months, ataxia and paraparesis become obvious. The pelvic limb spinal reflexes remain normal or become slightly hyperactive typical of a spinal cord lesion between T3-L3. As the disease progresses further, the patellar reflexes become depressed or absent due to degeneration of axons in the dorsal roots.[2] Affected dogs finally are unable to rise or walk in the pelvic limbs and develop urinary and fecal incontinence. Paraplegia typically develops within 6 months from the onset of signs. Thoracic limbs can then become progressively involved leading to quadriparesis and finally the animal develops respiratory paresis. Most animals are euthanized prior to this stage.

Since German Shepherds and other large breed dogs commonly develop Type II intervertebral disc disease (slow progressive disk protrusion) and lumbosacral degeneration (L7-S1 disk protrusion and spondylosis deformans), which can appear similarly, degenerative myelopathy must be differentiated from these spinal cord and cauda equina disorders. Some German Shepherds may have degenerative myelopathy concurrently with intervertebral disk disease and lumbosacral degeneration. If there is no evidence of spinal cord or cauda equina compression on the MRI, then degenerative myelopathy is strongly suspected, especially in German Shepherds, Boxers and Welsh/Pembroke Corgis with chronic progressive paraparesis. Since the long-term prognosis is generally poor and the disease continues to slowly progress, dogs are often referred for TCVM treatments. There is one case report of a dog with degenerative myelopathy that was treated with EA, DN, Aqua-AP and Chinese herbal medicine and although the neurological deficit continued to worsen, the treatments most likely slowed the course of the disease as he was maintained for 2 years after the diagnosis.[38] Further clinical studies of the response of dogs with degenerative myelopathy to TCVM are needed. The primary TCVM patterns associated with degenerative myelopathy and suggested TCVM treatments can be found in Tables 2, 3, 8.[6,38] Food therapy and *Tui-na* treatments are outlined in Tables 5-7.[20,28]

Etiology and Pathology

As our conventional understanding of degenerative myelopathy has grown, it has been shown primarily to affect specific pure breed dogs and involves premature degeneration (aging) of the spinal cord, often as early as 5-7 years old, which is typical of Kidney *Jing* Deficiency. The initial manifestation of degenerative myelopathy is difficulty rising due to weakness, which from the TCVM perspective is *Wei* syndrome.[5,8] *Wei* syndrome is typically associated with Spleen *Qi* Deficiency. As the disease progresses, pelvic limb paresis and paralysis become apparent, which are typical of *Tan-Huan* syndrome associated with Kidney *Qi* Deficiency.[8] As the disease progresses even further, either Kidney *Yang* Deficiency, Kidney *Yin* Deficiency or both develop, depending on the basic constitution of the dog.[38] In any chronic disease, when Kidney *Yin* Deficiency develops, Liver *Yin* Deficiency shortly follows, based on the pathological cycle of a "sick Mother creates a sick Child" from Five Element Theory. Besides TCVM treatments to support Kidney *Jing, Qi, Yin* and *Yang*, TCVM treatment to support Spleen *Qi* is needed to promote strong post-natal *Jing* and spare the pre-natal Kidney *Jing* as much as possible to halt or delay the progression of the disease. Applying the basic TCVM theories of *Yin/Yang*, Eight Principles, Five Treasures, Five Elements and *Zang Fu* physiology and pathology to make a TCVM diagnosis, there are four primary patterns associated with degenerative myelopathy in dogs (Table 2):

1. **Kidney *Jing*, Spleen *Qi* and Kidney *Qi* Deficiencies**
   Kidney *Jing* Deficiency results in premature degeneration (aging) of the thoracolumbar spinal cord in middle-aged dogs. The strong breed predisposition also suggests a *Jing* Deficiency related disorder, although the exact conventional etiology is unknown. The initial signs of *Wei* syndrome are associated with Spleen *Qi* Deficiency. Since the spinal cord and pelvic limbs are associated with the Kidney, as paraparesis or paraplegia (Grades 2-5 neurological deficits) develops, Kidney *Qi* Deficiency becomes apparent. Serial neurological and TCVM examinations are important, as evidence of one of the other underlying TCVM patterns (e.g. Kidney/Liver *Yin* or *Yang* Deficiency) may appear and also need to be treated.

2. **Kidney *Jing*, Spleen *Qi* and Kidney *Yang* Deficiencies**
   Kidney *Jing* Deficiency results in premature degeneration (aging) of the thoracolumbar spinal cord in middle-aged dogs. The strong breed predisposition also suggests a *Jing* Deficiency related disorder. The initial signs of *Wei* syndrome are associated with Spleen *Qi* Deficiency. Since the spinal cord and pelvic limbs are associated with the Kidney, as paraparesis or paraplegia (Grades 2-5 neurological deficits) develops Kidney *Qi* Deficiency becomes apparent. Evidence of Cold is found on the TCVM examination. When animals with Kidney *Qi* Deficiency develop clinical signs of Cold, the pattern becomes Kidney *Yang* Deficiency (*Qi* Deficiency plus Cold = *Yang* Deficiency). Kidney *Yang* Deficiency develops due to the underlying *Jing* Deficiency and chronic stress, illness or poor nutrition especially in *Yin* animals (Earth, Metal and Water constitutions).

3. **Kidney *Jing*, Spleen *Qi*, Kidney *Qi* and Kidney/Liver *Yin* Deficiencies**
   Kidney *Jing* Deficiency results in premature degeneration (aging) of the thoracolumbar spinal cord in middle-aged dogs. The strong breed predisposition also suggests a *Jing* Deficiency related disorder. The initial signs of *Wei* syndrome are associated with Spleen *Qi* Deficiency. Since the spinal cord and pelvic limbs are associated with the Kidney, as paraparesis or paraplegia (Grades 2-5 neurological deficits) develops Kidney *Qi* Deficiency becomes apparent. Clinical evidence of Heat on the TCVM examination is typical of a concurrent *Yin* Deficiency. The pattern then becomes Kidney *Jing*, Spleen *Qi*, Kidney *Qi* and Kidney/Liver *Yin* Deficiencies. Kidney/Liver *Yin* Deficiency occurs due to the underlying Kidney *Jing* Deficiency and chronic stress, illness or poor nutrition especially in *Yang* animals (Wood and Fire constitutions).

4. **Kidney *Jing*, Spleen *Qi*, Kidney *Yang* and Kidney/Liver *Yin* Deficiencies**
   Kidney *Jing* Deficiency results in premature degeneration (aging) of the thoracolumbar spinal cord in middle-aged dogs. The strong breed predisposition also suggests a *Jing* Deficiency related disorder. The initial signs of *Wei* syndrome are

associated with Spleen *Qi* Deficiency. Since the spinal cord and pelvic limbs are associated with the Kidney, as paraparesis or paraplegia (Grades 2-5 neurological deficits) develops Kidney *Qi* Deficiency becomes apparent. Kidney *Qi* Deficiency and clinical signs of Cold are typical of Kidney *Yang* Deficiency. Clinical evidence of Heat is found if Kidney *Yin* Deficiency is also present. The TCVM pattern then becomes Kidney *Jing* Deficiency with both Kidney *Yin* and *Yang* Deficiencies. Kidney *Yin* and *Yang* Deficiencies occur from Kidney *Jing* Deficiency and chronic stress, illness or poor nutrition.

Pattern Differentiation and Treatment

1. Kidney *Jing*, Spleen *Qi* and Kidney *Qi* Deficiencies

Clinical Signs:
- German Shepherd, Boxer or Welsh/Pembroke Corgi and a few other pure breed dogs
- 5 years of age or older
- Difficulty rising and muscle weakness in the pelvic limbs
- Chronic progressive paraparesis
- Usually Grades 2-4 neurological deficits
- Not painful unless has concurrent *Bi* syndrome
- Tongue- pale, wet
- Pulses- deep, weak, worse right

TCVM Diagnosis:
   The breed predisposition is associated with *Jing* Deficiency. Initial difficulty rising and muscle weakness is typical of *Wei* syndrome associated with Spleen *Qi* Deficiency. A diagnosis of paresis or paralysis or *Tan-Huan* syndrome (Grades 2-5 neurological deficits) is typical of Kidney *Qi* Deficiency. The pale, wet tongue is associated with Kidney *Jing*, Spleen *Qi* and Kidney *Qi* Deficiencies. The deep, weak pulses worse on the right reflect the Spleen *Qi* and Kidney *Qi* Deficiencies.

Treatment Principles:
- Tonify Kidney *Jing* to nourish the spinal cord and strengthen the pelvic limbs
- Tonify Spleen *Qi* to and strengthen the muscles
- Tonify Kidney *Qi* to strengthen the pelvic limbs

Acupuncture treatment:
   EA is more effective than DN to promote nerve regeneration and deter further degeneration. Although degenerative myelopathy is not a painful disease, many dogs have concurrent *Bi* Syndrome so the EA protocol recommended is: 20 Hz (cycles/sec) for 10-15 minutes then 80-120 Hz alternating frequencies for 10-15 minutes. EA is combined with DN and Aqua-AP. For Aqua-AP inject 0.25-0.5 ml vitamin B12 into the acupoint after *Tui-na*. Acupuncture treatments may be weekly or every other week for 5-7 times, then reduced to once a month long-term.

Acupoints recommended
- EA: Select appropriate acupoints in Table 3 for thoracolumbar lesions
- DN: Select acupoints in Table 3 plus BL-20, BL-21, BL-23, KID-3
- Aqua-AP: BL-20, BL-23, *Hua-tuo-jia-ji*

Pertinent acupoint actions
- See Table 3 for indications and actions of acupoints useful for EA and DN and location of classical acupoints
- BL-20 is the Back *Shu* Association point for the Spleen to support the production of post-natal *Jing* to reduce the use of pre-natal Kidney *Jing* and also a local acupoint to support the thoracolumbar spinal cord
- BL-21 is the Back *Shu* Association point for the Stomach to support the production of post-natal *Jing* to reduce the use of pre-natal Kidney *Jing* and also a local acupoint to support the thoracolumbar spinal cord
- BL-23 is the Back *Shu* Association point for the Kidney which tonifies the Kidney *Qi* to nourish the spinal cord and improve or delay progression of the paraparesis and also a local acupoint to support the thoracolumbar spinal cord
- KID-3 is the *Yuan* Source point for the Kidney which tonifies the Kidney *Qi* to nourish the spinal cord and improve or delay progression of the paraparesis

Herbal Medicine:
- Epimedium Formula (JT)[a] 0.5gm/10-20# twice daily orally to tonify and nourish Kidney *Jing* and *Yin* and tonify Kidney *Yang* and *Qi* and halt or slow the progression of the paraparesis
- Combine with *Bu Yang Huan Wu* (JT)[a] 0.5gm/10-20# twice daily orally to tonify *Qi* and halt or slow the progression of the paraparesis
- Administer herbs long-term to slow disease progression and improve the quality of life
- A description of all the ingredients of the Chinese herbal medicine listed is beyond the scope of this text, but can be found elsewhere.[7,8]

Food Therapy:
The purpose of the Food therapy is to tonify Kidney *Jing* and Spleen and Kidney *Qi* to promote nerve regeneration and delay degeneration in the affected region and strengthen the pelvic limbs. Foods that are too Cold or Hot are avoided.[28]
- Foods to tonify *Jing*: Liver, kidneys, fish, bone and bone marrow, millet, quinoa, spelt, wheat, almonds, black sesame, microalgae (e.g. chlorella, spirulina, wild blue-green algae), barley, wheat grass, black soy beans, black beans, kidney beans, seaweed, sea salt, mulberries, raspberries, strawberries, almonds, black sesame, clarified butter (ghee), royal jelly, bee pollen
- Foods to tonify Spleen and Kidney *Qi*: Beef, chicken, sardines, egg, potato, yam, sweet potato, rice, oats, millet, lentils, carrots, squash, microalgae, dates, figs, molasses, royal jelly

- Cold foods to avoid: Turkey, duck, duck eggs, conch, clams, mussels, yogurt, millet, barley, spinach, broccoli, celery, egg plant, kelp, alfalfa, cucumbers, pears, bananas, white radishes, watermelon
- Hot foods to avoid: Lamb, shrimp, corn-fed beef, chicken, trout, squash, turnips, sweet rice, basal, caraway, cherries, chilies, cinnamon, ginger, rosemary, sage

Tui-na Procedures:

The purpose of the *Tui-na* is to keep *Qi* and Blood flowing to promote nerve regeneration and delay degeneration in the affected spinal cord region. The descriptions and indications of each technique are outlined in more detail in Chapter 1 Table 8.[20]

- A *Tui-na* protocol for degenerative myelopathy is outlined in Table 6

Daily Life Style Recommendation for Owner Follow-up

- *Moo-fa* (Daubing or massaging) of the back for 3 minutes once or twice daily
- *Ca-fa* (Rubbing) of back for a few minutes until it feels warm, once or twice daily
- *Ba-shen-fa* (Stretching) of the pelvic limbs for 12 times once or twice daily
- Maintain excellent nutrition
- Maintain a low stress environment
- Daily physical therapy of walking or swimming has been shown to reduce progression of the pelvic limb paresis
- Walk with a harness
- Assist to walk with a sling if needed
- Swim with support and supervision
- If Grades 3-5 paresis or paralysis, move every 4-6 hours to prevent decubitus ulcers
- Keep on padding to avoid decubitus ulcers on the hips or tuber ischii
- Keep dry and clean of feces and urine

Comments:

Expect that the disease progression will be slowed and that the animal will maintain a high quality of life.

2. Kidney *Jing,* Spleen *Qi* and Kidney *Yang* Deficiencies

Clinical Signs:

- German Shepherd, Boxer or Welsh/Pembroke Corgi and a few other pure breed dogs
- 5 years of age or older
- Difficulty rising and muscle weakness in the pelvic limbs
- Chronic progressive paraparesis
- Grades 2-4 neurological deficits
- Not painful unless has concurrent *Bi* syndrome
- Seeks Heat
- Cold ears, back, feet
- Tongue- pale or purple, wet or swollen
- Pulses- deep, slow, weak, weaker on right

TCVM Diagnosis:

The breed predisposition is associated with *Jing* Deficiency. Initial difficulty rising and muscle weakness is typical of *Wei* syndrome associated with Spleen *Qi* Deficiency. A diagnosis of paresis or paralysis or *Tan-Huan* syndrome (Grades 2-5 neurological deficits) is typical of Kidney *Qi* Deficiency, but with clinical evidence of Cold, the pattern becomes Kidney *Yang* Deficiency (*Qi* Deficiency plus Cold = *Yang* Deficiency). Evidence of Cold is based on the Heat seeking behavior and cold ears, back and feet. A pale, wet or swollen tongue and weak pulses worse on the right reflect the Spleen *Qi* Deficiency. A purple tongue and slow, weak pulses worse on the right reflect the Kidney *Yang* Deficiency.

Treatment Principles:
- Tonify Kidney *Jing* to nourish the spinal cord and strengthen the pelvic limbs
- Tonify Spleen *Qi* to strengthen the muscles
- Tonify Kidney *Yang* to strengthen the pelvic limbs

Acupuncture treatment:

EA is more effective than DN to promote nerve regeneration and deter further degeneration. Although degenerative myelopathy is not a painful disease, many dogs have concurrent *Bi* Syndrome so the EA protocol recommended is: 20 Hz (cycles/sec) for 10-15 minutes then 80-120 Hz alternating frequencies for 10-15 minutes. EA is combined with DN and Aqua-AP. For Aqua-AP inject 0.25-0.5 ml vitamin B12 into the acupoint after *Tui-na*. Acupuncture treatments may be weekly or every other week for 5-7 times, then reduced to once a month long-term.

Acupoints recommended
- EA: Select appropriate acupoints for thoracolumbar lesions in Table 3
- DN: Select acupoints in Table 3 plus BL-20, BL-23, KID-3
- Moxibustion: GV-3, GV-4, *Bai-hui, Shen-shu, Shen-peng, Shen-jiao*
- Aqua-AP: GV-4, BL-23, *Hua-tuo-jia-ji*

Pertinent acupoint actions
- See Table 3 for indications and actions of acupoints useful for EA and DN and location of classical acupoints
- BL-20 is the Back *Shu* Association point for the Spleen to support the production of post-natal *Jing* to reduce the use of pre-natal Kidney *Jing* and also a local acupoint to support the thoracolumbar spinal cord
- BL-21 is the Back *Shu* Association point for the Stomach to support the production of post-natal *Jing* to reduce the use of pre-natal Kidney *Jing* and also a local acupoint to support the thoracolumbar spinal cord
- BL-23 is the Back *Shu* Association point for the Kidney which tonifies the Kidney *Qi* to nourish the spinal cord and improve or delay progression of the paraparesis and also a local acupoint to support the thoracolumbar spinal cord
- KID-3 is the *Yuan* Source point for the Kidney to treat *Qi* Deficiency and nourish the spinal cord

- GV-3 and GV-4 are useful to treat Kidney *Yang* and *Qi* Deficiency with pelvic limb paresis or paralysis
- *Shen-shu* (one *cun* lateral to *Bai-hui*), *Shen-peng* (one *cun* cranial to *Shen-shu*) and *Shen-jiao* (one *cun* caudal to *Shen-shu*) are useful to treat Kidney *Qi* and *Yang* Deficiency and pelvic limb paresis or paralysis

Herbal Medicine:
- *You Gui Wan* (JT)[a] 0.5gm/10-20# twice daily orally to replenish Kidney *Jing* and marrow and warm and nourish Kidney *Yang* to halt or slow the progression of the paraparesis
- As an alternative administer: *Jin Gui Shen Qi Wan* (JT)[a] 0.5gm/10-20# twice daily orally to warm and tonify Kidney *Yang* and halt or slow the progression of the paraparesis
- As another alternative administer: *Ba Ji San* (JT)[a] 0.5gm/10-20# twice daily orally to warm and tonify Kidney *Yang* and halt or slow the progression of the paraparesis
- Administer herbs long-term to slow disease progression and improve the quality of life
- A description of all the ingredients of the Chinese herbal medicine listed is beyond the scope of this text, but can be found elsewhere.[7,8]

Food Therapy:
The initial purpose of the Food therapy is to tonify Kidney *Yang* to clear false Cold. Later foods can be supplemented to tonify the underlying Kidney *Jing* and Spleen and Kidney *Qi* to promote nerve regeneration and delay degeneration in the affected region and strengthen the pelvic limbs. Foods that are Cold are avoided.[28]
- Foods to tonify Kidney *Yang*: Chicken, lamb, corn fed beef, corn, millet, oats, brown rice, microalgae, pumpkin, squash, rutabaga, shiitake mushrooms, yams, sweet potatoes, winter squash, cherries, dates, figs, hawthorn fruit, lychees, molasses, royal jelly
- Foods to tonify *Jing*: Liver, kidneys, fish, bone and bone marrow, millet, quinoa, spelt, wheat, almonds, black sesame, microalgae (e.g. chlorella, spirulina, wild blue-green algae), barley, wheat grass, black soy beans, black beans, kidney beans, seaweed, sea salt, mulberries, raspberries, strawberries, almonds, black sesame, clarified butter (ghee), royal jelly, bee pollen
- Foods to tonify Spleen and Kidney *Qi*: Beef, chicken, sardines, egg, potato, yam, sweet potato, rice, oats, millet, lentils, carrots, squash, microalgae, dates, figs, molasses, royal jelly
- Cold foods to avoid: Turkey, duck, duck eggs, conch, clams, mussels, yogurt, millet, barley, spinach, broccoli, celery, egg plant, kelp, alfalfa, cucumbers, pears, bananas, white radishes, watermelon

Tui-na Procedures:
The purpose of the *Tui-na* is to keep *Qi* and Blood flowing to promote nerve regeneration and delay degeneration in the affected spinal cord region. The descriptions and indications of each technique are outlined in more detail in Chapter 1 Table 8.[20]
- A *Tui-na* protocol for degenerative myelopathy is outlined in Table 6

Daily Life Style Recommendation for Owner Follow-up
- *Moo-fa* (Daubing or massaging) of the back for 3 minutes once or twice daily

- *Ca-fa* (Rubbing) of back for a few minutes until it feels warm, once or twice daily
- *Ba-shen-fa* (Stretching) of the pelvic limbs for 12 times once or twice daily
- Maintain excellent nutrition
- Maintain a low stress environment
- Daily physical therapy of walking or swimming has been shown to reduce progression of the pelvic limb paresis
- Walk with a harness
- Assist to walk with a sling if needed
- Swim with support and supervision only in warm water; avoid chilling the body and stressing *Yang* further
- If Grades 3-5 paresis or paralysis, move every 4-6 hours to prevent decubitus ulcers
- Keep on padding to avoid decubitus ulcers on the hips or tuber ischii
- Keep dry and clean of feces and urine
- For severely *Yang* Deficient dogs, select clients may be taught to administer moxibustion at GV-3, GV-4, *Bai-hui, Shen-shu, Shen-peng, Shen-jiao* in-between veterinary visits

Comments:

Expect that the disease progression will be slowed and that the animal will maintain a high quality of life.

3. Kidney *Jing*, Spleen *Qi*, Kidney *Qi* and Kidney/Liver *Yin* Deficiencies

Clinical Signs:
- German Shepherd, Boxer or Welsh/Pembroke Corgi and a few other pure breed dogs
- 5 years of age or older
- Difficulty rising and muscle weakness in the pelvic limbs
- Chronic progressive paraparesis
- Usually Grades 2-4 neurological deficits
- Not painful unless has concurrent *Bi* syndrome
- Seeks Cool
- Warm ears, back, feet
- Panting
- Dry skin
- Tongue- pale or red and dry, cracked
- Pulses- deep, rapid, thready, weak on both sides or weaker on left

TCVM Diagnosis:

The breed predisposition is associated with *Jing* Deficiency. Initial difficulty rising and muscle weakness is typical of *Wei* syndrome associated with Spleen *Qi* Deficiency. A diagnosis of paresis or paralysis or *Tan-Huan* syndrome (Grades 2-5 neurological deficits) is typical of Kidney *Qi* Deficiency. The cool seeking behavior, panting episodes, warm ears, back and feet and dry skin are typical of a *Yin* Deficiency. The tongue characteristics can vary depending on which pattern is primarily reflected. A pale tongue reflects the Kidney *Jing* and *Qi* Deficiencies. The red and dry tongue reflects the Kidney/Liver *Yin* Deficiency. The tongue may be cracked, if the *Yin*

Deficiency is chronic. The pulses can vary and may be deep and weak on both sides reflecting the combination of *Yin* and *Qi* Deficiency or be weaker on the left reflecting the Kidney/Liver *Yin* Deficiency.

Treatment Principles:
- Tonify Kidney *Jing* to nourish the spinal cord and strengthen the pelvic limbs
- Tonify Spleen *Qi* to and strengthen the muscles
- Tonify Kidney/Liver *Yin* to nourish the spinal cord
- Tonify Kidney *Qi* to and strengthen the pelvic limbs

Acupuncture treatment:

EA is more effective than DN to promote nerve regeneration and deter further degeneration. Although degenerative myelopathy is not a painful disease, many dogs have concurrent *Bi* Syndrome so the EA protocol recommended is: 20 Hz (cycles/sec) for 10-15 minutes then 80-120 Hz alternating frequencies for 10-15 minutes. EA is combined with DN and Aqua-AP. For Aqua-AP inject 0.25-0.5 ml vitamin B12 into the acupoint after *Tui-na*. Acupuncture treatments may be weekly or every other week for 5-7 times, then reduced to once a month long-term.

Acupoints recommended
- EA: Select appropriate acupoints in Table 3 depending on the lesion location
- DN: Select acupoints in Table 3 plus BL-18, BL-20, BL-21 BL-23, KID-3, KID-6, SP-6
- Aqua-AP: BL-20, BL-23 and *Hua-tuo-jia-ji*

Pertinent acupoint actions
- See Table 3 for indications and actions of acupoints useful for EA and DN and location of classical acupoints
- BL-18 is the Back *Shu* Association point for the Liver to nourish Liver *Yin*
- BL-20 is the Back *Shu* Association point for the Spleen to support the production of post-natal *Jing* to reduce the use of pre-natal Kidney *Jing* and also a local acupoint to support the thoracolumbar spinal cord
- BL-21 is the Back *Shu* Association point for the Stomach to support the production of post-natal *Jing* to reduce the use of pre-natal Kidney *Jing* and also a local acupoint to support the thoracolumbar spinal cord
- BL-23 is the Back *Shu* Association point for the Kidney which tonifies the Kidney *Qi* to nourish the spinal cord and improve or delay progression of the paraparesis and also a local acupoint to support the thoracolumbar spinal cord
- KID-3 is the *Yuan* Source point for the Kidney which tonifies the Kidney *Qi* to nourish the spinal cord and improve or delay progression of the paraparesis
- KID-6 is the confluent point with the *Yin Qiao* Extraordinary Channel useful to treat *Yin* Deficiencies
- SP-6 tonifies *Yin* and Blood

Herbal Medicine:
- *Hu Qian Wan* (JT)[a] 0.5gm/10-20# twice daily orally to tonify Kidney *Jing*, *Qi* and *Yin* and strengthen the pelvic limbs; can administer for 6 months or longer as needed
- As an alternative administer: Hind Quarter Weakness (JT)[a] 0.5gm/10-20# twice daily orally to tonify Kidney *Qi* and strengthen the pelvic limbs; can administer for 6 months or longer as needed
- A description of all the ingredients of the Chinese herbal medicine listed is beyond the scope of this text, but can be found elsewhere.[7,8]

Food Therapy:
The initial purpose of the Food therapy is to tonify Kidney/Liver *Yin* to clear false Heat. Later foods can be supplemented to tonify the underlying Kidney *Jing* and Spleen and Kidney *Qi* to promote nerve regeneration and delay degeneration in the affected region and strengthen the pelvic limbs. Foods that are Hot are avoided.[28]
- Foods to tonify Kidney/Liver *Yin*: Turkey, pork, duck, clams, crab, eggs, rice, wheat, wheat germ, wheat berries, Belgian endive, string beans, peas, kidney beans, sweet potatoes, yams, tomato, spinach, tofu, kiwi, lemons, rhubarb, pears, bananas, watermelon, sesame, seaweed
- Foods to tonify Kidney *Jing*: Liver, kidneys, fish, bone and bone marrow, millet, quinoa, spelt, wheat, almonds, black sesame, microalgae (e.g. chlorella, spirulina, wild blue-green algae), barley, wheat grass, black soy beans, black beans, kidney beans, seaweed, sea salt, mulberries, raspberries, strawberries, almonds, black sesame, clarified butter (ghee), royal jelly, bee pollen
- Foods to tonify Spleen and Kidney *Qi*: Beef, chicken, sardines, egg, potato, yam, sweet potato, rice, oats, millet, lentils, carrots, squash, microalgae, dates, figs, molasses, royal jelly
- Hot foods to avoid: Lamb, shrimp, corn-fed beef, chicken, trout, squash, turnips, sweet rice, basal, caraway, cherries, chilies, cinnamon, ginger, rosemary, sage

Tui-na Procedures:
The purpose of the *Tui-na* is to keep *Qi* and Blood flowing to promote nerve regeneration and delay degeneration in the affected spinal cord region. The descriptions and indications of each technique are outlined in more detail in Chapter 1 Table 8.[20]
- A *Tui-na* protocol for degenerative myelopathy is outlined in Table 6

Daily Life Style Recommendation for Owner Follow-up
- *Moo-fa* (Daubing or massaging) of the back for 3 minutes once or twice daily
- *Ca-fa* (Rubbing) of back for a few minutes until it feels warm, once or twice daily
- *Ba-shen-fa* (Stretching) of the pelvic limbs for 12 times once or twice daily
- Maintain excellent nutrition
- Maintain a low stress environment
- Daily physical therapy of walking or swimming has been shown to reduce progression of the pelvic limb paresis
- Do not allow the animal to become overheated and further stress the body's *Yin*
- Walk with a harness

- Assist to walk with a sling if needed
- Swim with support and supervision only in cool water to support the body's *Yin*
- If Grades 3-5 paresis or paralysis, move every 4-6 hours to prevent decubitus ulcers
- Keep on padding to avoid decubitus ulcers on the hips or tuber ischii
- Keep dry and clean of feces and urine

Comments:

Expect that the disease progression will be slowed and that the animal will maintain a high quality of life.

4. Kidney *Jing*, Spleen *Qi*, Kidney *Yang* and Kidney/Liver *Yin* Deficiencies

Clinical Signs:
- German Shepherd, Boxer or Welsh/Pembroke Corgi and a few other pure breed dogs
- 5 years of age or older
- Difficulty rising and muscle weakness in the pelvic limbs
- Chronic progressive paraparesis
- Usually Grades 2-4 neurological deficits
- Not painful unless has concurrent *Bi* syndrome
- May have warm or cool ears, back, feet
- Cool or Heat seeking
- May or not pant
- Tongue- red, dry, cracked or pale purple and wet
- Pulses- deep, weak both sides

TCVM Diagnosis:

The breed predisposition is associated with *Jing* Deficiency. Initial difficulty rising and muscle weakness is typical of *Wei* syndrome associated with Spleen *Qi* Deficiency. A diagnosis of paresis or paralysis or *Tan-Huan* syndrome (Grades 2-5 neurological deficits) is typical of Kidney *Qi* Deficiency, clinical evidence of both Heat and Cold may be present. The animal may at times have panting episodes, warm ears, back and feet and dry skin, typical of a Kidney/Liver *Yin* Deficiency. Warm ears and front feet and cold back and hind feet may be present and reflect the combination of *Yin* and *Yang* Deficiency patterns. The paresis or paralysis with cold ears, back or feet is typical of Kidney *Yang* Deficiency. The tongue characteristics can vary depending on which pattern is primarily reflected. A red and dry tongue reflects the Kidney/Liver *Yin* Deficiency. The tongue may be cracked, if *Yin* Deficiency is chronic. A pale purple and wet tongue reflects the Kidney *Yang* Deficiency. The pulses are usually deep and weak on both sides reflecting the combination of *Yin* and *Qi* Deficiency.

Treatment Principles:
- Tonify Kidney *Jing* to nourish the spinal cord and strengthen the pelvic limbs
- Tonify Spleen *Qi* to strengthen the muscles
- Tonify Kidney/Liver *Yin* to nourish the spinal cord
- Tonify Kidney *Yang* to strengthen the pelvic limbs

Acupuncture treatment:

EA is more effective than DN to promote nerve regeneration and deter further degeneration. Although degenerative myelopathy is not a painful disease, many dogs have concurrent *Bi* Syndrome so the EA protocol recommended is: 20 Hz (cycles/sec) for 10-15 minutes then 80-120 Hz alternating frequencies for 10-15 minutes. EA is combined with DN and Aqua-AP. For Aqua-AP inject 0.25-0.5 ml vitamin B12 into the acupoint after *Tui-na*. Acupuncture treatments may be weekly or every other week for 5-7 times, then reduced to once a month long-term.

Acupoints recommended

- EA: Select appropriate acupoints in Table 3 depending on the lesion location
- DN: Select acupoints in Table 3 plus BL-18, BL-20, BL-21, BL-23, KID-3, KID-6, SP-6, GV-3, GV-4, *Bai-hui, Shen-shu, Shen-peng, Shen-jiao,* BL-62
- Moxibustion: Do not perform moxibustion because of the concurrent *Yin* Deficiency
- Aqua-AP: BL-23 and *Hua-tuo-jia-ji*

Pertinent acupoint actions

- See Table 3 for indications and actions of acupoints useful for EA and DN and location of classical acupoints
- BL-18 is the Back *Shu* Association point for the Liver to nourish Liver *Yin*
- BL-20 is the Back *Shu* Association point for the Spleen to support the production of post-natal *Jing* to reduce the use of pre-natal Kidney *Jing* and also a local acupoint to support the thoracolumbar spinal cord
- BL-21 is the Back *Shu* Association point for the Stomach to support the production of post-natal *Jing* to reduce the use of pre-natal Kidney *Jing* and also a local acupoint to support the thoracolumbar spinal cord
- BL-23 is the Back *Shu* Association point for the Kidney which tonifies the Kidney *Qi* to nourish the spinal cord and improve or delay progression of the paraparesis and also a local acupoint to support the thoracolumbar spinal cord
- KID-3 is the *Yuan* Source point for the Kidney which tonifies the Kidney *Qi* to nourish the spinal cord and improve or delay progression of the paraparesis
- KID-6 is the confluent point with the *Yin Qiao* Extraordinary Channel useful to treat *Yin* Deficiencies
- SP-6 tonifies *Yin* and Blood
- GV-3 and GV-4 are useful to treat Kidney *Yang* and *Qi* Deficiency and nourish the spinal cord and improve or delay progression of the paraparesis
- *Shen-shu* (one *cun* lateral to *Bai-hui*), *Shen-peng* (one *cun* cranial to *Shen-shu*) and *Shen-jiao* (one *cun* caudal to *Shen-shu*) are useful to treat Kidney *Qi* and *Yang* Deficiency and nourish the spinal cord and improve or delay progression of the paraparesis

- BL-62 is the confluent point with the *Yang Qiao* Extraordinary Channel useful to treat *Yang* Deficiency and improve ataxia, paraparesis and paraplegia

Herbal Medicine:
- *Di Huang Yin Zi* (JT)[a] 0.5gm/10-20# twice daily orally to tonify Kidney *Jing*, *Yin* and *Yang* and strengthen the pelvic limbs
- Administer herbal formula up to 6 months or longer as needed
- A description of all the ingredients of the Chinese herbal medicine listed is beyond the scope of this text, but can be found elsewhere.[7,8]

Food Therapy:
The purpose of the Food therapy is to tonify Kidney *Jing* and Spleen and Kidney *Qi* to support nerve regeneration and delay degeneration in the affected region. Since both Kidney *Yin* and Kidney *Yang* are Deficient, foods that are too Cold or Hot are avoided.[28]
- Foods to supplement to tonify Kidney *Jing*: chicken egg, crab, sweet rice, peaches, carrots, coriander, squash, turnips
- Foods to tonify Spleen and Kidney *Qi*: Beef, chicken, sardines, egg, potato, yam, sweet potato, rice, oats, millet, lentils, carrots, squash, microalgae, dates, figs, molasses, royal jelly
- Cold foods to avoid: Turkey, duck, duck eggs, conch, clams, mussels, yogurt, millet, barley, spinach, broccoli, celery, egg plant, kelp, alfalfa, cucumbers, pears, bananas, white radishes, watermelon
- Hot foods to avoid: Lamb, shrimp, corn-fed beef, chicken, trout, squash, turnips, sweet rice, basal, caraway, cherries, chilies, cinnamon, ginger, rosemary, sage

Tui-na Procedures:
The purpose of the *Tui-na* is to keep *Qi* and Blood flowing to promote nerve regeneration and delay degeneration in the affected spinal cord region. The descriptions and indications of each technique are outlined in more detail in Chapter 1 Table 8.[20]
- A *Tui-na* protocol for degenerative myelopathy is outlined in Table 6

Daily Life Style Recommendation for Owner Follow-up
- *Moo-fa* (Daubing or massaging) of the back for 3 minutes once or twice daily
- *Ca-fa* (Rubbing) of back for a few minutes until it feels warm, once or twice daily
- *Ba-shen-fa* (Stretching) of the pelvic limbs for 12 times once or twice daily
- Maintain excellent nutrition
- Maintain a low stress environment
- Daily physical therapy of walking or swimming has been shown to reduce progression of the pelvic limb paresis
- Do not let the body become overheated or chilled to avoid further stress of the *Yin* and *Yang* respectively
- Walk with a harness
- Assist to walk with a sling if needed
- Swim with support and supervision, don't let the body become too hot or too cold

- If Grades 3-5 paresis or paralysis, move every 4-6 hours to prevent decubitus ulcers
- Keep on padding to avoid decubitus ulcers on the hips or tuber ischii
- Keep dry and clean of feces and urine

Comments:

Expect that the disease progression will be slowed and that the animal will maintain a high quality of life.

ATLANTOAXIAL MALFORMATION

Atlantoaxial (C1-C2) subluxation is usually associated with agenesis or hypogenesis of the dens and surrounding ligaments in toy breed dogs such as Toy Poodles, Yorkshire terriers and Pomeranians under one year of age.[3-5] Occasionally dogs may be a few years old before subluxation occurs, following a seemingly insignificant traumatic event such as falling from a low piece of furniture or playing with another animal. Periodic syncope-like episodes have been noted, presumably from the abnormal dens compressing the ventrally located basilar artery and reducing the blood flow to the brain. Acute subluxation can cause severe spinal cord injury (Grade 3-5 neurological deficits).

Pain is usually elicited in the high cervical region on cervical palpation. Ataxia of all four limbs, quadriparesis (Grades 2-3 neurological deficits) or quadriplegia (Grade 4 neurological deficit) is present and the thoracic limbs are often worse than the pelvic limbs. Spinal reflexes are normal to hyperactive and crossed extensor reflexes may be present in all four limbs. The diagnosis can usually be confirmed based a lateral radiograph of the cervical spine, which shows an abnormal separation of the dorsal arch of the atlas and the dorsal spinous process of the axis. Syringomyelia may occur and can be seen on an MRI of the region.

The treatment of choice is ventral surgical fusion of the atlantoaxial joint. The prognosis for functional recovery following surgery is usually fair to good, if there is no paralysis of respiration in the first 24 hours. Dogs with neck pain, ataxia and mild quadriparesis (Grades 1-2 neurological deficits) may be presented for TCVM treatment prior to surgery, but non-ambulatory dogs with Grades 3-4 neurological deficits may be presented for TCVM treatment post-operatively. TCVM may help avoid surgery in mildly affected cases or shorten the recovery time and improve the degree of functional recovery post-operatively, as has been seen in other forms of spinal cord injury.[10-17]

Etiology and Pathology

As with all congenital vertebral malformations in TCVM, an underlying Kidney *Jing* Deficiency is responsible for the lack of development of the dens and instability of C1-C2 (Table X).[23] Spinal cord trauma results in Stagnation of *Qi*/Blood flow and *Qi* Deficiency locally affecting the Spinal Cord. The Deficiency and Stagnation of *Qi* and bleeding, associated with the spinal cord contusion, depletes Blood and *Gu Qi* that nourish the neurons and other cells of the region and degeneration and demyelination occurs. Kidney *Qi* Deficiency is also present, if the animal develops quadriparesis (*Tan-Huan* syndrome).

1. **Spinal cord *Qi*/Blood Stagnation and Kidney *Jing* and *Qi* Deficiencies**

    Kidney *Jing* Deficiency results in malformation of the C2 causing C1-C2 (atlantoaxial) instability. The atlantoaxial instability initially causes pain due to *Qi*/Blood Stagnation in External Channels of the high cervical region affecting vertebral and paravertebral structures. If acute C1-C2 subluxation occurs, the spinal cord is traumatized causing contusion and further *Qi*/Blood Stagnation and local *Qi* Deficiency. The local spinal cord *Qi* Deficiency causes loss of spinal cord function and quadriparesis or quadriplegia. Since the spinal cord belongs to the Kidney, quadriparesis or quadriplegia is associated with Kidney *Qi* Deficiency. Combining the individual components, the complete diagnosis then becomes Spinal cord *Qi*/Blood Stagnation with Kidney *Jing* and *Qi* Deficiencies.

Pattern Differentiation and Treatment

1. Spinal cord *Qi*/Blood Stagnation and Kidney *Jing* and *Qi* Deficiencies

Clinical Signs:
- Neck pain
- Acute Grades 2-5 ataxia, paresis or paralysis
- Tongue- pale, purple
- Pulses- deep, weak or wiry

TCVM Diagnosis:
The conventional diagnosis of malformation of the dens with atlantoaxial instability is usually known and forms the basis for the diagnosis of Kidney *Jing* Deficiency. Spinal cord *Qi*/Blood Stagnation with Kidney *Qi* Deficiency is the source of paresis or paralysis. The tongue will be purple reflecting the *Qi*/Blood Stagnation or may be also be pale reflecting the Kidney *Jing* Deficiency. The pulses are usually wiry reflecting the *Qi*/Blood Stagnation.

Treatment Principles:
- Tonify Kidney *Jing*
- Resolve *Qi*/Blood Stagnation to return proper *Qi*/Blood flow, relieve pain and resolve quadriparesis
- Tonify Kidney *Qi* and resolve quadriparesis

Acupuncture treatment:
EA is more effective than DN to resolve *Qi*/Blood Stagnation and promote nerve regeneration. Since most dogs have neck pain before or after surgery for EA use 20 Hz for 10-15 minutes followed by 80-120 Hz alternating frequencies for 10-15 minutes. EA is combined with DN and Aqua-AP. For Aqua-AP inject 0.25-0.5 ml vitamin B12 into the acupoint after *Tui-na*. If pain is severe or for post-op treatment of non-ambulatory dogs (Grade 3-5 neurological deficits), EA and DN should be administered every 3 days for 3-5 times, depending on the patient's response, then reduced to once every 1-2 weeks until ambulatory. For mildly affected cases, the acupuncture treatments may be weekly or every other week. Most dogs that have had surgery will have a large neck brace with bandages that often extends from GV-22 or GV-23 caudal to GV-11 or GV-12 encompassing both thoracic limbs to the elbows. Therefore GB-20, GB-21, SI-9, SI-16 and *Jing-jia-jia* and other cervical acupoints will not be accessible for at least 6-8 weeks.

Acupoints recommended
- EA: If there is a neck brace, perform EA at GV-8/GV-24, TH-10/TH-23 and GB-14/GB-25; If there is no neck brace, select acupoints in Table 3 described for cervical lesions
- DN: Select acupoints in Table 3 plus BL-20, BL-21, BL-23, KID-7, KID-3
- Aqua-AP: BL-23

Pertinent acupoint actions
- See Table 3 for indications and actions of acupoints useful for EA and DN
- GV-8 is connected to GV-24 for EA to stimulate *Qi* flow through the Governing Vessel over the lesion (when a brace is blocking other points typically selected)
- TH-10 is connected to TH-23 for EA to stimulate *Qi* flow through the Triple Heater that traverses near the lesion (when a brace is blocking other points typically selected)
- GB-14 is connected to GB-25 to stimulate *Qi* flow through the Gall bladder Channel that traverses near the lesion (use when a brace is blocking other points typically selected)
- GB-25 is also a tonification acupoint for the Kidney
- BL-20 is the Back *Shu* Association point for the Spleen to support the production of post-natal *Jing* to reduce the use of pre-natal Kidney *Jing*
- BL-21 is the Back *Shu* Association point for the Stomach to support the production of post-natal *Jing* to reduce the use of pre-natal Kidney *Jing*
- BL-23 is the Back *Shu* Association point for the Kidney to support Kidney *Jing* and *Qi* and resolve paresis or paralysis and nourish the spinal cord
- KID-7 is the Mother (Metal) point on the Channel useful to treat Kidney *Qi* Deficiency and resolve paresis and paralysis
- KID-3 is the *Yuan* Source point useful to treat Kidney *Jing* and *Qi* Deficiency and resolve paresis and paralysis

Herbal Medicine:
- For Grades 2-5 paresis or paralysis administer Double P II (JT)[a] 0.5gm/10-20# twice daily orally to move *Qi* and Blood and eliminate Stagnation and pain
- Combine with Cervical Formula (JT)[a] 0.5gm/10-20# twice daily orally to activate Blood, move *Qi*, eliminate Stagnation and pain
- Add Epimedium Formula (JT)[a] 0.5gm/10-20# twice daily orally to support Kidney *Jing* when the Double P II is discontinued
- Administer Double P II for 1-3 months then continue Cervical Formula and Epimedium Formula until recovered up to 6 months or longer if needed
- A description of all the ingredients of the Chinese herbal medicine listed is beyond the scope of this text, but can be found elsewhere.[7,8]

Food Therapy:

The purpose of the Food therapy is to resolve *Qi*/Blood Stagnation and tonify Kidney *Jing* and Kidney *Qi* to promote nerve regeneration in the affected region and strengthen limbs. Foods that are too Cold or Hot are avoided.[28]

- Foods to supplement to promote *Qi* and Blood circulation include: chicken egg, crab, sweet rice, peaches, carrots, coriander, squash, turnips
- Foods to tonify *Jing*: Liver, kidneys, fish, bone and bone marrow, millet, quinoa, spelt, wheat, almonds, black sesame, microalgae (e.g. chlorella, spirulina, wild blue-green algae), barley, wheat grass, black soy beans, black beans, kidney beans, seaweed, sea salt, mulberries, raspberries, strawberries, almonds, black sesame, clarified butter (ghee), royal jelly, bee pollen
- Foods to tonify Kidney *Qi*: Beef, chicken, sardines, egg, potato, yam, sweet potato, rice, oats, millet, lentils, carrots, squash, microalgae, dates, figs, molasses, royal jelly
- Cold foods to avoid: Turkey, duck, duck eggs, conch, clams, mussels, yogurt, millet, barley, spinach, broccoli, celery, egg plant, kelp, alfalfa, cucumbers, pears, bananas, white radishes, watermelon
- Hot foods to avoid: Lamb, shrimp, corn-fed beef, chicken, trout, squash, turnips, sweet rice, basal, caraway, cherries, chilies, cinnamon, ginger, rosemary, sage

Tui-na Procedures:

The purpose of the *Tui-na* is to stimulate *Qi* and Blood flow to relieve pain and promote nerve regeneration in the affected region. The descriptions and indications of each technique are outlined in more detail in Chapter 1 Table 8.[20]

- Avoid manipulation of the neck and back
- *An-fa* pressing of SI-3, LI-4, TH-5 and LU-7 for 5-10 seconds per acupoint
- *Nian-fa* holding and kneading each of the digits and distal extremities repeat 12 times

Daily Life Style Recommendation for Owner Follow-up:

- If Grades 3-5 paresis or paralysis, turn (if in lateral recumbency) or move every 4-6 hours to prevent lung atelectasis and decubitus ulcers
- *Nian-fa* holding and kneading each of the digits and distal extremities repeat 12 times twice daily
- Keep on padding to avoid decubitus ulcers on shoulders, hips or tuber ischii
- Keep dry and clean of feces and urine
- Assist to walk with a sling if needed
- Swim with support and supervision once the brace is removed
- Remove all collars and only walk with a harness
- Once recovered avoid jumping on and off furniture and rough play

Comments:

Based on clinical experiences and current research, the TCVM treatments should shorten the recovery time and improve the degree of functional recovery.

MENINGITIS AND MENINGOMYELITIS

Meningitis is inflammation of the outer coverings of the spinal cord (meninges). Myelitis is inflammation of the spinal cord alone. Meningomyelitis is inflammation of the meninges and spinal cord. Meningitis can cause neck or back pain in dogs and cats with no other neurological deficits. (Grade 1).[1-3] Meningomyelitis causes neck and/or back pain along with Grades 2-5 neurological deficits. Pain may be worse in the cervical region, but can be multifocal or extend along the entire vertebral column. Dogs with meningitis and meningomyelitis are often lethargic, anorexic and may or may not be febrile. They may also have a concurrent meningoencephalitis and the conventional diagnosis then becomes meningoencephalomyelitis. Like meningoencephalitis, bacteria, viruses, fungi, protozoa, rickettsial organisms and immune-mediated processes may cause meningitis and meningomyelitis. Most of the inflammatory diseases of the brain discussed above (see **MENINGOENCEPHALITIS AND ENCEPHALITIS** in the **DEMENTIA, STUPOR AND COMA** section above) can also cause focal cervical, thoracolumbar or multifocal meningomyelitis. Like meningoencephalitis the diagnosis is based on finding a leukocytic pleocytosis and elevated protein levels in the CSF. Serum and CSF immunoassays for specific organisms may be help identify causative agents. An inflammatory focus may be visible on MRI. A steroid responsive meningitis/arteritis (SRMA) and granulomatous meningoencephalitis (GME) are suspected immune mediated disorders that can affect the meninges and spinal cord and are usually conventionally treated with corticosteroids or other immunosuppressive drugs.

TCVM treatments can be integrated with conventional treatments for organisms and immune-mediated processes to control pain, support the immune system and promote regeneration of the spinal cord. There are no clinical studies of the use of TCVM in the treatment of meningitis or meningomyelitis, but TCVM patterns and treatment recommendations from clinical practice are outlined in Tables 2-4.[5-8]

Etiology and Pathology

When *Zheng Qi* is weakened from poor nutrition, chronic illness, environmental stress or age, the *Wei Qi* portion of *Zheng Qi* that protects the body's exterior becomes weak and external pathogens such as Wind, Heat, Damp and/or Heat Toxins gain entrance.[2] Heat Toxins are often invasion of conventional organisms like viruses, fungi or other infectious agent. When pain is present meningeal *Qi*/Blood Stagnation has occurred. As paresis or paralysis of the limbs occurs Kidney *Qi* Deficiency is present. Like meningoencephalitis infectious diseases of the spinal cord may also be viewed from another diagnostic system called the Four Stages or Four levels of Disease. Based on the Four Stages the disease progresses from superficial levels to deeper levels and becomes more difficult to treat the deeper it goes. The Four Stages or Levels are: 1) the *Wei* stage (Exterior level), 2) *Qi* stage (next level), 3) *Ying* stage (nutrient level, level of the central nervous system) and 4) the *Xue* stage (Blood level) is the deepest level of all. Organisms (Heat Toxins) causing meningomyelitis are generally located at the *Ying* stage, so has already invaded the body relatively deeply to Interior levels. Disease at this level may require intensive and prolong treatment to ensure recovery. Applying the basic TCVM theories of *Yin/Yang*, Eight Principles, TCVM pathogens, Five Treasures, Five Elements and *Zang Fu* physiology and pathology to make a TCVM diagnosis, there is currently one basic pattern associated with meningomyelitis (Table X).

1. **Damp-Heat of the Spinal Cord with *Qi*/Blood Stagnation and Kidney *Qi* Deficiency (Heat in the *Ying* Stage)**
   Inflammation of the brain is due to a weak *Zheng Qi* and the invasion of the exterior pathogens Wind/Damp/Heat and Heat Toxins resulting in Damp Heat in the meninges and/or spinal cord. The External Pathogens cause *Qi*/Blood Stagnation and neck or back pain. If paresis or paralysis develops, then Kidney *Qi* Deficiency is present. Damp-Heat in the meninges and/or spinal cord can also be described as Heat in the *Ying* Stage using the Four Stages or Levels diagnostic system.

Pattern Differentiation and Treatment

1. **Damp-Heat of the Spinal Cord with *Qi*/Blood Stagnation and Kidney *Qi* Deficiency (Heat in the *Ying* Stage)**

Clinical Signs:
- Acute neck or back pain
- Grade 2-5 neurological deficits
- Lethargy
- Dementia, stupor or seizures if the brain is also affected
- May or not have fever
- Panting
- Warm ears, back and feet
- Tongue- red, yellow coating and dry
- Pulses- superficial, strong, forceful and rapid

TCVM Diagnosis:
The diagnosis of Heat Toxin is based on the evidence of Heat on the TCVM examination with a possible fever and warm ears, back and feet and panting. A red tongue with a yellow coating also reflects Heat in the body. The superficial, strong, forceful and rapid pulses are typical of Excess Heat and the wiry nature of the pulse reflects the *Qi*/Blood Stagnation causing the clinical signs of pain, paresis or paralysis

Treatment Principles:
- Clear Damp Heat and Heat Toxin
- Resolve *Qi*/Blood Stagnation to control pain
- Tonify Kidney *Qi* to strengthen the limbs
- Tonify *Zheng Qi*

Acupuncture treatment:
Acupuncture may be combined with conventional medications to treat pain, inflammation and specific organisms. Acupuncture is useful to promote spinal cord regeneration and balance the immune system. If the animal has no evidence of brain involvement, EA is recommended combined with DN as EA resolves *Qi*/Blood Stagnation better than DN alone. If seizures are induced by EA, discontinue and the seizures often will immediately cease. Because pain is common with meningomyelitis, EA 20 Hz (cycles/second) for 10-15 minutes followed by 80-120

Hz alternating frequencies for 10-15 minutes is recommended. Some acupoints may be too painful to treat initially, so less painful acupoints are selected to avoid undue patient stress. Treat both sides. If pain is severe or animals are acutely non-ambulatory (Grade 3-5 neurological deficits), EA and DN should be administered every 3-5 days for 3-5 times, depending on the patient's response, then reduced to once every 1-2 weeks until ambulatory. In less severely affected animals, acupuncture may be administered weekly for 3-5 treatments, then every 2-4 weeks for 6-8 treatments or longer if needed. For Aqua-AP inject 0.25-0.5 ml vitamin B12 into the acupoint.

Acupoints recommended
- EA: Select appropriate acupoints in Table 3 depending on the lesion location; avoid acupoints in the immediate area of the lesion as it may be too painful
- DN: Select acupoints in Table 3 plus GV-14, LI-11, *Er-jian*, *Wei-jian*
- Aqua-AP: GV-14

Pertinent acupoint actions
- See Table 3 for indications and actions of acupoints useful for EA and DN
- GV-14, LI-11, *Er-jian* (ear tip) and *Wei-jian* (tail tip) are all useful to clear Heat
- GV-14 and LI-11 are also useful to balance the immune system and support *Zheng Qi*

Herbal Medicine:
- Administer *Wu Wei Xiao Du Yin* (JT)[a] 0.5gm/10# twice daily orally to Clear Heat and remove Heat Toxins combined with conventional medications as needed for immunosuppression, organisms and/or pain control
- Continue *Wu Wei Xiao Du Yin* for 1 month
- Then switch to *Zhi Bai Di Huang* (JT)[a] 0.5gm/10-20# twice daily orally to tonify *Yin* and clear Heat until the animal recovers up to 6-9 months
- A description of all the ingredients of the Chinese herbal medicine listed is beyond the scope of this text, but can be found elsewhere.[7,8]

Food Therapy:
The purpose of the Food therapy is to clear Heat and Damp and promote *Qi*/Blood circulation and nerve regeneration. Cooling foods are prescribed and Damp producing and Hot foods are avoided.[28]
- Foods to supplement to clear Heat: Turkey, duck, duck eggs, conch, clams, mussels, yogurt, millet, barley, spinach, broccoli, celery, egg plant, kelp, alfalfa, cucumbers, pears, bananas, white radishes, watermelon
- Foods to supplement to Drain Damp: Eel, mackerel, quail, corn, barley, rye, blueberries, celery, mushrooms
- Foods to promote *Qi*/Blood circulation: Crab, sweet rice, peaches, carrots, coriander, turnips
- Damp producing foods to avoid: Eggs, milk, cheese, yoghurt, ghee, bananas, sugar

- Hot foods to avoid: Lamb, shrimp, corn-fed beef, chicken, trout, squash, turnips, sweet rice, basal, caraway, cherries, chilies, cinnamon, ginger, rosemary, sage

Tui-na Procedures:
The purpose of the *Tui-na* is to stimulate *Qi* and Blood flow to relieve pain and promote nerve regeneration in the affected regions. If pain is severe, avoid *Tui-na* in the region of the pain until acupuncture and Chinese herbal medicine have relieved the pain. The descriptions and indications of each technique are outlined in more detail in Chapter 1 Table 8.[20]

- Initially pain is usually severe and manipulation of the neck and back are avoided
- *An-fa* pressing of SI-3, LI-4, TH-5 and LU-7 for 5-10 seconds per acupoint
- *Nian-fa* holding and kneading each of the digits and distal extremities repeat 12 times
- Later can select techniques outlined in Tables 5 and 6 useful to treat cervical or thoracolumbar *Qi*/Blood Stagnation

Daily Life Style Recommendation for Owner Follow-up:
- Delay *Tui-na* until the pain is controlled
- Gentle *Moo-fa* (Daubing or massaging) of the neck or back for 3 minutes
- Gentle *Ca-fa* (Rubbing) of neck or back for a few minutes until it feels warm, once daily for 14-21 days
- *Ba-shen-fa* (Stretching) and range of motion exercises of all the limbs for 12 times twice daily until can walk
- Assist to walk with a sling if needed
- Avoid collars and walk with a harness

Comments:
Disease in the *Ying* Stage may require intensive and prolong treatment to ensure recovery. Combine TCVM and conventional treatments initially for 2 months if needed then continue TCVM alone for total of 6 months.

SPINAL CORD TUMORS
Vertebral tumors like osteosarcoma initially cause extreme neck or back pain (Grade 1 neurological deficits).[1-3] As the vertebral tumors enlarge they narrow the spinal canal and compress the spinal cord causing paresis or paralysis (Grades 2-5 neurological deficits) of all four limbs (cervical tumors) or the pelvic limbs alone (thoracolumbar tumors). Meningiomas and peripheral nerve sheath neoplasms most commonly affect the spinal cord of dogs.[1-3] Gliomas and ependymomas are the most frequent primary intramedullary spinal cord tumors. Hemangiosarcoma, adenocarconomas from mammary glands and the prostate may metastasize to spinal cord. Lymphoma is the most common spinal tumor of cats and can cause progressive painful paraparesis as there is predilection for the lymphoma to be localized in the thoracic and lumbar vertebral canal.[2,3]

Tumors are best visualized with MRI, but tumor aspiration, biopsy or resection is necessary to determine the tumor type. The immediate goal of therapy is to relieve the pain and the effects of spinal cord compression with conventional pain medications, corticosteroids and in some cases decompression surgery. Chemotherapy and radiation also may be available for some tumor types.[2,3]

TCVM may be combined with conventional medications to further control pain, reduce the mass size, support the immune system and improve the quality and length of life.[35,39] An overview of the diagnosis and treatment of spinal cord tumors is outlined in Tables 8 and 3.[5-8] Acupoints in the immediate area of the tumor are avoided and only distant acupoints on the Channels that traverse the lesion and those with special effects are suggested. Generally dogs or cats with vertebral and spinal cord neoplasia have a poor long-term prognosis, but in some cases with the integration of TCVM their quality of life may be increased for a longer period. There are currently no case reports of the treatment of spinal cord tumors with TCVM and clinical studies are needed.

Etiology and Pathology

Chronic environmental toxins, poor nutrition and emotional stress weaken *Zheng Qi* and allow Phlegm to accumulate or Blood to become stagnant in the vertebrae and spinal cord and both can create tumors.[2] Unlike tumors in the brain, tumors on the surface of the spinal cord like meningiomas, lymphosarcomas and other metastatic tumors are very painful and reflect the presence of local *Qi*/Blood Stagnation. Tumors within the spinal cord parenchyma are usually not painful. Tumors due to Phlegm or Blood Stagnation can cause local *Qi*/Blood Deficiency in the spinal cord and loss of function (Table 2). Paresis or paralysis results due to Kidney *Qi* Deficiency.

1. **Spinal Cord Phlegm and Kidney *Qi* Deficiency with or without *Qi*/Blood Stagnation**
   Meningiomas, gliomas and ependymomas and non-blood origin metastatic tumors are considered Excess patterns of spinal cord Phlegm. As the Phlegm mass enlarges local *Qi*/Blood Deficiency develops and affects spinal cord function. The result is ataxia, paresis or paralysis. Since the spinal cord belongs to the Kidney, the paresis or paralysis is associated with Kidney *Qi* Deficiency.

2. **Blood Stagnation of the Spinal Cord with Kidney *Qi* Deficiency**
   When tumors associated with blood such as lymphosarcoma and hemangiosarcoma occur in the spinal cord, the result is Blood Stagnation. As the Blood Stagnation mass enlarges local *Qi*/Blood Deficiency develops and affects spinal cord function. The result is ataxia, paresis or paralysis. Since the spinal cord belongs to the Kidney, the paresis or paralysis is associated with Kidney *Qi* Deficiency.

Pattern Differentiation and Treatment

1. Spinal Cord Phlegm and Kidney *Qi* Deficiency with or without *Qi*/Blood Stagnation

Clinical Signs:
- Usually middle age to geriatric animals
- May or not have neck or back pain (Grade 1 neurological deficits)
- Quadriparesis, quadriplegia, paraparesis or paraplegia (Grades 2-5 neurological deficits)
- Tongue- pale, greasy coat or purple
- Pulses- slippery or wiry

TCVM Diagnosis:

The diagnosis of Spinal Cord Phlegm is supported by knowledge that the tumor is of non-blood origin. The paresis or paralysis is associated with Kidney *Qi* Deficiency. A pale tongue with a white greasy coat and slippery pulses are found in animals with Phlegm. If the animal is in pain, because the tumor has resulted in local *Qi*/Blood Stagnation, the tongue may be purple and the pulses wiry.

Treatment Principles:
- Expel Phlegm to shrink the mass
- Support *Wei Qi* and balance the immune system to reduce further mutation and tumor growth
- Tonify Kidney *Qi* to nourish the spinal cord and strengthen the limbs
- Relieve secondary *Qi*/Blood Stagnation to relieve pain

Acupuncture treatment:

EA is more effective than DN to resolve *Qi*/Blood Stagnation and promote nerve regeneration. For EA use 20 Hz (cycles/sec) for 10-15 minutes then 80-120 Hz alternating frequencies for 10-15 minutes. Do not perform EA across the tumor or select Governing Vessel, Back *Shu* Association points or *Hua-tuo-jia-ji* or *Jing-jia-ji* acupoints in the area of the tumor. EA is combined with DN and Aqua-AP. For Aqua-AP inject 0.25-0.5 ml vitamin B12 into the acupoint after *Tui-na*. Do not treat local acupoints in the area of the tumor, but instead select distant acupoints on the Governing Vessel and other Channels near the tumor. Acupoints that help control pain, balance the immune system and tonify *Qi* are also recommended. Treat every 1-2 weeks as needed to control pain and strengthen limbs. Combine acupuncture with conventional medication to control pain and secondary spinal cord edema if necessary.

Acupoints recommended
- EA: In non-ambulatory paresis or paralysis (Grades 3-5 neurological deficits) treat bilateral limb points connecting left and right acupoints like ST-36/ST-36, LI-10/LI-10, PC-8/PC-8, KID-1/KID-1 (No EA across or near the tumor)
- DN cervical tumors: GV-20, GV-1, TH-5, LI-4, LI-11, LIV-3, ST-36, LI-10, LIV-3, LU-7, ST-40, SP-6, SP-9, BL-23, KID-3
- DN thoracic and lumbar tumors: GV-20, GV-1, TH-5, LI-4, LI-11, LIV-3, ST-36, LI-10, ST-40, SP-6, SP-9, BL-40, KID-3
- Aqua-AP: ST-40, LI-11

Pertinent acupoint actions
- GV-20 and GV-1 are useful to calm the animal but also are distant points on the Governing Vessel that courses over the tumor region
- TH-5, LI-4, LI-11 and ST-36 are useful to balance the immune system for *Wei Qi* Deficiency
- LI-4 and LIV-3 are useful to control pain if present
- LI-4 and LU-7 are Master points for the neck useful for cervical tumors
- ST-36 and LI-10 are *Qi* tonic acupoints useful for Kidney *Qi* Deficiency
- ST-40 is the Influential point for Phlegm useful to dispel Phlegm

- SP-6 and SP-9 are useful to reduce Damp contained in Phlegm
- BL-23 is the Back *Shu* Association Kidney to nourish the Kidney and strengthen the limbs (select only in cervical tumors)
- KID-3 is the *Yuan* Source point for the Kidney to nourish the Kidney and strengthen the limbs
- BL-40 is the Master point for the pelvic limbs and especially useful for thoracolumbar tumors

Herbal Medicine:
- Max's Formula (JT)[a] 0.5 gm/10-20# twice daily orally to soften the hardness, clear nodules and transform Phlegm
- If there is no response after 30 days or the animal has non-ambulatory paresis or paralysis administer Stasis Breaker (JT)[a] 0.5 gm/10-20# twice daily orally as an alternative to remove Blood Stasis, soften hardness and clear masses
- Combine either of the above formulas with *Wei Qi* Booster (JT)[a] 0.5 gm/10-20# orally twice daily orally to tonify *Qi*, boost *Wei Qi* and inhibit mutation
- Administer both formulas for up to 6 months, then as needed for maintenance
- A description of all the ingredients of the Chinese herbal medicine listed is beyond the scope of this text, but can be found elsewhere.[7,8]

Food Therapy:

The purpose of the Food Therapy is to support Spleen *Qi* to resolve Phlegm and support Kidney *Qi* to strengthen the limbs. Damp producing foods and food that are too Hot or too Cold should be avoided.[28]

- Foods to supplement to support the Spleen and transform Phlegm: Chicken, oats, glutinous rice, brown rice, pumpkin, squash, sweet potato, almond, garlic, ginger, pear, radish, seaweed, thyme
- Foods to tonify Spleen and Kidney *Qi*: Beef, chicken, sardines, egg, potato, yam, sweet potato, rice, oats, millet, lentils, carrots, squash, microalgae, dates, figs, molasses, royal jelly
- Damp producing foods to avoid: Pork, eggs, milk, cheese, yoghurt, ghee, bananas, sugar
- Hot foods to avoid: Lamb, shrimp, corn-fed beef, chicken, trout, squash, turnips, sweet rice, basal, caraway, cherries, chilies, cinnamon, ginger, rosemary, sage
- Cold foods to avoid: Turkey, duck, duck eggs, conch, clams, mussels, yogurt, millet, barley, spinach, broccoli, celery, egg plant, kelp, alfalfa, cucumbers, pears, bananas, white radishes, watermelon

Tui-na Procedures:

The purpose of *Tui-na* therapy is to promote *Qi*/Blood circulation and nerve regeneration in the affected region. The descriptions and indications of each technique are outlined in more detail in Chapter 1 Table 8.[20]

- Avoid manipulation of the neck and back
- *Nian-fa* holding and kneading each of the digits and distal extremities for 12 times
- *Ba-shen-fa* stretching the front and rear limbs for 12 times
- *Dou-fa* shaking each limb for 12 times

- *Yi-zhi-chan* and *Rou-fa* single thumb and rotary kneading at ST-40 or BL-40, KID-1 and LIV-3 for 12 times each
- *An-fa* pressing of SI-3, LI-4, TH-5 and LU-7 for 5-10 seconds per acupoint

Daily Life Style Recommendation for Owner Follow-up:
- *Nian-fa* holding and kneading each of the digits and distal extremities repeat 12 times twice daily
- Feed nutritious easily digestible food
- Keep in a low stress environment
- Take for short walks daily
- If Grades 3-5 paresis or paralysis, turn (if in lateral recumbency) or move every 4-6 hours to prevent lung atelectasis and decubitus ulcers
- Keep on padding to avoid decubitus ulcers on shoulders, hips or tuber ischii
- Keep dry and clean of feces and urine
- Assist to walk with a sling if needed
- Swim with support and supervision, if not painful

Comments:
The overall prognosis for most vertebral and spinal tumors is poor, but TCVM can be very useful to balance the immune system, support the constitution, relieve pain and generally improve the quality of the life of the animal.[19,35,39] More experience is needed using TCVM to treat spinal tumors, before an accurate prognosis can be provided.

2. Blood Stagnation of the Vertebra and/or Spinal Cord with Kidney *Qi* Deficiency

Clinical Signs:
- Usually middle age to geriatric animals
- Neck or back pain (Grade 1 neurological deficits)
- Quadriparesis, quadriplegia, paraparesis or paraplegia (Grades 2-5 neurological deficits)
- Tongue- purple
- Pulses- wiry

TCVM Diagnosis:
The diagnosis of Blood Stagnation of the vertebrae or spinal cord is supported by knowledge that the tumor is of bone or blood origin. The paresis or paralysis is due to Kidney *Qi* Deficiency. The purple tongue and wiry pulses reflect the Blood Stagnation.

Treatment Principles:
- Resolve Blood Stagnation to shrink the mass and control the pain
- Support *Wei Qi* and balance the immune system to reduce further mutation and tumor growth
- Tonify Kidney *Qi* to nourish the spinal cord and strengthen the limbs

Acupuncture treatment:

EA is more effective than DN to resolve *Qi*/Blood Stagnation and promote nerve regeneration. For EA use 20 Hz (cycles/sec) for 10-15 minutes then 80-120 Hz alternating frequencies for 10-15 minutes. Do not perform EA across the tumor or select Governing Vessel, Back *Shu* Association points or *Hua-tuo-jia-ji* or *Jing-jia-ji* acupoints in the area of the tumor. EA is combined with DN and Aqua-AP. For Aqua-AP inject 0.25-0.5 ml vitamin B12 into the acupoint after *Tui-na*. Do not treat local acupoints in the area of the tumor, but instead select distant acupoints on the Governing Vessel and other Channels near the tumor. Acupoints that help control pain, balance the immune system and tonify *Qi* are also recommended. Treat every 1-2 weeks as needed to control pain and strengthen limbs. Combine acupuncture with conventional medication to control pain and secondary spinal cord edema if necessary.

Acupoints recommended
- EA: In non-ambulatory paresis or paralysis (Grades 3-5), treat bilateral limb points connecting left and right acupoints like ST-36/ST-36, LI-10/LI-10, PC-8/PC-8, KID-1/KID-1 (No EA across or near the tumor)
- DN cervical tumors: GV-20, GV-1, TH-5, LI-4, LI-11, ST-36, LI-10, LIV-3, LU-7, BL-23, KID-3, BL-17, SP-10
- DN thoracic and lumbar tumors: GV-20, GV-1, TH-5, LI-4, LI-11, LIV-3, ST-36, LI-10, BL-40, KID-3, SP-10

Pertinent acupoint actions
- GV-20 and GV-1 are useful to calm the animal but are also distant points on the Governing Vessel that courses over the tumor region
- TH-5, LI-4, LI-11 and ST-36 are useful to balance the immune system for *Wei Qi* Deficiency
- LI-4 and LIV-3 are useful to control pain if present
- LI-4 and LU-7 are Master points for the neck and useful for cervical tumors
- ST-36 and LI-10 are *Qi* tonic acupoints useful for Kidney *Qi* Deficiency
- BL-23 is the Back *Shu* Association Kidney and useful to nourish the Kidney and strengthen the limbs (select only in cervical tumors)
- KID-3 is the *Yuan* Source point for the Kidney and useful to nourish the Kidney and strengthen the limbs
- BL-40 is the Master point for the pelvic limbs, useful for thoracolumbar tumors
- BL-17 is the Influential point for Blood, useful to move Blood and break-up Blood Stasis to shrink the mass (select for cervical tumors only)
- SP-10 is the "Sea of Blood", useful to move Blood and break-up Blood Stasis to shrink the mass

Herbal Medicine:
- Stasis Breaker (JT)[a] 0.5 gm/10-20# twice daily orally to remove Blood Stasis, soften hardness and clear masses
- Combine with *Wei Qi* Booster (JT)[a] 0.5 gm/10-20# twice daily orally to tonify *Qi*, boost *Wei Qi* and inhibit mutation

- Administer both formulas for up to 6 months, then as needed for maintenance
- A description of all the ingredients of the Chinese herbal medicine listed is beyond the scope of this text, but can be found elsewhere.[7,8]

Food Therapy:

The purpose of the Food therapy is to further promote *Qi*/Blood circulation and tonify *Qi* to support nerve regeneration in the affected region. Foods that are Cold or Hot are avoided.[28]

- Foods to supplement to promote *Qi* and Blood circulation include: chicken egg, crab, sweet rice, peaches, carrots, coriander, squash, turnips
- Foods to tonify *Qi*: Beef, chicken, sardines, egg, potato, yam, sweet potato, rice, oats, millet, lentils, carrots, squash, microalgae, dates, figs, molasses, royal jelly
- Cold foods to avoid: Turkey, duck, duck eggs, conch, clams, mussels, yogurt, millet, barley, spinach, broccoli, celery, egg plant, kelp, alfalfa, cucumbers, pears, bananas, white radishes, watermelon
- Hot foods to avoid: Lamb, shrimp, corn-fed beef, chicken, trout, squash, turnips, sweet rice, basal, caraway, cherries, chilies, cinnamon, ginger, rosemary, sage

Tui-na Procedures:

The purpose of *Tui-na* therapy is to promote *Qi*/Blood circulation and nerve regeneration in the affected region. The descriptions and indications of each technique are outlined in more detail in Chapter 1 Table 8.[20]

- Avoid manipulation of the neck and back
- *Nian-fa* holding and kneading each of the digits and distal extremities for 12 times
- *Ba-shen-fa* stretching the front and rear limbs for 12 times
- *Dou-fa* shaking each limb for 12 times
- *Yi-zhi-chan* and *Rou-fa* single thumb and rotary kneading at SP-10, BL-40, KID-1 and LIV-3 for 12 times each
- *An-fa* pressing of SI-3, LI-4, TH-5 and LU-7 for 5-10 seconds per acupoint

Daily Life Style Recommendation for Owner Follow-up:

- *Nian-fa* holding and kneading each of the digits and distal extremities repeat 12 times twice daily
- Feed nutritious easily digestible food
- Keep in a low stress environment
- Take for short walks daily
- If Grades 3-5 paresis or paralysis, turn (if in lateral recumbency) or move every 4-6 hours to prevent lung atelectasis and decubitus ulcers
- Keep on padding to avoid decubitus ulcers on shoulders, hips or tuber ischii
- Keep dry and clean of feces and urine
- Assist to walk with a sling if needed
- Swim with support and supervision, if not painful

Comments:

The overall prognosis for most vertebral and spinal tumors is poor, but TCVM can be very useful to balance the immune system, support the constitution, relieve pain and generally improve the quality of the life of the animal.[19,35,39] More experience is needed using TCVM to treat spinal tumors, before an accurate prognosis can be provided.

Footnotes:

[a] (JT) = *Jing Tang* Herbal www.tcvmherbal.com; Reddick, FL
[b] (P) =Patented formula available through *Jing Tang* Herbal www.tcvmherbal.com; Reddick, FL

References:

1. De Lahunta A, Glass E. Veterinary Neuroanatomy and Clinical Neurology 3nd Ed. Philadelphia, PA:WB Saunders 2008:95-113,14.
2. Chrisman C, Mariani C, Platt S, Clemmons R. Neurology for the Small Animal Practitioner. Jackson Wy: Teton NewMedia 2003:125-167.
3. Platt S, Olby N (ed). BSAVA Manual of Canine and Feline Neurology 5th Ed. Gloucester, UK:BSAVA Publications 2012:1-500.
4. Kline KL, Caplan ER, Joseph RJ. Acupuncture for neurological disorders. In Schoen AM (ed) Veterinary Acupuncture 2nd Ed. St Louis, Mo: Mosby Publishing 2001:179-192.
5. Xie H, Priest V. Xie's Veterinary Acupuncture. Ames, Iowa:Blackwell Publishing 2007:585.
6. Xie H. Personal communications
7. Xie H, Preast V. Xie's Chinese Veterinary Herbology. Ames. IA:Wiley-Blackwell 2010:305-347, 486-510, 387,449-460.
8. Xie H, Preast V. Chinese Veterinary Herbal Handbook 2nd Ed. Reddick, FL: Chi Institute of Chinese Medicine 2008:305-585.
9. Janssens LA. Acupuncture for thoracolumbar and cervical disk disease. Veterinary Acupuncture 2nd Ed. Schoen A (ed). St Louis, Mo:Mosby Publishing 2001:193-198.
10. Tangjitjaroen W. Acupuncture for the treatment of spinal cord injuries. American Journal of Traditional Chinese Veterinary Medicine 2011; 6(2)37-43.
11. Choi DC, Lee JY, Moon YJ et al. Acupuncture-mediated inhibition of inflammation facilitates significant functional recovery after spinal cord injury. Neurobiology of Disease 2010; 39(3):272-82.
12. Yang JW, Jeong SM, Seo KM et al. Effects of corticosteroid and electroacupuncture on experimental spinal cord injury in dogs. Journal of Veterinary Science 2003; 4(1):97-101.
13. Hayashi AM and Matera JM. Evaluation of electroacupuncture treatment for thoracolumbar intervertebral disk disease in dogs. Journal of the American Veterinary Medical Association 2007; 231(6):913-918.
14. Joaquim JG, Luna SP, Brondani JT et al. Comparison of decompressive surgery, electroacupuncture, and decompressive surgery followed by electroacupuncture for the treatment of dogs with intervertebral disk disease with long-standing severe neurologic deficits. Journal of the American Veterinary Medical Association 2010; 36(11):1225-9.
15. Han HJ, Yoon HY, Kim JY et al. Clinical effect of additional electroacupuncture on thoracolumbar intervertebral disc herniation in 80 paraplegic dogs. American Journal of Chinese Medicine 2010; 38(6):1015-25.
16. Li WJ, Pan SQ, Zeng YS et al. Identification of acupuncture-specific proteins in the process of electro-acupuncture after spinal cord injury. Neurosci Res 2010; 67:307-316.
17. Xie H, Priest V. Traditional Chinese Veterinary Medicine. Reddick, FL: Jing Tang Publishing 2002:209-293,307-380,409-419.

18. Cassu RN, Luna SP, Clark RM, Kronka SN. Electroacupuncture analgesia in dogs: is there a difference between uni- and bi-lateral stimulation? Veterinary Anaesthesia and Analgesia 2008; 35(1):52-61.
19. Kenney JD. Acupuncture for the treatment of pain. American Journal of Traditional Chinese Veterinary Medicine 2010; 5(2):37-53.
20. Xie H, Ferguson B, Deng X. Application of *Tui-na* in Veterinary Medicine 2nd Ed. Reddick, FL:Chi Institute 2007:1-94,129-132.
21. Yu JN, Ma XJ, Liu ZS et al. Effect of electroacupuncture at "Ciliao"(BL 32) on c-fos expression in the sacral segment of spinal cord in rats with detrusor hyperreflexia. Zhen Ci Yan Jiu 2010; 35(3):204-7. (in Chinese)
22. Shin BC, Lee MS, Kong JC et al. Acupuncture for spinal cord injury survivors in the Chinese literature: a systematic review. Complementary Therapies in Medicine 2009; 17(5-6):316-327.
23. Scaglia M, Delaini G, Destefano I et al. Fecal incontinence treated with acupuncture- a pilot study. Autonomic Neuroscience 2009; 145(1-2):89-92.
24. Chen A, Wang H, Zhang J et al. BYHWD rescues axotomized neurons and promotes functional recovery after spinal cord injury in rats. Journal of Ethnopharmacolology 2008; 117(3):451-6.
25. Wang L and Jiang DM. Neuroprotective effect of *Buyang Huanwu* decoction on spinal ischemia/reperfusion injury in rats. Journal of Ethnopharmacology 2009; 124(2), 219-23
26. Seo TB, Baek K, Kwon KB. *Shengmai-san*-mediated enhancement of regenerative responses of spinal cord axons after injury in rats. Journal of Pharmacological Science 2009; 110(4):483-92.
27. Huang YM, Zhao YQ and Tian W. Experimental study on the effect of *Suifukang* in promoting repair and regeneration of nerve fibers in spinal cord. Chinese Journal of Integrated Traditional and Western Medicine 2007; 27(8):724-7.
28. Leggett D. Helping Ourselves: A Guide to Traditional Chinese Food Energetics. Totnes, England: Meridian Press 2005:21-36.
29. Xie H. How to use TCVM for the treatment of thoracolumbar intervertebral disk disease. Traditional Chinese Veterinary Medicine, Empirical Techniques to Scientific Validation. Reddick, FL:Jing Tang Publishing 2010:189-192.
30. Sun Z, Li X, Su Z et al. Electroacupuncture-enhanced differentiation of bone marrow stromal cells into neuronal cells. Journal of Sports Rehabilitation 2009; 18(3):398-406.
31. Yan Q, Ruan JW, Ding Y et al. Electro-acupuncture promotes differentiation of mesenchymal stem cells, regeneration of nerve fibers and partial functional recovery after spinal cord injury. Experimental Toxicology and Pathology 2011; 63(1-2):151-6.
32. Sumano H, Bermudez E, Obregon K. Treatment of wobbler syndrome in dogs with electroacupuncture. Deutsche Tierarztliche Wochenschrift 2000; 107(6):231-5.
33. Xie H, Rimar T. Effect of a combination of acupuncture and herbal medicine on wobbler syndrome in dogs and horses. Traditional Chinese Veterinary Medicine- Empirical Techniques to Scientific Validation. Reddick, FL:Jing Tang Publishing 2010:103-114.
34. Medina C. An integrative approach for the treatment of suspected fibrocartilaginous embolism of the spinal cord in a dog. American Journal of Traditional Chinese Veterinary Medicine 2010; 5(2):55-60.
35. Feng BB, Zhang JH, Chen H. Mechanisms of actions of Chinese herbal medicine in the prevention and treatment of cancer. American Journal of Traditional Chinese Veterinary

Medicine 2010; 5(1):37-47.
36. Sánchez-Araujo M, Puchi A. Acupuncture enhances the efficacy of antibiotics treatment for canine otitis crises. Acupunct Electrother Res 1997; 22(3-4):191-206.
37. Sánchez-Araujo M, Puchi A. Acupuncture prevents relapses of recurrent otitis in dogs: a 1-year follow-up of a randomised controlled trial. Acupunct Med 2011; 29(1):21-26.
38. Xie H. How to treat degenerative myelopathy (DM)? Traditional Chinese Veterinary Medicine- Empirical Techniques to Scientific Validation. Reddick, FL:Jing Tang Publishing 2010:197-202.
39. Lu W, Dean-Clower E, Doherty-Gilman A, Rosenthal DS. The value of acupuncture in cancer care. Hematol Oncol Clin North Am 2008; 22(4):631-48.

Acupuncture Helps Dog With Vertebral Fracture Return to Near Normal Function

Elisa Katz, DVM, CVA

Abstract

A 7 month old male Bergamasco Sheepdog was referred for acupuncture treatment to help with spinal cord compression and nerve damage due to an L6 vertebral fracture sustained in an automobile accident. The spinal cord compression and inflammation resulting from the fracture led to pain, stasis of blood, and interfered with nerve function. A combination of acupuncture, Class IV laser therapy[a], NSAIDS, and restricted activity over the next several weeks helped him return to near normal function.

History

Two weeks prior to presentation, the dog had been riding in an automobile when it swerved and overturned. He had been thrown from the vehicle, lost in the woods for a week, and then finally reunited with his family. When he was found, he had wire entwined around his hind legs. Since being home, he was noted to have a non-weight-bearing paresis of the right hind limb. There was no history of prior health issues.

Clinical Signs and Diagnosis Conventional (Western)

Examination findings by the referring veterinarian were non-weight-bearing paresis and muscle atrophy of the right hind limb. The dog was prescribed Rimadyl (carprofen) 75 mg ½ tablet twice daily for 4 days, then ½ tablet once daily thereafter (body weight was 40 lbs). Radiographs of the right hind limb were unremarkable. However, radiographs of the lumbar spine showed an overriding, comminuted (3 pieces), and displaced compression fracture of the L6 vertebral body (see initial radiographs). The radiologist's report also noted, "significant foreshortening of the vertebral body and dorsal and cranial displacement of the caudal segment" and, "there appears to be significant compromise to the spinal canal". See radiographs figures 1 and 2. Magnetic resonance imaging was recommended but the owners elected not to pursue further diagnostics. Surgery was not considered though it was suggested.

On initial physical examination, both the patella reflex and cranial tibial reflexes appeared to be decreased. The dog had positive withdrawl reflex and good anal tone with no problems defecating or continence issues. These findings were consistent with an injury involving the femoral nerve (L4-L6) and possibly the obturator nerve (L4-L6) and peroneal (L6-S2) portion of the sciatic nerve.[1]

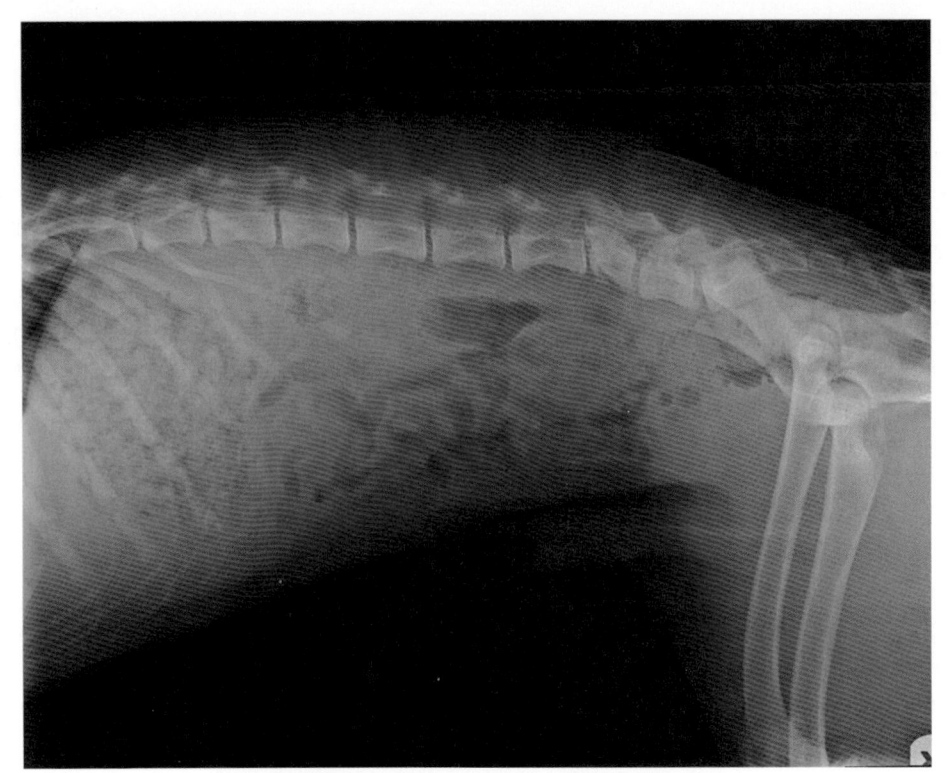

Figure 1: Initial lateral radiograph

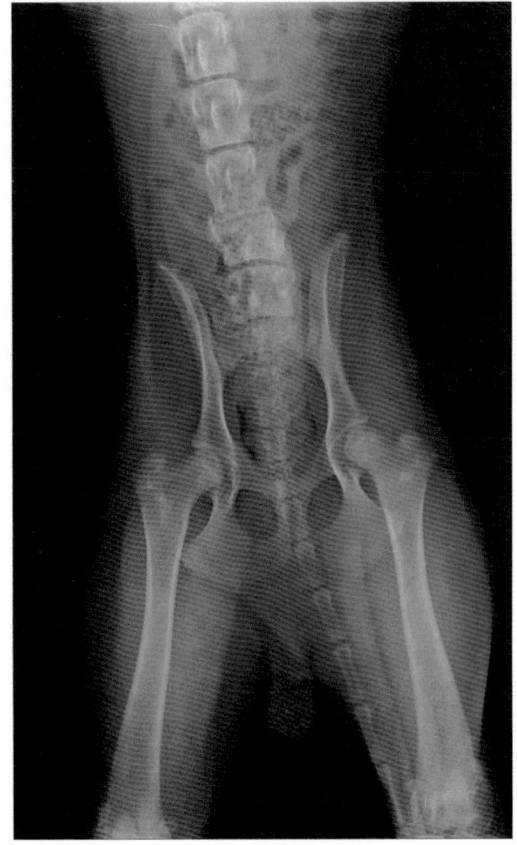

Figure 2: Initial V-D radiograph

Clinical Signs and Diagnosis – TCVM/Eastern

On initial evaluation, the dog would not bear weight on his right hind leg. He was painful on palpation of L6-L7 and had mild warmth palpable in the area of BL 26-27. His tongue color was a slightly dark red with a moist coating. His pulses were superficial and slightly bounding with a normal rate of 120 pulse beats per minute. The dog had a very friendly and relaxed temperament and was considered to be an earth constitution. These findings led to a TCVM diagnosis of Blood Stasis of the Bladder channel as a result of trauma and heat (inflammation) with potential for Dampness and Phlegm (in the form of arthritis) at the site of the injury.

Western/Conventional Treatment: The only Western treatment used was Rimadyl (Carprofen) 75 mg, ½ tablet given every 12 hours for 4 days, then ½ tablet every 24 hours for approximately 2 weeks.

Eastern/TCVM Treatment

Treatment goals were to move *Qi* and Blood in the Bladder (*Tai Yang*) channel in order to relieve pain and to strengthen kidney and bone in order to help speed healing. A longer term goal was to help the patient regain as much nerve function as possible. The owner's hope was to enable him to show as he had been bred from champion blood lines. Class IV laser[a] therapy was used as an adjunct to help with pain and inflammation and assist with healing.

Acupuncture was performed twice weekly for the first 1 ½ weeks. Then, due to owner's schedule 2 weeks were skipped, then weekly treatments were performed for a total of 9 treatments.

At each session Carbo needles were used of the size 0.25 x 25 mm for most points and 0.22 x 13 mm for points with shallow connective tissue or in sensitive areas such as KI1 and ST36. Needles were placed just about to the handle (13 mm to 25 mm) and inserted with a clockwise twist. See chart for all points used and locations. Electro-stimulation (ES) was applied at each session with a little variation in the points stimulated. ES was applied to one or more of the following combinations of points: BL 23 – Lumbar *Bai-hui*, BL-54 (R) – ST-36 (R), BL-54 (R) – BL-40 (R), BL-26 – BL-35, Lumbar *Bai-hui* – BL-40, BL-26 – BL-27. The duration of ES was 4 minutes for the first 3 sessions, 5 minutes for session 4, then increased to 6 minutes duration for subsequent sessions. A Pantheon® 6c Pro electrostimulator[b] was used on the mixed frequency setting with alternation between 1 Hz and 5 Hz. The power level used ranged from 1.5 to 2.5 volts. A class IV therapy laser treatment was administered to the area of injury at lumbar vertebrae 5-7 after the first 4 treatments and after the 7th and 9th treatments. The setting was 6 watts and a protocol for acute trauma was used with a total energy delivery of 1.077 joules at each treatment.

After the first treatment, the owners noted some mild improvement stating that the patient appeared to be using the right hind limb a little more and not fatiguing as easily. By the 5th treatment, the owners stated that the patient had significantly improved and was almost 100% sound on the right hind. According to a recheck radiograph at the referring veterinarian the fracture was healing though it appeared that there would be a permanent shortening of the L6 vertebral body (see radiographs figures 3 and 4). As of the last treatment, the patient was ambulating very well and able to run. It was discernable at a walk that he had a barely noticeable altered gait in the right hind limb.

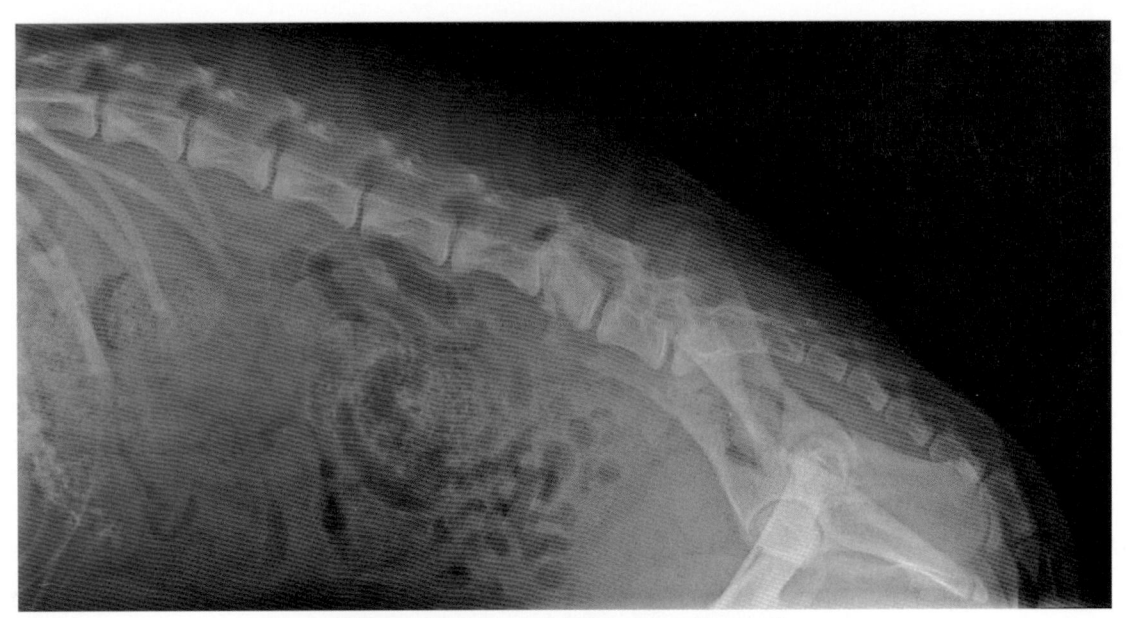

Figure 3: One month lateral radiograph

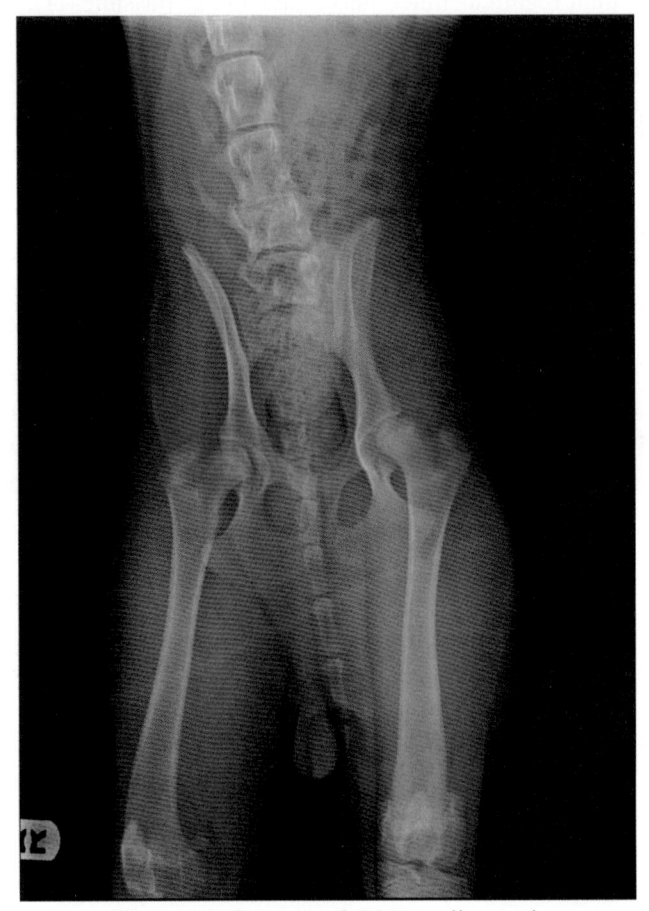

Figure 4: One month V-D radiograph

Table 1: Name, location and indications of points used[3]

IVAS Name/Chinese Name	Anatomical Location	Indication
GV-20/*Bai-hui*	Dorsal midline of skull, in the notch between the sagittal and frontal crest	Calming point, benefits *Yang* meridians
BL-11/*Da-zhu*	1.5 cun lateral to the caudal border of the spinous process of the 1st thoracic vertebra, midway from the spinous process to the medial border of the scapula	Influential point for bone, nourish Blood and ease pain, helpful for any disorder of bone
BL-23/*Shen-shu*	1.5 cun lateral to the caudal border of the spinous process of the 2nd lumbar vertebra	Kidney *Shu* point, strengthens bone, bone marrow, and caudal back
BL 26/*Guan-chang-shu*	1.5 cun lateral to the caudal border of the spinous process of L6 vertebra	Used as a local point
BL-27/*Xiao-chang-shu*	1.5 cun lateral to the caudal border of the spinous process of L7 vertebra	Used as a local point
BL-35/*Hui-yang*	In the crease on either side of the tail head	Paresis of hind limbs
BL-40/*Wei-zhong*	Knee – in the center of the popliteal crease	BL lower *He*-sea point, helps with hind limb paralysis
BL-54/*Zhi-bian*	Dorsal to the greater trochanter of the femur	Hind limb paresis
BL 60/*Kun-lun*	In the depression between the lateral malleolus and the common calcanean tendon level with the tip of the malleolus, opposite and slightly dorsal to KI 3	Remove obstructions from the Bladder channel, helps with weakness/paralysis of hind limbs
KID-1/*Yang quan*	On the plantar surface of the hind paw between MT 2 and 3 proximal to the MTP joint under the pad	Paralysis/paresis of hind limbs
KID-3/*Tai xi*	In the depression between the medial malleolus and the common calcanean tendon, level with the tip of the malleolus, opposite and slightly ventral to BL 60	Tonifies the Kidney and helps with pelvic limb paralysis
Bai-hui (lumbar)	On the dorsal midline between L7 and S1 vertebrae	Helpful for pelvic limb paralysis
ST-36/*Hou-san-li*	3 cun distal to ST 35, distal to tibial tuberosity and lateral to cranial border of tibia in depression approximately in the middle of the cranial tibial muscle	Pelvic limb paralysis, especially that involving tibial and fibular nerves
SP-6/*San-yin-jiao*	3 cun directly above the tip of the medial malleolus on the caudal border of the tibia on line drawn from medial malleolus to SP 9	General tonification point

Discussion

At presentation, the patient was noted to have had a significant gait abnormality of the right hind limb so much that he was unable to bear weight on it. The patient also had pain upon palpation of the caudal lumbar area. After several acupuncture treatments this gait abnormality was significantly reduced and the patient's pain had resolved.

This dog's signs were caused by an acute injury. Acute injury causes can lead to *Qi* and Blood stasis.[4] This is manifested as pain, swelling, and bruising. Stasis results in the generation of Heat in the form of inflammation at the site of the injury. In this case, these factors as well as the dorsal and cranial displacement of the vertebral body all appeared to play a role in the patient's nerve damage, pain, and gait abnormality.

Acupuncture points were selected to elicit both a local and generalized effect. The desired local effects being to expedite healing, regain nerve function, and control pain and the desired generalized effects being to support the processes and organs necessary to help heal bone and tonify the patient. BL-11 and BL-23 were both selected to help strengthen and heal the bones. BL-26, BL-27, BL 35, and BL-54 were all chosen as local points. BL-40, BL-60, KID-1, KID-3, lumbar *Bai-hui*, and ST-36 were all used because they can help with pelvic limb paresis and weakness. SP 6 was used as a general tonification point as well as a local point. GV-20 was used to help relax the patient. Electro-acupuncture was performed locally to assist with bone healing and to decrease pain.[5] Points for electro-stimulation varied a little but included BL-26 – BL-35, BL-26 – BL-27, BL-54 – BL-40, BL-54 – ST-36. A mixed frequency setting that alternated between 1 and 5 Hz was used. Because the primary goal was to regain as much function in the right hind limb as possible and speed healing, the lower frequencies were chosen as they are determined to be better for tonification.[6]

Electro-acupuncture has been demonstrated to be especially useful in cases of spinal nerve injury.[7] Though most of the research that has been done involves intervertebral disc disease, in this case it was never proven whether or not intervertebral discs were involved in the injury because an MRI was not pursued. Protrusion of any material that may impinge on the spinal cord, be it disc material or a displaced piece of vertebra can be expected to result in similar signs and therefore respond to a similar treatment (with the exception being tumor).

Despite the vertebral fracture healing with a slight displacement, after being treated with acupuncture and laser, the patient seems to have done quite well.

Footnotes:

[a.] 6 Watt Companion Class IV Therapeutic Laser® by Litecure, 250 Corporate Boulevard, Suite B, Newark, DE 19702. Companiontherapylaser.com

[b.] Pantheon 6c. Pro Electro-Acupuncture Stimulator. Pantheon Research 626-A Venice Boulevard, Venice, CA 90291. PantheonResearch.com

References:

1. Oliver, John E. Jr., and Lorenz, Michael D. Handbook of Veterinary Neurology, Second Edition. Philadelphia, PA: W. B. Saunders Co.1993: 116-119
2. Dyce, K. M., Sack, W. O., and Wensing, C. J. G. Textbook of Veterinary Anatomy, Second Edition. Philadelphia, PA: W. B. Saunders Co. 1996: 317
3. Course Notes: IVAS Basic Course on Veterinary Acupuncture, 2007-2008
4. Xie, Huisheng and Preast, Vanessa Traditional Chinese Veterinary Medicine Volume 1: Fundamental Principles. Beijing, China: Jing Tang 2005: 226-227

5. Schoen, Allen M. Veterinary Acupuncture: Ancient Art to Modern Medicine, Second Edition. St. Louis, MO: Mosby, Inc. 2001: 102
6. Schoen, Allen M. Veterinary Acupuncture: Ancient Art to Modern Medicine, Second Edition. St. Louis, MO: Mosby, Inc. 2001: 104-105
7. Hayashi, A.M. and Mater, J.M. Evaluation of electroacupuncture treatment for thoracolumbar intervertebral disc disease in dogs. Journal of the American Veterinary Medical Association 2007; 231: 913-918

Canine Intervertebral Disk Disease Treated with Aquapuncture and Chinese Herbal and Western Medicine

Chi Hsien Chien, DVM, PhD

The prevalence of canine thoracolumbar intervertebral disk disease (IVDD) is increasing recently in small animal practice. The causes of the IVDD are calcification and/or protrusion of the cartilaginous intervertebral disk and vertebral spondylosis in multifocal vertebral segment mostly. The diagnosis is basically on plan radiographically and advanced with computerized tomography.

Chief complain of IVDD are walk slowly, reluctant to jump or climbing, back pain, hindlimbs paresis or ataxia and weakness or loss of proprioception. The severity is grade I and II according to Janssens (2001). These disorders are known as "Bi syndrome" in traditional Chinese veterinary medicine. (Xie 2007)

About 50 cases of canine IVDD were present in our clinic from 2008 to 2010. The treatment is an integrated aquapuncture with vitamin B1, herbal and western medicine. Acupoints selected are local bladder meridian according to the lesion sites, Bai Hui (GV 20), and *Hou-san-li* (ST 36). Herbal medicine prescribed are *Xue Fu Zhu Yu Tang, Tao Hong Si Wu Tang, Bu Yang Huan Wu Tang, Liu Wei Di Huang Wan and Huang Qi Tang* (Astragalus decoction), alternatively. Western medicines used are NSAID analgesics, muscle relaxant, and occasionally a long tern effect of steroid injection at the first visit.

Significant improvement in mobility, proprioception, and spinal posture were noticed within the first two weeks of treatment. About 80% of patients were able to rise, walk and recovered to the normal activity four weeks after the sudden onset of the IVDD. The results suggested that the integrated treatment is an acceptable, and satisfied medical maneuver prior to surgical intervention.

References:
1. Luc A.A. Janssens Acupuncture for thoracolumbar and cervical disk disease 2001 in Veterinary Acupuncture p.193-198
2. Choi K.H. and S.A.Hill. Case repont acupuncture treatment for feline multifocal intervertebral disc disease 2009. Journal of Feline Medicine and Surgery. 11: 706-710.
3. Wynn S.G. and S. Marsden Intervertebral disk disease 2003 in Therapies for neurologic disorders. p.466-469
4. Xie H and V Preast Acupuncture for treatment of musculoskeletal and neurological disorder 2007 in Xie's Veterinary Acupuncture p.247-265
5. Xie H, M.S. Kim and C Chrisman Herbs to tonify deficiency 2010 in Xie's Chinese veterinary Herbology

An Effective and Simple Protocol to Treat Intervertebral Disk Disease Associated with a *Qi*-Deficient/Stagnation Pattern

Bruce Ferguson, DVM, MS, CVA, CVCH, CVTP, CVFT

Overview

Intervertebral Disk Disease (IVDD) TCVM Patterns will be reviewed (see Table 1). Then this paper will focus on Clinical Signs of *Qi* Deficiency with Stagnation Pattern. Following that, we will Review the role of the Governing Vessel (see Table 2). Next we will briefly review the use and functions of moxibustion. Lastly this paper will introduce a simple protocol for *Qi* Deficiency pattern of IVDD.

IVDD TCVM Patterns

Table 1: Patterns and Primary Clinical Signs of TCVM IVDD

TCVM Pattern	Clinical Signs
Wind-Cold-Damp	Very painful on palpation Acute onset without traumatic injury
Blood Stagnation	Very sensitive on palpation Acute onset May be caused by traumatic injury
Cervical IVDD	Paresis or paralysis Wobbler's syndrome
Thoracic or Lumbar Area	Very sensitive on palpation Radiographic evidence
Heat Toxin	Discospondylitis Red tongue, rapid pulse
Qi/Yang Deficiency	Lethargy or depression Heat-seeking Pale moist tongue Deep weak pulse
Yin Deficiency	Panting, restless, cool-seeking Red dry tongue Thin rapid pulse

Introduction

Qi-deficient type intervertebral disk disease (IVDD) with local stagnation is the most common Pattern of IVDD seen in my practice in Western Australia. A strategy to tonify and invigorate the patient and resolve local stagnation which leads to consistently good outcomes will be described using moxibustion, acupuncture and the TCM herbal formula *Bu Yang Huan Wu Tang*. Moreover, a novel acupuncture point combination to regulate the Governing Vessel unique to quadrupeds will be introduced. Lastly, the role of multiple Governing Vessel points in IVDD and other spinal cord diseases will be emphasized.

Qi Deficiency with Stagnation Pattern: Multiple Thoracolumbar IVDD patients have come to me in Western Australia with the same clinical signs. They tend to have a pale, usually moist tongue with occasional lavender hue; they have a deep weak pulse which is always weaker on the right; the patients always present with right hind-end weaker than left. Further they have a cool nose and ears, cool feet, cool lumbus and ventral abdomen, +/- pain on IVDD area upon palpation.

Governing Vessel

Increase Your Use of Governing Vessel! Why choose the Governing Vessel? The *Huang Di Nei Jing* states "Treat wilting solely by choosing the *Yang Ming*". (Su Wen: Wei Lun). Presumably this is because the *Yang Ming* channels are abundant in *Qi* and Blood. Thus one might select such points as LI-4, 10, 11, 15, ST-41, 36.

Wang Le-Ting used the *Yang Ming* for hundreds of clinical cases and had poor results. After experimentation and then clinical application, Dr. Wang began to say "First select the governing vessel"[1]. The *Du Mai* governs all "stirring" in the body and *Yang Qi*. *Yang Qi* empowers movement; movement is lost with IVDD. According to Dr. Wang, clinical applications of the GV include all of the following: Paralysis and wilting, Traumatic spinal cord injury, Wei syndrome, Hemiplegia, Central and peripheral infarcts, and Wind-Cold-Damp *Bi*, especially chronic issues with underlying deficiency.

Table 2: Functions of Select GV Points according to Dr. Wang Le-ting[1]

Point Name	Point Location	Point Function(s)
Bai-hui, GV-20	On the dorsal midline of the skull at the level of the center of the ears	Supplement the true *Yang*
Feng-fu, GV-16	Immediately caudal to occipital protuberance	Arouse the brain and open the portals
Da-zhui, GV-14	Cranial to T1	Functions to diffuse and free the flow of all kinds of *Yang*
Tao-dao, GV-13	Caudal to T1	Supplements *Yang* and strengthens the spine
Shen-zhu, GV-12	Caudal to T3	Strengthens the lower back, relieves pain, quiets the *Shen*
Shen-dao, GV-11	Caudal to T5	Fortifies the brain and frees the flow of the vessels
Zhi-yang, GV-9	Caudal to T7	Frees the flow of *Qi* and promotes *Yang*
Jin Suo, GV-8	Caudal to T10	Strengthens the low back and softens the sinews
Ji-zhong, GV-6	Caudal to T12	Strengthens and fortifies the lumbar spine; calms the *Shen*
Xuan-shu, GV-5	Caudal to L1	Strengthens the lumbar spine and fortifies the SP and ST

Ming-men, GV-4	Caudal to T2	Supplements *Yang* and boosts the Kidneys
Yao-yang-guan, GV-3	Caudal to the largest depression of T4, T5, or T6	Benefits turning the low back, strengthens and fortifies the lumbar spine, supplements *Yang* and boosts the Kidneys
Hou-hai, GV-1	Dorsal to the external anal sphincter	Foundation and Root of the Governing Vessel

Moxibustion

Moxibustion is a method by which moxa punk or other herbs are burned on or above the skin near acupuncture points. The heat and herbal essence warms the *Qi* and Blood in the channels and collaterals and thus increases the flow during times of Stasis. Moxibustion also invigorates the *Yang Qi* and dispels internal Cold and Dampness as well as eliminates some forms of local Heat Toxin[2]. Moxibustion according to Wang Le-Ting: "Acupuncture and moxibustion each have their limits and abilities and therefore should mutually assist and mutually support each other". According to Dr. Wang, moxibustion has the following functions: Warming action and supports *Yang*, Course and free the flow of the channels and network vessels, Move the *Qi* and quicken the Blood, Dispel Dampness and expel Cold, Disperse swelling and scatter nodulation, and Secure *Yang* and stem counterflow[1].

Protocol for *Qi* Deficiency IVDD

The protocol is quite simple. First, combine SI-3 and BL-65 unilaterally to open and seal the Governing Vessel. Then add multiple GV points cranial to, at the lesion, and caudal to area of tissue trauma. Use Needle Moxibustion at area of tissue trauma. I prefer the stick-on "mini-moxa" cones with hollow center. Finally, use the herbal formula *Bu Yang Huan Wu Tang* to Tonify *Qi*, nourish Blood, invigorate Blood, and dredge the Stagnation (see Table 3).

Table 3: *Bu Yang Huan Wu Tang* Ingredients[3]

English Name	*Pin Yin* Name	Action
Astragalus	*Huang Qi*	Warm and tonify *Qi*
Angelica	*Dang Gui*	Nourish Blood
Paoenia	*Bai Shao*	Nourish Blood and *Yin*, soothe Liver *Yang*
Earthworm	*Di Long*	Break Blood stagnation
Ligusticum	*Chuan Xiong*	Activate Blood and relieve pain
Carthamus	*Hong Hua*	Break stasis and relieve pain
Persica	*Tao Ren*	Break stasis and relieve pain

References:
1. Yu Hui-chan and Han Fu-ru. Golden Needle Wang Le-Ting: A 20th Century Master's Approach to Acupuncture, Blue Poppy Press, 2001 Boulder, CO, USA.
2. Ferguson, B. Acupuncture and Moxibustion Techniques, in Traditional Chinese Veterinary Medicine, Volume 2, Elesevier, edited by Xie, Huisheng. 2007.
3. Xie, H.S. Chinese Veterinary Herbal Handbook. Chi Institute of Chinese Medicine, Reddick, FL. 2004.

Acupuncture for the Treatment of Spinal Cord Injuries

Weerapongse Tangjitjaroen DVM, PhD

Reprinted with permission from AJTCVM volume 6, number 2, August 2011

From: The Department of Companion Animals and Wildlife Clinic, Faculty of Veterinary Medicine, Chiang Mai University, Thailand

ABSTRACT

Spinal cord injuries with or without vertebral fractures cause neurological deficits associated with spinal cord concussion, compression, contusion, laceration or a combination of these. The diagnosis is based on the history, clinical signs and diagnostic imaging. The prognosis for spinal cord injuries varies with the type of injury and the severity of neurological deficits. If no radiographic evidence of vertebral fracture or luxation are present, the prognosis may be better, but the severity of the neurological deficits and improvement of these deficits over the following 1-2 months best determines the prognosis. From a tradtional Chinese Veterinary Medicine perspective, spinal cord injuries are due to *Qi* and Blood Stagnation with *Qi* Deficiency below the site of Stagnation. In experimental studies of spinal cord injury, electro-acupuncture has been shown to reduce cell death, promote neuronal plasticity and enhance cellular regeneration. Clinical research has shown that electro-acupuncture and dry needle acupuncture combined with conventional treatments is significantly more effective to treat spinal cord injury from intervertebral disk herniation, than conventional therapy alone. Current acupuncture treatment recommendations for animals with spinal cord injuries have been based on the clinical experiences of different individuals. Further studies are needed to determine the most effective acupoints, acupuncture techniques and duration and frequency of acupuncture treatments to develop the optimum standards of care for acupuncture treatment of spinal cord injuries in animals.

Key words: acupuncture, electro-acupuncture, spinal cord injury, veterinary, small animals

ABBREVIATIONS

TCVM	Traditional Chinese veterinary medicine
AP	Acupuncture
DN	Dry needle acupuncture
EA	Electro-acupuncture

The spinal cord is part of the central nervous system, located within a protective bony canal formed by the the vertebral column.[1] Acute spinal cord injury commonly occurs in dogs and cats when the vertebral column is injured from automobile accidents, falls, fights and gunshot wounds and or when intervertebral disks protrude or herniate into the spinal canal.[1,2] Chronic repeated spinal cord injury can occur from vertebral instabilty as in "Wobbler Syndrome" (cervical spondylomelopathy).[1] Spinal cord injury results in neurological deficits due to concussion, compression, contusion, laceration or a combination of these.[1,2]

Injury to the spinal cord results in mild to severe neurological deficits. Vertebral fractures and luxations and acute intervertebral disk herniation occur in the cervical, thoracic, lumbar regions and often result in an immediate onset of neurological deficits. Cervical injuries may cause neck pain, ataxia, quadriparesis or quadriplegia with paralysis of the respiratory muscles and death. Thoracolumbar spinal cord injuries often cause local pain, pelvic limb proprioceptive deficits, paraparesis, paraplegia, loss of voluntary control of urination and defecation and loss of deep pain sensation from the toes.[1] Lesions between T3-L3 commonly cause hyperactive pelvic limb spinal reflexes and lesions between L4-S2 cause depressed or absent pelvic limb spinal cord reflexes in dogs and cats.[2] Injury of the spinal cord at the thoracolumbar region in dogs and cats results in paraplegia and thoracic limb hyperextension (Schiff-Sherrington phenomenon). Although the Schiff-Sherrington phenomenon indicates acute severe injury, if deep pain is still present in the pelvic limb toes and remains present over the next few days, the prognosis may still be good for recovery.

Clinical signs associated with spinal cord injury generally occur immediately after the injury and are generally non-progressive even though progessive pathophysiological changes occur locally at the site of the lesion.[1] In some patients with spinal cord injury, an ascending and descending myelomalacia develops from the original site of injury within 2-4 days. When this occurs, paraplegic dogs with a T3-L3 injury and intact pelvic limb spinal cord reflexes will lose the spinal cord reflexes over the next few days, as the lesion progressively descends. As the lesion progressively ascends, the spinal cord segments and nerves to intercostal and diaphragm muscles become affected and respiration function is depressed. The prognosis for ascending and descending myelomalcia is grave.[1] Hemorrhage, edema, ischemia, laceration, degeneration, necrosis, demyelination and focal and ascending and descending malacia of the neuronal tissues can be seen on histological examination of spinal cord injury of patients at necropsy. When the injury involves a fracture of the vertebral column, sequestered bone fragments may be lodged in the vertebral canal and can cause compression, inflammation and degeneration further damaging the spinal cord.

The diagnosis of spinal cord injury is based on the history, clinical signs and diagnostic imaging. An obvious fracture or dislocation of the vertebral column may be seen on routine radiographs, but computerized axial tomography (CT) and magnetic resonance imaging (MRI) are needed to visualize spinal cord lesions.[1] A therapeutic plan should be implemented as soon as possible. Delay of the treatment can dramatically prolong the recovery period and may decrease the success of any treatment, affect the long-term survival and quality of life of the animal. In quadriplegic and paraplegic animals high dose methylprednisolone sodium succinate is recommended as soon as possible, but not after 8 hours.[1,2] Oral analgesic drugs are also administered and surgical decompression of the spinal cord is performed as soon as the patient is stable.[1,2] Although the prognosis is often considered poor in patients with no deep pain sensation, many animals if properly treated anyway, show a return of sensation and improvement of function in 4-6 weeks. Improvement may continue over the next 1-2 years.

Spinal Cord Injury from a TCVM Perspective

In traditional Chinese veterinary medicine (TCVM), spinal cord injuries are due to *Qi* and Blood Stagnation.[3] Paresis and paralysis are due to *Qi* Deficiency below the site of Stagnation. The *Qi* and Blood Stagnation may cause pain around the injury site. Deficiency and Stagnation of *Qi* depletes Blood and *Gu Qi* that nourish the neurons and other cells and degeneration and demyelination occurs.

Spondylosis, other forms of vertebral degeneration and intervertebral disk disease are classified as Bony *Bi* syndrome in TCVM.[3,4] If left untreated, animals suffering from Wind *Bi*, Cold *Bi*, Damp *Bi* and Heat *Bi* syndromes will progress to Bony *Bi* syndrome. Bony *Bi* is most commonly associated with Kidney *Yang* Deficiency, Kidney *Yin* Deficiency or Kidney *Yang* or *Yin* Deficiency plus Kidney *Qi* Deficiency. The treatment strategy for Bony *Bi* syndrome includes expelling or eliminating the pathogenic factors (Wind, Cold, Damp and/or Heat), eliminating the Stagnation of *Qi* and Blood (cause of painful sensations) and nourishing the Kidney.[3,4]

In TCVM, the brain and spinal cord are included in the Extraordinary *Fu* organs and are referred to as Brain and Marrow, respectively.[4] The Extraordinary *Fu* organs possess anatomical characteristics similar to those of the *Fu* organs (tubular in structure), but possess TCVM physiological functions similar to those of the *Zang* organs (store essential substances).[4] The Extraordinary *Fu* organs store Kidney *Jing*, Marrow, Blood or Bile. The functions of the Extraordinary *Fu* organs are directly or indirectly related to the Kidney.

The Brain is located in the highest point of the body and is referred to as the "Sea of the Marrow", "House of the Mind" and *Shen*.[4] Therefore, the Brain controls memory, consciousness, thought processes, the spirit of the animal and the all the activities of the body. Normal functions of the Brain require nourishment from Kidney *Jing* and Heart Blood. The Marrow is the substance that can be found within the brain, spinal cord and bone marrow. The Kidney is the origin of Essence that is essential for Marrow production. The major function of Marrow is to replenish, nourish and replenish the substances in the brain, spinal cord and bone marrow.[4]

Acupuncture (AP) treatment of spinal cord injury includes controlling pain (*Hua-tuo-jia-ji*, LI-4, LIV-3), alleviating incontinence (SP-6, BL-32, BL-39, BL-40, KID-1, CV-3, CV-4), facilitating repair of the neuronal tissues (*Bai-hui*, GV-14, GV-4, GV-1, *Wei-jian*), alleviating *Qi* and Blood Stagnation (LIV-3, BL-17, SP-10), nourishing Kidney (BL-23, KID-3, *Shen-shu, Shen-peng, Shen-jiao*) and improving the general *Qi* levels and immune function of the animal (ST-36, LI-10, LI-11). Acupoints BL-30, BL-36, BL-37, BL-40, BL-60, GB-21, and GB-34 can also be used along with others (Table 1).[3] Details of the anatomical locations and indications of the acupoints commonly used to treat spinal cord injuries are outlined in Table 1.

In spinal cord injuries with severe neurological deficits and spinal cord compression, surgical decompression and stabilization of the fractured vertebrae (when present) should be performed as soon as the patient is stable. After the surgery, a combination of electro-acupuncture (EA) and dry needle acupuncture (DN) should also be initiated as soon as possible. Acupoints on the incision site are not used. Electro-acupuncture of Governing Vessel, *Hua-tuo-jia-ji* or Bladder Channel acupoints above and below the lesion site is recommended and EA and DN of other acupoints may also be performed (Table 1). Local EA at 2-4 milliampere and 2-20 Hertz for 30 minutes is usually recommended.[3] Acupuncture may be administered two to three times per week for several weeks initially in patients with severe neurological deficits, but the treatment interval can be increased to once or twice a month for four to six months depending on the neurological status of the patient.

Table 1: The location, attributes, indications of actions of acupuncture points suggested to treat spinal cord injuries[3]

Acupoint	Anatomical location	Attributes, Indications, and Actions
Bai-hui	Dorsal midline between L7-S1	Pelvic limb paresis or paralysis, lumbosacral pain, intervertebral disk disease over lumbosacral region
Hua-tuo-jia-ji	On dorsolateral region of back, 0.5 *cun* lateral to dorsal spinous process of each vertebra from T1 to L7	Thoracic and lumbar pain, intervertebral disk disease
Wei-jian	At tip of tail	Paralysis of the tail, pelvic limb weakness
Shen-shu	On dorsolateral caudal lumbar region, 1.5 *cun* lateral to *Bai-hui*	Kidney *Yin/Qi* Deficiency, urinary incontinence, thoracolumbar pain
Shen-peng	On dorsolateral caudal lumbar region, 1.5 *cun* cranial to *Shen-shu*	Pelvic limb paresis or paralysis, lumbosacral pain, lumbosacral intervetebral disk disease
BL-17	On dorsolateral aspect of spine, 1.5 *cun* lateral to caudal border of dorsal spinous process of T7	Influential point for Blood
BL-23	On dorsolateral aspect of spine, 1.5 *cun* lateral to caudal border of dorsal spinous process of L2	Kidney *Yin* and *Qi* Deficiency, urinary incontinence, thoracolumbar intervertebral disk disease, pelvic limb weakness
BL-36	Ventral to lateral border of tuber ischii in groove between biceps femoris and semitendinosus muscles	Lumbosacral pain, pelvic limb paresis or paralysis
BL-39	On lateral end of popliteal crease, on medial border of biceps femoris muscle tendon	Urinary incontinence, thoracolumbar intervertebral disk disease
BL-40	In center of popliteal crease	Master point of the caudal back and coxofemoral joint, urinary incontinence, and pelvic limb paresis or paralysis
CV-3	Ventral midline 4 *cun* caudal to umbilicus	Urinary incontinence
CV-4	Ventral midline 3 *cun* caudal to umbilicus	Urine retention, urinary incontinence, dysuria
GV-14	Dorsal midline in intervertebral space of C7-T1	*Yin* Deficiency, cervical pain, intervertebral disk disease
GV-4	Dorsal midline in intervertebral space of L2-L3	Thoracolumbar pain, intervertebral disk disease
LIV-3	Proximal to metatarsopharyngeal joint between second and third metatarsal bones	*Qi* Stagnation, pelvic limb paresis or paralysis

SP-10	When stifle is flexed, SP10 is located 2 *cun* proximal and medial to patella, in depression cranial to sartorius muscle	Blood Deficiency, pelvic limb paresis or paralysis
KID-1	On volar side of pelvic limb between third and fourth metatarsals underneath central pad	Dysuria and urinary incontinence
KID-3	On caudomedial aspect of pelvic limb in thin fleshy tissue between medial maleolus of tibia and calcaneus level with tip of medial maleolus	Thoracolumbar intervertebral disk disease
ST-36	On craniolateral aspect of pelvic limb 3 *cun* distal to ST35 and 0.5 *cun* lateral to cranial aspect of tibial crest, in cranial tibialis muscle	General *Qi* tonic, generalized weakness, hind limb weakness
LI-10	On craniolateral aspect of thoracic limb, 2 *cun* distal to LI11, in groove between extensor carpiradialis and common digital extensor muscles.	Generalized or hind limb weakness, lameness or paresis or paralysis of thoracic limb.
LI-11	On lateral side of thoracic limb at lateral end of cubital crease, halfway between lateral epicondyle of humerus and biceps tendon with elbow flexed	Paresis or paralysis of thoracic limb.
GB-34	On lateral side of pelvic limb at stifle, in small depression cranial and distal to head of fibula	Influential point for tendon and ligaments, weakness, paresis and paralysis

Acupuncture Mechanisms of Action for Spinal Cord Injuries

Acupuncture has been used extensively for pain management and a useful adjunct for pain associated with vertebral and spinal cord injuries.[4,5] Endogenous opioids such as endorphin have been shown to be involved in acupuncture analgesia at both peripheral and central nervous system levels.[5-7] Dynorphin, an important endogenous opioid, acts at the spinal cord level and is another important mechanism of acupuncture analgesia.[8] Acupuncture modulation of pain is complex and involves many ascending and descending spinal cord and brainstem pathways.[5]

The benefit of EA has been studied in rats after partial surgical removal of the dorsal root ganglia.[9] In this animal model, EA significantly promoted collateral sprouting of the spared nerve fibers and neuronal plasticity. It was shown using microarray analysis that EA modulated the expression of several genes. For example, the ciliary neurotrophic factor was upregulated at 1 day after injury, the fibroblast growth factor (FGF)-1, insulin-like growth factor (IGF) 1 receptor, neuropeptide Y and FGF-13 were upregulated at 7 days after injury and the calcitonin gene related peptide was upregulated at 14 days injury.[9]

In another experimental study of spinal cord injury in rats, five 30-minute DN sessions using acupoints GV-26 and GB-34 were performed beginning immediately after the injury and then once a day for 4 days. Rats were then euthanitized and tissues collected for analysis.[10] Acupuncture at the two acupoints significantly reduced spinal cord ventral motor neuron loss compared to the sham acupuncture control group. The combination of acupoints GV-26 and GB-34 resulted in less neuronal loss compared to rats receiving DN at only one of the acupoints. The group receiving the two point acupuncture had significantly reduced death of neurons and oligodendrocytes associated with reduced caspase-3 activation as compared to the sham acupuncture control group. Rats receiving acupuncture at GV-26 and GB-34 also significantly reduced expressions of the pro-inflammatory cytokines and inflammatory mediators tumor necrosis factor-α (TNF-α), interleukin-1β (IL-1β), interleukin-6 (IL-6), nitric oxide (NO) synthase, cyclooxygenase-2 (COX-2) and metric metalloproteases-9 (MMP9) levels compared to the control group.[10] Traumatic injury to the spinal cord causes not only the immediate mechanical damage but a cascade of secondary degenerative processes over the following days that greatly impact functional recovery.[1,10] In another group of rats, the extent of spinal cord tissue loss was compared 38 days after injury in rats receiving DN and those receiving sham acupuncture. The total lesion volume was significantly less in the DN treated group. Functional recovery of rats with and without AP following spinal cord injury was also compared in rats that were maintained for 35 days. Rats receiving AP had a significantly improved function on day 35 post-injury compared to and the sham AP control group.[10]

In another experiment of spinal cord injury in rats, neural specific proteins associated with EA treatment of acupoints on the Governing Vessel above and below the lesion were studied.[11] A pair of 0.35 mm diameter stainless steel acupuncture needles were inserted into acupoints GV-6 (midline between T11-12 in rats) and GV-9 (midline between T7-T8 in rats) and the spinal cord injury lesion was at T10. Connected together to a standard EA machine, a dense and disperse technique was used that provided ≤ 1 milliampere, 60 Hz alternating for 1.05 and 2.8 seconds for 20 minutes. Most groups of rats were treated with EA beginning on the 7th day after injury when they were stable and then were treated daily for 7 days. The neural specific proteins Annexin-A5 (ANXA5) and collapsing response mediator proteins-2 (CRMP2), known to be beneficial to neuronal survival and axonal regeneration, were increased in the group receiving EA at GV-6 and GV-9 compared to the control non-acupoint electrical stimulation group. Besides these proteins, other proteins in the spinal cord associated with inflammation, cell adhesion, cell migration, signal transduction and cell apoptosis were also altered significantly to favor neuroprotection and regeneneration in the group receiving EA at GV-6 and GV-9. In another group *Hua-tuo-jia-ji* acupoints lateral to GV-6 and GV-9 were stimulated with EA. The amount of ANXA5 and CRMP was higher in rats receiving EA at GV-6 and GV-9 than those receiving EA at *Hua-tuo-jia-ji*, indicating that in this parameter of neuroprotection, EA of GV acupoints may be superior to EA of *Hua-tuo-jia-ji* acupoints.

The effects of EA on the survival of transplanted bone marrow mesenchymal stem cells (MSCs) into the transected spinal cord of rats were studied in another experiment. Electro-acupuncture was administered at GV-6, GV-9, GV-1 and GV-2 in rats with a T10 spinal cord lesion once every other day for 7 weeks using the same dense and disperse ≤ 1 milliampere, 60 Hz technique described above.[12] After EA treatment for 2-8 weeks, increased levels of neurotrophin-3 (NT-3), cyclic adenosine monophosphate (cAMP), differentiated MSCs and 5-hydroxytryptamine (5-HT) positive and the calcitonin related peptide (CGRP) positive nerve fibers were increased in the lesion and nearby tissues compared to the untreated control groups.[12]

In a subsequent study by the same group, the same protocol for EA and transplantation of MSCs resulted in significant improvements in pelvic limb function using a standard scoring system compared to a non-treated group, one receiving only transplantation of MSCs and another receiving only EA treatment without MSCs.[13] Although further studies are needed for confirmation, EA plus transplantation of MSCs may improve the prognosis for recovery of function in severe spinal cord injuries in other species.

Aquaporin-4 (AQP4) is an integral membrane protein that transports water through the cell membrane. In the central nervous system, it is found in astrocytes and is increased by insults to central nervous system tissues.[14] Electro-acupuncture of GV-4 and GV-14 with 20 Hz significantly reduced the expression of AQP4 in rats with experimental spinal cord injury compared to controls.[15] The reduction in AQP4 expression was in conjunction with improvement of neurological function. It was suggested that the mechanism of action of low frequency EA may be due partly to a reduction of spinal cord edema, alleviating secondary spinal cord injury.[14,15]

In an experimental spinal cord compression study in dogs, the recovery time was compared in dogs receiving corticosteroids alone, EA alone, corticosteroids plus EA or no treatment.[16] Acupoints GV-4, GV-3, BL-23, BL-24, GB-30, GB-34, ST-36, ST-40 and ST-41 were electrically stimulated with 2 volts, 25 Hertz for 20 minutes every other day. Dogs that received either corticosteroids or EA treatment alone had shorter recovery times (21.2 and 19.8 days, respectively) compared to untreated dogs (46.6 days), but dogs receiving a combination of corticosteroid and EA treatment had significantly shorter recovery times (8.2 days) than all other groups.[16] In another experimental study in dogs with spinal cord compression, the recovery time of dogs receiving decompression surgery alone was compared to those receiving decompression plus EA treatment. Dogs receiving decompression plus EA recovered significantly faster than those receiving decompression alone.[17]

In an experimental study where the dorsal root ganglia at L1-L5 and L7-S2 was removed, cats receiving 98 Hz of EA at ST-32, ST-36, GB-39 and SP-6 showed a significant increase in the number of cells expressing nerve growth factor (NGF), neurotrophin-3 (NT-3) and a brain derived neurotrophic factor (BDNF) in the the spared L6 dorsal root ganglia ipsilateral to the treatment side.[19] Similar EA stimulation in a normal cat showed significantly increased expressions of mRNA of these neurotrophic factors in a dorsal root ganglia ipsilateral to the treatment side as compared to the non-treatment side providing further evidence for the promotion of nerve regeneration by EA.[18,19]

Clinical Studies of Electro-acupuncture for Spinal Cord Injuries

For many years, EA and DN have been used alone and in conjunction with surgical decompression and corticosteroid therapy for animals with spinal cord injury from intervertebral disk disease.[3,20-22] In one clinical study, 50 dogs with intervertebral disk disease and varying degrees of neurological deficits greater than 48 hours duration were randomly divided into two groups.[23] One group received a combination of EA and DN combined with decreasing doses of prednisone and tramadol for pain control as needed. The other group received only prednisone and tramadol. Acupoints used in this study included SI-3, BL-62, BL-20, BL-23, BL-25, BL-60, ST-36, KID-3, GV-1, *Bai-hui*, LI-4 and GB-30.[23] These acupoints were electrically stimulated with 3 Hz alternated with 100 Hz for 3 seconds each. Total stimulation time was 20 minutes. The combination of EA and conventional medical therapy significantly increased the success rate of treatment (88.5%) for dogs with all grades of dysfunction when compared to the success rate of treatment for dogs receiving only the conventional medical therapy (58.3%). Time to recover ambulation in dogs receiving EA integrated with conventional medical treatments was also significantly shorter than in dogs receiving conventional medical treatment alone.

In another clinical study, 40 dogs with confirmed thoracolumbar intervertebral disk disease and severe neurological deficits (Grades 4 or 5 out of 5) were treated with either prednisone alone, prednisone and decompressive surgery alone, prednisone and EA/DN (electro-acupuncture plus dry needle acupuncture) or prednisone, decompressive surgery and EA/DN.[24] The acupoints treated varied slightly with the location of the spinal cord lesion. The EA was performed connecting BL-18 to BL-23 and ST-36 to GB-34 on each side.[24] Alternating current EA with frequencies of 2 to 15 Hz were used for 20 minutes. The voltage was increased until muscle twitching was observed. Dry needle acupuncture was performed at BL-40, KID-3 and GB-30. The EA/DN treatment was performed once per week for 1 to 6 months. Treatment was discontinued when dogs improved from Grade 4 or 5 to Grade 1 or 2 neurological deficits. At six months after the initiation of the experiment, the dogs receiving prednisone and EA/DN alone had the best clinical recovery of all the groups.[24]

In a retrospective study of the outcome of 80 paraplegic dogs with intact deep pain and intervertebral disk herniation, 37 dogs were treated with prednisone alone and 43 dogs were treated with prednisone plus EA. Acupoints GV-7 and GV-2 were treated with EA at 0.5-2.5 millivolts and mixed frequencies of 2 and 15 Hz for 30 minutes. Acupoints on the Bladder Channel near the lesion and bilaterally at GB-30, GB-34 and ST-36 were treated with DN for 30 minutes. The combination of EA/DN with prednisone was more effective than prednisone treatment alone to recover ambulation, relieve back pain and decrease relapses.[25]

The successful use of DN and EA for spinal cord injury recovery has also been documented in human clinical case reports.[26-27] When DN and EA were used to treat humans with acute spinal cord injury, the long-term neurological recovery including motor, sensory and bowel/bladder functions was improved. Patients that received EA at CV-3 and BL-32 with 30-50 milliampere, 20 Hertz pulses for 15 minutes for 4-5 treatments per week regained their bladder control within a significantly shorter period than did the non-treatment group.[28] Electro-acupuncture was been reported to be useful to manage chronic pain associated with spinal cord inuries.[29] No adverse side effects of EA and DN were seen in these studies.[26,27]

As shown in this review, there is growing scientific support from controlled basic science studies that EA and DN have neuroprotective effects, shorten the recovery times and improve outcomes in animals with experimental spinal cord injuries.[9-19] Clinical research has further shown that EA and DN combined with conventional treatments is significantly more effective to treat spinal cord injury from intervertebral disk herniation and other causes, than conventional treatments alone.[23-29] At least in rats EA of GV acupoints above and below the lesion were more effective than *Hua-tuo-jia-ji* acupoints at the same level.[11] Current acupuncture treatment recommendations for animals with spinal cord injuries have been based on the clinical experiences of different individuals.[3,4,20-25] Further studies are needed to determine the most effective acupoints, acupuncture techniques and duration and frequency of acupuncture treatments to develop the optimum standards of care for acupuncture treatment of spinal cord injuries in animals.

References:
1. Platt SR, Olby NJ. BSAVA Manual of Canine and Feline Neurology. 3rd ed. Gloucester, UK:BSAVA 2004:320-325,4-22,24-25,70-83.

2. Kube SA, Olby NJ. Managing acute spinal cord injuries. Compend Contin Educ Vet 2008;30:496-504.
3. Xie H, Preast V. Xie's Veterinary Acupuncture. Ames, Iowa:Blackwell Publishing 2007: 247-266, 129-234.
4. Xie H, Preast V. Traditional Chinese Veterinary Medicine. Reddick, FL:Jing Tang 2002:105-132.
5. Kenney J. Acupuncture for pain management. American Journal of Traditional Chinese Veterinary Medicine 2010; 5(2):37-53.
6. Zhu L, Li C, Ji C, et al. The role of OLS in peripheral acupuncture analgesia in arthritic rats. Zhen Ci Yan Jiu 1993; 18:214-218. (in Chinese)
7. Bragin EO, Popkova EV, Vasilenko GF. Effects of repeated acupuncture action on pain sensitivity and beta-endorphin contents of the hypothalamus and midbrain of the rat. Biull Eksp Biol Med 1989;107:59-61.
8. Han JS, Xie GX. Dynorphin: important mediator for electroacupuncture analgesia in the spinal cord of the rabbit. Pain 1984; 18:367-376.
9. Wang XY, Li XL, Hong SQ et al. Electroacupuncture induced spinal plasticity is linked to multiple gene expressions in dorsal root deafferented rats. J Mol Neurosci 2009; 37:97-110.
10. Choi DC, Lee JY, Moon YJ, et al. Acupuncture-mediated inhibition of inflammation facilitates significant functional recovery after spinal cord injury. Neurobiol Dis 2010; 39:272-282.
11. Li WJ, Pan SQ, Zeng YS et al. Identification of acupuncture-specific proteins in the process of electro-acupuncture after spinal cord injury. Neurosci Res 2010; 67:307-316.
12. Ding Y, Yan Q, Ruan JW et al. Electro-acupuncture promotes survival, differentiation of the bone marrow mesenchymal stem cells as well as functional recovery in the spinal cord-transected rats. BMC Neurosci 2009; 10:35.
13. Ding Y, Yan Q, Ruan JW et al. Bone marrow mesenchymal stem cells and electro-acupuncture downregulate the inhibitor molecules and promote the axonal regeneration in the transected spinal cord of rats. Cell Transplant 2010 (Epub ahead of print).
14. Nesic O, Lee J, Ye Z et al. Acute and chronic changes in aquaporin-4 expression after spinal cord injury. Neuroscience 2006; 143:779-792.
15. Xie J, Fang J, Feng X et al. Effect of electroacupuncture at acupoints of the governor vessel on aquaporin-4 in rat with experimental spinal cord injury. J Tradit Chin Med 2006; 26:148-152.
16. Yang JW, Jeong SM, Seo KM, Nam TC. Effects of corticosteroid and electroacupuncture on experimental spinal cord injury in dogs. Journal Veterinary Science 2003; 4:97-101.
17. Kim SY, Kim MS, Seo KM, Nam TC. Effect of the combination of electroacupuncture and surgical decompression on experimental spinal cord injury in dogs. Journal of Veterinary Clinics 2005; 22(4):297-301.
18. Chen J, Qi JG, Zhang W et al. Electro-acupuncture induced NGF, BDNF and NT-3 expression in spared L6 dorsal root ganglion in cats subjected to removal of adjacent ganglia. Neurosci Res 2007; 59:399-405.
19. Wang TH, Wang XY, Li XL et al. Effect of electroacupuncture on neurotrophin expression in cat spinal cord after partial dorsal rhizotomy. Neurochem Res 2007; 32:1415-1422.
20. Buchli R. Successful acupuncture treatment of a cervical disc syndrome in a dog. Vet Med Small Anim Clin 1975; 70:1302.

21. Janssens LA, Rogers PA. Acupuncture versus surgery in canine thoracolumbar disc disease. Vet Rec 1989; 124:283.
22. Janssens LA. Acupuncture for the treatment of thoracolumbar and cervical disc disease in the dog. Problems Veterinary Medicine 1992; 4:107-116.
23. Hayashi AM, Matera JM, Fonseca Pinto AC. Evaluation of electroacupuncture treatment for thoracolumbar intervertebral disk disease in dogs. J Am Vet Med Assoc 2007; 231:913-918.
24. Joaquim JG, Luna SP, Brondani JT, et al. Comparison of decompressive surgery, electroacupuncture, and decompressive surgery followed by electroacupuncture for the treatment of dogs with intervertebral disk disease with long-standing severe neurologic deficits. J Am Vet Med Assoc 2011; 236:1225-1229.
25. Han HJ, Yoon HY, Kim JY, Jang HY, Lee B, Choi SH, Jeong SW. Clinical effect of additional electroacupuncture on thoracolumbar intervertebral disc herniation in 80 paraplegic dogs. Am J Chin Med. 2010;38(6):1015-25.
26. Dorsher PT, McIntosh PM. Acupuncture's Effects in Treating the Sequelae of Acute and Chronic Spinal Cord Injuries: A Review of Allopathic and Traditional Chinese Medicine Literature. Evid Based Complement Alternat Med 2009:1-8.
27. Shin BC, Lee MS, Kong JC, et al. Acupuncture for spinal cord injury survivors in Chinese literature: a systematic review. Complement Ther Med 2009;17:316-327.
28. Cheng PT, Wong MK, Chang PL. A therapeutic trial of acupuncture in neurogenic bladder of spinal cord injured patients--a preliminary report. Spinal Cord 1998;36:476-480.
29. Cardenas DD, Jensen MP. Treatments for chronic pain in persons with spinal cord injury: A survey study. J Spinal Cord Med 2006;29:109-117.

How I Treat Degenerative Myelopathy

RM Clemmons, DVM, PhD, CVA, CVFT

Degenerative Myelopathy (DM) was first described as a specific degenerative neurologic disease in 1973.[1-7] Since then, much has been done to understand the processes involved in the disease and into the treatment of DM. Hopefully, this will help you understand the problem and to explain further the steps that can be taken to help dogs afflicted with DM.

The age at onset is 5 to 14 years, which corresponds to the third to sixth decades of human life. Although a few cases have been reported in other large breeds of dogs, the disease appears with relative frequency only in the German Shepherd breed, suggesting that there is a genetic predisposition for German Shepherd dogs (GSD) in developing DM. The work presented here and by others on the nature of DM has been performed in the German Shepherd breed. Care must be taken in extrapolating this information to other breeds of dogs. It is currently not known whether the exact condition exists in other breeds of dogs. Many dogs may experience a spinal cord disease (myelopathy) which is chronic and progressive (degenerative); but, unless they are caused by the same immune-related disease which characterizes DM of GSD, the treatments described herein may be ineffectual.

The gross pathologic examination of dogs with DM generally is not contributory toward the diagnosis. The striking features being the reduction of rear limb and caudal axial musculature. The microscopic neural tissue lesions consist of widespread demyelination of the spinal cord, with the greatest concentration of lesions in the thoracolumbar spinal cord region. In severely involved areas, there is also a reduced number of axons, an increased number of astroglial cells and an increased density of small vascular elements. In the thoracic spinal cord, nearly all funiculi are vacuolated. Similar lesions are occasionally seen scattered throughout the white matter of the brains from some dogs, as well. Many patients have evidence of plasma cell infiltrates in the kidneys on throughout the gastrointestinal tract, providing a hint to the underlying immune disorder causing DM.

I have studied this disease over the last 37 years and continue to do so. The current program (http://dog2doc.com/neuro/DM_Web/DMofGS.htm) is unique and designed to improve the diagnosis of GSDM and offer a sensible treatment for GSDM based upon what we know of the underlying cause of the disease. From that work and the genetic data available on GSDM, we believe the evidence says that GSDM is an animal model of Primary Progressive Multiple Sclerosis in human beings. So, at least, we think we know what GSDM is when we separate those who do have it from those who do not.

Part of the program is the diagnosis of the condition. Unfortunately, it is correct that the only current method to be absolutely sure is with a necropsy, which does not help patients before death. We have established criteria that help us make accurate diagnosis. I think that we do better than what has been reported by some authors where only 25% of the patients enrolled in the study were found to have the disease. The complicating factors which confused the diagnosis in that study would have been found by our diagnostic criteria. So, what do we do. Basically, they are routine clinical test, but applied in a specific sequence to help us find out all of the patient's problems. First, is the clinical examination that includes looking at who the patient is. If the patient is a German Shepherd, then there is a higher probability that a chronic progressive spinal cord problem might be due to GSDM. If it is not a German Shepherd, it may have a myelopathy, but it may be from another cause. We are not sure that the disease in the Corgi or in the Boxer is related to the disease in the German Shepherd. On the other hand, we can distinguish the disease that Corgis and Boxers get from GSDM based upon genetic aspects that these breeds have that related to their form of DM. Since these diseases are genetically different, applying our treatment to these breeds may not do any good. The second criterion is based upon the EMG (electromyogram), which evaluates the muscle-nerve connection. The EMG and all peripheral tests of neuromuscular function are normal in uncomplicated GSDM. On the other hand, the spinal cord evoked potential evaluated over C1 is abnormal in GSDM. This indicates that there are problems in the white matter of the spinal cord. We also look at the difference between the cerebrospinal fluid (CSF) collected from the cisterna magnum and the lumbar cistern. The latter shows elevations of CSF protein without concurrent increases in CSF cell counts. While many of these proteins are inflammatory in nature, one of the ones that can be measured easily is CSF cholinesterase. The CSF cholinesterase is elevated in the lumbar CSF (above 300 IU/ml) in most cases. Unfortunately, this change is not specific for GSDM, only for inflammation (GSDM is one of the inflammatory disease of the spinal cord). Titers for infectious diseases are normal or, at least, do not indicate another disease process. Finally, we look at special imaging to evaluate the structure of the spinal column and whether there is evidence of spinal cord compression from some disease process. This does not rule-out GSDM, rather imaging rules-in complications. The former criteria are what help diagnose GSDM: the clinical picture, the EMG with spinal evoked potential, and the CSF analysis with cholinesterase. The imaging only looks for a surgical disease (or its absence). Depending upon the condition and clinical signs, we do myelography plus or minus CT scan or MRI scans to help us determine whether there is a local compressive disease.

The other part of our program is the treatment outlined on our web site. It includes exercise, diet, supplements and medications. Each of these has an impact upon health and upon the disease. The components of the treatment work together to reduce the progression of GSDM. They target the processes THAT we have uncovered as the causes of the pathologic changes we see. We have seen few side effects (mostly GI upset) in the patients we diagnose and treat. There are things that can happen as rare occurrences when using any drug. If the complications resolve on stopping the drug and return on re-introduction, then it is probably drug related. If your veterinarians feel there is a problem, then the medications should be stopped until it is determined whether they are the cause or not. Many times it is discovered that some other disease is present rather than the medications. All of the medications have been used in dogs for many years (not just for treating GSDM) so they are not new. Only the application is new. N-acetylcysteine is the newest and we have used it for over 10 years. On the other hand, we do not like to use medications unless we know what we are treating.

So, we do not treat without reaching a diagnosis. The two parts of our program, diagnosis and treatment, work together. We diagnose early and treat early, which is why we have success. In the past, most patients progressed to posterior paralysis in 3-6 months. This would progress to all 4 legs in another 3-6 months with death from brainstem failure (in those patients allowed to progress that far without intervention) 9-18 months from the first diagnosis of GSDM. That has changed now. In our hands, most GSDM patients will remain functional for 12 months, while many outlive their disease.

TCM Diagnosis and Treatment:

From a TCVM perspective, GSDM and probably BM (Boxer Myelopathy) are *Wei* syndromes. Most of the patients we evaluate are combined *Qi* and *Yin* deficient. Of course, there is a spectrum and we, therefore, need to assess each patient to find their pattern. Dr. Xie's formulas appear to help several; but, in general, acupuncture and herbs are palliative and designed to improve quality of life rather than to achieve a cure. Cures seem to put the diagnosis in question; whereas we do see dogs that outlive GSDM. If the standard TCVM therapies do not work, the formulas that I prefer to use in GSDM and BM patients (both diseases are closer from TCVM pattern diagnosis than Western diagnosis) are *Hu Qian Tang* and *Di Huang Yin Zi Tang*. These are available from Jing Tang.[a]

Wei Zheng (flaccidity syndrome) in Western medicine is any disorder of the PNS (Peripheral Nervous System) that may cause weakness or numbness, such as MS (multiple sclerosis or spinal and muscular disorders). This leads of flaccidity of muscles, paralysis, hemiplegia, and muscular atrophy of the limbs. TCVM patterns include excess and deficiency causes, but those that we tend to see in DM patients are chronic deficiencies. The root cause of these problems lies in Kidney *Jing* deficiency, since the problems are now known to have a genetic basis (even though they take years to develop). Generally, the patterns recognized are:
1) Spleen/Kidney *Qi* Deficiency; 2) *Qi* and *Yin* Deficiency; and 3) *Yin* and *Yang* Deficiency. This is also the apparent order in which the signs progress to an extent as well.

Deficiency of *Qi*: Signs include muscular flaccidity or atrophy of the limbs with motor impairment, marked by lassitude, listlessness, short breath, weak voice, sweating on slight exertion, dizziness, palpitation, pale-wet tongue, and weak pulses.

Deficiency of *Qi* and *Yin*: Signs are mostly seen in elderly people. Typically symptoms are muscular flaccidity of the limbs come on slowly, a mild to moderate amount of motor weakness in the legs, accompanied with soreness and weakness of the loin and knees, dizziness and blurring of vision, impotence or seminal emission, red-dry tongue, and thready-rapid pulse.

Deficiency of *Yin* and *Yang*: Signs are a combination of the aforementioned processes with the addition of Cold signs. The tongue may be pale or red while the pulses are deep and weak.

Local AP points: *Hua-tuo-jia-ji*, GV-14, *Bai-hui*

Special AP points: BL-62, BL-64, SI-3, *Er-yan*, *Liu-feng*

TCVM herbal medicine: *Hu Qian Wan* (Table 1); *Di Huang Yin Zi* (Table 2)

Table 1: Ingredients and Actions of *Hu Qian Wan*

Pin Yin Name	English Name	Actions
Bai Shao Yao	Paeonia	Nourish Blood
Chen Pi	Citrus	Move *Qi* and Relieve Pain
Gan Jiang	Zingiberis	Strengthen Stomach and Promote Appetite
Gui Ban	Plastrum	nourish *Yin*, anchors *Yang*, tonify Blood, Nourish Heart
Huang Bai	Phellodendron	Clear Heat, Nourish *Yin*
Niu Xi	Achyranthes	Strengthens the Kidney and Benefit the Knees

Shu Di Huang	Rehmannia	Nourish *Yin*, Blood and *Jing*
Suo Yang	Cynomorium	Tonify *Yang* and *Jing*, Nourish Blood, Strengthen Sinews
Zhi Mu	Anemarrhena	Nourish *Yin*, Clear Heat

Table 2: Ingredients and Actions of *Di Huang Yin Zi*

Pin Yin Name	English Name	Actions
Ba Ji Tian	Morinda	Tonify Kidney, Strengthen *Yang*
Fan Shi Hu	Descurainiae Herba	Nourish *Yin*, Clear Deficient Heat, Nourish Stomach *Yin*
Fu Ling	Poria	Drain Damp, Strengthen Spleen
Fu Zi	Aconite	Warm Spleen
Mai Men Dong	Ophiopogon	Nourish *Yin*
Rou Cong Rong	Cistanche	Tonify Kidney, Strengthen *Yang*
Rou Gui	Cinnamomum	Tonify Kidney *Yang*
Shan Zhu Yu	Cornus	Nourish *Yin*
Shi Chang Pu	Acorus	Open Orifices, Transform Phlegm, Calm Spirit, Harmonize Middle Burner
Shu Di Huang	Rehmannia	Nourish Blood and *Yin*
Wu Wei Zi	Schisandra	Consolidate and Nourish Lung *Yin*
Yuan Zhi	Polygala	Calm Spirit, Quiet Heart, Clear Orifices

Footnotes:

[a] (JT) = *Jing Tang* Herbal www.tcvmherbal.com; Reddick, FL

References:

1. Xie H: Common Disease. In: H Xie (ed), Traditional Chinese Veterinary Medicine, Beijing, Beijing Agricultural University Press, pp. 427-428, 1994.
2. Clemmons RM: Degenerative myelopathy. In: RW Kirk (ed), Current Veterinary Therapy X, Philadelphia, WB Saunders, pp. 830-833, 1989.
3. Clemmons RM: Degenerative myelopathy. Vet Clin N Am, 22:965-971, 1992.
4. Clemmons RM: Degenerative myelopathy. In: MJ Bojrab (ed), Disease Mechanisms in Small Animal Surgery, Philadelphia, Lea & Febiger, pp. 984-986, 1993.
5. Clemmons RM, Wheeler S, LeCouteur RA: How Do I Treat? Degenerative Myelopathy. Prog Vet Neruol, 6:71-72, 1995.
6. Dewey CW: Myelopathies: Disorders of the Spinal Cord. In: CW Dewey (ed), A Practical Guide to Canine and Feline Neurology, Ames, Wiley-Blackwell, pp. 344-345, 2008.
7. Xie H: How to Treat Degenerative Myleopathy (DM)? Proc 12th Chi Instit Ann Conf, 197-202, 2010.

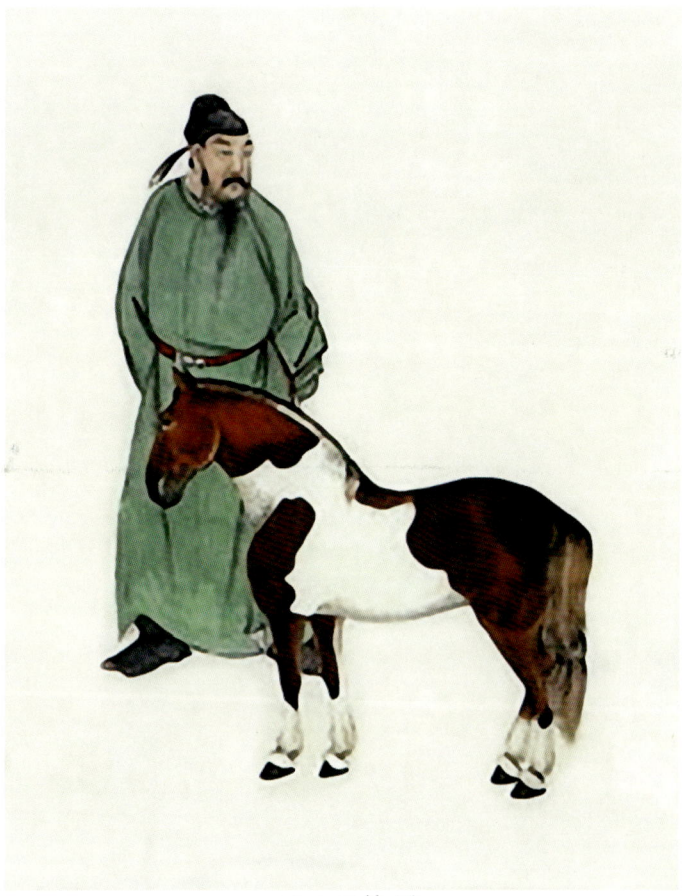

BO LE伯乐

Bo Le was the most famous equine specialist who lived during the *Qing-mu-gong* period (659-621 BCE). His expertise was treating horses and identifying a *Qian-li-ma* or a good racehorse. *Bo Le* was a part of the title of the first veterinary acupuncture text, which is called *Bo Le Zhen Jing* (Bole's Canon of Veterinary Acupuncture). *Qian-li-ma* refers to horses that are able to run 1,000 Chinese miles (approximately 312 American miles) without stopping. All Chinese people are familiar with the saying: "*Qian-li-ma* horses are always there, unfortunately, they are recognized by only one, *Bo Le*", or in other words "exceptional resources are never deficient, but they may not be identified because of a lack of *Bo Le*". *Zhuang Zi,* an ancient text (circa 300 CE) contains a chapter entitled "*Ma Ti Lun*" (Dissertation of Equine Hooves) that described aspects of traditional equine health care including acupuncture and moxibustion attributed to *Bo Le*. Although *Bo Le* was his official identification, his real name was *Sun Yang*.

Bo Le Zhen Jing (Bo Le's Canon of Veterinary Acupuncture) is considered the first veterinary acupuncture text. One cannot say exactly when this book was published, but *Si Mu An Ji Ji* (Simu's Collection of Equine Medicine) included the whole text of "*Bo Le Zhen Jing*". *Li Shi* wrote *Si Mu An Ji Ji* during the *Tang* dynasty (618-907 CE). *Li Shi*'s high rank as a government official helped his book gain popularity and keep it well preserved. This book systematically presents the basic theories, diagnoses and treatment techniques of Traditional Chinese Veterinary Medicine. The book describes acupuncture methods including tonification and sedation, needling depth and angle, loci and indications of 77 acupuncture points in horses.

CHAPTER 5

Neuromuscular Disorders

Generalized Neuromuscular Disorders

Cheryl L Chrisman DVM, MS, EdS, DACVIM-Neurology, CVA

Generalized neuromuscular disorders include polyneuropathies, myasthenia gravis and polymyositis and the underlying conventional cause is often immune-mediated. Since traditional Chinese medicine can be useful to balance the immune system, acupuncture, Chinese herbal medicine, *Tui-na* and Food therapy may be useful to promote remission and recovery of these devastating diosrders.

POLYNEUROPATHY

Acute polyradiculoneuritis (sometimes referred to as "coonhound paralysis" in dogs and Guillain-Barre syndrome in humans) is the most common polyneuropathy of dogs and cats.[1-3] Affected animals have quadriplegia with depressed or absent spinal reflexes in all four limbs (flaccid quadriplegia) that develops over a 24-48 hour period. If intercostal muscles and the diaphragm become involved, mechanical ventilation is necessary to prevent death. Some dogs and cats also have pharyngeal and laryngeal paresis, so swallowing becomes difficult and aspiration of food can also lead to death. Acute polyradiculoneuritis is an immune-mediated disorder and since the spinal nerve roots (radicles) are significantly affected, the name includes them instead of being simply referred to as polyneuritis. There is no effective conventional medication for acute polyradiculoneuritis and only physical therapy and nursing care are provided.[2,3] Affected animals take months to recover and often have residual weakness and muscle atrophy. Recurrences are also seen.

In one experimental study of acute polyradiculoneuritis in a rabbit model, the nerve conduction was significantly improved with acupuncture.[4] In a small clinical trial of humans with acute polyradiculoneuritis, a polyglycoside extract of the Chinese herbal medicine *Lei Gong Teng* (Tripterygium), known to clear Heat and resolve Stagnation, positively affected the immune parameters and hastened recovery significantly more than corticosteroids.[5] Although further randomized controlled clinical trails are needed, based on preliminary data, acupuncture and Chinese herbal medicine should shorten recovery time, improve the degree of recovery and reduce the recurrence rates in animals with acute polyradiculoneuritis.[4,5]

Polyneuropathy is often associated with diabetes mellitus in humans and cats.[2,3,6,7] Diabetic cats often become irritable and avoid physical contact, because of a painful sensory polyneuropathy or walk plantigrade in the pelvic limbs from a motor neuropathy. In several human clinical studies of diabetic neuropathy, acupuncture significantly relieved pain and improved conduction of both sensory and motor nerves, compared to no treatment and conventional drugs.[7-9] *Liu Wei Di Huang* has been useful to treat diabetic neuropathy in humans.[10] Further studies on the use of acupuncture and Chinese herbal medicine to treat the pain and neuroloficl deficits of diabetic polyneuropathy of cats is warranted.[11]

Chronic progressive or recurrent intermittent paraparesis and quadriparesis can occur from more chronic forms of polyneuropathy. From a conventional perspective the underlying etiology is often unknown, but in some animals is suspected to be immune-mediated. Because of the ability of TCVM to balance the immune system and promote nerve regeneration, further exploration of the use of TCVM in the treatment of these chronic polyneuropathies is also warranted.[12-15] An overview of the currently known TCVM patterns, diagnosis and treatment of polyneuropathies is listed in Tables 1 and 2.[16-18] Food therapy and *Tui-na* techniques are outlined under each TCVM pattern.[20,21]

Table 1: Common conventional diagnoses and traditional Chinese veterinary medicine (TCVM) patterns and examination findings associated with generalized neuromuscular disorders[6,16-19]

		Generalized Peripheral Nerve and Muscle Disorders		
Conventional Diagnosis	**TCVM Pattern**	**Clinical Findings**	**Tongue**	**Pulses**
Polyneuropathy	Wind-Heat Invasion causing *Qi*/Blood Stagnation and Generalized *Qi* Deficiency	Often *Yang* animals Acute onset quadriplegia Reduced/absent spinal reflexes +/- Generalized pain +/-Facial paresis/paralysis +/-Laryngeal paresis/paralysis +/- Pharyngeal paresis/paralysis Panting Warm ears, back and feet	Red, dry, purple or pale	Superficial, forceful, rapid or wiry
	Wind-Cold Invasion causing *Qi*/Blood Stagnation and Generalized *Qi* Deficiency	Often *Yin* animals Acute onset quadriplegia Reduced/absent spinal reflexes +/- Generalized pain +/-Facial paresis +/-Laryngeal paresis +/- Pharyngeal paresis Cold ears, back, feet	Purple, pale, wet	Superficial, forceful, slow or wiry
	Kidney *Yin* and *Qi* Deficiency with Blood Stagnation	Diabetes mellitus Generalized pain or sensitivity Pelvic limb paresis with a plantigrade stance Cool seeking Panting Warm ears, back and feet Dry skin	Red, dry or pale	Deep, weak, worse on left, rapid and thready or worse on right

	Spleen *Qi* and Kidney *Qi* Deficiency	Acute onset Quadriplegia (Grade 4 deficits) Depressed or absent spinal reflexes in all 4 limbs +/-Facial paresis +/-Laryngeal paresis +/- Pharyngeal paresis	Pale, wet	Deep, weak, worse on right
Myasthenia gravis	Spleen *Qi* and Kidney *Qi* Deficiencies	Chronic Generalized muscle weakness worse with exercise Megaesophagus +/-Facial paresis +/-Laryngeal paresis +/- Pharyngeal paresis	Pale, wet	Deep, weak, worse on right
Polymyositis	Wind-Heat invasion causing *Qi*/Blood Stagnation and Generalized *Qi* Deficiency	Acute onset Regurgitation Megaesophagus Muscle weakness worse with exercise Stiff, stilted gait Painful muscles Cool seeking Panting Warm ears, back and feet	Red, purple or pale	Superficial, forceful, rapid or wiry
	Spleen *Qi* and Kidney *Qi* Deficiencies	Chronic progressive onset Regurgitation Megaesophagus Muscle weakness worse with exercise Stiff, stilted gait Painful muscles	Pale, wet	Deep, weak, worse on right

Table 2: Treatment strategy, acupuncture points and Chinese herbal medicine used to treat generalized neuromuscular disorders[16-19]

Generalized Peripheral Nerve and Muscle Disorders				
Conventional Diagnosis	**TCVM Pattern**	**Acupuncture points and Techniques**	**Chinese Herbal Medicine**	**Comments**
Polyneuropathy	Wind-Heat Invasion causing	**EA:** GV-3/GV-14, SI-9/SI-9, BL-54/BL-54, *Liu-feng/Liu-feng* or	Double P II and *Pu Ji Xiao Du*	For acute paralysis, repeat acupuncture every 3-5 days for 3-5 times then

	Qi/Blood Stagnation and Generalized Qi Deficiency	PC-8/KID-1, LI-10/ST-36, BL-40/BL-40	Yin	reduce to every 1-2 weeks for 6-8 treatments or until ambulatory; Use herbal formulae 2-4 months as needed
		DN: GB-20, LI-4, Er-jian, Wei-jian		
	Wind-Cold Invasion causing Qi/Blood Stagnation and Generalized Qi Deficiency	EA: GV-3/GV-14, SI-9/SI-9, BL-54/BL-54, Liu-feng/Liu-feng or PC-8/KID-1, LI-10/ST-36, BL-40/BL-40	Double P II and Shu Jin Huo Lou	For acute paralysis, repeat acupuncture every 3-5 days for 3-5 times then reduce to every 1-2 weeks for 6-8 treatments or until ambulatory; Use herbal formulae 2-4 months as needed
		DN: GB-20, LI-4, Moxibustion: BL-10, Bai-hui		
	Kidney Yin and Qi Deficiency with Blood Stagnation	EA: GV-3/GV-14, SI-9/SI-9, PC-8/KID-1, LI-10/ST-36, BL-40/BL-40	Jiang Tang Cha and Body Sore	Repeat acupuncture weekly every 1-2 weeks for 6-8 treatments or longer if needed; Use herbal formulae for up to 6 months
		DN: BL-23, KID-3, BL-60, KID-6		
	Spleen Qi and Kidney Qi Deficiency	EA: GV-3/GV-14, SI-9/SI-9, BL-54/BL-54, LI-10/ST-36, BL-40/BL-40; can add Liu-feng/Liu-feng or PC-8/KID-1 if needed	Bu Yang Huan Wu Add Body Sore if painful (reduce dose of others to 0.5 gm/20# twice daily)	Repeat acupuncture weekly for 3-5 treatments then every 2-4 weeks for 6-8 treatments or longer if needed; Use herbal formulae for up to 6 months
		DN: BL-20, BL-21, BL-23, KID-3, SP-3		
Myasthenia gravis	Spleen Qi and Kidney Qi Deficiencies	DN Moxibustion: Bai-hui, BL-20, BL-21, BL-23;	Bu Yang Huan Wu	Repeat acupuncture weekly every 1-2 weeks for 6-8 treatments or longer if needed; Use herbal formulae for up to 6 months
		DN regular: Bai-hui, BL-20, BL-21, BL-23, GV-14, LI-10, ST-36, BL-40, BL-54, SI-9, LI-4, KID-3, SP-3		
Polymyositis	Wind-Heat invasion causing Qi/Blood Stagnation and generalized Qi Deficiency	EA: GV-3/GV-14, SI-9/SI-9, BL-54/BL-54, BL-40/BL-40	Wu Wei Xiao Du Yin	Repeat acupuncture weekly for 3-5 treatments then every 2-4 weeks for 6-8 treatments or longer if needed; Use herbal formula 2-4 months as needed
		DN: GB-20, Er-jian, Wei-jian, LI-4, LI-11, ST-36, LI-10, Bai-hui, KID-1, PC-8		

		EA: GV-3/GV-14, SI-9/SI-9, BL-54/BL-54, LI-10/ST-36, BL-40/BL-40	*Bu Yang Huan Wu*	Repeat acupuncture weekly for 3-5 treatments then every 2-4 weeks for 6-8 treatments or longer if needed; Use Body Sore for 1-2 months if needed for pain and use herbal formula up to 6 months
	Spleen *Qi* and Kidney *Qi* Deficiencies	DN: BL-20, BL-21, BL-23, KID-3, SP-3	Body Sore	

The number of acupoints selected and treatment frequency will vary with the animal's condition and response to treatment; Chinese herbal medicine doses are generally 0.5 gm/10-20# orally twice daily; EA=electro-acupuncture, DN=dry needle acupuncture; All Chinese herbal formulas available from Jing Tang Herbal:www.tcvmherbal.com except *Wu Wei Xiao Du Yin*, which is available from Mayway Herbal www.mayway.com.

Etiology and Pathology

When *Zheng Qi* is weakened from poor nutrition, chronic illness, environmental stress or age, the *Wei Qi* portion of *Zheng Qi* that protects the body's exterior becomes weak and external pathogens such as Wind-Heat or Wind-Cold gain entrance.[22] In general, the constitution of the animal can affect their susceptibility to invasion of either Wind/Cold or Wind/Heat. When *Zheng Qi* is weakened, *Yin* animals such as Water, Metal and Earth constitutions tend to be more susceptible to Wind-Cold invasion while *Yang* animals like Wood and Fire constitutions are more susceptible to Wind-Heat invasion.[22] More experience is needed to see if this holds true for animals with acute polyradiculoneuritis.

In acute polyradiculoneuritis, the limb Channels are primarily affected. Wind-Heat or Wind-Cold invasion results in *Qi*/Blood Stagnation and local *Qi* Deficiency. Some animals exhibit limb pain from the *Qi*/Blood Stagnation, but the primary clinical signs are quadriparesis (Grades 3-4 neurological deficits are most common) with or without cranial neuropathies due to *Qi* Deficiency causing dysfunction of the peripheral nerves.

Overeating of carbohydrates and fats as occurs in many obese cats leads to Stagnation of Food (a secondary TCVM pathogen) that generates internal Fire and Heat and damages Body Fluids and Kidney *Yin*.[22] Kidney *Yin* Deficiency can be manifested as diabetes mellitus. The dry Internal Heat associated with chronic Kidney *Yin* Deficiency can consume *Qi* causing Kidney *Qi* Deficiency and pelvic limb weakness (standing and walking plantigrade). Since *Qi* is necessary for normal Blood flow, Blood movement through the Channels become Stagnant and results in generalized limb and body pain and hypersensitivity as seen with diabetic polyneuropathy. The TCVM pattern then becomes Kidney *Yin* and *Qi* Deficiency with Blood Stagnation

Chronic immune-mediated disorders (*Zheng Qi* disorders) may be associated with chronic Spleen *Qi* and Kidney *Qi* Deficiencies.[22] Over time a poor quality diet, underfeeding or overfeeding, chronic illness and environmental stress can weaken the Spleen and negatively impact normal transformation and transportation functions. The result is Spleen *Qi* Deficiency with reduced *Gu Qi* (Food *Qi*) and *Ying Qi* (Nutrient *Qi*) needed to regenerate *Qi* and Blood. *Gu Qi* is essential for a normal functioning. *Zheng Qi* (immune system) and immune-mediated disorders can result from Spleen *Qi* Deficiency. Prolonged Spleen *Qi* Deficiency and reduced post-natal *Jing* can stress prenatal Kidney *Jing* and cause Kidney *Qi* Deficiency. A manifestation of Spleen *Qi* Deficiency is *Wei* syndrome or generalized weakness and muscle atrophy. A manifestation of Kidney *Qi* Deficiency is *Tan-Huan* syndrome or paresis or paralysis of all four limbs. Together Spleen *Qi* and Kidney *Qi* Deficiencies can result in chronic progressive or intermittent paresis or paralysis and muscle atrophy, as nerve and muscles become progressively affected. Applying the basic TCVM theories of *Yin/Yang*, Eight Principles, Five Treasures, Five Elements and *Zang Fu* physiology and pathology to make a TCVM diagnosis, there are currently four patterns associated with polyneuropathy in dogs and cats, but with more experience other TCVM patterns with different diagnostic features and requiring different treatment may be found:

1. **Wind-Heat invasion causing *Qi*/Blood Stagnation and generalized *Qi* Deficiency**
   Wei Qi may become weak due to poor nutrition, chronic illness, environmental stress and aging and Wind-Heat can invade the Channels of the limbs, especially in *Yang* animals (Wood and Fire constitutions). *Qi*/Blood Stagnation results and causes Deficiency of *Qi* flow to local tissues and loss of peripheral nerve function. The result is acute generalized paralysis with loss of spinal reflexes of all four limbs.

2. **Wind-Cold invasion causing *Qi*/Blood Stagnation and generalized *Qi* Deficiency**
   Wei Qi may become weak due to poor nutrition, chronic illness, environmental stress and aging and Wind-Cold can invade the Channels of the limbs, especially in *Yin* animals (Earth, Metal and Water constitutions). *Qi*/Blood Stagnation results and causes Deficiency of *Qi* flow to local tissues and loss of peripheral nerve function. The result is acute generalized paralysis with loss of spinal reflexes of all four limbs.

3. **Kidney *Yin* and *Qi* Deficiency with Blood Stagnation**
   Overeating fats and carbohydrates, chronic illness and environmental stress can result in Kidney *Yin* and *Qi* Deficiencies. *Qi* Deficiency leads to Blood Stagnation in the Channels and generalized pain.

4. **Spleen *Qi* and Kidney *Qi* Deficiency**
   Over time, poor nutrition, chronic illness or environmental stress can result in Spleen *Qi* and Kidney *Qi* Deficiencies. The result is a generalized reduction of *Qi* flow to superficial tissues including nerves and chronic progressive generalized paresis or paralysis with reduced or absent spinal reflexes of all four limbs associated with a polyneuropathy.

Pattern Differentiation and Treatment

1. Wind-Heat invasion causing *Qi*/Blood Stagnation and generalized *Qi* Deficiency

Clinical Signs:
- Often *Yang* animals (Wood and Fire constitutions)
- Acute onset quadriplegia (Grades 3-4 neurological deficits are most common)
- Depressed or absent spinal reflexes in all 4 limbs
- +/- Generalized pain
- +/-Facial paresis or paralysis
- +/-Laryngeal paresis or paralysis
- +/- Pharyngeal paresis or paralysis
- Paralysis of the diaphragm and intercostal muscles can lead to death

- Panting
- Warm ears, back and feet
- Tongue- red, dry, purple or pale
- Pulses- Superficial, forceful, rapid or wiry

TCVM Diagnosis:
The acute onset of clinical signs is typical of an Excess pattern with invasion of an External pathogen and *Qi*/Blood Stagnation. The diagnosis of Wind-Heat invasion causing *Qi*/Blood Stagnation and local *Qi* Deficiency is based on the clinical findings. The panting and warmth of the ears, back and feet are typical of a Heat pattern. The tongue color will vary with the stage of the process. The tongue is red and dry from the Wind-Heat, purple if *Qi*/Blood Stagnation is most prominent and pale if *Qi* Deficiency is most prominent. The pulses may be forceful and rapid from the Heat or wiry from the *Qi*/Blood Stagnation.

Treatment Principles:
- Clear Wind-Heat
- Resolve *Qi*/Blood Stagnation
- Promote local *Qi* flow and recovery of nerve function

Acupuncture treatment:
For EA use 80-120 Hz alternating frequencies for 15-30 minutes, as EA is more effective to resolve Stagnation than DN alone. If animals seem painful, change the EA protocol to 20 Hz for 10-15 minutes and 80-120 Hz alternating frequencies for 10-15 minutes. Treat both sides. For acute paralysis, repeat acupuncture every 3-5 days for 3-5 times then reduce to every 1-2 weeks for 6-8 treatments or until ambulatory. For Aqua-AP inject 0.25-0.5 ml vitamin B12 into the acupoint.

Acupoints recommended
- EA: GV-3/GV-14, SI-9/SI-9, BL-54/BL-54, *Liu-feng*/*Liu-feng* or PC-8/KID-1, LI-10/ST-36, BL-40/BL-40
- DN: GB-20, LI-4, *Er-jian*, *Wei-jian*
- Aqua-AP: GB-20, GV-14

Pertinent acupoint actions
- During EA, GV-3 can be connected to GV-14 to stimulate the Governing Vessel and *Qi* Flow in all the spinal nerve roots
- GV-14 is also useful to clear Heat and balance the immune system
- SI-9 is a local acupoint near the brachial plexus nerve roots useful to stimulate *Qi*/Blood flow to the region
- BL-54 is a local acupoint near the sciatic nerve useful to stimulate *Qi*/Blood flow to the region
- *Li-feng* acupoints (at the skin fold on the dorsal aspect of the metacarpophalangeal and metatarsophalangeal joints of all four feet) between digits 2-3, 3-4 and 4-5) are useful to treat limb paralysis

- KID-1 and PC-8 are the "four roots" and are also useful to treat limb paralysis
- LI-10 and ST-36 tonify *Qi* and stimulate *Qi* flow in the Channels
- ST-36 is also useful to balance the immune system
- BL-40 is the master point for the pelvic limbs
- GB-20 is useful to Dispel Wind
- LI-4 is useful to Clear Heat and balance *Zheng Qi*
- *Er-jian* (ear tip) and *Wei-jian* (tail tip) are useful to clear Heat

Herbal Medicine:

- Double P II (JT)[a] 0.5gm/10# twice daily orally to relieve *Qi*/Blood Stagnation causing paralysis
- Combine with *Pu Ji Xiao Du Yin* (JT)[a] 0.5gm/10# twice daily orally to clear Heat and disperse Wind-Heat
- Administer herbal formulae 2-4 months as needed
- A description of all the ingredients of the Chinese herbal medicine listed is beyond the scope of this text, but can be found elsewhere.[18,19]

Food Therapy:

The purpose of the Food therapy is to clear Heat and promote *Qi*/Blood circulation, so cooling foods are prescribed and Hot foods are avoided.[21]

- Foods to supplement to cleat Heat: Turkey, duck, duck eggs, conch, clams, mussels, yogurt, millet, barley, spinach, broccoli, celery, egg plant, kelp, alfalfa, cucumbers, pears, bananas, white radishes, watermelon
- Foods to promote *Qi*/Blood circulation: Chicken egg, crab, sweet rice, peaches, carrots, coriander, turnips
- Foods to avoid: Lamb, shrimp, corn-fed beef, chicken, trout, squash, turnips, sweet rice, basal, caraway, cherries, chilies, cinnamon, ginger, rosemary, sage

Tui-na Procedures:

The purpose of the *Tui-na* is to stimulate *Qi* and Blood flow to relieve pain and promote nerve regeneration in the affected region. The descriptions and indications of each technique are outlined in more detail in Chapter 1 Table 8.[20]

- *Ca-fa* rubbing along the back from GV-2 to GV-20 to relieve nerve root *Qi* Stagnation
- *Moo-fa* massaging using the palms or fingers from the shoulder to the paw and the hip to the paw for 3-5 minutes each leg
- *Nie-fa* holding and pinching the skin and muscle in the main muscle groups of each limb for 30 seconds each
- *An-fa* and *Rou-fa* pressing and rotary kneading at LI-10, LI-11, SI-9, TH-14 and GB-21 for the thoracic limb and ST-36, BL-40, GB-34, GB-31, BL-54 for 30 seconds per acupoint
- *Ca-fa* rubbing from the scapula to the carpus and then from the hip to the tarsus on each side for 1 minute on each limb
- *Dou-fa* gently shaking for 12 times, *Ba-shen-fa* stretching for 12 times and *Ban-fa* flexing and extending joints for 12 times; perform on each limb

Daily Life Style Recommendation for Owner Follow-up:
- *Moo-fa* massaging up and down the back and all the muscles of the limbs for 3-5 minutes in each area twice daily until recovers function to improve *Qi*/Blood flow to the peripheral nerves
- *Dou-fa* gently shaking, *Ba-shen-fa* stretching, and *Ban-fa* flexing and extending joints on each limb for 12 times twice daily until recovers to improve *Qi*/Blood flow to the peripheral nerves
- While in lateral recumbency, turn every 4-6 hours to avoid lung atelectasis and decubitus ulcers
- Keep on padding to avoid decubitus ulcers especially on shoulders and hips
- Keep clean of urine and feces and dry to avoid skin lesions
- Feed a high quality soft diet to support *Zheng Qi*
- In the first 7-10 days ensure swallowing is normal and food does not collect in the pharynx
- Keep in a low stress environment to support *Zheng Qi* and avoid Liver *Qi* Stagnation which can increase Internal Heat
- When some movement returns can begin daily supervised swimming
- When some movement returns can begin walking with a sling that supports the neck and thoracic and pelvic limbs

Comments:
Based on experimental and clinical studies of the positive effects of TCVM treatments on immune disorders and nerve regeneration, further clinical studies of TCVM for the treatment of acute polyradiculoneuritis are warranted.[4,5,12-15] Expect TCVM treatments to shorten the recovery time, improve the degree of recovery and reduce the recurrence rate.

2. Wind-Cold invasion causing *Qi*/Blood Stagnation and generalized *Qi* Deficiency

Clinical Signs:
- Often *Yin* animals (Earth, Metal and Water constitutions)
- Acute onset quadriplegia (Grades 3-4 neurological deficits are most common)
- Depressed or absent spinal reflexes in all 4 limbs
- +/- Generalized pain
- +/-Facial paresis or paralysis
- +/-Laryngeal paresis or paralysis
- +/- Pharyngeal paresis or paralysis
- Paralysis of the diaphragm and intercostal muscles can lead to death
- Cool ears, back and feet
- Tongue- purple or pale, wet
- Pulses- Superficial, forceful, slow or wiry

TCVM Diagnosis:
The acute onset of clinical signs is typical of an Excess pattern with invasion of an External pathogen and *Qi*/Blood Stagnation. The diagnosis of Wind-Cold invasion causing *Qi*/Blood Stagnation and local *Qi* Deficiency is based on the clinical findings. The coolness of the ears, back and feet are typical of a Cold pattern. The tongue color will vary with the stage of the process. The tongue is purple if the Wind-Cold and *Qi*/Blood Stagnation are most prominent and pale if *Qi* Deficiency is most prominent. The pulses are superficial, strong forceful, but slow reflecting the Cold or wiry reflecting the *Qi*/Blood Stagnation.

Treatment Principles:
- Clear Wind-Cold
- Resolve *Qi*/Blood Stagnation
- Promote local *Qi* flow and recovery of nerve function

Acupuncture treatment:
For EA use 80-120 Hz alternating frequencies for 15-30 minutes, as EA is more effective to resolve Stagnation than DN alone. If animals seem painful, change the EA protocol to 20 Hz for 10-15 minutes and 80-120 Hz alternating frequencies for 10-15 minutes. Treat both sides. For acute paralysis, repeat acupuncture every 3-5 days for 3-5 times then reduce to every 1-2 weeks for 6-8 treatments or until ambulatory. For Aqua-AP inject 0.25-0.5 ml vitamin B12 into the acupoint.

Acupoints recommended
- EA: GV-3/GV-14, SI-9/SI-9, BL-54/BL-54, *Liu-feng/Liu-feng* or PC-8/KID-1, LI-10/ST-36, BL-40/BL-40
- DN: GB-20, LI-4
- Moxibustion: BL-10, *Bai-hui*
- Aqua-AP: GB-20, BL-54

Pertinent acupoint actions
- During EA, GV-3 can be connected to GV-14 to stimulate the Governing Vessel and *Qi* Flow in all the spinal nerve roots
- GV-14 is also useful to balance the immune system
- SI-9 is a local acupoint near the brachial plexus nerve roots useful to stimulate *Qi*/Blood flow
- BL-54 is a local acupoint near the sciatic nerve useful to stimulate *Qi*/Blood flow
- *Li-feng* acupoints (at the skin fold on the dorsal aspect of the metacarpophalangeal and metatarsophalangeal joints of all four feet) between digits 2-3, 3-4 and 4-5) are useful to stimulate *Qi*/Blood flow and treat limb paralysis
- KID-1 and PC-8 are the "four roots" and are also useful to stimulate *Qi*/Blood flow and treat limb paralysis
- LI-10 and ST-36 tonify *Qi* and stimulate *Qi* flow in the Channels
- ST-36 is also useful to balance the immune system

- BL-40 is the master point for the pelvic limbs to strengthen the pelvic limbs
- GB-20 is useful to Dispel Wind
- LI-4 is useful to balance *Zheng Qi*
- BL-10 is are useful to clear Wind-Cold and moxibustion is useful to warm the Cold in the thoracic limbs
- *Bai-hui* (midline between L7-S1) moxibustion is useful to warm the Cold in the pelvic limbs

Herbal Medicine:
- Double P II (JT)[a] 0.5gm/10# twice daily orally to relieve *Qi*/Blood Stagnation causing paralysis
- Combine with *Shu Jin Huo Lou* (JT)[a] 0.5gm/10# twice daily orally to dispel Wind-Cold, warm the Channels and further relieve *Qi*/Blood Stagnation
- Administer herbal formulae 2-4 months as needed
- A description of all the ingredients of the Chinese herbal medicine listed is beyond the scope of this text, but can be found elsewhere.[18,19]

Food Therapy:
The purpose of the Food therapy is to clear Cold and promote *Qi*/Blood circulation so warming foods are prescribed and cooling foods are avoided.[21]
- Foods to supplement to clear Cold: Lamb, shrimp, corn-fed beef, chicken, trout, squash, turnips, sweet rice, basal, caraway, cherries, chilies, cinnamon, ginger, rosemary, sage
- Foods to supplement to promote *Qi*/Blood circulation: Chicken egg, crab, sweet rice, peaches, carrots, coriander, squash, turnips
- Foods to avoid: Turkey, duck, clams, white fish, mussels, yogurt, millet, barley, spinach, broccoli, celery, cucumber

Tui-na Procedures:
The purpose of the *Tui-na* is to stimulate *Qi* and Blood flow to relieve pain and promote nerve regeneration in the affected region. The descriptions and indications of each technique are outlined in more detail in Chapter 1 Table 8.[20]
- *Ca-fa* rubbing along the back from GV-2 to GV-20 to relieve nerve root *Qi* Stagnation
- *Moo-fa* massaging using the palms or fingers from the shoulder to the paw and the hip to the paw for 3-5 minutes each leg
- *Nie-fa* holding and pinching the skin and muscle in the main muscle groups of each limb for 30 seconds each
- *An-fa* and *Rou-fa* pressing and rotary kneading at LI-10, LI-11, SI-9, TH-14 and GB-21 for the thoracic limb and ST-36, BL-40, GB-34, GB-31, BL-54 for 30 seconds per acupoint
- *Ca-fa* rubbing from the scapula to the carpus and then from the hip to the tarsus on each side for 1 minute on each limb
- *Dou-fa* gently shaking for 12 times, *Ba-shen-fa* stretching for 12 times and *Ban-fa* flexing and extending joints for 12 times; perform on each limb

Daily Life Style Recommendation for Owner Follow-up:
- *Moo-fa* massaging up and down the back and all the muscles of the limbs for 3-5 minutes in each area twice daily until recovers function to improve *Qi*/Blood flow to the peripheral nerves
- *Dou-fa* gently shaking, *Ba-shen-fa* stretching, and *Ban-fa* flexing and extending joints on each limb for 12 times twice daily until recovers to improve *Qi*/Blood flow to the peripheral nerves
- While in lateral recumbency, turn every 4-6 hours to avoid lung atelectasis and decubitus ulcers
- Keep on padding to avoid decubitus ulcers especially on shoulders and hips
- Keep clean of urine and feces and dry to avoid skin lesions
- Feed a high quality soft diet to support *Zheng Qi*
- In the first 7-10 days ensure swallowing is normal and food does not collect in the pharynx
- Keep in a low stress environment to support *Zheng Qi*
- When some movement returns can begin daily supervised swimming
- When some movement returns can begin walking with a sling that supports the neck and thoracic and pelvic limbs

Comments:
Based on experimental and clinical studies of the positive effects of TCVM treatments on immune disorders and nerve regeneration, further clinical studies of TCVM for the treatment of acute polyradiculoneuritis are warranted.[4,5,12-15] Expect TCVM treatments to shorten the recovery time, improve the degree of recovery and reduce the recurrence rate.

3. Kidney *Yin* and *Qi* Deficiency

Clinical Signs:
- Diabetes mellitus
- Irritable due to generalized sensitivity or pain
- Pelvic limb paresis with a plantigrade stance
- Cool seeking
- Panting
- Warm ears, back and feet
- Dry skin
- Tongue- red, dry or pale
- Pulses- deep, rapid weak worse on the left, thready or weak worse on right

TCVM Diagnosis:
The diagnosis of a Deficiency disease is based on the chronicity of the signs and the deep weak pulses. The pelvic limb weakness is associated with Kidney *Qi* Deficiency. Cool seeking, panting, warm ears, back and feet, dry skin, a red, dry tongue and deep, weak, thready pulses, weaker on the left, reflect Kidney *Yin* Deficiency. A pale tongue and weak pulses worse on the right reflect Kidney *Qi* Deficiency.

Treatment Principles:
- Tonify Kidney *Yin*
- Tonify Kidney *Qi*
- Promote local *Qi* flow and restore nerve function

Acupuncture treatment:
Some acupoints may be too painful to treat initially. Because the animal is usually painful, use EA at 20 Hz (cycles/second) for 10-15 minutes followed by 80-120 Hz alternating frequencies for 10-15 minutes. Combine with DN and Aqua-AP and treat both sides. Repeat acupuncture weekly every 1-2 weeks for 6-8 treatments or longer if needed. For Aqua-AP inject 0.25-0.5 ml vitamin B12 into the acupoint.

Acupoints recommended
- EA: GV-3/GV-14, SI-9/SI-9, PC-8/KID-1, LI-10/ST-36, BL-40/BL-40
- DN: BL-23, KID-3, BL-60, KID-6
- Aqua-AP: BL-40, BL-23 (may be too painful to administer during first few treatments)

Pertinent acupoint actions
- During EA, GV-3 can be connected to GV-14 to stimulate the Governing Vessel and *Qi*/Blood Flow in all the peripheral to reduce generalized pain and stimulate regeneration
- SI-9 is a local acupoint near the brachial plexus nerve roots useful to stimulate *Qi*/Blood flow and reduce pain in the thoracic limbs
- BL-40 is the Master point of the pelvic limbs and useful to stimulate *Qi*/Blood flow, reduce pain and strengthen the pelvic limbs
- BL-54 is a local acupoint near the sciatic nerve useful to stimulate *Qi*/Blood flow and reduce pain and strengthen the pelvic limbs
- LI-10 and ST-36 tonify *Qi* and stimulate *Qi* flow in the Channels to reduce pain and promote nerve regeneration
- BL-40 is the Master point of the pelvic limbs and useful to stimulate *Qi*/Blood flow, reduce pain and strengthen the pelvic limbs
- BL-23 is the Back *Shu* Association point for Kidney and is useful to support the Kidney in Deficiency disorders
- KID-3 is the *Yuan* source point for the Kidney and is useful to support the Kidney in Deficiency disorders
- BL-60 is useful to promote *Qi*/Blood flow and reduce pain
- KID-6 is the confluent point of the *Yin Qiao* Extraordinary Channel useful to treat *Yin* Deficiency

Herbal Medicine:
- *Jiang Tang Cha* (JT)[a] 0.5gm/10# twice daily orally to Clear Heat and tonify Kidney *Yin* and *Qi*
- Combine with Body Sore (JT)[a] 0.5gm/10# twice daily orally to relieve pain

- Administer herbal formula for up to 6 months
- Can administer herbs in combination with conventional medications for diabetes mellitus
- A description of all the ingredients of the Chinese herbal medicine listed is beyond the scope of this text, but can be found elsewhere.[18,19]

Food Therapy:

The purpose of Food therapy is to clear false Heat and tonify Kidney *Yin* and tonify Kidney *Qi*. Foods that are Hot are avoided.[21]
- Foods to Cool and tonify *Yin*: Turkey, pork, duck, clams, crab, eggs, rice, wheat, wheat germ, wheat berries, Belgian endive, string beans, peas, kidney beans, sweet potatoes, yams, tomato, spinach, tofu, kiwi, lemons, rhubarb, pears, bananas, watermelon, sesame, seaweed
- Foods to tonify *Qi*: Beef, chicken, sardines, egg, potato, yam, sweet potato, rice, oats, millet, lentils, carrots, squash, microalgae, dates, figs, molasses, royal jelly
- Hot foods to avoid: Lamb, shrimp, corn-fed beef, chicken, trout, squash, turnips, sweet rice, basal, caraway, cherries, chilies, cinnamon, ginger, rosemary, sage

Tui-na Procedures:

The purpose of the *Tui-na* therapy is to stimulate *Qi* and Blood flow to relieve pain and promote nerve regeneration in the affected region, but *Tui-na* may have to be delayed, until the acupuncture and Chinese herbal medicine control the pain. The techniques descriptions and indications are outlined in more detail in Chapter 1 Table 8.[20]
- *Ca-fa* rubbing along the back from *Bai-hui* to GV-20 to relieve nerve root *Qi* Stagnation
- *Moo-fa* massaging using the palms or fingers from the shoulder to the paw and the hip to the paw for 3-5 minutes each leg
- *An-fa* and *Rou-fa* pressing and rotary kneading at LI-10, LI-11, SI-9, TH-14 and GB-21 for the thoracic limb and ST-36, BL-40, GB-34, GB-31, BL-54 for 30 seconds per acupoint
- *Ca-fa* rubbing from the scapula to the carpus and then from the hip to the tarsus on each side for 1 minute on each limb
- *Dou-fa* gently shaking for 12 times, *Ba-shen-fa* stretching for 12 times and *Ban-fa* flexing and extending joints for 12 times; perform on each limb

Daily Life Style Recommendation for Owner Follow-up:
- Continue conventional medications to control diabetes, but monitor closely as may need less
- Once pain has been controlled, home *Tui-na* may begin
- Gentle *Moo-fa* massaging up and down the back and all the muscles of the limbs for 3-5 minutes twice daily to improve *Qi*/Blood flow to the peripheral nerves
- *Dou-fa* gently shaking, *Ba-shen-fa* stretching, and *Ban-fa* flexing and extending joints on each limb for 12 times twice daily until recovers to improve *Qi*/Blood flow to the peripheral nerves
- Reduce simple carbohydrate intake
- Reduce weight if overweight, but do slowly and do not stress the animal

- Keep in a low stress environment to avoid Liver *Qi* Stagnation and Liver *Yang* rising so Kidney *Yin* is not stressed further

Comments:
Based on experimental studies of the positive effects of TCVM for diabetic polyneuropathy, further clinical studies of TCVM are warranted.[7-10] Expect TCVM treatments to improve control of the diabetes mellitus and resolve pain and paresis.[11]

4. Spleen *Qi* and Kidney *Qi* Deficiency

Clinical Signs:
- Chronic progressive or intermittent recurrent onset
- Paraparesis, quadriparesis, quadriplegia (Grades 3-5 deficits neurological deficits)
- Depressed or absent patellar reflexes
- +/- Generalized sensitivity or pain
- +/- Depression or absence of other limb reflexes
- +/-Facial paresis
- +/-Laryngeal paresis
- +/- Pharyngeal paresis
- Tongue- pale, wet
- Pulses- deep, weak worse on the right

TCVM Diagnosis:
The diagnosis of a Deficiency disease is based on the chronicity of the signs and the deep weak pulses. Weakness and muscle atrophy (*Wei* syndrome) are characteristic of Spleen *Qi* Deficiency and paresis or paralysis (*Tan-Huan* syndrome) is characteristic of Kidney *Qi* Deficiency. A pale, wet tongue and pulses weaker on the right are typical of Spleen *Qi* and Kidney *Qi* Deficiencies.

Treatment Principles:
- Tonify Spleen *Qi*
- Tonify Kidney *Qi*
- Promote local *Qi* flow and restore nerve function

Acupuncture treatment:
If the animal is painful (rare) use EA 20 Hz (cycles/second) for 10-15 minutes followed by 80-120 Hz alternating frequencies for 10-15 minutes. If not painful, use EA at 80-120 Hz for 20-30 minutes. Combine with DN and Aqua-AP and treat both sides. Repeat acupuncture weekly for 3-5 treatments then every 2-4weeks for 6-8 treatments or longer if needed. For Aqua-AP inject 0.25-0.5 ml vitamin B12 into the acupoint.

Acupoints recommended
- EA: GV-3/GV-14, SI-9/SI-9, BL-54/BL-54, LI-10/ST-36, BL-40/BL-40; can add *Liu-feng/Liu-feng* or PC-8/KID-1 if non ambulatory (Grades 3-5 neurological deficits)

- DN: BL-20, BL-21, BL-23, KID-3, SP-3
- Aqua-AP: GV-14, BL-20, BL-21, BL-23

Pertinent acupoint actions
- During EA, GV-3 can be connected to GV-14 to stimulate the Governing Vessel and *Qi* Flow in all the spinal nerve roots
- GV-14 is also useful to balance the immune system
- SI-9 is a local acupoint near the brachial plexus nerve roots useful to stimulate *Qi*/Blood flow to the region and stimulate nerve regeneration
- BL-54 is a local acupoint near the sciatic nerve useful to stimulate *Qi*/Blood flow to the region useful to stimulate *Qi*/Blood flow to the region and stimulate nerve regeneration
- LI-10 and ST-36 tonify *Qi* and stimulate *Qi* flow in the Channels
- ST-36 is also useful to balance the immune system
- BL-40 is the master point for the pelvic limbs
- *Li-feng* acupoints (at the skin fold on the dorsal aspect of the metacarpophalangeal and metatarsophalangeal joints of all four feet) between digits 2-3, 3-4 and 4-5) are useful to treat limb paralysis
- KID-1 and PC-8 are the "four roots" and are also useful to treat limb paralysis
- LI-4 is useful to balance the immune system (*Zheng Qi*)
- BL-20 is the Back *Shu* Association point for Spleen and is useful to support the Spleen in Deficiency disorders
- BL-21 is the Back *Shu* Association point for Stomach and is useful to support the Spleen and Stomach in Deficiency disorders
- BL-23 is the Back *Shu* Association point for Kidney and is useful to support the Kidney in Deficiency disorders
- KID-3 is the *Yuan* source point for the Kidney and is useful to support the Kidney *Qi* in Deficiency disorders
- SP-3 is the *Yuan* source point for the Spleen and is useful to support the Spleen *Qi* in Deficiency disorders

Herbal Medicine:
- *Bu Yang Huan Wu* (JT)[a] 0.5gm/10# twice daily orally to tonify Kidney *Qi*
- If the animal has generalized pain (rare), add Body Sore (JT)[a] 0.5gm/10# twice daily orally to resolve *Qi*/Blood Stagnation and pain
- Administer Body Sore for 1-2 months or longer if needed
- Administer *Bu Yang Huan Wu* for up to 6 months
- A description of all the ingredients of the Chinese herbal medicine listed is beyond the scope of this text, but can be found elsewhere.[18,19]

Food Therapy:
The purpose of the Food therapy is to tonify Spleen and Kidney *Qi* to support nerve regeneration. Foods that are Cold or Hot are avoided.[21]

- Foods to supplement to tonify Spleen and Kidney *Qi*: Beef, chicken, sardines, egg, potato, yam, sweet potato, rice, oats, millet, lentils, carrots, squash, microalgae, dates, figs, molasses, royal jelly
- Cold foods to avoid: Turkey, duck, duck eggs, conch, clams, mussels, yogurt, millet, barley, spinach, broccoli, celery, egg plant, kelp, alfalfa, cucumbers, pears, bananas, white radishes, watermelon
- Hot foods to avoid: Lamb, shrimp, corn-fed beef, chicken, trout, squash, turnips, sweet rice, basal, caraway, cherries, chilies, cinnamon, ginger, rosemary, sage

Tui-na Procedures:

The purpose of the *Tui-na* therapy is to stimulate *Qi* and Blood flow in the affected region, relieve pain if present and promote regeneration of nerves. If the animal has generalized pain, delay *Tui-na* therapy until the pain has subsided. The descriptions and indications of each technique are outlined in more detail in Chapter 1 Table 8.[20]

- *Ca-fa* rubbing along the back from GV-2 to GV-20 to relieve nerve root *Qi* Stagnation
- *Moo-fa* massaging using the palms or fingers from the shoulder to the paw and the hip to the paw for 3-5 minutes on each side
- *Nie-fa* holding and pinching the skin and muscle in the main muscle groups of each limb for 30 seconds each
- *An-fa* and *Rou-fa* pressing and rotary kneading at LI-10, LI-11, SI-9, TH-14 and GB-21 for the thoracic limb and ST-36, BL-40, GB-34, GB-31, BL-54 for 30 seconds per acupoint
- *Ca-fa* rubbing from the scapula to the carpus and then from the hip to the tarsus on each side for 1 minute on each limb
- *Dou-fa* gently shaking for 12 times, *Ba-shen-fa* stretching for 12 times and *Ban-fa* flexing and extending joints for 12 times; perform on each limb

Daily Life Style Recommendation for Owner Follow-up:

- If painful, delay *Tui-na* therapy until the pain has subsided otherwise begin immediately
- *Moo-fa* massaging up and down the back and all the muscles of the limbs for 3-5 minutes in each area twice daily until recovers function to improve *Qi*/Blood flow to the peripheral nerves
- *Dou-fa* gently shaking, *Ba-shen-fa* stretching, and *Ban-fa* flexing and extending joints on each limb for 12 times twice daily until recovers to improve *Qi*/Blood flow to the peripheral nerves
- If in lateral recumbency, turn every 4-6 hours to avoid lung atelectasis and decubitus ulcers
- Keep on padding to avoid decubitus ulcers especially on shoulders and hips
- Keep clean of urine and feces and dry to avoid skin lesions
- Feed a high quality soft diet to support *Zheng Qi*
- Ensure swallowing is normal and food does not collect in the pharynx
- Keep in a low stress environment to reduce the chances of Liver *Qi* Stagnation and over-control of the Spleen further weakening the Spleen
- If the animal has movement allow supervised swimming 3-5 times weekly

- If the animal is able stand and walk with a sling that supports the neck and thoracic and pelvic limbs

Comments:
Based on experimental and clinical studies of the positive effects of TCVM treatments on immune disorders and nerve regeneration, further clinical studies of TCVM for the treatment of chronic and recurring polyneuropathies are warranted.[12-15,26] Expect TCVM treatments to shorten the recovery time, improve the degree of recovery and reduce the recurrence rate.

MYASTHENIA GRAVIS

Myasthenia gravis in dogs and cats commonly presents as episodic or exercise-induced weakness due to impaired transmission of acetylcholine at the neuromuscular junctions of skeletal muscles.[1-3] Other clinical presentations of myasthenia gravis include: dysphagia, laryngeal paresis, regurgitation, paraparesis and quadriparesis. Acquired myasthenia gravis is associated with an immune-mediated or paraneoplastic process. Antibodies are formed against the acetylcholine receptors of skeletal muscles and the resulting immune complexes interfere with normal muscle contraction. With exercise, affected animals will develop a progressive shortened stride that progresses to total fatigue and inability to walk. Strength returns after a brief rest and the animal will again be able to ambulate for a short distance. The palpebral and sometimes patellar reflexes will fatigue with repeated testing and in other animals continual facial nerve paresis or paralysis is present. Despite profound weakness, conscious proprioception and other spinal reflexes are usually normal. Megaesophagus and dysphagia are common and can result in excessive salivation, regurgitation, aspiration pneumonia and death. A definitive diagnosis can be made with serology documenting elevated acetylcholine receptor (AchR) antibodies in the serum. As some cases may be falsely seronegative, re-testing is important in all weak animals suspected to have myasthenia gravis. The severity of clinical signs may not correspond with the degree of elevation of AchR antibody titers.

Megaesophagus and aspiration pneumonia may be seen on thoracic radiographs. In paraneoplastic myasthenia gravis, a thymoma may be seen as a cranial mediastinal mass on thoracic radiographs. Thorough physical and radiographic examinations including abdominal ultrasonography should be performed to search for neoplasia. Some dogs with myasthenia gravis have concurrent hypothyroidism and weakness will not improve until both disorders are treated. In hypothyroid animals, the serum total T4 or free T4 levels are usually reduced and TSH levels are usually elevated. Myasthenia gravis and polymyositis may also occur concurrently and serum creatine kinase levels may be elevated. An electromyogram is often normal in cases of myasthenia gravis except for a decremental evoked muscle response on repetitive nerve stimulation of 5/second.

Initial conventional therapy usually consists of the administration of oral pyridostigmine bromide (Mestinon) 0.5-3 mg/kg every 8-12 hours with food. A liquid formulation of pyridostigmine bromide is recommended, so that the dose can be easily adjusted to the level needed to control the clinical signs. With high doses, weakness may occur as a result of a cholinergic crisis and therefore a low dose of pyridostigmine is initially given, then slowly increased until weakness is resolved. Oral famotidine (Pepcid AC) 5 mg/kg/day may reduce the nausea and gastrointestinal irritation from the pyridostigmine bromide. Concurrent hypothyroidism is treated with levothyroxine sodium (Soloxine). Although spontaneous remissions occur, so do disease recurences. Since there are adverse side effects to conventional medications and they do not treat the underlying cause, TCVM may offer support for the effective resolution of myasthenia gravis.

The diagnosis and treatment of the most likely TCVM pattern associated with myasthenia gravis is outlined in Tables 1 and 2. There are some clinical studies in humans and an experimental study in rats that support the use of acupuncture and Chinese herbal medicine for their immunomodulating effects on clinical and experimental myasthenia gravis, so further studies in veterinary medicine are warranted.[23-26] Since spontaneous remission occurs, well controlled studies are needed to ensure TCVM treatments actually enhance remission and resolution of signs.

Etiology and Pathology

Some chronic immune-mediated disorders (*Zheng Qi* imbalance) like myasthenia gravis, may be associated with chronic Spleen *Qi* and Kidney *Qi* Deficiencies.[22] Since myasthenia gravis is common in German Shepherds, Golden Retrievers and other large pure breed dogs, an underlying Kidney *Jing* Deficiency may make these breeds more likely to develop Kidney and Spleen *Qi* Deficiency. As with chronic polyneuropathies, over time poor nutrition, chronic illness and environmental stress can also weaken the Spleen and negatively affect normal transformation and transportation functions in any dog or cat. The result is Spleen *Qi* Deficiency with reduced *Gu Qi* (Food *Qi*) and *Ying Qi* (Nutrient *Qi*) necessary to regenerate *Qi* and Blood. *Gu Qi* is also essential for a normal functioning *Zheng Qi* (immune system) and immune imbalances can be associated with Spleen *Qi* Deficiency. Prolonged Spleen *Qi* Deficiency and reduced post-natal *Jing* can stress prenatal Kidney *Jing* and cause Kidney *Qi* Deficiency. A manifestation of Spleen *Qi* Deficiency is *Wei* syndrome, generalized weakness and weakness worse on exercise. A manifestation of Kidney *Qi* Deficiency is fatigue and *Tan-Huan* syndrome or paresis of the pelvic limbs alone or all four limbs. Together Spleen *Qi* and Kidney *Qi* Deficiencies can result in *Zheng Qi* imbalance and fatigue and exercise induced weakness as seen in myasthenia gravis. Applying the basic TCVM theories of *Yin/Yang*, Eight Principles, Five Treasures, Five Elements and *Zang Fu* physiology and pathology to make a TCVM diagnosis, there is currently one primary pattern associated with the typical presentation of myasthenia in dogs and cats. With more critical examination and experience, other TCVM patterns with different diagnostic features and requiring different treatments may be found:

1. **Spleen *Qi* and Kidney *Qi* Deficiency**
Over time, poor nutrition, chronic illness or environmental stress can result in Spleen *Qi* and Kidney *Qi* Deficiencies. The result is reduction of *Qi* flow to superficial tissues including nerves and muscles producing fatigue and exercise intolerance.

Pattern Differentiation and Treatment

1. Spleen *Qi* and Kidney *Qi* Deficiency

<u>Clinical Signs:</u>
- Episodic weakness worse with exercise
- Normal conscious proprioception
- Eyelid paresis with repetitive touching to stimulate closure
- Depressed patellar reflexes after repetitive stimulation to elicit the reflex

- Muscles are not painful unless has concurrent polymyositis
- Megaesophagus
- +/-Facial paresis
- +/-Laryngeal paresis
- +/- Pharyngeal paresis
- Tongue- pale, wet
- Pulses- deep, weak worse on the right

TCVM Diagnosis:

The diagnosis of a Deficiency disease is based on the chronicity of the signs and the deep, weak pulses. Fatigue, exercise intolerance and muscle weakness (*Wei* syndrome) are characteristic of Spleen *Qi* Deficiency and fatigue, exercise intolerance and paresis or paralysis (*Tan-Huan* syndrome) are characteristic of Kidney *Qi* Deficiency. A pale, wet tongue and pulses weaker on the right are typical of Spleen *Qi* and Kidney *Qi* Deficiencies.

Treatment Principles:
- Tonify Spleen *Qi*
- Tonify Kidney *Qi*
- Promote local *Qi* flow and restore nerve function

Acupuncture treatment:

Since repetitive nerve stimulation can cause muscle fatigue to worsen, EA should be avoided until there is more experience treating this disease with acupuncture. Based on the clinical studies in humans, moxibustion (warming of needles and keep warm not hot for 3-5 minutes at each site) is recommended along with regular DN for 20-30 minutes. Repeat acupuncture weekly every 1-2 weeks for 6-8 treatments or longer if needed. For Aqua-AP inject 0.25-0.5 ml vitamin B12 into the acupoint.

Acupoints recommended
- DN moxibustion (warm needles for 3-5 minutes each): *Bai-hui,* BL-20, BL-21, BL-23
- DN regular: *Bai-hui,* BL-20, BL-21, BL-23, GV-14, LI-10, ST-36, BL-40, BL-54, SI-9, LI-4, KID-3, SP-3
- Aqua-AP: BL-20, BL-21, BL-23

Pertinent acupoint actions
- *Bai-hui* (midline at the lumbosacral junction) is useful to support Kidney and strengthen the pelvic limbs
- BL-20 is the Back *Shu* Association point for Spleen and is useful to support the Spleen in Deficiency disorders
- BL-21 is the Back *Shu* Association point for Stomach and is useful to support the Spleen and Stomach in Deficiency disorders
- BL-23 is the Back *Shu* Association point for Kidney and is useful to support the Kidney in Deficiency disorders
- GV-14 is also to balance the immune system

- LI-10 and ST-36 tonify *Qi* and stimulate *Qi* flow in the Channels
- ST-36 is also useful to balance the immune system
- KID-1 and PC-8 are the "four roots" and are also useful to treat limb weakness
- BL-40 is the Master point for the pelvic limbs
- BL-54 is a local acupoint near the sciatic nerve is useful to treat pelvic limb weakness
- SI-9 is a local acupoint near the brachial plexus useful to treat thoracic limb weakness
- LI-4 is useful to balance *Zheng Qi*
- KID-3 is the *Yuan* source point for the Kidney and is useful to support the Kidney *Qi* in Deficiency disorders
- SP-3 is the *Yuan* source point for the Spleen and is useful to support the Spleen *Qi* in Deficiency disorders

Herbal Medicine:
- *Bu Yang Huan Wu* (JT)[a] 0.5gm/10# twice daily orally to tonify Kidney *Qi*
- Administer *Bu Yang Huan Wu* up to 6 months
- A description of all the ingredients of the Chinese herbal medicine listed is beyond the scope of this text, but can be found elsewhere.[18,19]

Food Therapy:
The purpose of the Food therapy is to tonify Spleen and Kidney *Qi* to support neuromuscular regeneration. Foods that are Cold or Hot are avoided.[21]
- Foods to tonify Spleen and Kidney *Qi*: Beef, chicken, sardines, egg, potato, yam, sweet potato, rice, oats, millet, lentils, carrots, squash, microalgae, dates, figs, molasses, royal jelly
- Cold foods to avoid: Turkey, duck, duck eggs, conch, clams, mussels, yogurt, millet, barley, spinach, broccoli, celery, egg plant, kelp, alfalfa, cucumbers, pears, bananas, white radishes, watermelon
- Hot foods to avoid: Lamb, shrimp, corn-fed beef, chicken, trout, squash, turnips, sweet rice, basal, caraway, cherries, chilies, cinnamon, ginger, rosemary, sage

Tui-na Procedures:
The purpose of the *Tui-na* therapy is to stimulate *Qi* and Blood flow to promote regeneration of the neuromuscular junction region, tonify Spleen and Kidney *Qi* and balance the immune system. The descriptions and indications of each technique are outlined in more detail in Chapter 1 Table 8.[20]
- *Ca-fa* rubbing along the back from GV-2 to GV-20
- *Moo-fa* massaging using the palms or fingers from the shoulder to the paw and the hip to the paw for 3-5 minutes on each side
- *Nie-fa* holding and pinching the skin and muscle in the main muscle groups of each limb for 30 seconds each

- *An-fa* and *Rou-fa* pressing and rotary kneading along the back at BL-20, BL-21, BL-23, at LI-10, LI-11, SI-9, TH-14 and GB-21 for the thoracic limb and ST-36, BL-40, GB-34, GB-31, BL-54 for 30 seconds per acupoint; treat back and all four legs
- *Ca-fa* rubbing from the scapula to the carpus and then from the hip to the tarsus on each side for 1 minute on each limb
- *Ba-shen-fa* stretching and *Dou-fa* gently shaking each limb for 12 times

Daily Life Style Recommendation for Owner Follow-up:
- *Moo-fa* massaging up and down the back and all the muscles of the limbs for 3-5 minutes in each area to improve *Qi*/Blood flow to the nerves and muscles
- *Ba-shen-fa* stretching and *Dou-fa* gently shaking each limb for 12 times twice daily until recovers to improve *Qi*/Blood flow to the nerves and muscles
- Feed a high quality soft diet to support *Zheng Qi*
- Feed with head held elevated and for 10 minutes after eating until megaesophagus has resolved
- Ensure swallowing is normal to avoid choking
- Keep in a low stress environment to reduce the changes of Liver *Qi* Stagnation and over-control of the Spleen
- Begin slow walking but go slowly with adequate rest periods so muscles do not fatigue; can increase duration and speed as animal becomes stronger

Comments:

Based on the limited clinical and experimental studies of the positive effects of TCVM on myasthenia gravis and other immune mediated disorders, further clinical studies of TCVM treatments for myasthenia gravis in animals are warranted.[23-26] Expect TCVM treatments to shorten the recovery time, improve the degree of recovery of neuromuscular junction function and reduce recurrences.

POLYMYOSITIS

Polymyositis is a generalized inflammatory process of the muscles, most commonly due to an idiopathic process that may be immune-mediated in adult dogs and cats.[2,3] The clinical findings include acute or chronic exercise intolerance and muscle weakness, which can be continuous or episodic. Anorexia, dysphagia and weight loss may also occur. Some dogs are presented with recurrent bouts of aspiration pneumonia secondary to dysphagia and megaesophagus. A stiff and stilted gait and muscle pain and atrophy are often present. The musculature of the the head is antigenically different than the limb and back muscles so is rarely affected in polymyositis.

A CBC may be normal or have leukocytosis. Serum creatine kinase is often elevated. Serum immunoassays for Neospora caninum or Toxoplasma gondii should be performed to rule out a muscle infection from one of these organisms. A serum anti-nuclear antibody (ANA) assay may be positive, supporting an immune-mediated process, but is often normal in other animals suspected to have immune-mediated polymyositis. Histological evidence of muscle inflammation is found on examination of a muscle biopsy. A thorough evaluation for neoplasia should be performed including thoracic and abdominal radiographs and abdominal ultrasound. If an underlying disease process such as neoplasia or infection is found then that must also be treated.

Corticosteroids and other immunosuppressive drugs are the conventional treatment for idiopathic polymyositis, but recurrences can occur when the medication is discontinued.

The diagnosis and treatment of common TCVM patterns associated with polymyositis are outlined in Tables 1 and 2. One study of the TCVM treatment of experimental polymyositis in guinea pigs showed a positive response with Chinese herbal medicine.[27] There are currently no case studies using TCVM treatments for polymyositis in the human or veterinary literature. Because of the long-term adverse effects of immunosuppressive therapy, possibility of disease recurrence and the therapeutic effects of TCVM treatments in other immune-mediated diseases, further studies of the TCVM treatments for polymyositis are warranted.[26]

Etiology and Pathology

Once again, when *Zheng Qi* is weakened from poor nutrition, chronic illness, environmental stress or age, the *Wei Qi* portion of *Zheng Qi* that protects the body's exterior becomes weak and external pathogens such as Wind-Heat or Wind-Cold gain entrance.[2] In general, the basic constitution of the animal can affect their susceptibility to invasion of either Wind/Cold or Wind/Heat. When *Zheng Qi* is weakened, *Yin* animals like Water, Metal and Earth constitutions tend to be more susceptible to Wind-Cold invasion, while *Yang* animals like Wood and Fire constitutions are more susceptible to Wind-Heat invasion.[22] More experience is needed to determine if this holds true for animals with polymyositis.

More chronic forms of polymyositis may be associated with Spleen *Qi* and Kidney *Qi* Deficiencies and result in a *Zheng Qi* imbalance (immune-mediated disease).[2] As previously stated, a poor quality diet, chronic illness and environmental stress can weaken the Spleen and negatively impact normal transformation and transportation functions over time. The result is Spleen *Qi* Deficiency and reduced *Gu Qi* (Food *Qi*) and *Ying Qi* (Nutrient *Qi*) needed to regenerate *Qi* and Blood. *Gu Qi* is essential for a normal functioning *Zheng Qi* (immune system) and immune imbalances can result from Spleen *Qi* Deficiency. Prolonged Spleen *Qi* Deficiency and reduced post-natal *Jing* can stress prenatal Kidney *Jing* and cause Kidney *Qi* Deficiency. A manifestation of Spleen *Qi* Deficiency is *Wei* syndrome, weakness and atrophy from reduced *Qi* flow in the muscles. Since *Qi* is necessary to carry Blood, Blood can become Stagnant and cause muscle pain. A manifestation of Kidney *Qi* Deficiency is *Tan-Huan* syndrome or paresis of the pelvic limbs alone or all four limbs. Together Spleen *Qi* and Kidney *Qi* Deficiencies can result in fatigue and exercise induced weakness. Applying the basic TCVM theories of *Yin/Yang*, Eight Principles, Five Treasures, Five Elements and *Zang Fu* physiology and pathology to make a TCVM diagnosis, there are currently two primary patterns associated with the acute and chronic forms of polymyositis in dogs and cats, but with more experience other TCVM patterns like Wind-Cold invasion, with different diagnostic features and requiring different treatment, may be found:

1. **Wind-Heat invasion causing *Qi*/Blood Stagnation and generalized *Qi* Deficiency**
   When *Wei Qi* becomes weak due to poor nutrition, chronic illness or environmental stress, Wind-Heat invades the Channels of the limbs causing *Qi*/Blood Stagnation that results in Deficiency of *Qi* flow to local tissues including muscles. The result is muscle pain and weakness.

2. Spleen *Qi* and Kidney *Qi* Deficiency with Blood Stagnation

Over time poor nutrition, chronic illness or environmental stress can result in Spleen *Qi* and Kidney *Qi* Deficiencies. The result is a reduction of *Qi* flow to superficial tissues including muscles resulting weakness and exercise intolerance. Blood Stagnation occurs because *Qi* is needed to move the Blood and the muscles become painful.

Pattern Differentiation and Treatment

1. Wind-Heat invasion causing *Qi*/Blood Stagnation and generalized *Qi* Deficiency

Clinical Signs:
- Acute onset
- Regurgitation
- Megaesophagus
- Muscle weakness worse with exercise
- Stiff, stilted gait
- Painful muscles
- Normal conscious proprioception
- Normal spinal reflexes
- Cool seeking
- Panting
- Warm ears, back and feet
- Tongue- red, dry or purple
- Pulses- Superficial, forceful, rapid or wiry

TCVM Diagnosis:

The acute onset of clinical signs is typical of an Excess pattern with invasion of an External pathogen and *Qi*/Blood Stagnation. The diagnosis of Wind-Heat invasion causing *Qi*/Blood Stagnation and local *Qi* Deficiency is based on the clinical findings. The warmth of the ears, back and feet are typical of a Heat pattern. The tongue color will vary with the stage of the process. The tongue is red and dry from the Wind-Heat, purple if *Qi*/Blood Stagnation is most prominent and pale if *Qi* Deficiency is most prominent. The pulses may be forceful and rapid from the Heat or wiry from the *Qi*/Blood Stagnation.

Treatment Principles:
- Clear Wind-Heat
- Resolve *Qi*/Blood Stagnation
- Promote local *Qi* and Blood flow to the muscles

Acupuncture treatment:

Because muscle pain is common with polymyositis, use EA 20 Hz (cycles/second) for 10-15 minutes followed by 80-120 Hz alternating frequencies for 10-15 minutes. Some acupoints in muscle bellies may be too painful to treat initially so choose less painful acupoints to avoid undue patient stress. Combine with DN and Aqua-AP and treat both sides. Repeat acupuncture weekly for 3-5 treatments then every 2-4 weeks for 6-8 treatments or longer if needed. For Aqua-AP inject 0.25-0.5 ml vitamin B12 into the acupoint

Acupoints recommended
- EA: GV-3/GV-14, SI-9/SI-9, BL-54/BL-54, BL-40/BL-40
- DN: GB-20, *Er-jian*, *Wei-jian*, LI-4, LI-11, ST-36, LI-10, *Bai-hui*, KID-1, PC-8
- Aqua-AP: GB-20

Pertinent acupoint actions
- During EA, GV-3 can be connected to GV-14 to stimulate the Governing Vessel and *Qi* Flow in all the paravertebral muscles
- GV-14 is also useful to clear Heat and balance the immune system
- SI-9 is a local acupoint useful to stimulate *Qi*/Blood flow in the muscles of the region
- BL-54 is a local acupoint useful to stimulate *Qi*/Blood flow to muscles of the region
- BL-40 is the Master point for the pelvic limbs
- GB-20 is useful to dispel Wind
- *Er-jian* (ear tip) and *Wei-jian* (tail tip) are useful to clear Heat
- LI-4 and LI-11 are also useful to clear Heat and balance the immune system
- LI-10 and ST-36 tonify *Qi* and stimulate *Qi* flow in the Channels
- ST-36 is also useful to balance the immune system
- *Bai-hui* (midline at the lumbosacral junction) is useful to strengthen the pelvic limbs
- KID-1 and PC-8 are the "four roots" and are also useful to treat limb weakness

Herbal Medicine:
- *Wu Wei Xiao Du Yin* (MW)[b] 0.5gm/10# twice daily orally to clear Heat and disperse Wind-Heat
- Administer *Wu Wei Xiao Du Yin* for 2-4 months as needed
- A description of all the ingredients of the Chinese herbal medicine listed is beyond the scope of this text, but can be found elsewhere.[18,19]

Food Therapy:
The purpose of the Food therapy is to clear Heat and promote *Qi*/Blood circulation, so cooling foods are prescribed and Hot foods are avoided.[21]
- Foods to supplement to cleat Heat: Turkey, duck, duck eggs, conch, clams, mussels, yogurt, millet, barley, spinach, broccoli, celery, egg plant, kelp, alfalfa, cucumbers, pears, bananas, white radishes, watermelon
- Foods to promote *Qi*/Blood circulation: Chicken egg, crab, sweet rice, peaches, carrots, coriander, turnips
- Foods to avoid: Lamb, shrimp, corn-fed beef, chicken, trout, squash, turnips, sweet rice, basal, caraway, cherries, chilies, cinnamon, ginger, rosemary, sage

Tui-na Procedures:

Delay *Tui-na* treatments until muscle pain has been controlled. The purpose of the *Tui-na* is to stimulate *Qi* and Blood flow in the affected region to relieve pain and promote muscle regeneration and function. The technique descriptions and indications are outlined in more detail in Chapter 1 Table 8.[20]

- *Ca-fa* rubbing along the back from GV-2 to GV-20
- *Moo-fa* massaging using the palms or fingers from the shoulder to the paw and the hip to the paw for 3-5 minutes on each side
- *Nie-fa* holding and pinching the skin and muscle in the main muscle groups of each limb for 30 seconds each
- *An-fa* and *Rou-fa* pressing and rotary kneading along the neck and back at GB-20, GV-14 and *Bai-hui*, on the thoracic limb at LI-10, LI-11, SI-9, TH-14 and GB-21 and the pelvic limbs at ST-36, BL-40, GB-34, GB-31, BL-54 for 30 seconds per acupoint; treat back and all four legs
- *Ca-fa* rubbing from the scapula to the carpus and then from the hip to the tarsus on each side for 1 minute on each limb
- *Ba-shen-fa* stretching and *Dou-fa* gently shaking each limb for 12 times

Daily Life Style Recommendation for Owner Follow-up:

- Delay *Tui-na* treatments until muscle pain has been controlled
- *Moo-fa* massaging up and down the back and all the muscles of the limbs for 3-5 minutes in each area to improve *Qi*/Blood flow to the nerves and muscles
- *Ba-shen-fa* stretching and *Dou-fa* gently shaking each limb for 12 times twice daily until recovers to improve *Qi*/Blood flow to the nerves and muscles
- Feed a high quality soft diet to support *Zheng Qi*
- Feed with head held elevated and for 10 minutes after eating until megaesophagus has resolved
- Ensure swallowing is normal to avoid choking
- Keep in a low stress environment to further balance *Zheng Qi*
- Once pain is controlled, begin walking or supervised swimming, but go slowly with adequate rest periods so muscles do not fatigue; can increase duration and speed as animal becomes stronger

Comments:

Based on clinical and experimental studies of the positive effects of TCVM to control pain and for other immune-mediated disorders, further clinical studies of TCVM treatments for polymyositis are warranted.[11,26,27] Expect TCVM treatments to relieve pain, shorten the recovery time, improve the degree of recovery and reduce recurrences.

1. Spleen *Qi* and Kidney *Qi* Deficiency with Blood Stagnation

Clinical Signs:

- Episodic weakness worse with exercise

- Stiff, stilted gait
- May have muscle atrophy
- Normal conscious proprioception
- Normal spinal reflexes
- Muscles are painful on palpation
- Megaesophagus
- Tongue- pale, wet or purple
- Pulses- deep, weak worse on the right or wiry

TCVM Diagnosis:
The diagnosis of a Deficiency disease is based on the chronicity of the signs and the deep, weak pulses. Fatigue, exercise intolerance and muscle weakness and atrophy (*Wei* syndrome) are characteristic of Spleen *Qi* Deficiency and fatigue, exercise intolerance and paresis (*Tan-Huan* syndrome) are characteristic of Kidney *Qi* Deficiency. A pale, wet tongue and pulses weaker on the right are typical of Spleen *Qi* and Kidney *Qi* Deficiencies. If pain is severe the tongue may be purple and the pulses may be wiry from *Qi*/Blood Stagnation.

Treatment Principles:
- Tonify Spleen *Qi*
- Tonify Kidney *Qi*
- Resolve *Qi*/Blood Stagnation
- Promote local *Qi* flow to restore muscle function and regenerate muscles

Acupuncture treatment:
Because muscle pain is common with polymyositis, use EA 20 Hz (cycles/second) for 10-15 minutes followed by 80-120 Hz alternating frequencies for 10-15 minutes. Some acupoints in muscle bellies may be too painful to treat initially, so choose less painful acupoints to avoid undue patient stress. Combine EA with DN and Aqua-AP and treat both sides. Repeat acupuncture weekly for 3-5 treatments then every 2-4 weeks for 6-8 treatments or longer if needed. For Aqua-AP inject 0.25-0.5 ml vitamin B12 into the acupoint.

Acupoints recommended
- EA: GV-3/GV-14, SI-9/SI-9, BL-54/BL-54, LI-10/ST-36, BL-40/BL-40
- DN: BL-20, BL-21, BL-23, KID-3, SP-3
- Aqua-AP: GV-14, BL-20, BL-21, BL-23

Pertinent acupoint actions
- During EA, GV-3 can be connected to GV-14 to stimulate the Governing Vessel and *Qi* Flow in all the paravertebral muscles
- GV-14 is also useful to balance the immune system
- SI-9 is a local acupoint useful to stimulate *Qi*/Blood flow in the muscles of the region
- BL-54 is a local acupoint useful to stimulate *Qi*/Blood flow to muscles of the region

- LI-10 and ST-36 tonify *Qi* and stimulate *Qi* flow in the Channels and muscles of the region
- ST-36 is also useful to balance the immune system
- BL-40 is the master point for the pelvic limbs to strengthen the muscles
- LI-4 is useful to balance *Zheng Qi*
- BL-20 is the Back *Shu* Association point for Spleen and is useful to support the Spleen in Deficiency disorders
- BL-21 is the Back *Shu* Association point for Stomach and is useful to support the Spleen and Stomach in Deficiency disorders
- BL-23 is the Back *Shu* Association point for Kidney and is useful to support the Kidney in Deficiency disorders
- KID-3 is the *Yuan* source point for the Kidney and is useful to support the Kidney *Qi* in Deficiency disorders
- SP-3 is the *Yuan* source point for the Spleen and is useful to support the Spleen *Qi* in Deficiency disorders

Herbal Medicine:
- *Bu Yang Huan Wu* (JT)[a] 0.5gm/10# twice daily orally to tonify Kidney *Qi*
- Combine with Body Sore (JT)[a] 0.5gm/10# twice daily orally to treat Blood Stagnation while painful
- Administer Body Sore for 1-2 months or longer if needed
- *Bu Yang Huan Wu* up to 6 months
- A description of all the ingredients of the Chinese herbal medicine listed is beyond the scope of this text, but can be found elsewhere.[18,19]

Food Therapy:

The purpose of the Food therapy is to tonify Spleen and Kidney *Qi* to support neuromuscular regeneration. Foods that are Cold or Hot are avoided.[21]
- Foods to tonify Spleen and Kidney *Qi*: Beef, chicken, sardines, egg, potato, yam, sweet potato, rice, oats, millet, lentils, carrots, squash, microalgae, dates, figs, molasses, royal jelly
- Cold foods to avoid: Turkey, duck, duck eggs, conch, clams, mussels, yogurt, millet, barley, spinach, broccoli, celery, egg plant, kelp, alfalfa, cucumbers, pears, bananas, white radishes, watermelon
- Hot foods to avoid: Lamb, shrimp, corn-fed beef, chicken, trout, squash, turnips, sweet rice, basal, caraway, cherries, chilies, cinnamon, ginger, rosemary, sage

Tui-na Procedures:

Delay *Tui-na* treatments until muscle pain has been controlled. The purpose of the *Tui-na* is to stimulate *Qi* and Blood flow in the affected region to relieve pain and promote muscle regeneration and function. The technique descriptions and indications are outlined in more detail in Chapter 1 Table 8.[20]
- *Ca-fa* rubbing along the back from GV-2 to GV-20
- *Moo-fa* massaging using the palms or fingers from the shoulder to the paw and the hip to the paw for 3-5 minutes on each side

- *Nie-fa* holding and pinching the skin and muscle in the main muscle groups of each limb for 30 seconds each
- *An-fa* and *Rou-fa* pressing and rotary kneading along the back at BL-20, BL-21, BL-23, at LI-10, LI-11, SI-9, TH-14 and GB-21 for the thoracic limb and ST-36, BL-40, GB-34, GB-31, BL-54 for 30 seconds per acupoint; treat back and all four legs
- *Ca-fa* rubbing from the scapula to the carpus and then from the hip to the tarsus on each side for 1 minute on each limb
- *Ba-shen-fa* stretching and *Dou-fa* gently shaking each limb for 12 times

Daily Life Style Recommendation for Owner Follow-up:
- Delay *Tui-na* treatments until muscle pain has been controlled
- *Moo-fa* massaging up and down the back and all the muscles of the limbs for 3-5 minutes in each area to improve *Qi*/Blood flow to the nerves and muscles
- *Ba-shen-fa* stretching and *Dou-fa* gently shaking each limb for 12 times twice daily until recovers to improve *Qi*/Blood flow to the nerves and muscles
- Feed a high quality soft diet to support *Zheng Qi*
- Feed with head held elevated and for 10 minutes after eating until megaesophagus has resolved
- Ensure swallowing is normal to avoid choking
- Keep in a low stress environment to avoid Liver *Qi* Stagnation and over control of the Spleen
- Once pain is controlled, begin walking or supervised swimming, but go slowly with adequate rest periods so muscles do not fatigue; can increase duration and speed as animal becomes stronger

Comments:
Based on clinical and experimental studies of the positive effects of TCVM to control pain and for other immune-mediated disorders, further clinical studies of TCVM treatments for polymyositis are warranted.[11,26,27] Expect TCVM treatments to relieve pain, shorten the recovery time and improve the degree of recovery.

Footnotes:
[a] (JT) = *Jing Tang* Herbal www.tcvmherbal.com; Reddick, FL
[b] (MW)= Mayway Herbs www.mayway.com; Oakland, CA

References:
1. De Lahunta A, Glass E. Veterinary Neuroanatomy and Clinical Neurology 3nd Ed. Philadelphia, PA:WB Saunders 2008:95-113,14.
2. Chrisman C, Mariani C, Platt S, Clemmons R. Neurology for the Small Animal Practitioner. Jackson Wy: Teton NewMedia 2003:125-167.
3. Platt S, Olby N (ed). BSAVA Manual of Canine and Feline Neurology 5th Ed. Gloucester, UK:BSAVA Publications 2012:1-500.
4. Wang HF, Dong GR. Effects of electroacupuncture at shu-points of the five zang-organs on electrophysiologic function of sciatic nerve in the rabbit of Guillain-Barre syndrome. Zhongguo Zhen Jiu 2008; 28(6):433-5. (in Chinese)

5. Hughes RA, Pritchard J, Hadden RD. Pharmacological treatment other than corticosteroids, intravenous immunoglobulin and plasma exchange for Guillain Barré syndrome. Cochrane Database Syst Rev 2011; 16(3):CD008630.
6. Kline KL, Caplan ER, Joseph RJ. Acupuncture for neurological disorders. In Schoen AM (ed) Veterinary Acupuncture 2nd Ed. St Louis, Mo: Mosby Publishing 2001:179-192.
7. Ji XQ, Wang CM, Zhang P et al. Effect of spleen-stomach regulation-needling on nerve conduction activity in patients with diabetic peripheral neuropathy. Zhen Ci Yan Jiu 2010; 35(6):443-7. (in Chinese)
8. Tong Y, Guo H, Han B. Fifteen-day acupuncture treatment relieves diabetic peripheral neuropathy. J Acupunct Meridian Stud 2010; 3(2):95-103.
9. Zhang C, Ma YX, Yan Y. Clinical effects of acupuncture for diabetic peripheral neuropathy. J Tradit Chin Med 2010; 30(1):13-4.
10. Poon TY, Ong KL, Cheung BM Review of the Traditional Chinese Medicine formula, Rehmannia Six Formula, on diabetes mellitus and its complications. J Diabetes 2011: Epub.
11. Kenney JD. Acupuncture for the treatment of pain. American Journal of Traditional Chinese Veterinary Medicine 2010; 5(2):37-53Feng BB, Zhang JH, Chen H. Mechanisms of actions of Chinese herbal medicine in the prevention and treatment of cancer. American Journal of Traditional Chinese Veterinary Medicine 2010; 5(1):37-47.
12. Hao J, Zhao C, Cao S et al (1995) Electric acupuncture treatment of peripheral nerve injury. Journal of Traditional Chinese Medicine 1995; 15(2):114-7.
13. Xiao GR, Hao H, Zhao QL et al. Observation on the therapeutic effect of electroacupuncture combined with functional training for treatment of peripheral nerve incomplete injury of upper limbs. Chinese Acupuncture and Moxibustion2007; 27(5):329-32.
14. Wei SY, Zhang PX, Yang DM et al. Traditional Chinese medicine and formulas for improving peripheral nerve regeneration. Zhongguo Zhong Yao Za Zhi 2008; 33(17), 2069-72.
15. Shu B, Li XF, Xu LQ et al. Effects of *Yiqi Huayu* decoction on brain-derived neurotrophic factor expression in rats with lumbar nerve root injury. Zhong Xi Yi Jie He Xue Bao 2010; 8(3), 280-6.
16. Xie H, Priest V. Xie's Veterinary Acupuncture. Ames, Iowa:Blackwell Publishing 2007:585.
17. Xie H. Personal communications
18. Xie H, Preast V. Xie's Chinese Veterinary Herbology. Ames. IA:Wiley-Blackwell 2010:305-347, 486-510, 387,449-460.
19. Xie H, Preast V. Chinese Veterinary Herbal Handbook 2nd Ed. Reddick, FL: Chi Institute of Chinese Medicine 2008:305-585.
20. Xie H, Ferguson B, Deng X. Application of *Tui-na* in Veterinary Medicine 2nd Ed. Reddick, FL:Chi Institute 2007:1-94,129-132.
21. Leggett D. Helping Ourselves: A Guide to Traditional Chinese Food Energetics. Totnes, England: Meridian Press 2005:21-36.
22. Xie H, Priest V. Traditional Chinese Veterinary Medicine. Reddick, FL: Jing Tang Publishing 2002:209-293,307-380,409-419.
23. Xu FQ, Li HX, Huang T. Observation on therapeutic effect of warming needle moxibustion combined with medicine on 128 cases of myasthenia gravis. Zhongguo Zhen Jiu 2006; 26(5):339-41. (in Chinese)
24. Liu P, Ding XF, Zhang YY, Qiao J. Modulation of Jianjining Recipe on differential protein expression in rats with experimental autoimmune myasthenia gravis. Zhong Xi Yi Jie He Xue

Bao 2007; 5(6):642-6. (in Chinese)

25. Niu GH, Sun X, Zhang CM. Effect of compound astragalus recipe on lymphocyte subset, immunoglobulin and complements in patients with myasthenia gravia. Zhongguo Zhong Xi Yi Jie He Za Zhi 2009; 29(4):305-8. (in Chinese)

26. Feng BB, Zhang JH, Chen H. Mechanisms of actions of Chinese herbal medicine in the prevention and treatment of cancer. American Journal of Traditional Chinese Veterinary Medicine 2010; 5(1):37-47.

27. Chu X, Hou X. Experimental study on therapeutical effect of Chinese medicine on polymyositis in guinea pigs. Zhongguo Zhong Xi Yi Jie He Za Zhi 1998; 18(6):356-8. (in Chinese)

Acupuncture and *Tui-na* Treatment of Generalized Tetanus in a Dog

Margaret Fowler, DVM, CVA CVCH, CVTP, CVTFT

Introduction

Tetanus is an acute and often fatal disease of the nervous system caused by the obligate anaerobic spore forming organism *Clostridium tetani* which only occasionally affects dogs.[1] It can result from contaminated wounds, particularly punctures, and is more common in working and hunting breeds. After infection, a potent neurotoxin is released, travels up the nerves, and affects the neuromuscular junction by interfering with the release of neurotransmitters from the pre-synaptic nerve endings. This causes the voluntary muscles to continuously tighten into severe contractions and spasms, leading to a spastic paralysis.[2] Dogs often initially present with stiffness and rigidity in the wounded limb which progresses to the other limb, masseter muscles and hindend resulting in ambulatory difficulties due to a stiff gait. The disease may advance to a generalized state with facial and limb muscle spasms, arching of the back, incoordination and possible seizures. Complications can include temporomandibular and shoulder dislocations, long bone fractures and vertebral fractures. Recovery from generalized tetanus is prolonged (2-4 months) and requires physical therapy to re-gain full use of the limbs and to prevent permanent muscle contracture from shortening and tightening of muscles and tendons caused by constant spasms.[3] Little is published on the physical therapy requirements for dogs and no references to the acupuncture or *Tui-na* treatment of tetanus could be found in the medical literature.

Background

A six year old Short Haired Pointer presented with a history of generalized tetanus which had been treated by the referring veterinarian one month prior with wound flushing, antibiotics, anti-spasmodics, anti-toxin and hospitalization. The tetanus resulted from a severe raccoon attack with multiple bite wounds on the face and both front legs. The dog still had a few muscle tremors involving the face and front limbs. He had a stiff stilted gait with a shortened stride of the front limbs. Lumbar back pain was easily elicited and muscle atrophy was pronounced over the temporal area of the head and both shoulders. Extensive trigger points were palpated in both triceps and both front limbs had severely restricted range of motion especially on extension. The dog was referred for evaluation as an acupuncture and rehabilitative therapy candidate.

TCVM Evaluation

A TCVM evaluation revealed a Water personality. Although the dog was alert, he was obviously very anxious, fearful and distrustful, and tried to hide behind his owner. He had no temperature preferences, his tongue was purple and his pulses were wiry. An excess pattern of *Qi*/Blood Stagnation was identified along with an unbalanced Water personality.

Treatment Principles

The treatment principles were to re-establish the flow of *Qi* and Blood and re-balance the Water constitution. Acupuncture, aquapuncture and *Tui-na* were chosen to achieve these goals.

Treatment

Six treatment sessions were performed over the next four months. Fifteen minutes before each session, 6cc of Vitamin B12 diluted with saline were injected at each of the classical points behind the ears, *An-shen*. This was done to provide a *Shen* calming effect. Dry sterile filiform one inch needles were inserted in acupuncture points from the following list with not all points being used in each session: *Da-feng-men* (calming effect, head tremors), *Long-hui* (calming, facial atrophy), *Nao-shu* (*Shen* disturbances, location in atrophied temporalis muscles), and *Tai-yang* (facial paralysis and atrophy). Points were chosen from the following list and used in various combinations for electro-acupuncture: Seven points consisting of *Bai-hui, Shen-shu, Shen-peng,* and *Shen-jiao* (lumbar pain), GB-21, *Bo-lan, Fei-men* and *Fei-pan* (shoulder lameness, restriction and atrophy), SI-9 (shoulder lameness and restriction, master point for the front limb), TH-14, LI-15 (shoulder lameness and restriction), LI-11, TH-10, *Zhou-shu* (elbow lameness and restriction), KID-3 (*Yuan* source point to support Water element, back pain), and BL-23 (Kidney association point to support Water element, local back pain).[4] Electro-acupuncture was performed for 10 minutes at 20 hertz and 10 minutes at 80 + 120 hertz. At the end of each session aquapuncture with 1000 mcg per ml of Vitamin B12 was performed at SI-9 and the extensive triceps trigger points. The triceps are one of the several known areas to develop trigger points in the dog and injection treatments are effective at alleviating spasms and lameness.[5]

The owner was then instructed in the use of *Tui-na* with the goals of relieving anxiety and calming *Shen* and to serve as physical therapy for the contracting and atrophied muscles particularly in the front end. Because of the *Shen* issues, the introductory technique selected was *Moo-fa* (Daubing) along the GV channel over the nose and head, *Nao-Shu* and ending at *An-shen*. This technique is calming, non-threatening and feels good. The second technique was *Rou-fa* (Rotary Kneading) over the atrophied head, shoulder and sore back only to the point of comfort. *Rou-fa* unblocks stagnated *Qi* and Blood and relieves pain. Next, range of motion exercise or *Ba-shen-fa* (Stretching) was performed on the neck, shoulders and elbows paying particular attention to stretching the contacted extensor muscles of the front limbs. *Ba-shen-fa* is often used to stretch the tendons and muscles and regulates the channels. The last technique performed was *Dou-fa* (Shaking) because it regulates *Qi* and Blood and is effective in muscle atrophy. The owner was instructed to perform these techniques for a minimum of 30 minutes daily.[6]

Outcome

After just the first session, the dog displayed decreased anxiety, a less stilted gait, and increased muscle in the shoulder area. After the second session the tongue returned to a pink color, the pulses were less wiry, the back pain had improved, and more muscle in the face and shoulders had returned. After the third session, the pulses were normal, the back pain had completely resolved and the front limbs had significantly increased mobility and extension. The dog no longer displayed anxiety when arriving for a treatment and actually seemed to enjoy the sessions. By the time of the last and sixth session, both forelimbs could be extended fully, the trigger points had resolved, the dog had a normal gait, and over 90% of the atrophied muscles in the head and forelimbs had returned.

Conclusion

This case is significant and unique in that it demonstrates how effective TCVM therapy is in a severe neuromuscular life threatening and functionally disabling disease such as generalized tetanus. It is also important in that it establishes Acupuncture and *Tui-na* as effective rehabilitative therapy techniques in the treatment of tetanus in animals. No other literature references other than herbal could be found in TCM or TCVM recommended tetanus treatments in humans or animals.

References:
1. Tilley, Larry, DVM and Smith, Francis, DVM. The Five Minute Veterinary Consult, Canine and Feline, 3rd Edition. Lippincott Williams and Wilkins, 2004, pg 1255.
2. Kahn, Cynthia and Line, Scott. Merck Veterinary Manual, 10th Edition. Merck and Co, Inc., 2010.
3. Dire, Daniel, MD, Clinical Professor, Dept of Emergency Medicine, University of Texas-Houston. Medscape Clinical Reference, 2010.
4. Xie, Huisheng, DVM and Preast, Vanessa, DVM. Traditional Chinese Veterinary Medicine, Vol 1, Fundamental Principles. Jing Tang, 2002, pg various.
5. Shoen, Allen, DVM. Veterinary Acupuncture, 2nd Edition. Mosby, 2001, pg 201-203.
6. Xie, Huisheng, DVM and Ferguson, Bruce, DVM and Deng, Xiaolin, OMD. Application of *Tui-na* in Veterinary Medicine, 2nd Edition. Chi Institute of Chinese Medicine, 2006, pg 29-31, 16, 81-90, 47-49.

Idiopathic Phrenic Neuropathy in a Cria

Joan D. Winter, DVM, CVA, CVCH, CVTP

Abstract

In a paper by Nader Kamangar, MD, FACP, FCCP, FAASM, the author reports that the human respiratory system functions as a vital pump that moves air in and out of the lung gas-exchange units. The respiratory pump consists of central respiratory centers, the spinal cord, peripheral nerves, neuromuscular junctions, and respiratory muscles. The diaphragm is the most important muscle of ventilation. A functional diaphragm allows negative intra-thoracic pressure leading to the start of ventilation. In humans, the diaphragm muscle is innervated by the cervical motor neurons, C3-C5, via the phrenic nerve. The diaphragm muscle is described as cone shaped and during inspiration it contracts expanding the rib cage, and facilitates air into the lungs.

In people, diaphragmatic paralysis has been described as unilateral diaphragmatic paralysis (UDP) involving a single leaflet, and bilateral diaphragmatic paralysis (BDP) involving both leaflets.

Normal ventilation in people, requires the simultaneous contraction of the diaphragm and the respiratory accessory muscles including the scalene, parasternal portion of the internal and external intercostal muscles, sternocleidomastoid, and trapezius. In people with bilateral diaphragmatic paralysis, the respiratory accessory muscles assume some or all of the work of breathing. The muscles contract more intensely and increased effort to breathe may cause fatigue of the accessory respiratory muscles and lead to ventilatory failure.

Human patients with BDP are usually symptomatic. When symptoms are so severe or in the presence of underlying lung disease, people may develop ventilatory failure without medical intervention. Most cases of UDP are found incidentally during imaging studies, and many people have no symptoms. The people that do have symptoms with UDP have underlying lung disease and decreased quality of life. The frequency of UDP and BDP are unknown within the United States.

The most common cause of people having UDP is a malignant lesion causing compression of the phrenic nerve. Many times though, the etiology is unknown. Other causes in people include herpes zoster, cervical spondylosis, or trauma. BDP occurs most often secondary to motor neuron disease, amyotrophic lateral sclerosis and post polio syndrome. Also, BDP causes include thoracic trauma, multiple sclerosis, myopathies and muscular dystrophy.

"Annabelle," a cria (baby alpaca) was born in August of 2007. She was presented to the UC Davis, School of Veterinary Medicine, Teaching Hospital, on November 7, 2007, for two week duration of respiratory distress. The referring veterinarian, Dr. Jana Smith, had treated "Annabelle" with Naxcel, Amikacin and Dexamethasone. "Annabelle" did not respond to treatment. She was referred to UC Davis for further diagnostics.

On physical examination, "Annabelle" had increased respiratory effort and breathing characterized as "abdominal." Slight increased lung sounds were asculted in the cranial lung fields, which were louder during expiration. No crackles or wheezes were asculted. The rest of the physical exam was within normal limits.

Venous blood work resulted in a pH=7.389 with a pCO2 61.3mmHG and HCO3 of 36.2 mEq/L. "Annabelle" was described as hypo ventilating in the presence of being tachypneic. "Annabelle" had respiratory acidosis with metabolic compensation. Pulse oximetry revealed 98%

saturation. Overnight therapy included oxygen insufflation, Naxcel and Vitamin E. The CBC and blood chemistries were unremarkable. A fecal floatation was negative.

"Annabelle's" thoracic radiographs were within normal limits. Fluoroscopy showed minimal movement of the diaphragm, and, the diaphragm moved cranial on inspiration (paradoxical Movement). The clinicians of UC Davis teaching hospital, headed by Dr. Gary Magdesian concluded that these findings are consistent with idiopathic phrenic neuropathy of camelids associated with phrenic nerve degeneration. This syndrome may have a variable course. Some camelids deteriorate over time. Crias appear to have a better prognosis. Some crias have recovered in weeks to a month's time.

"Annabelle's" therapy discontinued oxygen insufflations after 12 hours of treatment. Her respiratory distress did not change. "Annabelle" was compensating for her respiratory distress and did not require supplemental oxygen. "Annabelle" remained afebrile, had an excellent appetite and was passing normal feces.

"Annabelle" was sent home November 12, 2007, under the observation and guidance of her referral veterinarian, Dr. Jana Smith. UC Davis recommended that "Annabelle" be re-checked every 2-3 weeks by her veterinarian. "Annabelle" continued to receive Naxcel antibiotic for 3 more days in light of the long trailer haul (1.6cc=80 mg Naxcel under the skin once daily until November 15, 2007). Vitamin E therapy, 1000 IU orally once daily, was to be continued for 3 months. A dust free environment was recommended to decrease respiratory stress. Monitor for respiratory distress and call immediately if occurs.

On November 26, 2007, I examined the cria named "Annabelle" formerly seen by UC Davis, for the first time. The owner pleaded with me to work on "Annabelle" having contacted several veterinarians unwilling to acupuncture a camelid. The farm was at least 1½ hours away due to distance and traffic. I remember Dr. Xie teaching his students that a veterinarian acupuncturist should not turn away an animal because of one's unfamiliarity with the species. So, November 26, 2007, became another exciting adventure for me as a mixed animal veterinarian.

On physical examination, I found "Annabelle" easy to handle! Rightly so with lung *Qi* deficiency! Her nose was moist, tongue black (usual pigment for an alpaca), no tail or femoral pulses taken due to possible incurred stress, tachypnea with 80 breaths per minute. I decided on electro acupuncture as a therapy for "Annabelle's" bilateral phrenic nerve paralysis. I researched and found that the phrenic nerve is associated with C5-C6-C7, unlike the human (C4-C5-C6). I needled between cervical para-vertebral (on each side of the cervical vertebrae) spaces and attached my wires to my needles from left to right, and, cranial to caudal on each side (cranial left to caudal left and, cranial right to caudal right). I used amplitude of 2 with a frequency set at 4/0 × 10, then, 8/12 × 10. I also utilized *Bai Hui* (for Hundred Crossings, *Yang* deficiency and lumbosacral intervertebral disk disease), *Shen Shu* (for Kidney *Qi* deficiency) and Back *Shu* Lung Association Points (BL-13 for Lung *Qi* deficiency), Back-*Shu* Kidney Association Points (BL-23 for *Jing* deficiency), and KID-1 (Kidney controls spinal cord and peripheral nerves), BL-60 (cervical stiffness and husband to Kidney) and BL-40 (Husband to Kidney).

I returned December 6, 2007, and, found "Annabelle" respiratory rate above normal and abdominal in character with no abnormal lung sounds asculted. She was described as bright and alert. In my opinion, her tail and femoral pulses were poor in character. I again used electro acupuncture between the cervical facets, *Bai Hui*, *Shen Shu*, Back *Shu* Lung Association Points, LU-1 (Alarm point for lung) and KID-27 (house of association points, can be used for multiple organ complaints, heaves). I used the same amplitude and frequency as above for 10 minutes at each frequency.

On December 13, 2007, I introduced one small scoop of *Breath Easier B* given orally twice daily for deficient Lung and Kidney *Qi*. I repeated the same electro acupuncture pattern.

Table 1: Ingredients and Actions of Breathe Easier B

Pin Yin Name	English Name	Actions
Bai He	Lily	Moisten the Lung
Dang Shen	Codonopsis	Tonify *Qi*
Jie Geng	Platycodon	Open the Lung and eliminate phlegm
Mai Men Dong	Ophiopogon	Nourish Lung *Yin*
Qian Hu	Peucedanum Root	Transform phlegm, stop asthma
Rou Gui	Cinnamomum	Warm Kidney and dispel Cold
Wu Wei Zi	Schisandra	Consolidate and nourish Lung *Yin*
Xing Ren	Armeniaca	Stop cough and asthma
Zhe Bei Mu	Fritillaria	Eliminate phlegm and clear Lung Heat
Zi Su Zi	Perillae	Descend *Qi* to stop asthma, transform phlegm to stop cough

Manufactured and distributed by Jing-tang Herbal, Inc., Reddick, FL

On December 28, 2007, I was delighted to return to the farm to find that "Annabelle's" respiration rate was normal (compared to other cria's on the farm). Her pulses were still difficult for me to palpate-due to her deficiency or my lack of expertise in that species? I repeated the electro acupuncture in the same fashion.

January 3 of 2008, was a new year! "Annabelle's" respiratory rate remained normal at 24 breaths per minute and achieved 30 breaths per minute now resisting to the electro acupuncture. I repeated the electro acupuncture in the same fashion, but for only a short time. "Annabelle's" *Shen* was great and started jumping around dislocating my wires!

I reported back to Dr. Gary Magdesian. I was very accepting of "Annabelle's" recovery. Yet, he reminded me that some crias's get better without treatment. As a scientist, I know more cases are needed. The owner and I rejoiced at such an outcome. I spoke with the owner November 2010. He reported that "Annabelle" is doing well with a newborn cria by her side!

References:
1. Jana Smith, DVM. Referring veterinarian to UC Davis
2. Gary Magdesian, DVM. Diplomate ACVIM, ACVECC, ACVCP
3. Jamie Higgins, DVM, Resident UC Davis
4. Ellie Tortosa, UC Davis student
5. Nader Kamamgar, MD, FACP, FCCP, FAASM
6. Shahriar, MD
7. Sat Sharma, MD, FRCPC

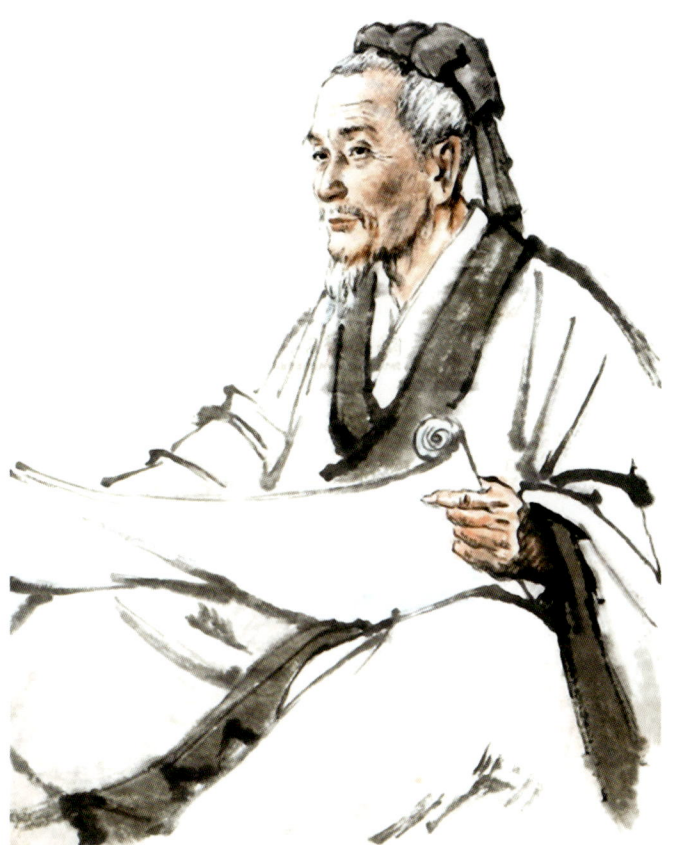

ZHANG ZHONGJING 张仲景

Zhang Zhongjing (150 – 219 CE) was born in Nanyang, Henan Province of the Eastern Han dynasty (25-220 CE). His formal name was Zhang Ji. He is honored as the father of Traditional Chinese Medicine (TCM) because of his establishment of the system of *Bian Zheng Lun Zhi* (treatment based on pattern differentiation), which is the core of TCM and Traditional Chinese Veterinary Medicine (TCVM).

In his early years, Zhang Zhongjing was a high-ranking officer who served at the Changsha government. Unfortunately, an epidemic claimed the lives of millions during the later years of the Eastern Han Dynasty. Most of Zhang's family members died in the epidemic. In order to save his family and other people, he started to learn medicine from other physicians and the medical literature of the time. Zhang Zhongjing was gifted in medicine and grasped it quickly. On the basis of his clinical findings, Zhang Zhongjing believed that the febrile disease responsible for the epidemic was caused by pathogenic "cold" factor and developed a series of herbal prescription for different stages and patterns of this disease. The epidemic was finally controlled using his methods. How to diagnose and treat epidemic diseases prevalent during his era was well documented in his masterpiece *Shang Han Za Bing Lun* (*Treatise on Cold Pathogenic and Miscellaneous Diseases*). In addition, this work developed the process of treatment based upon pattern differentiation or *Bian Zheng Lun Zhi* system. This text has been used as an important TCM and TCVM reference ever since. His other book *Jin Gui Yao Lue* (Essential Prescriptions of the Golden Coffer) is also a highly influential doctrine. These two books are used as classical texts for the study of TCM and TCVM in China.

CHAPTER 6

Peripheral Nerve Injuries

Peripheral Spinal Nerve Injuries

Cheryl L Chrisman DVM, MS, EdS, DACVIM-Neurology, CVA

Peripheral spinal nerve injury is the most common cause of acute monoparesis or monoplegia.[1-4] Neurapraxia is the failure of nerve function in the absence of structural change due to blunt trauma, stretching, compression or ischemia and recovery occurs within a few days to weeks.[2] Axonotmesis is the disruption of the axon and myelin sheath, but with preservation of the connective tissue elements that form the neural sheath.[2] The axon distal to the injury site degenerates (Wallerian degeneration). Although nerves with axonotmesis can regenerate, the distance between the nerve injury site and muscle must also be considered in the prognosis. Nerves grow approximately 2.5 cm/month, but after approximately six months neural sheath shrinkage and neurogenic muscle atrophy may inhibit further growth and improvement of function. Nerves injured greater than 15 cm proximal to the muscle previously innervated may not be able to regenerate far enough to make anatomic contact with the muscle and if they do their distal conduction times may be so slow that function is greatly reduced. Neurotmesis is partial or complete severance of a nerve, with disruption of the axon, its myelin sheath and the connective tissue nerve sheath, necessary to form the pathway for nerve regeneration to the appropriate muscle fibers.[2] Axonal regeneration cannot occur unless the nerve segments are surgically reattached. Most nerve injuries are due to neurapraxia or a combination of neurapraxia and axonotmesis and initially they can all cause monoplegia with loss of superficial and deep pain sensations. If deep pain is present from all the digits, then the nerve is intact and chances for recovery are good. Since the prognosis varies with the nerve injured and the type of injury, referral to a neurologist for electromyography can be useful to localize which nerves have been injured and differentiate between the types of nerve injury.

TCVM may be useful to promote nerve regeneration and nerve injuries are effectively treated using TCVM methods. There are many laboratory animal studies of peripheral nerve injuries that report significant positive effects of EA and/or Chinese herbal medicine to reduce pain and self mutilation and promote nerve regeneration, but no clinical studies have been performed in veterinary medicine.[5-8] In one study of 54 humans with peripheral nerve injuries, the EA treatment group had significantly improved recovery compared to the control group.[5] In a another human clinical study of 90 cases of peripheral nerve injury, the combination of EA and physical therapy resulted in significantly improved recovery and quality of life compared to either treatment alone.[6] Experimental studies of peripheral nerve injury have shown positive effects of Chinese herbal medicines to promote nerve regeneration.[7,8] Further clinical studies of peripheral nerve injuries in dogs and cats could confirm the benefits of adding these TCVM treatments to currently recommended rehabilitation regimes. An overview of the TCVM diagnosis and treatment of peripheral nerve injuries is outlined in Tables 1 and 2.[9,10]

Table 1: Common conventional diagnoses and traditional Chinese veterinary medicine (TCVM) patterns and examination findings associated with peripheral spinal nerve injuries[9,10]

		Focal Spinal Nerve Injuries		
Conventional Diagnosis	**TCVM Pattern**	**Clinical Findings**	**Tongue**	**Pulses**
Brachial plexus injury	Nerve *Qi*/Blood Stagnation with local *Qi* Deficiency	History or physical evidence of trauma Paresis or paralysis of a thoracic limb Reduced sensation Atrophy of affected muscles	Purple or pale	Wiry, later may be weak
Sciatic nerve injury	Nerve *Qi*/Blood Stagnation with local *Qi* Deficiency	History or physical evidence of trauma Can support weight on pelvic limb, but not flex and extend to walk Reduced sensation Atrophy of affected muscles	Purple or pale	Wiry, later may be weak
Cauda equina injury	Nerve *Qi*/Blood Stagnation with local *Qi* Deficiency	History or physical evidence of trauma Dilated unresponsive anal sphincter with fecal incontinence Large overflow bladder and urinary incontinence or dysuria (cats) Paralysis of the tail	Purple or pale	Wiry, later may be weak

Table 2: Treatment strategy, acupuncture points and Chinese herbal medicine used to treat peripheral spinal nerve injuries[9,10]

		Focal Spinal Nerve Injuries		
Conventional Diagnosis	**TCVM Pattern**	**Acupuncture points and Technique**	**Chinese Herbal Medicine**	**Comments**
Brachial plexus injury	Nerve *Qi*/Blood Stagnation with	EA: *Liu-feng/Liu-feng* (connect 4-6	Double P II and Cervical	For acute paralysis, repeat acupuncture

	local *Qi* Deficiency	points), LI-4/LI-15 on affected side, SI-9/SI-9, GB-21/GB-21	Formula initially (1-4 months) then Cervical Formula and *Qi* Performance (up to 6 months)	every 3-5 days for 3-5 times, then reduce to every 1-2 weeks for 6 months.
		DN: LI-10, ST-36, GB-34		
Sciatic nerve injury	Nerve *Qi*/Blood Stagnation with local *Qi* Deficiency	**EA:** *Liu-feng/Liu-feng* (connect 4 acupoints), *Bai-hui*/GV-1, ST-36/*Shen-shu* on the side of the paralysis, BL-40/BL-40, BL-54/BL-54	Double P II or Body Sore combined with *Qi* Performance	For acute injuries, repeat acupuncture every 3-5 days for 3-5 times, then reduce to every 1-2 weeks for 6 months.
		DN: LI-10		
Cauda equina injury	Nerve *Qi*/Blood Stagnation with local *Qi* Deficiency	**EA:** GV-1/GV-3, CV-1/CV-3, BL-39/BL-39, BL-54/BL-54, BL-36/BL-36	Double P II or Body Sore combined with *Qi* Performance	For acute injuries, repeat acupuncture every 3-5 days for 3-5 times, then reduce to every 1-2 weeks for 6 months.
		DN: BL-40, BL-36, ST-36		

The number of acupoints selected and treatment frequency will vary with the animal's condition and response to treatment; Chinese herbal medicine doses are generally 0.5 gm/10-20# orally twice daily; EA=electro-acupuncture, DN=dry needle acupuncture; All Chinese herbal formulas available from Jing Tang Herbal:www.tcvmherbal.com except *Wu Wei Xiao Du Yin*, which is available from Mayway Herbal www.mayway.com.

BRACHIAL PLEXUS INJURY

Injury of the brachial plexus and subsequent paralysis of one thoracic limb is the most common type of trauma and is frequently seen after encounters with automobiles[1-4] Other causes of injury include falls, animal fights and human interactions that involve severe over-stretching of a thoracic limb, scapular blows or fracture and gun shots. If the nerve roots of the brachial plexus (C6-T2) are torn from the spinal cord (brachial plexus avulsion), a Horner's syndrome (ptosis, miosis and enophthalmos) of the eye is usually present on the same side as the limb paralysis. In some cases of brachial plexus injury, the musculocutaneous nerve is spared and the limb is held flexed at the elbow. An examination of the motor abilities, spinal reflexes, sensation and muscles atrophied can be useful to determine which nerves are affected (Table 3). The TCVM diagnosis and treatment of brachial plexus injuries is outlined in Tables 1, 2 and 4.

Table 3: Thoracic limb peripheral nerves and associated signs of dysfunction[2]

Nerve Affected	Neurological Deficits	Can support weight?	Decreased or Absent Spinal Reflexes	Muscles Atrophied	Area of Reduced or Absent Sensation
Suprascapular	Loss of shoulder extension	Yes	None	Supraspinatus Infraspinatus	None
Axillary	Loss of shoulder flexion	Yes	Flexor of shoulder	Deltoid	Dorsolateral surface shoulder to elbow
Musculocutaneous	Loss of elbow flexion	Yes	Biceps, flexor of elbow	Biceps	Medial surface shoulder to elbow
Radial	Loss of elbow, carpus and digits extension	No	Triceps and extensor carpi radialis	Triceps, Extensor carpi radialis, and digital extensors	Front of limb from elbow to toes
Median	Loss of carpus and digits flexion	Yes	Flexor of carpus	Superficial and deep digital flexors	Back of limb from elbow to toes
Ulnar	Loss of carpus and digits flexion	Yes	Flexor of carpus	Deep digital flexors	Fifth digit
Brachial Plexus	All of the above signs; complete or partial loss	No	All or variations of the above	All or variations of the above	All or variations of the above

Table 4: A 20-30 minute *Tui-na* treatment for brachial plexus injuries[11]

Name	Technique	Duration or Number of Repetitions
Moo-fa	Massaging using the palms or fingers from the shoulder to the paw	For 3-5 minutes
Nie-fa	Holding and pinching the skin and muscle in the atrophied areas	For 3 minutes
Yi-zhi-chan and *Tui-fa*	Single thumb and pushing on the affected side	For 1 minute
An-fa and *Rou-fa*	Pressing and rotary kneading at LI-10, LI-11, SI-9, TH-14 and GB-21	30 seconds per acupoint
Ca-fa	Rubbing from the top of the scapula to the carpus	For 1 minute

Nie-fa and *Na-fa*	Holding and pinching the skin and pulling from the shoulder to the carpus	For 1 minute
Dou-fa	Gently shake the thoracic limb	20-30 seconds
Ba-shen-fa and *Ban-fa*	Stretch, flex and extend the thoracic limb	Repeat 12 times

Etiology and Pathology

From a TCVM perspective, trauma to the brachial plexus results in Stagnation of *Qi*/Blood, loss of *Qi*/Blood flow and *Qi* Deficiency locally that affects the function of one or more peripheral nerves to the thoracic limb.[9,10,12] The Deficiency and Stagnation of *Qi* and bleeding, associated with the trauma, depletes Blood and *Gu Qi* that nourish the neurons and other cells of the region and nerve degeneration occurs. Applying the basic TCVM theories of *Yin/Yang*, Eight Principles, Five Treasures, Five Elements and *Zang Fu* physiology and pathology to make a TCVM diagnosis, there is one main TCVM pattern associated with trauma to the brachial plexus:

1. **Brachial plexus *Qi*/Blood Stagnation with local *Qi* Deficiency**
   Trauma induces *Qi*/Blood Stagnation at the site of injury that causes *Qi* Deficiency of local tissues including nerves. The result is the acute onset of paresis or paralysis of the thoracic limb.

Pattern Differentiation and Treatment

1. Brachial plexus Blood/*Qi* Stagnation with local *Qi* Deficiency

Clinical Signs:
- Acute onset
- Paresis or paralysis of a thoracic limb
- Inability to flex or extend the shoulder, elbow, carpus or digits to support weight or walk on the limb
- Loss of sensation below the elbow
- Loss of thoracic limb spinal reflexes
- Atrophy of all the thoracic limb muscles
- Horner's syndrome (ptosis, miosis and enophthalmos of the eye on the same side as the paralysis is usually present in severe injuries
- May be able to flex the elbow, if the musculocutaneous nerve has been spared
- In partial or incomplete injuries the motor and sensory deficits, spinal reflex changes and muscles atrophied vary with the nerve(s) involved (Table 3)
- Tongue- purple, then pale
- Pulses- wiry, then deep and weak

TCVM Diagnosis:

The diagnosis of *Qi*/Blood Stagnation and local *Qi* Deficiency is based on a history or physical evidence of trauma and acute onset of paresis or paralysis of the thoracic limb. The tongue color is purple from the *Qi*/Blood Stagnation and the pulses wiry from the Stagnation. Later the tongue may become pale and pulses deep and weak if *Qi* Deficiency becomes chronic.

Treatment Principles:
- Resolve *Qi*/Blood Stagnation
- Tonify local *Qi* Deficiency
- Promote peripheral nerve regeneration

Acupuncture treatment:
EA is more effective to resolve *Qi*/Blood Stagnation and promote nerve regeneration than DN alone. For EA use 80-120 Hz alternating frequencies for 15-30 minutes. Treat normal and abnormal sides. For acute paralysis, repeat acupuncture every 3-5 days for 3-5 times, then reduce to every 1-2 weeks for 6 months. If paresthesias develop and the animal tries to mutilate the paw, change the EA protocol to 20 Hz for 10-15 minutes, followed by 80-120 Hz alternating frequencies for 10-15 minutes. For Aqua-AP inject 0.25-0.5 ml vitamin B12 into the acupoint.

Acupoints recommended
- EA: Thoracic limb *Liu-feng*/*Liu-feng* (connect 4-6 points), LI-4/LI-15 on affected side, SI-9/SI-9, GB-21/GB-21
- DN: LI-10, ST-36, GB-34
- Aqua-AP: SI-9, LI-10 on affected side

Pertinent acupoint actions
- *Li-feng* acupoints (at the skin fold on the dorsal aspect of the metacarpophalangeal and metatarsophalangeal joints of all four feet) between digits 2-3, 3-4 and 4-5) are useful to treat limb paralysis; the left to right connection is made to bring *Qi* from the normal side to the *Qi* Deficient side
- LI-4 can be connected to LI-15 to restore *Qi* flow from the digits to the shoulder region to resolve *Qi*/Blood Stagnation
- SI-9 is a local acupoint near the radial nerve useful to stimulate *Qi*/Blood flow to the region; the left to right connection is made to bring *Qi* from the normal side to the *Qi* Deficient side
- GB-21 is a local acupoint near the brachial plexus useful to stimulate *Qi*/Blood flow to the region; the left to right connection is made to bring *Qi* from the normal side to the *Qi* Deficient side
- LI-10 and ST-36 tonify *Qi* and stimulate *Qi* flow in the Channels
- GB-34 is useful for *Qi* Stagnation and an acupoint on the pelvic limb to balance the treatment

Herbal Medicine:
- If injury is severe, administer Double P II (JT)[a] 0.5gm/10# twice daily orally to move *Qi* and Blood to resolve Stagnation
- Combine with Cervical Formula (JT)[a] 0.5gm/10# twice daily orally to further move *Qi* and Blood to resolve Stagnation in the C6-T2 region

- When Double P II is discontinued after 1-4 months, combine *Qi* Performance (JT)[a] 0.5gm/10# twice daily orally with Cervical formula (JT)[a] to tonify *Qi*
- Administer Double P II (JT)[a] for up to 4 months
- Can administer Cervical Formula (JT) and *Qi* Performance (JT)[a] for 6 months if needed
- A description of all the ingredients of the Chinese herbal medicine listed is beyond the scope of this text, but can be found elsewhere.[10,13]

Food Therapy:

The purpose of the Food therapy is to further promote *Qi*/Blood circulation and tonify *Qi* to support nerve regeneration in the affected region. Foods that are too Cold or Hot are avoided.[14]

- Foods to supplement to promote *Qi* and Blood circulation include: chicken egg, crab, sweet rice, peaches, carrots, coriander, squash, turnips
- Foods to tonify *Qi*: Beef, chicken, sardines, egg, potato, yam, sweet potato, rice, oats, millet, lentils, carrots, squash, microalgae, dates, figs, molasses, royal jelly
- Cold foods to avoid: Turkey, duck, duck eggs, conch, clams, mussels, yogurt, millet, barley, spinach, broccoli, celery, egg plant, kelp, alfalfa, cucumbers, pears, bananas, white radishes, watermelon
- Hot foods to avoid: Lamb, shrimp, corn-fed beef, chicken, trout, squash, turnips, sweet rice, basal, caraway, cherries, chilies, cinnamon, ginger, rosemary, sage

Tui-na Procedures:

Tui-na therapy is performed to promote *Qi*/Blood circulation to the limb and peripheral nerve regeneration. A description of each technique and their actions can be found in Chapter 1 Table 8.[11]

- An example of a 20-30 *Tui-na* treatment for paralysis of one thoracic limb is outlined in Table 4

Daily Life Style Recommendation for Owner Follow-up:

- Gentle *Moo-fa* massaging up and down the affected limb for 3-5 minutes twice daily to improve *Qi*/Blood flow to the peripheral nerves
- *Dou-fa* gently shaking, *Ba-shen-fa* stretching, and *Ban-fa* flexing and extending all joints, including the digits, on the affected thoracic limb for 12 times each, twice daily to improve *Qi*/Blood flow to the peripheral nerves and promote nerve regeneration
- Feed a high quality diet to increase *Gu Qi* for nerve regeneration
- May place the limb in a sling to reduce dragging that causes paw abrasions; do not compromise Blood circulation
- Do not bandage the limb or apply a tight splint that could reduce Blood circulation further
- Do not allow the animal to lick or chew the limb (apply an Elizabethan Collar if needed)
- Animals with paresthesias (tingling or itching sensations) in the paw, might chew off their toes
- As function returns, supervised swimming may be begun and continued until recovered

Comments:

If the nerve roots of the brachial plexus are torn from the spinal cord, recovery is unlikely. Begin TCVM treatments as soon as possible. If there is some sensation or return of sensation on serial neurological examinations within 4-6 weeks, then expect TCVM treatments to reduce the recovery time and increase the degree of recovery of nerve function. If there is no improvement within 6 months, the prognosis is poor.

SCIATIC NERVE INJURY

The spinal nerve roots of L4-S2 form the lumbosacral plexus.[1-3] As with brachial plexus injuries, the lumbosacral plexus may be injured due to automobile encounters, falls, animal fights and human interactions that result in severe over-stretching of a pelvic limb, pelvic and hip fractures and gun shot wounds. An examination of the pelvic limb motor abilities, spinal reflexes, sensation and muscles atrophied can be useful to determine, which nerves are affected and need to be treated (Table 5). When all the nerves of the lumbosacral plexus are injured the animal is unable to support weight or walk on the limb.

Table 5: Pelvic limb peripheral nerves and associated signs of dysfunction[2]

Nerve Affected	Neurological Deficits	Can support weight?	Decreased or Absent Spinal Reflexes	Muscles Atrophied	Area of Reduced or Absent Sensation
Obturator	None (Adduction of hip)	Yes	None	Pectineus Gracillus	None
Cranial and Caudal Gluteal	Reduced hip flexion	Yes	Reduced flexor of the hip	Gluteals	None
Femoral	Loss of extension of the stifle	No	Patellar	Quadriceps	Inside of thigh and leg
Sciatic	Loss of extension of the hip, hock, tarsus and digits and flexion of the stifle, hock, tarsus and digits	Yes	Flexor, sciatic, cranial tibial and gastrocnemius	Biceps femoris Semimembranosus Semitendinosus Cranial tibial Gastrocnemius	Entire limb except inside of thigh and leg
Peroneal (Fibular)	Loss of extension of the hock, tarsus and digits	Yes	Cranial tibial	Cranial tibial	Front of leg below the stifle
Tibial	Loss of flexion of the hock, tarsus and digits	Yes	Flexor of hock and tarsus and gastrocnemius	Gastrocnemius	Back of leg below the stifle

The most common peripheral nerve injury of the pelvic limb involves the sciatic nerve with sparing of the femoral nerve.[1-3] The L6-S2 nerve roots that form the sciatic nerve exit the lumbosacral vertebral column in the pelvic region. The sciatic nerve then passes between the greater trochanter of the hip and the ischiatic tuberosity (tuber ischium) of the pelvis, courses along the caudal femur and just proximal to the stifle, it splits into the tibial and peroneal (fibular) nerves.[1] The sciatic nerve is subject to injury associated with pelvic and hip fractures, accidental stretching or ligation during hip surgery and injections into the caudal thigh muscles. The sciatic nerve innervates all extensor muscles of the pelvic limb, except the stifle, and all flexor muscles except the hip. With sciatic nerve injury alone, the animal may be able to partially support weight on the limb, because of the preserved ability to extend the stifle, but will be walk knuckled on the paw and drag the limb, unable to actively extend the other joints or flex any joint except the hip. Sensation to the limb will be depressed or absent except for the strip of skin on the inner side of the limb innervated by the femoral nerve. All muscles of the limb will be atrophied except for the gluteal and quadriceps muscles. If only the tibial or peroneal (fibular) branches of the sciatic nerve are affected, the neurological examination findings will vary (Table 7). The TCVM diagnosis and treatment of sciatic nerve injury are outlined in Tables 1, 2 and 6.[9-11] The treatment protocol is the same for other less common pelvic limb peripheral nerve injuries.

Table 6: A 20-30 minute *Tui-na* treatment for sciatic nerve injuries[11]

Name	Technique	Duration or Number of Repetitions
Moo-fa	Massaging using the palms or fingers from the shoulder to the paw	For 3-5 minutes
Nie-fa	Holding and pinching the skin and muscle in the atrophied areas	For 3 minutes
Yi-zhi-chan and *Tui-fa*	Single thumb and pushing on the affected side	For 1 minute
An-fa and *Rou-fa*	Pressing and rotary kneading at LI-10, LI-11, SI-9, TH-14 and GB-21	30 seconds per acupoint
Ca-fa	Rubbing from the top of the hip to the tarsus	For 1 minute
Nie-fa and *Na-fa*	Holding and pinching the skin and pulling from the hip to the tarsus	For 1 minute
Dou-fa	Gently shake the thoracic limb	20-30 seconds
Ba-shen-fa and *Ban-fa*	Stretch, flex and extend the pelvic limb	Repeat 12 times

Etiology and Pathology

From a TCVM perspective, as with other peripheral nerve trauma, sciatic nerve injury results in Stagnation of *Qi*/Blood flow with *Qi* Deficiency locally that affects the function of one or more of the peripheral nerves to the pelvic limb.[9-12] The Deficiency and Stagnation of *Qi* and bleeding, associated with trauma, locally depletes Blood and *Gu Qi* that nourish the nerves and other tissues of the region and nerve degeneration occurs. Applying the basic TCVM theories of *Yin/Yang*, Eight Principles, Five Treasures, Five Elements and *Zang Fu* physiology and pathology to make a TCVM diagnosis, there is one main TCVM pattern associated with sciatic nerve trauma:

3. Sciatic nerve Blood/*Qi* Stagnation and Local *Qi* Deficiency

Trauma induces *Qi*/Blood Stagnation at the site of injury that causes *Qi* Deficiency of local tissues including nerves. The result is the acute onset of paralysis of the pelvic limb.

Pattern Differentiation and Treatment

1. Sciatic nerve Blood/*Qi* Stagnation with local *Qi* Deficiency

Clinical Signs:
- Acute onset
- Loss of extension of the hip, hock, tarsus and digits and flexion of the stifle, hock, tarsus and digits
- Loss of limb sensation except medial side
- Atrophy of biceps femoris, semimembranosus, semitendinosus, cranial tibial and gastrocnemius muscles
- Animal is able to support weight on the limb and has sensation on the medial aspect of the limb, if the femoral nerve is intact
- Motor and sensory deficits of individual nerves of the lumbosacral plexus vary with the nerve(s) involved (Table 7)
- Tongue- purple, then pale
- Pulses- wiry, then deep and weak

TCVM Diagnosis:

The diagnosis of *Qi*/Blood Stagnation and local *Qi* Deficiency is based on a history or physical evidence of trauma and acute onset of paresis or paralysis of the pelvic limb. The tongue color is purple from the *Qi*/Blood Stagnation and the pulses wiry from the Stagnation. Later the tongue may become pale and pulses deep and weak, if *Qi* Deficiency becomes chronic.

Treatment Principles:
- Resolve *Qi*/Blood Stagnation
- Tonify local *Qi* Deficiency
- Promote peripheral nerve regeneration

Acupuncture treatment:

EA is more effective to resolve *Qi*/Blood Stagnation and promote nerve regeneration than DN alone. For EA use 80-120 Hz alternating frequencies for 15-30 minutes. Treat normal and abnormal sides. For acute paralysis, repeat acupuncture every 3-5 days for 3-5 times and then reduce to every 1-2 weeks for 6 months. If paresthesias develop and the animal tries to mutilate the paw, change the EA protocol to 20 Hz for 10-15 minutes, followed by 80-120 Hz alternating frequencies for 10-15 minutes. For Aqua-AP inject 0.25-0.5 ml vitamin B12 into the acupoint.

Acupoints recommended
- EA: Pelvic limb *Liu-feng/Liu-feng* (connect 4 acupoints), *Bai-hui*/GV-1, ST-36/*Shen-shu* on the side of the paralysis, BL-40/BL-40, BL-54/BL-54
- DN: LI-10

- Aqua-AP: BL-40, ST-36 on affected side

Pertinent acupoint actions
- *Liu-feng* acupoints (at the skin fold on the dorsal aspect of the metacarpophalangeal and metatarsophalangeal joints of all four feet) between digits 2-3, 3-4 and 4-5) are useful to treat limb paralysis
- *Bai-hui* (dorsal midline at L7-S1) can be connected to GV-1 to stimulate *Qi* flow in the L7-S2 nerve roots supplying the sciatic nerve
- ST-36 is useful to tonify *Qi* and connected to *Shen-shu* (one *cun* lateral to *Bai-hui*) can stimulate *Qi* flow through the area of the sciatic nerve
- BL-40 is the Master point for the pelvic limbs
- BL-54 is a local acupoint near the sciatic nerve useful to stimulate *Qi*/Blood flow to the region
- LI-10 is useful to tonify *Qi* and can balance the treatment since it is located on the thoracic limb

Herbal Medicine:
- If injury is severe, administer Double P II (JT)[a] 0.5gm/10# twice daily orally to move *Qi* and Blood to resolve Stagnation
- If injury is less severe, administer Body Sore (JT)[a] 0.5gm/10# twice daily orally to move *Qi* and Blood to resolve Stagnation instead of Double P II
- Combine either formula with *Qi* Performance (JT)[a] 0.5gm/10# twice daily orally to tonify *Qi*
- Administer Double P II (JT)[a] for up to 4 months
- Can administer Body Sore (JT)[a] and *Qi* Performance (JT)[a] for 6 months if needed
- A description of all the ingredients of the Chinese herbal medicine listed is beyond the scope of this text, but can be found elsewhere.[10,13]

Food Therapy:
The purpose of the Food therapy is to further promote *Qi*/Blood circulation and tonify *Qi* to support nerve regeneration in the affected region. Foods that are Cold or Hot are avoided.[14]
- Foods to supplement to promote *Qi* and Blood circulation include: chicken egg, crab, sweet rice, peaches, carrots, coriander, squash, turnips
- Foods to tonify *Qi*: Beef, chicken, sardines, egg, potato, yam, sweet potato, rice, oats, millet, lentils, carrots, squash, microalgae, dates, figs, molasses, royal jelly
- Cold foods to avoid: Turkey, duck, duck eggs, conch, clams, mussels, yogurt, millet, barley, spinach, broccoli, celery, egg plant, kelp, alfalfa, cucumbers, pears, bananas, white radishes, watermelon
- Hot foods to avoid: Lamb, shrimp, corn-fed beef, chicken, trout, squash, turnips, sweet rice, basal, caraway, cherries, chilies, cinnamon, ginger, rosemary, sage

Tui-na Procedures:
Tui-na therapy is performed to promote *Qi*/Blood circulation to the limb and peripheral nerve regeneration. A description of each technique and their actions can be found in Chapter 1 Table 8.[11]

- An example of a 20-30 *Tui-na* treatment for paralysis of the pelvic limb is outlined in Table 6

Daily Life Style Recommendation for Owner Follow-up:
- Gentle *Moo-fa* massaging up and down the pelvic limb for 3-5 minutes twice daily to improve *Qi*/Blood flow to the peripheral nerves
- *Dou-fa* gently shaking, *Ba-shen-fa* stretching, and *Ban-fa* flexing and extending all joints, including the digits, on the affected pelvic limb for 12 times each, twice daily to improve *Qi*/Blood flow to the peripheral nerves and promote nerve regeneration
- Feed a high quality diet to increase *Gu Qi* for nerve regeneration
- Avoid rough surfaces as dragging will cause paw abrasions
- Can protect the foot with a small child's sock, but keep dry, clean and well aerated
- Do not bandage the limb or apply a tight splint that could reduce Blood circulation further
- Do not allow the animal to lick or chew the limb (apply an Elizabethan Collar if needed)
- Animals with paresthesias (tingling or itching sensations) in the paw, might chew off their toes
- As function returns, supervised swimming may be begun and continued until recovered

Comments:

If the sciatic nerve is only stretched (neurapraxia or axonotmesis), recovery is likely. Begin TCVM treatments as soon as possible. If there is some return of function on serial neurological examinations within 4-6 weeks, then expect TCVM treatments to further reduce the recovery time and increase the degree of recovery of nerve function. If there is no improvement within 6 months, the prognosis for recovery is poor.

CAUDA EQUINA INJURY

The cauda equina consists primarily of the L7, S1-S3 and Cd-1 nerve roots.[1-3] Acute nerve root trauma most commonly results from encounters with automobiles or aggressive animals and humans that result in vertebral fracture, luxation, or subluxation of the lumbosacral, sacral or sacrocaudal vertebrae or gun shot wounds.[1-3] Fracture and/or luxation at the sacrocaudal junction may occur in animals that try to escape or run away, when their tail is caught by something. This is particularly common in cats. Cauda equina injuries result in paralysis of the tail and urinary and fecal incontinence. With lumbosacral fractures, there may be mild pelvic limb weakness that appears similar to mild bilateral sciatic nerve dysfunction, but often the anus, bladder and tail are primarily affected. While dogs have a flaccid urinary bladder that is easy to express, the bladder may be difficult to manually express in cats. Two radiographic views are imperative to assess the degree of displacement at the site of a fracture in most cases. CT can be useful to better visualize bone fragments in the spinal canal. Surgical decompression and stabilization may be required for lumbosacral injuries.

Conventional management consists of manual expression of the bladder and fecal evacuation if necessary. Low-dose oral propanolol 1.25 mg total dose every 8-12 hours may facilitate bladder expression in cats after several days of therapy. The prognosis is better if tail and perineal sensation are preserved. Sacrocaudal luxations typically have a better prognosis for the return of bowel and bladder function than do lumbosacral luxations. The tail may be permanently paralyzed and may eventually have to be amputated due to soiling or mutilation.

Lumbosacral degeneration, common in large breed dogs, can cause progressive cauda equina compression and injury.[2-4] Chronic joint instability and subluxation, proliferation of the surrounding ligaments and other soft tissues and a Type II intervertebral disk protrusion at L7-S1 produce a stenotic lumbosacral spinal canal compressing the nerve roots. Affected dogs initially have lumbosacral pain and low tail carriage and may have difficulty rising or jumping into the car or onto furniture. As the disease progresses, paresis or paralysis of the tail and fecal or urinary incontinence often develop. Some dogs also show tail and leg biting and genital licking that may be due to paresthesias. Conscious proprioceptive deficits and pelvic limb paresis are rarely present. Lumbosacral radiographs and MRI show profound changes in animals with urinary and fecal incontinence. Surgical decompression of nerve roots result in significant improvement, if diagnosed early, but improvement is less once urinary or fecal incontinence develops.

From a TCVM perspective cauda equina trauma is *Qi*/Blood Stagnation with local *Qi* Stagnation, while lumbosacral degeneration is typical of intervertebral disk disease *Bi*-syndrome and has *Qi*/Blood Stagnation combined with Kidney *Yin*, *Qi*, and /or *Yang* Deficiencies. The EA and *Tui-na* treatments for cauda equina injury from trauma and lumbosacral degeneration are the same as described below, but the correct DN, Aqua-AP, Chinese herbal medicine and Food therapy for lumbosacral degeneration will vary with the additional TCVM patterns besides *Qi*/Blood stagnation and local *Qi* Deficiency (see TCVM diagnosis and treatment in the **INTERVERTEBRAL DISK DISEASE** section above). Information in this section will focus on traumatic cauda equina injury. There are currently no case or clinical studies specific for lumbosacral, sacral or sacrocaudal injury, but based on the evidence for the effectiveness of acupuncture and Chinese herbal medicine for the treatment of peripheral nerve injuries in other areas and for fecal incontinence, treatment of clinical cases and clinical studies in veterinary medicine are warranted.[5-8,15] An overview of the TCVM diagnosis and treatment of cauda equina injury is outlined in Tables 1 and 2.[9,10]

Etiology and Pathology

From a TCVM perspective, as with other peripheral nerve trauma, injuries of the cauda equina result in local *Qi*/Blood Stagnation, reduced *Qi*/Blood flow and *Qi* Deficiency that affects cauda equina function and results in fecal and urinary incontinence and tail paralysis.[9,12] The Deficiency and Stagnation of *Qi* and bleeding, associated with trauma, locally depletes Blood and *Gu Qi* that nourish the nerves and other tissues of the region and nerve degeneration occurs. Applying the basic TCVM theories of *Yin/Yang*, Eight Principles, Five Treasures, Five Elements and *Zang Fu* physiology and pathology to make a TCVM diagnosis, there is one main TCVM pattern associated with cauda equina nerve root trauma:

1. Blood/*Qi* Stagnation with local *Qi* Deficiency of the sacrocaudal nerve roots

Trauma induces *Qi*/Blood Stagnation at the site of injury that results in *Qi* Deficiency of local tissues including nerves. The result is the acute onset of paralysis of anus, bladder and tail with normal or minimally weak pelvic limbs.

Pattern Differentiation and Treatment

1. Blood/*Qi* Stagnation with local *Qi* Deficiency of the sacrocaudal nerve roots

Clinical Signs:
- Acute onset
- Flaccid tail
- Loss of anal tone and sensation
- Large easily expressed bladder that drips when full or dysuria in cats
- May have lumbosacral or sacrocaudal pain
- Tongue- purple, then pale
- Pulses- wiry, then deep and weak

TCVM Diagnosis:
The diagnosis of *Qi*/Blood Stagnation and local *Qi* Deficiency is based on a history or physical evidence of trauma and acute onset of paresis or paralysis of the anal sphincter, bladder and tail. The tongue color is purple from the *Qi*/Blood Stagnation and the pulses wiry from the Stagnation. Later the tongue may become pale and pulses deep and weak if *Qi* Deficiency becomes chronic.

Treatment Principles:
- Resolve *Qi*/Blood Stagnation
- Tonify local *Qi* Deficiency
- Promote peripheral nerve regeneration

Acupuncture treatment:
EA is more effective to resolve *Qi*/Blood Stagnation and promote nerve regeneration than DN alone. Since most animals with cauda equina injuries have sacral or sacrocaudal pain for fracture or dislocations, the EA protocol suggested is 20 Hz for 10-15 minutes, followed by 80-120 Hz alternating frequencies for 10-15 minutes. Combine EA with DN of other acupoints. Begin acupuncture as soon as possible. For acute injuries, repeat acupuncture every 3-5 days for 3-5 times, then reduce to every 1-2 weeks for 6 months. For Aqua-AP inject 0.25-0.5 ml vitamin B12 into the acupoint.

Acupoints recommended
- EA: GV-1/GV-3, CV-1/CV-3, BL-39/BL-39, BL-54/BL-54, BL-36/BL-36
- DN: BL-40, BL-36, ST-36
- Aqua-AP: GV-1 (thoroughly clean area first), BL-39, BL-40

Pertinent acupoint actions
- GV-1 connected to GV-3 for EA is useful to stimulate *Qi*/Blood flow across the injured site at the lumbosacral, sacral or sacrocaudal regions; GV-1 is also useful to stimulate *Qi*/Blood flow to the perineal area to promote regeneration of nerves to the anal sphincter and bladder
- CV-1 connected to CV-3 for EA is useful to stimulate *Qi*/Blood flow in the perineal area to promote nerve regeneration; CV-1 is also a local acupoint useful to stimulate *Qi*/Blood flow to the perineal area to promote regeneration of nerves to the anal sphincter and bladder

- BL-39 acupoints connected bilaterally for EA are useful for urinary incontinence
- BL-54 acupoints connected bilaterally for EA are local acupoints near the sacrum useful to stimulate *Qi*/Blood flow to the region to promote nerve regeneration
- BL-36 acupoints connected bilaterally for EA are local acupoints near the perineal area useful to stimulate *Qi*/Blood flow to the region to promote nerve regeneration
- BL-40 is the Master point for the pelvic limbs and is also useful to treat urinary incontinence
- ST-36 and LI-10 is useful to generally tonify *Qi*; LI-10 can balance the treatment since it is located on the thoracic limb

Herbal Medicine:
- If injury is severe, administer Double P II (JT)[a] 0.5gm/10# twice daily orally to move *Qi* and Blood to resolve Stagnation and control pain and treat paralysis
- If injury is less severe, administer Body Sore (JT)[a] 0.5gm/10# twice daily orally to move *Qi* and Blood to resolve Stagnation instead of Double P II
- Combine either formula with *Qi* Performance (JT)[a] 0.5gm/10# twice daily orally to tonify *Qi*
- Administer Double P II for up to 4 months
- Can administer Body Sore and *Qi* Performance for 6 months if needed
- A description of all the ingredients of the Chinese herbal medicine listed is beyond the scope of this text, but can be found elsewhere.[10,13]

Food Therapy:
The purpose of the Food therapy is to further promote *Qi*/Blood circulation and tonify *Qi* to support nerve regeneration in the affected region. Foods that are Cold or Hot are avoided.[14]
- Foods to supplement to promote *Qi* and Blood circulation include: chicken egg, crab, sweet rice, peaches, carrots, coriander, squash, turnips
- Foods to tonify *Qi*: Beef, chicken, sardines, egg, potato, yam, sweet potato, rice, oats, millet, lentils, carrots, squash, microalgae, dates, figs, molasses, royal jelly
- Cold foods to avoid: Turkey, duck, duck eggs, conch, clams, mussels, yogurt, millet, barley, spinach, broccoli, celery, egg plant, kelp, alfalfa, cucumbers, pears, bananas, white radishes, watermelon
- Hot foods to avoid: Lamb, shrimp, corn-fed beef, chicken, trout, squash, turnips, sweet rice, basal, caraway, cherries, chilies, cinnamon, ginger, rosemary, sage

Tui-na Procedures:
Tui-na therapy is performed before Aqua-AP to promote *Qi*/Blood circulation to the perineal region and promote regeneration of the nerves. Avoid *Tui-na* treatment of the tail and sacral region as manipulation may worsen fractures, dislocations and pain. Instead focus on increasing *Qi*/Blood circulation in the caudal thigh region and treatment of acupoints known to relieve incontinence. A description of each technique and their actions can be found in Chapter 1 Table 8.[11]

- Gentle *Moo-fa* massaging up and down the caudal pelvic limbs for 3-5 minutes (do not stretch the limbs)
- *An-fa* and *Rou-fa* pressing and rotary kneading at ST-36, BL-39, BL-40, KID-10, BL-54 (if not too painful), BL-36 (if not too painful) for 30 seconds per acupoint
- Gentle *Moo-fa* massaging up and down the tail for 3-5 minutes, if not too painful (do not stretch the tail)

Daily Life Style Recommendation for Owner Follow-up:
- Gentle *Moo-fa* massaging up and down the caudal pelvic limbs for 3-5 minutes twice daily to improve *Qi*/Blood flow to the peripheral nerves
- Feed a high quality diet to increase *Gu Qi* for nerve regeneration
- Make plenty of fresh water available
- Express Bladder every 4-6 hours (during the day)
- Monitor the urine for a foul odor (Heat) or Blood (Damp-Heat) as Bladder Damp Heat (cystitis) can occur and require treatment
- Bathe often to keep perineal area clean and dry
- The animal should wear protective diapers to avoid soiling the environment
- Do not allow to lick or chew the perineal or genital area (apply an Elizabethan collar if needed)
- Animals with paresthesias (abnormal tingling or itching sensations) in the genital region, might chew on their penis and bleed to death or mutilate the vulva and anal region

Comments:
The more caudal the lesion along the L7- Cd1 vertebrae, the better the prognosis. If the cauda equina is only stretched (neurapraxia or axonotmesis), even if the initial clinical signs are severe, recovery is likely, but may take 6 months of nursing care and TVM treatments. Begin TCVM treatments as soon as possible. If there is some return of function on serial neurological examinations within 4 weeks, then expect TCVM treatments to further reduce the recovery time and increase the degree of recovery of nerve function. If there is no improvement within 6 months, the prognosis for recovery is poor.

Footnotes:
[a] (JT) = *Jing Tang* Herbal www.tcvmherbal.com; Reddick, FL

References:
1. De Lahunta A, Glass E. Veterinary Neuroanatomy and Clinical Neurology 3nd Ed. Philadelphia, PA:WB Saunders 2008:95-113,14.
2. Chrisman C, Mariani C, Platt S, Clemmons R. Neurology for the Small Animal Practitioner. Jackson Wy: Teton NewMedia 2003:125-167.
3. Platt S, Olby N (ed). BSAVA Manual of Canine and Feline Neurology 5th Ed. Gloucester, UK:BSAVA Publications 2011:1-500.
4. Kline KL, Caplan ER, Joseph RJ. Acupuncture for neurological disorders. In Schoen AM (ed) Veterinary Acupuncture 2nd Ed. St Louis, Mo: Mosby Publishing 2001:179-192.
5. Hao J, Zhao C, Cao S et al (1995) Electric acupuncture treatment of peripheral nerve injury. Journal of Traditional Chinese Medicine 1995; 15(2):114-7.

6. Xiao GR, Hao H, Zhao QL et al. Observation on the therapeutic effect of electroacupuncture combined with functional training for treatment of peripheral nerve incomplete injury of upper limbs. Chinese Acupuncture and Moxibustion 2007; 27(5):329-32.
7. Wei SY, Zhang PX, Yang DM et al. Traditional Chinese medicine and formulas for improving peripheral nerve regeneration. Zhongguo Zhong Yao Za Zhi 2008; 33(17), 2069-72.
8. Shu B, Li XF, Xu LQ et al. Effects of *Yiqi Huayu* decoction on brain-derived neurotrophic factor expression in rats with lumbar nerve root injury. Zhong Xi Yi Jie He Xue Bao 2010; 8(3), 280-6.
9. Xie H, Priest V. Xie's Veterinary Acupuncture. Ames, Iowa:Blackwell Publishing 2007:585.
10. Xie H, Preast V. Chinese Veterinary Herbal Handbook 2nd Ed. Reddick, FL: Chi Institute of Chinese Medicine 2008:305-585.
11. Xie H, Ferguson B, Deng X. Application of *Tui-na* in Veterinary Medicine 2nd Ed. Reddick, FL:Chi Institute 2007:1-94,129-132.
12. Xie H. Personal communications
13. Xie H, Preast V. Xie's Chinese Veterinary Herbology. Ames. IA:Wiley-Blackwell 2010:305-347, 486-510, 387,449-460.
14. Leggett D. Helping Ourselves: A Guide to Traditional Chinese Food Energetics. Totnes, England: Meridian Press 2005:21-36.
15. Scaglia M, Delaini G, Destefano I et al. Fecal incontinence treated with acupuncture- a pilot study. Autonomic Neuroscience 2009; 145(1-2):89-92.

Neurological Case Studies Associated with Trauma

Han Wen Cheng, DVM

Head trauma and peripheral nerve injury are commonly seen in the clinical practice, but management of these traumas by the veterinarian is difficult due to the complex anatomy and function of the nervous system. Head trauma and/or peripheral nerve injury in animals often have a poor to grave prognosis. In this article, traditional Chinese veterinary medicine will be chosen individually or combined with western medicine to address these diseases.

HEAD TRAUMA CASE 1: "MAO QIU"

Signalment: 7 kg, 17 year-old, Female, Maltese

History and Complaint: Mao Qiu had fallen from the 7th to the 6th floor, the patient presented with insomnia and pacing at night. Atropine had been given by the previous veterinarian to control salivation; in addition, a neck brace was used to protect the neck.

Physical Examination: Mao Qiu had signs of head turning to left side, tight circling movement, head pressing, insomnia, purple tongue, and thin and wiry pulse.

TCVM Diagnosis: Head trauma with *Qi*/Blood stagnation and Phlegm obstruction in the upper orifices.

Treatment:[3]
- Western medicine: Furosemide, 14 mg IM; Sodium Prednisolone Succinate, 75 mg, IV.
- Herbal medicine: Dispel Stasis from the Mansion of Blood (*Xue Fu Zhu Yu Tang*) 10.8 gm+Pinellia, Atractylodes, and Gastrodia Decoction (*Ban Xia Bai Zhu Tian Ma Tang*) 9.6 gm, Tid Po for 4 days.
- Acupuncture: *Jing-jia-ji*: C_{1-3}, *An-shen*, HT-7 (*Shen-men*), ST-36 (*Hou-san-li*), and BL-60 (*Kun-lun*).

Results: Mao Qiu improved and was discharged from the clinic on the same day after being treated with a combination of Western medicine and TCVM.

Discussion: In Chinese medicine, the head is connected to the *Zang Fu* organs, the channels and meridians, *Qi*, Blood, and Body Fluids, these all have a physiological and pathological association with each other.[2] Physically, the brain controls the spiritual activity. The 'Simple Question' in chapter 17 says: 'The head is the palace of intelligence'. Li Shi Zhen said: 'The brain is the Palace of Original *Shen* '. Wang Qing Ren also said: 'Intelligence and Memory reside not in the heart but in the brain'. Thus the brain controls intelligence, consciousness, memory and thinking. Mind-Spirit (*Shen*) not only resides in the Heart but also relates to other organs, e.g. the Ethereal Soul (*Hun*) for the Liver, the Corporeal Soul (*Po*) for the Lungs, the Will-Power (*Zhi*) for the Kidneys, and the Intellect (*Yi*) for the Spleen.[2,7]

The brain controls memory and thinking, but it depends on the fullness and health of Marrow. Marrow, the common matrix of bone marrow and Brain, is produced by the Kidney *Jing* (essence), and it nourishes the Brain, spinal cord and bones, forming bone marrow. Marrow contributes to make Blood, but Blood is transformed by *Qi* and Body Fluids, as well as being regulated by the function of Heart, Spleen and Liver. The Brain is the Sea of Marrow and it controls the senses of seeing, hearing, smell and taste.[2,7]

The head is the convergence place of all *Yang* channels. The three *Yang* channels of the thoracic and pelvic limb travel up to the head. *Yang-ming* channels pass through the frontal area; *Shao-yang* channels move along the side of head; Thoracic limb *Tai-yang* channels go through the facial area; Pelvic limb *Tai-yang* pass over the top of head and the occipital area; in addition, Pelvic limb *Jue-yin* channels and Governing Vessel channels converge to the parietal area.[2,7]

Pathologically, head trauma may affect other organs and the Channels. For example, the Heart pattern presents as palpitation and insomnia; the Liver and Gall Bladder pattern presents as irritability, agitation, dizziness and seizure; the Spleen and Stomach pattern presents as poor appetite, vomiting, and abdominal fullness; the Kidney pattern presents as insomnia, deafness, and back pain with foot weakness; the pattern of thoracic and pelvic limb *Tai-yang* channels presents as neck stiffness and shoulder and arm pain. The pattern of thoracic and pelvic limb *Yang-ming* channels presents as retching and adverse flow of *Qi*; the pattern of *Qi*, Blood, and Body Fluids presents as *Qi* block, *Qi* desertion, *Qi* accumulation, adverse flow of *Qi*, *Qi* deficiency, Blood stasis, Blood deficiency, bleeding, and fluid depletion.[2,7]

Injury to the brain is usually caused by car accidents, animal bites, kicks, falls and malicious human behavior. In the initial or acute stage, head trauma manifests as an excess pattern presented with *Qi* accumulation and Blood stasis as well as stagnation in the upper orifice. In the late or chronic stage, it is characterized by Deficient Essence-Blood and loss of nourishment of brain marrow, which is a type of deficiency or deficiency mixed with excess. The treatment strategies in the initial or acute stage should focus on opening the sensory orifice, clear heat, stop bleeding, induce dieresis to reduce edema, and rescue the *Qi* from collapse due to devastated *Yang*. In the intermediate stage one need to focus on activating Blood, dispelling Stasis, removing Phlegm, calming the Liver and extinguishing Wind. During the late or chronic stage one must proceed to invigorate *Qi*, replenish Blood, nourish the essence-marrow, and move the lingering stagnation or stasis.[5,8,12,13]

The treatment strategies can be used to address the head trauma according to the pattern differentiation:

FOR THE INITIAL OR ACUTE STAGE [4, 10, 13]

1. **Open the sensory orifices**
    a. **Aromatic medicinals that open the sensory orifices:**
        a) Liquid Styrax Pill (*Su He Xiang Wan*) used for sudden collapse, loss of consciousness, and clenched jaw; abdominal fullness, pain; excessive mucus and saliva, cold extremities, pale tongue, submerged, slippery pulse.
    b. **Formulas that relieve convulsion and induce resuscitation:**
        a) Calm the Palace Pill with Cattle Gallstone (*An Gong Niu Huang Wan*) indicated for high fever, irritability and restlessness, impaired consciousness, convulsion, coma; dry mouth, parched tongue that is red

or scarlet, and rapid pulse.
- b) Greatest Treasure Special Pill (*Zhi Bao Dan*) served for fever, irritability and restlessness, impaired consciousness to the point of coma, spasms, convulsions; red or deep-red tongue with foul, greasy yellow coating, and slippery, rapid pulse.
- c. **Formulas that clear heat and open the sensory orifices:**
  - a) Purple Snow Special Pill (*Zi Xue Dan*) adequate for high fever, irritability and restlessness, impaired consciousness, spasms, convulsions; scarlet red tongue with dry, yellow coat, and forceful, wiry, and rapid pulse.

2. **Stop bleeding**: used to stop bleeding for moderate and severe cases
   a. *Yunnan Bai Yao*
   b. Agrimony Decoction (*Xian He Cao Tang*)

3. **Induce diuresis to reduce edema: given for acute brain edema:**
   a. Polyporus Decoction (*Zhu Ling Tang*)
   b. Dispel Stasis from the Mansion of Blood Decoction (*Xue Fu Zhu Yu Tang*)

4. **Clear heat and eliminate toxin**: used for controlling the secondary inflammatory infection due to trauma e.g. open wound:
   a. *Pu Ji Xiao Du Yin* (Universal Benefit Drink to Eliminate Toxin)
   b. *Chi Feng Qing Pu Tang* (Red peony, Selaginella, Isatis leaf, and Dandelion Decoction)

5. **Rescue *Qi* from collapse due to devastated *Yang*:**
   a. Unaccompanied Ginseng Decoction (*Du Shen Tang*): given for strengthening the exhausted *Qi* associated with acute, severe blood loss.
   b. Ginseng and Aconite Decoction (*Shen Fu Tang*): adequate for sudden collapse of *Yang Qi*.

FOR THE INTERMEDIATE STAGE[8,11,12]

1. **Activate Blood and dispel Stasis, ascend the clear and descend the turbid**: used in the internal accumulation of Phlegm and Stasis:
   a. Bupleurum and Asarum Decoction (*Chai Hu Xi Xin Tang*)

2. **Activate Blood and dispel Stasis, remove Phlegm and free the orifice**: used in the mutual binding of Phlegm and stagnation.
   a. Four-Substance Decoction with Safflower and Peach Pit (*Tao Hong Si Wu Tang*
   b. Pinellia, Atractylodes, and Gastrodia Decoction (*Ban Xia Bai Zhu Tian Ma Tang*)

3. **Calm the Liver and extinguish Wind, ascend the clear and descend the turbid:**
   a. Gastrodia and Uncaria Drink (*Tian Ma Gou Teng Yin*):

FOR THE LATE OR CHRONIC STAGE [4, 8, 13]

1. **Invigorate *Qi* and replenish Blood, and strengthen spleen and calm the mind:**
   a. Heavenly Emperor's Nourish the Heart Pill (*Tian Wan Bu Xin Dan*).
   b. Restore the Spleen Decoction (*Gui Pi Tang*): used for Heart and Spleen Deficiency.

2. **Tonify the *Qi* and Activate Blood, and Dispel stasis and unblock the channels**
   a. Tonify *Yang* to Restore Five-Tenths Decoction (*Bu Yang Huan Wu Tang*) : used for paresis

3. **Tonify the Kidney and nourish the Heart**
   a. Nourish the Heart Decoction (*Yang Xin Tang*)

HEAD TRAUMA CASE 2: "XUE XIAO KUI"

Signalment: 3.8 kg, $4^{1}/_{2}$ year-old, male, Mix

History and Complaint: Xue Xiao Kui had been hit by a car on the right side of the head and he presented with loss of consciousness 3 months before the current visit. He had been hospitalized in the clinic with IV infusion for 22 days (10 days in the special care, 12 days for regular care). Polyuira and polydipsea were noted after using steroids by the previous veterinarian. The owner reported sneezing with occasional runny nose.

Physical Examination: Xue Xiao Kui presented with myosis, blindness, internal strabismus of left eye, and tremor. He also had signs of forceful movement, ataxia, hypermetria with occasional uplifting head and turning a somersault and involuntary attempt to catch something in the air while walking. He did not sleep much at night. His tongue was pale, and the pulse was soft, and slow.

TCVM Diagnosis: Head trauma- *Qi* and Blood deficiency with Blood Stasis.

TCVM Treatment:
1. Herbal medicine
   - Dispel Stasis from the Mansion of Blood Decoction (*Xue Fu Zhu Yu Tang*)
   - Pinellia, Atractylodes, and Gastrodia Decoction (*Ban Xia Bai Zhu Tian Ma Tang*)
   - *Nao De Sheng Wan*
   - Five Worms Powder with additions and subtractions (*Wu Chong San Jia Jian*)

2. Electroacupuncture:[9]
   - ST-1 (*Cheng-qi*): 5 Hz, 10 mins
   - SI 18 (*Quan-liao*): 10 Hz, 10 mins

3. Dry needle:
   - GB-20 (*Feng-chi*)
   - *Bai-hui*

- BL-2 (*Zan-zhu*), GB-1 (*Tai-yang*)
- LI-4 (*He-gu*), TH-5 (*Wei-guan*)
- BL-23 (*Shen-shu*)ST-36 (*Hou-san-li*)+GB-34 (*Yang-ling-quan*).

Results: After treatment, Xue Xiao Kui slept much better, his vision improved, he didn't have signs of tremor, and walked better than before.

Discussion[9]:
1. ST-1 (*Cheng-qi*)
    - Location: In the center of the ventral border of the orbit, between the globe of the eye and the orbital rim (zygomatic arch).
    - Location Method: There is a small notch in the orbital rim. Also, directly below the center of the pupil between the eyeball and infraorbital ridge.
    - Characteristics: Local point that expels exterior and interior Wind from the eye.
    - Indications: Conjunctivitis, atrophy of the optic nerve, retinitis, cataract, any other eye disorder including intracranial blindnes, stroke.
    - Method of insertion: Press the eyeball dorsally, and insert the long needle gently to the depth of 0.5-2 cm. along the border of the orbit. This acupoint should be done only by experienced acupuncturist due to the danger of puncturing the eye! Good restraint of the dog is needed. For ischemic stroke therapy, one might go deep up to 5 cm until one hits the pterygopalatine bone.

2. ST-2 (*Si-bai*)
    - Location: Directly below ST-01.
    - Location Method: Directly below the pupil, ventral to the orbital ridge of the zygomatic bone.
    - Characteristics: Expels exterior and interior Wind from the eye. Relaxes tendons and muscles, smoothes *Qi* and Blood circulation.
    - Indications: Facial paralysis, conjunctivitis, mandibular myositis, maxillary teeth problems, gingivitis, intracranial blindness, stroke.
    - Method of insertion: Perpendicular insertion 0.5-2 cm, or up to 1 cm if with angular insertion. For ischemic stroke therapy, one might go deep up to 5 cm till one hits the pterygopalatine bone.

3. SI-18 (*Quan-liao*)
    - Location: Directly below the lateral eye canthus and below the lower border of zygomatic arch.
    - Characteristics: Expels exterior and interior Wind from the face and eye.
    - Indications: Facial paralysis, trigeminal neuralgia, conjunctivitis, mandibular myositis, maxillary teeth problems, gingivitis, intracranial blindness, stroke.
    - Method of insertion: Perpendicular insertion 0.2-0.5 cm, or up to 1 cm if with angular insertion. For ischemic stroke therapy might go deep up to 5 cm till you hit the pterygopalatine bone.

4. Suggested protocol
    - Treat the dogs for all the other conditions involved in the trauma.
    - Do a diagnosis of intracranial blindness by a certified veterinary ophthalmologist.
    - Treat the blindness by routine advised pharmacological methods (steroids etc) for ten days.
    - If the dog cannot see during and after ten days – consider performing electro acupuncture procedure.
    - The acupuncture points are ST-1(*Cheng-qi*) in a calm dog, but in a more active dog consider ST-2 (*Si-bai*), and the second acupuncture point is SI-18 (*Quan-liao*).
    - It means – we are going to use either ST-1 or ST-2 and the second point will be SI-18.
    - Insert the needles bi-laterally, begin with 1 Hz, elevate gradually up to 10 Hz, A/C mode, 5-10 Volts, 6 mA, intermittent mode for 20 minutes.
    - Evaluation of a successful insertion of the needles is done by evaluation of increased production of eye tears and nasal discharge – this can be seen after a few minutes of stimulation at levels above 5 Hz.
    - If no drops are seen – change location of needles.
    - Total time of stimulation is 20 minutes.
    - Re-evaluate the vision abilities during the next 48 hours.
    - If no improvement is seen during this period of time – re-treat the animal. Also, one can stimulate for 20 minutes, stop for 20 minutes, and re-stimulate. This procedure can be re-done a few times in the time period mentioned above (48 hours).

CERVICAL INJURY CASE STUDY 1: "XIAO BAI" [3]

Signalment: 2.3-kg, 5 ½ year-old, intact male, Pomeranian

History and Complaint: A bystander sent Xiao Bai to the animal shelter after being hit by a car. The current owner adopted him from the animal shelter two months ago. He was very active and often jumped up and down from the sofa. Two weeks ago, the patient reacted at the owner's touch and was unable to jump up to the sofa.

Physical Examination: Xiao Bei was presented with neck pain, root signature of left thoracic limb, arched back, reluctant to recumb, dislike walking, and sitting still most of time.

TCVM Diagnosis: He was diagnosed as atlantoaxial subluxation by x-ray. His tongue was purple and the pulse was wiry. The TCVM diagnosis was cervical *Bi* syndrome with Blood stagnation.

TCVM Treatment:
- Herbal medicine: Pueraria Root Decoction (*Ge Gan Tang*) 0.5 gm Tid Po + Drive Out Stasis from a painful Body Decoction (*Shen Tong Zhu Yu Tong*) 0.5 gm Tid Po
- Acupuncture: *Jing-jia-ji* C_{1-7}, *Hua-tuo-jia-ji* T_1 and *Bo-jian* (Scapula Tip), *Bo-lan* (Scapula Post), *Fei-men* (Lung Gate), LI-15 (*Jian-jing*), *Jian-wai-yu* (Shoulder Lateral Clavicale) and *Liu-feng* (Six Raphes) of thoracic limb.

Results: Xiao Bai received acupuncture once every two weeks for two treatments and herbal medicine for 3 weeks. The owner claimed Xiao Bai was walking longer than before and pain was 50 % decreased after the first treatment, 80 % improvement after the second treatment, and almost normal after the third treatment.

Discussion: Cervical *Bi* syndrome or cervical vertebral disease is caused by external pathogens (e.g. Wind, Cold and Dampness, and acute or chronic injury) and internal pathogens (e.g. congenital malformation of cervical vertebra, deficient Kidney *Jing*, and geriatric weakness). It appears that the neck may lose its Channel's function and proceeds to *Qi* accumulation and Blood Stasis or occurs following Liver and Kidney deficiency. In the early stage of disease, exuberant evil *Qi* mainly occurs, resulting in poor circulation of *Qi* and Blood in the Channels or blockage of meridians, or *Qi* accumulation and Blood stasis. With longstanding, the disease invades the interior from the exterior, into the *Zang fu* organs from the Channels, involving Kidney, Liver and Spleen, manifesting as dysfunction of *Zang fu* organs.[1,6]

Cervical *Bi* syndrome is characteristic of neck pain, difficulty in moving, pain in the shoulder and back, or lameness in one or two limbs or even all limbs, walking unstably, or muscle atrophy. It is often seen in middle age and geriatric patient. According to TCM, the disease can be categorized into four types: 1) sympathetic pattern, presenting as dizziness, pain in the area of cranial thorax, palpitation, deafness, and cold or heat of extremities; 2) nerve root or root signature pattern, presenting as pain of neck, shoulders and back, numbness, paresis, or pain in extremities; 3) cervical vertebral arterial pattern, presenting as positional dizziness or retching, limitation of movement in the neck; 4) spinal marrow pattern, presenting as numbness, paresis, stiffness of limbs, walking unstably or paralysis in severe case, and fecal and urinary incontinence.[1,6]

There are five differentiation patterns for the disease, including 1) the pattern of Greater *Tai-yang* channel *Qi* unable to flow smoothly: Pueraria Root Decoction (*Ge Gan Tang*) or Cinnamon Twig Decoction plus Pueraria Root (*Gui Zhi Jia Ge Gan Tang*), 2) the pattern of painful obstruction (*Bi* syndrome): Remove Painful Obstruction Decoction (*Juan Bi Tang*) or Drive Out Stasis from a painful Body Decoction (*Shen Tong Zhu Yu Tong*), 3) the pattern of *Qi* accumulation and blood stasis: Dispel Stasis from the Mansion of Blood Decoction (*Xue Fu Zhu Yu Tang*), 4) the pattern of internal accumulation of phlegm and stagnation: Guide Out Phlegm Decoction (*Dao Tan Tang*), 5) the pattern of Liver and Kidney deficiency: Six-Ingredient Pill with Rehmannia (*Liu Wei Di Huang Wan*).[1,6]

PERIPHERAL NERVE INJURY CASE STUDY 1: "TA BU"

Signalment: 4.8 kg, 10 year-old, male mixed cat

History and Complaint: Ta Bu was seen two weeks prior to this appointment and had blood chemistry test done. Heart murmur and increased glucose (150 mg/dl) were found. Ta Bu was presented to the veterinarian because of acute weakness of left thoracic limb.

Physical Examination: The patient couldn't extend any joint except the shoulder and couldn't bear weight. There was no sensation of deep pain in the ill limb. Horner's syndrome was noted in the left eye. The tongue was purple. The pulse couldn't be palpated.

TCVM Diagnosis: Radial paralysis or *Qi* stagnation of left thoracic limb was diagnosed.

Treatment:
- Western medicine
    - Prednisolone sodium succinate, 10 mg/kg IV
- Herbal medicine
    - *Da Huo Luo Dan*, 1/4 pill, Bid Po.
- Acupuncture
    - *Jing-Jia-Ji*: C_{5-7}; *Bo-Jian* (Scapula Tip), *Bo-Lan* (Scapula Post), *Fei-Men* (Lung Gate), LI-15 (*Jian -Jing*), Zhou-shu (Elbow Association point), LI-11 (*Qu-chi*), LI-10 (*Qian-san-li*), LI-4 (*He-gu*), and *Qian-liu-feng* (Six Raphes, fore limb); BL-1 (Bright Eye), ST-1 (*Cheng-qi*), and GB-1 (*Tai-yang*).

Results: Ta Bu could lift the ill limb on the second day. Wheelbarrowing was performed normally on the third day; Ta Bu could walk nearly normal on the fourth day. Horner's syndrome also recovered normally one month later.

Discussion: There are two pattern differentiations in the radial nerve paralysis. One is ascribed to Stagnation of Blood as well as obstruction of Channel vessel, caused by trauma and surgery, manifesting as purplish dark or normal tongue with whitish coating, and slow and choppy pulse. This type can be treated by *Da Huo Luo Dan* or Four-Substance Decoction with Safflower and Peach Pit (*Tao Hong Si Wu Tang*); the other one is ascribed to *Qi* and Blood Deficiency, caused by Deficient *Qi* unable to move Blood with subsequent numbness of muscle, manifesting as pale tongue, thin pulse, shortness of breathing, and weakness. This type can be treated by Eight-Treasure Decoction (*Ba Zhen Tang*) or All-Inclusive Great Tonifying Decoction (*Shi Quan Da Bu Tang*).[1, 13]

References:
1. Chen, Gui-Ting and Si-Shu Yang. Practical Diagnosis and Therapeutics of Integrated Traditional Disease and Western Medicine. Chinese Medical and Technological Press. 1991:803-805; 1587-1588.
2. Chen, Shao Dong. Golden Mirror of Knocks and Falls with Internal Injury. Chinese Medical Classics Publishing, China. 2004: 117-136.
3. Cheng, Han-Wen and Tzong-Fu Kuo. The Application of Jing-Jia-Ji and Hua-Tuo-Jia-Ji in Small Animals. Proceedings of the 34th International Congress on Veterinary Acupuncture. 2008: 85-92.
4. Dai, Xin-Min. Traumatology of Chinese Medicine. Qi Ye Books Company. 1991: 419-434.
5. Dewey, Curtis W, Steve C, Budsberg, and John E, Oliver, Jr. Principles of Head Trauma Management in Dogs and Cats─Part I & Part─II. In The Compendium Collection- Head and Neck Medicine & Surgery in Small Animal Practice. VLS. 1996: 257-277.
6. Hu, Yin-Qi and Zhi-Sui Chang. Bi Syndrome: Analysis of Experiences and Cases by Ancient and Modern Famous Doctors. Scientific Technology Publishing, China. 2006: 268-271.
7. Maciocia, Giovanni. The Foundations of Chinese Medicine. 2nd Edition. Elsevier. 2006:10, 100-101, 231-233.
8. Ren, Ji-Xue and Dian-Jun Sui. Emergency Medicine in TCM. Chinese Medical

Pharmacological Publishing, China. 2004: 606-611.
9. Sagiv, Ben-Yakir. Evidence-Based Acupuncture or the Full Answer Dr. Douglas H. Slatter was Waiting For. Lecture Notes of Integrative Medicine of Small Animal Practice in Taiwan. National Chia-Yi University. 2007.
10. Scheid, Volker, Dan Bensky, Andrew Ellis, and Randall Barolet. Chinese Herbal Medicine-Formulas & Strategies. 2nd Edition. Eastland Press. 2009: 485-502, 573.
11. Shi, Yang Shan and De Hua Qiu. Shi's Traumatology. People Health Publishing, China. 2008:165.
12. Wang, Yong-Yang and Bo-Li Zhang. Brain Medicine in TCM. People Health Publishing, China. 2007: 753-756.
13. Xie, Huisheng. Head Trauma: TCM Approaches. Xie's Notes in Integrative Medicine of Taipei-International Conference. 2007.
14. Xie, Huisheng and Vanessa Preast. Xie's Veterinary Acupuncture. Blackwell Publishing. 2007: 222, 226, 254.

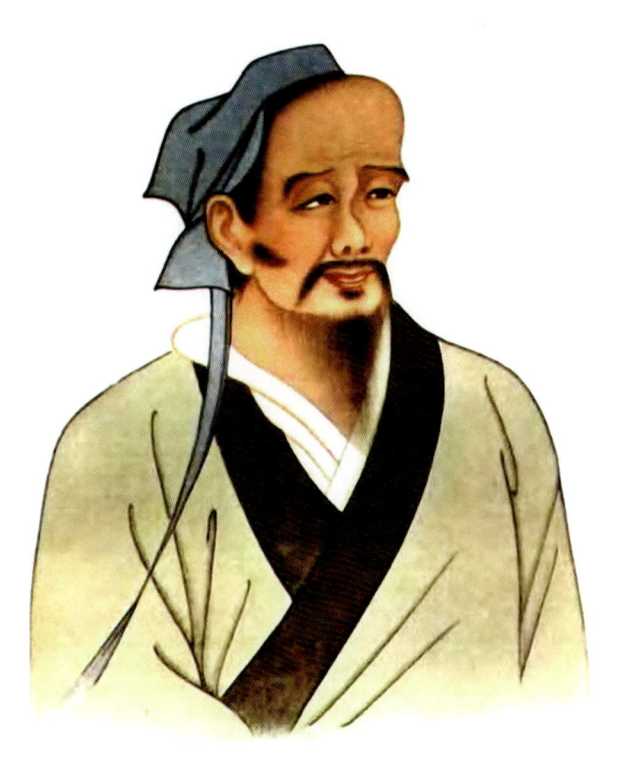

HUA TUO 华佗

Hua Tuo (110-207 CE) was a famous physician whose expertise included internal medicine, surgery, pediatrics and acupuncture during the Han Dynasty. He was born in Haoxian, Anhui province, which has become one of the four major centers of herb distribution in China. Historical records indicate that Hua Tuo created an herbal recipe called *Ma Fei San* to be used as a general anesthesic method during surgery. He found a set of 34 *Jia Ji* (paravertebral) acupoints to be safer and more effective than the acupoints of the Bladder and Governing Channels. In later times, *Hua Tuo Jia Ji* was named to honor his findings. He lived nearly 100 years, with perfect health. He created medical *Daoyin* (early form of *Qigong*) exercises and developed the *Wu Qin Xi* (Exercise of the Five Animals") to mimic natural movements of the tiger, deer, bear, monkey, and crane.

Very sadly, this great physician was executed by a politician Cao Cao in 207 CE, the governor of Wei, one of the Three Kingdoms. During that time, China was divided into three kingdoms, Wei, Shu and Wu. There were non-stop wars among these kingdoms during that time. The governor was suffering from chronic severe migraine attacks. Since his headache was relieved by Hua's acupuncture treatment, he ordered Hua to be his exclusive private physician, which Hua resented. Hua did not stay in the Wei Court for too long and always made excuses to return to his home near Wu. Cao was very angry and upset with Hua because of his disobedience and suggested he perform brain surgery that was perhaps considered an assassination attempt and finally Cao put Hua in jail. During Hua Tuo's time in prison, he wrote *Qing Nang Jing* (Green Gag Book) to record all his secret techniques and herbal formulations including *Ma Fei San*. When Hua Tuo was about to be executed he handed this book over to the jailer. Unfortunately, the jailer would not accept it as he was fearful of the law. At the end, Hua Tuo asked for a fire in which he burned the book.

CHAPTER 7

Equine Neurological Disorders

TCVM for Treatment of Equine Neurological Diseases

Huisheng Xie, DVM, MS, PhD

Neurological diseases can be seen in horses of all ages and breeds. The incidence of neurological diseases in horses is reported from 6.4% to 12.6%.[1,2] Of 565 equine neurological cases, the necropsy results indicated cervical stenotic myelopathy (31%), infectious/inflammatory diseases including equine protozoal myeloencephalitis (EPM) and West Nile virus (31%), trauma (22%), degenerative (11%), congenital (5%) and neoplastic (<1%).[1] Even though many neurological diseases present with similar symptoms, the conventional medical diagnostic tests including neurological examination, cerebrospinal fluid (CSF), radiography and magnetic resonance imaging (MRI), can often pinpoint the exact cause of symptoms and make a definitive diagnosis. However, it can be difficult and frustrating to treat equine neurologic diseases with conventional medicine alone.

Traditional Chinese Veterinary Medicine (TCVM), including acupuncture and herbal medicine, has been used effectively for the treatment of many equine neurological diseases, including laryngeal hemiplegia, radial paralysis, facial paralysis, tetanus, encephalitis, myelitis, meningitis and wobbler syndrome.[3-10] Conventional medicine and TCVM combine together to create a powerful tool for the diagnosis and treatment of neurologic problems in horses. This paper reviews TCVM etiology of neurological disorders and discusses treatment strategies for cervical stenotic myelopathy, equine protozoal myeloencephalitis, laryngeal hemiplegia, facial paralysis, radial paralysis, and encephalomyelitis. Each condition is followed by a case example from clinical practice.

TCVM Etiology and Pathology

The most common causes of neurologic etiologies are trauma, infection, degeneration and congenital defects (Table 1).

1) Trauma injury: Traumatic injury is the most common cause of neurologic problems in performance horses. Trauma causes *Qi*-Blood Stagnation, leading to pain. Chronic Stagnation of *Qi* will gradually cause a local *Qi* Deficiency that presents as paresis, paralysis or muscle atrophy.

2) Infections: When *Zheng Qi* is not strong enough to prevent the invasion of *Xie Qi*, pathogens including viruses (West Nile, Eastern equine encephalitis, Western equine encephalitis), bacteria (Streptococci and, *Escherichia coli* etc) and parasites (*Sarcocystis neurona*), will invade the body, spinal cord and even the brain causing myelitis, encephalitis, myeloencephalitis and meningitis resulting in incoordination (ataxia), weakness, paresis and paralysis.

3) Degeneration/Congenital defects: Degeneration due to aging and/or congenital defects is caused by Kidney *Jing* Deficiency, leading to vertebral malformation, spinal stenosis and arthritic changes.

Table 1: An overview of the common etiologies of neurological diseases in horses and basic treatments

Causes	Main Signs Tongue/Pulse	TCVM Pattern	Acupoints and Herbal Medicine	Herbal Medicine
Trauma	Pain in acute cases Muscle atrophy in chronic cases Purple/wiry	*Qi*-Blood Stagnation	LI-4, GB-21, BL-54, GB-44, LIV-3	Body Sore, or Double P#2[a]
Infection	Fever or no fever Paralysis or seizure Red/fast	Heat Toxin or Damp-Heat	LI-4, LI-11, LU-5, GV-14, *Bai-hui*, *Wei-jian*, *Er-jian*, *Tai-yang*	*Pu Ji Xiao Du Yin* or *Wu Wei Xiao Du Yin*
Degeneration/ Congenital defects	Development orthopedic diseases Pale/weak	Kidney *Jing* Deficiency	*Qi-hai-shu*, BL-26, *Shen-shu*, *Shen-peng*, *Shen-jiao*, KID-10, KID-27	Epimedium Formula[a]

CERVICAL VERTEBRAL STENOTIC MYELOPATHY

Cervical vertebral stenotic myelopathy (CVSM) or cervical vertebral compression myelopathy (CVCM) is caused by spinal cord compression at the cervical level. Its main clinical sign is an abnormal gait in the thoracic and/or pelvic limbs, thus it is referred to as "wobblers" or "wobbler" syndrome, as the affected horse often seems wobbly, when walking or exercising. CVSM is the most common spinal cord disease in young horses (6 months to 2 years).[2] Stallions and geldings are affected three times as often as mares.[11] Horses affected with lesions in the mid-cervical region (vertebrae C3–C5) are significantly younger than those exhibiting more caudal lesions (vertebrae C5–C7). The prevalence is usually higher in Thoroughbreds.[2] Clinical signs of CVSM include: ataxia, muscle tension lines along the cervical vertebra (LI-16 to LI-18), cervical stiffness, and paresis. The ataxia associated with CVSM is usually worse in the pelvic limbs. If it is worse in the thoracic limbs the lesion is most likely at the C6-C7 vertebrae.

In TCVM, CVSM belongs to the cervical *Bi* syndrome, which is often associated with *Qi*-Blood Stagnation in the neck region. A traumatic incident, such as a fall or collision, can cause a blockage of *Qi* flow leading to *Qi*-Blood Stagnation in the neck. Prolonged travel in a trailer results in a lack of cervical movement and exercise that can also lead to *Qi*-Blood Stagnation of the neck. An external pathogenic invasion of Wind-Damp-Cold can also cause *Qi*-Blood Stagnation in the neck. Patients with Kidney *Jing* Deficiency, who already have abnormal joints and soft tissues, are prone to cervical *Bi* syndrome. Cervical *Bi* syndrome (including wobbler syndrome) can be divided into three Patterns: Cervical *Qi* Stagnation, Cervical Blood Stagnation and Kidney *Jing* Deficiency. All seven *Yang* Channels (GV, GB, BL, TH, SI, LI, ST) course through the neck region, thus, they are involved in cervical stiffness and wobbler syndrome. TCVM can effectively treat CVSM. It has been shown in rats that acupuncture with moxibustion can effectively maintain cellular form and the microstructures of the nerve, as well as inhibit the release of inflammatory factors in a model of nerve root compression.[12] In a retrospective study of 19 dogs and horses with wobbler syndrome, the TCVM treatments completely resolved neurological signs in 10 animals (52.6%), partially resolved neurological signs in 8 animals (42.1%) and only 1 animal (5.3%) had no response to the TCVM. [6]

TCVM Pattern Differentiation and Treatment

1) Cervical *Qi* Stagnation:

Clinical Signs:
- mild neck pain on palpation / manipulation, or mild evidence of ataxia, possibly in only the hind limbs, cervical stiffness, but no abnormal radiographic evidence, purple, or pale purple tongue, and wiry pulse

Acupuncture:
- Dry needle: *Bai-hui, Shen-shu*
- Electro-acupuncture (20 Hz for 5 to 10 minutes then 80-120 Hz for 15 to 20 minutes) connecting the following pairs of acupoints:
  Left GB-20 + right GB-21
  Right GB-20 + left GB-21
  Jing-jia-ji (bilaterally)
  Jiu-wei (bilaterally)
- Aqua-acupuncture (Vitamin B12) at *Jing-jia-ji*, BL-62, SI-3, KID-6

Herbal Medicine:
- Cervical Formula[a]: 15 to 30 grams twice daily for 1 to 3 months. [13]

2) Cervical Blood Stagnation:

Clinical signs:
- obvious/severe evidence of ataxia of all 4 hind limbs (worse in pelvic limbs), neck pain on palpation/manipulation, cervical stiffness, abnormal radiographs as evidenced by narrow intervertebral disk spaces and sclerosis of the demi-facets, purple tongue, wiry or fast pulse

Acupuncture:
- Dry needle: *Bai-hui*, BL-23, LIV-3, GB-44, BL-67, LI-4, LU-7
- Electroacupuncture (20 Hz for 5 to 10 minutes + 80-120 Hz for 15 to 20 minutes) connecting the following pairs of acupoints:
  Left GB-20 + right GB-21
  Right GB-20 + left GB-21
  Jing-jia-ji (bilateral)
  Shen-shu + KID-1
  BL-10 + BL-11 in horses
- Aqua-acupuncture (Vitamin B12) at *Jing-jia-ji*, BL-62, SI-3, KID-6

Herbal Medicine: [13]
- Cervical Formula,[a] 15 g twice daily for 1 to 3 months
- Double P#2[a] (*Da Huo Luo Dan* modification), 15-30 g twice daily for 1 to 3 months

3) Kidney *Jing* Deficiency:

Clinical Signs:
- Wobbler syndrome that occurs in young animals (less than 2 years old).
- The horse may have other developmental orthopedic diseases (DOD). *Qi* or Blood Stagnation are also present.

Acupuncture:
- Dry needle: *Bai-hui*, BL-23, BL-24, BL-26
- Electro-acupuncture (20 Hz for 5 to 10 minutes + 80-120 Hz for 15 to 20 minutes) connecting the following pairs of acupoints:
  Left GB-20 + right GB-21
  Right GB-20 + left GB-21
  Jing-jia-ji (bilateral)
  Shen-shu + BL-21
  BL-10 + BL-11 in horses
- Aqua-acupuncture (Vitamin B12) at *Jing-jia-ji*, BL-62, SI-3, KID-6, KID-3, KID-10

Herbal Medicine:
- Use Cervical Formula or/and Double P#2 first. After clinical signs (ataxia and other neurological signs) are resolved, use Epimedium Formula (15 g twice daily for 3 to 6 months) to treat Kidney *Jing* Deficiency.

Other Herbal Treatments: [13]
- Body Sore[a] (*Shen Tong Zhu Yu* modification) is added for patients with severe neck pain of any patterns listed above.
- *Bu Yang Huan Wu* is added when *Qi/Yang* Deficiency was present (rear weakness, cold back, pale and wet tongue, and deep/weak pulse)
- Hindquarter Weakness[a] is added when *Qi+Yin* Deficiency was present (cool-seeking, rear weakness, red/dry tongue, and fast/thin pulse), was given orally.

Case example:

A 4-month thoroughbred colt presented with a 4-week history of pelvic limb ataxia. Recently his clinical signs were getting worse and he was diagnosed with wobbler syndrome. He was very ataxic in all four limbs, but worse in the pelvic limbs. He was restless. His tongue was pale and wet, and his pulse was deep and weak. He had a Fire constitution. His TCVM diagnosis was Blood Stagnation with Kidney *Jing* Deficiency. He was treated with aqua-acupuncture (vitamin B$_{12}$, 1 ml per point) at *Bai-hui*, BL-62 and SI-3 and electroacupuncture at *Shen-shu* (bilaterally), GB-21 (bilaterally), SI-16 + TH-16, *Jing-jia-ji* at C2/3, C4/5, C5/6, for one session per month for a total of 7 treatments. He also received 10 grams of Cervical Formula[a] orally twice daily for 3 months and then 10 grams of Epimedium Formula[a] twice daily for 4 months. He also received daily acupressure (*Tui-na, Dian-fa*) at GB-21 and *Jing-jia-ji*. His ataxia completely resolved after 7 months of TCVM treatment. He was sold for $350,000 at a yearling sale in Kentucky.

EQUINE PROTOZOAL MYELOENCEPHALITIS (EPM)

Equine protozoal myeloencephalitis (EPM) may be caused by four types of protozoa. *Sarcocystis neurona* is the major cause in > 50% EPM cases. Horses of all ages may be affected, however most are young horses 1 to 6 years old. The clinical presentation of EPM varies widely. Some horses have mild lameness for months while others can become recumbent within a day of the first signs of disease. Some horses have alternating limb lameness and others have facial paralysis or other focal neurological signs. The clinical signs of EPM are frequently unilateral, but can be bilateral and mimic cervical stenotic myelopathy, Eastern equine encephalitis or West Nile viruses. A full conventional diagnostic work up is recommended. With proper, quick and aggressive conventional medical treatment, 60% to 70% of horses make a significant or complete recovery.

TCVM Etiology and Pathology:

From a TCVM perspective, stress, travel, and immunosuppressive drugs negatively affect the *Zheng Qi*. *Zheng Qi* is not strong enough to dispel parasites, including protozoa and allows them to enter the body. The protozoal parasites eventually invade the Lower *Jiao* and Kidney system, where they spread to the spinal cord and brain leading to *Qi*-Blood stagnation, causing muscle loss, toe dragging and loss of coordination in the hind limbs (ataxia). The strength of the *Zheng Qi* is dependent on the strength of the *Yuan Qi, Gu Qi, Ying Qi* and *Wei Qi*. This is why conditions that deplete *Qi* such as prolonged illness, poor nutrition and stress make the horse more susceptible to EPM. A weakness of *Zheng Qi* stems from a Deficiency of all the components comprising it, so the overall pattern with EPM is a Global *Qi* Deficiency.

Clinical Signs:
- Acute onset of neurologic abnormalities including ataxia
- Mild to severe lameness
- Weakness, recumbency
- Muscle atrophy over the hindquarters
- Cranial nerve deficits or single limb paralysis, reflex loss
- Acupoint sensitivities on palpation including KID-27, GB-32, *Feng-long, Bai-cong-wo*
- Tongue: pale purple and wet
- Pulse: weak and deep

TCVM Diagnosis *Qi* Deficiency with *Qi* Stagnation

Acupuncture Treatment:
- Dry needle: *Bai-hui*, GV-14, *Qi-hai-shu*, BL-20, BL-23, BL-26, BL-54, LI-10, LI-4, GB-39, KID-6

- Electro-acupuncture (for ten minutes at 80 Hz and ten to twenty minutes at 120 to 200 Hz) at the following pairs:
  BL-21 + BL-21,
  Shen-shu + ST-36,
  BL-54 + BL-54,
  BL-62 + KID-1
- Aqua-acupuncture: KI-27, LI-11, GV-14, *Bai-hui,* GB-32 with B12 or the horse's own blood to stimulate the *Zheng Qi*

Herbal treatment:
- *Qing Hao San,*[a] 15-30 g twice daily for 2 to 6 months can be used in conjunction with other medications; tonifies *Qi*, kills parasites, and tonifies *Zheng Qi*

Case example

A seven year old Thoroughbred colt named Calvin had a history of having tripping problems of rear limbs. He also began to show some muscle atrophy in the hind end 4 months ago. Calvin was shipped to the local university animal hospital 3 months ago. The myelogram and MRI ruled out any compression of the cervical vertebrae. And the CSF confirmed the EPM diagnosis. Calvin had sulfa/pyramethamine and Baycox for 3 months. After 3-month medication, Calvin became more active and experienced less tripping (about 50% improvement), but he continued tripping on both rear limbs occasionally, and had muscle atrophy in the hind end. He was then recommended for a TCVM assessment and treatment. On the first TCVM visit on March 7, 2001, Calvin was noticed to have weakness at both hind limbs with high sensitivity at LI-17/18, SI-16, BL-16 to *Qi-hai-shu*, BL-54/*Lu-gu, Shen-shu* on palpation. His tongue was pale purple, pulse was deep weak (worse at the right side). His personality was Wood.
The following acupuncture points were sensitive on palpation

	Left	Right
LI-17/18, SI-16	+4	+5
BL-16 to *Qi-hai-shu*	+4	+4
BL-54/*Lu-gu, Shen-shu*	+5	+4

His TCVM Pattern was *Qi* Deficiency with local stagnation at the back and hip areas. The TCVM treatments were as follows.

Acupuncture Treatment:
- Dry needle: *Yan-chi*, BL-23, BL-62, SI-3
- Electro-acupuncture at the following pairs (20Hz 15 min + 80-120Hz 15 min)
  Bai-hui +GV-9
  Shen-shu, bilateral
  BL-16, bilateral
  Qi-hai-shu, bilateral
  Left BL-53 +BL-54
  Left *Lu-gu* +BL-40
  Right BL-54 + BL-53

Aquacupuncture of his own blood at KID-27, LI-11, GV-14 (3 cc per point)

Herbal Medicine:
- *Qing Hao San*, 15 grams twice daily orally for 4 weeks; and
- Body Sore,[a] 15 grams twice daily orally for 4 weeks.

On the second visit on April 11, 2001, the trainer reported that his rear weakness and tripping were 40-50% better. On palpation, he had sensitivity only at BL-54/*Lu-gu*. His tongue was slightly pale and pulse was deep. A similar acupuncture treatment was given. *Qing Hao San*, 30 grams twice daily was given orally. Body Sore[a] was discontinued.

On the third visit on May 16, 2001, the owner reported that he walked and trotted with 100% normal gait, and showed slight ataxia when he galloped. His activity and attitude were great. He enjoyed training. On palpation, no sensitivity at any acupoints was noticed. His *Shen* looked great with normal tongue and pulse.

LARYNGEAL HEMIPLEGIA

Laryngeal hemiplegia in horses is characterized by paresis or paralysis of the arytenoid cartilage and vocal fold. It is also known as "roaring" because of the characteristic inspiratory noise heard during intense exercise. Laryngeal hemiplegia is most commonly seen on the left side, in male horses typically Thoroughbreds and Draft horses, although other breeds are affected. The main problems caused by this disease are the lack of adequate oxygen intake during maximal exercise and the accompanying roaring sound. Surgical correction is a common treatment, but still leaves 30-40% of the horses with exercise intolerance or respiratory noise.[14] Acupuncture is a good alternative for horse with Grades I to III. In one retrospective study 13 out of 18 thoroughbred racehorses with laryngeal hemiplegia (Grades I to III) became normal via endoscopy examination, after 3-7 acupuncture treatments and the other 5 cases improved their Grades after acupuncture treatments.[15]

TCVM Etiology and Pathology:

The normal functions of the larynx and airway are associated with Lung *Qi*. The cause of laryngeal hemiplegia is degeneration or traumatic damage to the laryngeal nerve. Degeneration is often associated with Kidney *Jing* Deficiency, which can gradually cause Lung *Qi* Deficiency, leading to a lack of adequate oxygen intake. Damage to the local nerve causes local *Qi*-Blood Stagnation, leading to roaring. Thus, laryngeal hemiplegia can be diagnosed as Local *Qi*-Blood Stagnation with Kidney *Jing* and Lung *Qi* Deficiency.

Clinical Signs:
- Hoarse, raspy respiratory sounds, particularly during inspiration
- Exercise intolerance
- Dyspnea, inspiratory stridor or an inspiratory noise ("roaring")
- Coughing or gagging, or hoarse voice or unable to vocalize
- Tongue: normal or pale purple
- Pulse: normal, or deep, weaker on the right side

TCVM Diagnosis: Local *Qi*-Blood Stagnation with Kidney *Jing* and Lung *Qi* deficiency.

Acupuncture Treatment: 3 to 6 treatments, 1 to 4 weeks apart.
- Dry needle: *Bai-hui*, LI-4, LU-7, LI-10, SI-3
- Electro-acupuncture: 20 Hz 15 min and 80-120 Hz 15 min (total: 30 min) at the following acupuncture paired-points:
    - GB-21 + CV-23 a or CV-23 b (CV-23 a and CV-23 b are located 0.5 cun lateral to CV-23)
    - LI-18 +LI-17, bilateral
    - CV-23 + LI-15
    - LI-16 + *Hou-bi*
    - SI-17 bilateral
    - ST-9 + *Hou-shu*
    - Other points: CV-24, TH-17

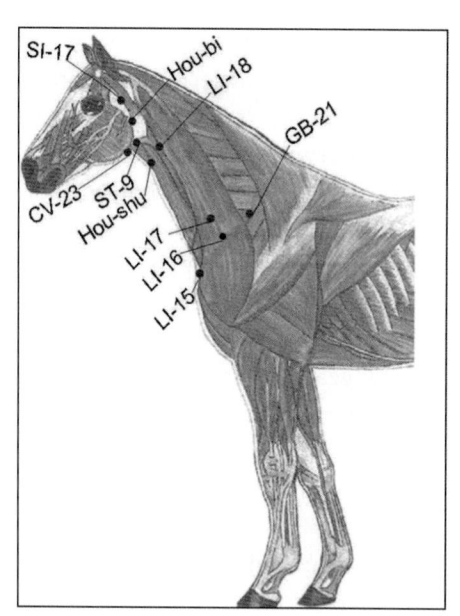

Figure 1: Acupuncture points used in Laryngeal Hemiplegia

Herbal Medicine:
- Four Gentlemen[a] (*Si Jun Zi Tang*), 15 g twice daily for 1 to 3 months.

Case Example:

A 1 year old thoroughbred colt presented with left laryngeal hemiplegia (Grade II). His tongue and pulse were normal. No other abnormal clinical signs were found. He was a Wood constitution. He was treated with acupuncture therapy, which included dry needle at *Bai-hui*, SI-3 and LU-7 and electro-acupuncture at ST-9 (bilaterally), SI-17 (bilaterally), left LI-17 + CV-23, left GB-21 + CV-23a, *Hou-shu* + CV-24, LI-18 (bilaterally). His laryngeal muscles returned to normal function after 7 acupuncture treatments (one session every 2 to 4 weeks). He was sold for $560,000 at a 2-year-old sale in Kentucky.

FACIAL PARALYSIS

Facial paralysis refers to motor function loss of the muscles, innervated by the facial nerve. This condition is characterized by acute onset, in any season and at any age. Unilateral facial paralysis is most common in horses and usually caused by trauma. The facial nerve is very superficial as it runs across the facial crest. Damage can be from a blow, such as a kick from another horse or from pressure, usually the halter while the horse is lying down or if the horse pulls back while tied. The trauma blocks the flow of *Qi* and Blood leading to a deficiency in the local tissues. TCVM calls this condition *Wai-zui-feng*, Deviating Mouth Wind. As indicated by its name, facial paralysis is also associated with invasion of Wind. The main Channels involved in facial paralysis are ST, LI and SI as they are located in this region. In a study on human facial nerve paralysis, using acupuncture and electro-acupuncture, in the treatment group the recovery rate was 94.6-98.6%, while in the control group it was 72.1%. [16]

TCVM Etiology and Pathology:

When *Zheng Qi* is not strong enough due to overwork and stress, the weakened *Wei Qi* allows invasion of Wind-Cold or Wind-Heat to the face and Channels. This leads to blockage of *Qi*-Blood and failure of *Qi*-Blood circulation to nourish the local muscles. Trauma can also cause local *Qi*-Blood stagnation. Thus, the consequence is facial paralysis. The three *Yang* Channels, including LI, ST and SI, are the ones primarily involved.

Clinical Signs:
- Mouth, eyelids and ear may droop on the affected side
- May have pain on palpation
- Excessive salivation
- General weakness or exercise intolerance
- Tongue: pale purple
- Pulse: normal or weak on right

TCVM Diagnosis: *Qi* Deficiency with Local *Qi*-Blood Stagnation

Acupuncture Treatment:
- Electro-acupuncture: Choose 5 pairs of the points below. Apply 80-120 Hz for 20-30 minutes once every 1 to 2 weeks for 3 to 5 treatments
- Aqua-puncture: Choose 8 to 10 of the points below. Use 3 ml vitamin B_{12}, per point once every 2 to 3 days for 5 to 10 treatments.
- Points: ST-4, ST-5, ST-6, ST-7, ST-36, LI-18, LI-10, LI-4, SI-19, SI-18, GV-26, *Fen-shui*, CV-24.

ST, LI and SI are three main Channels which distribute *Qi* and Blood in the face. Therefore, they are the key Channels to treat facial paralysis. ST-4, ST-5, ST-6, ST-7, LI-18, SI-18 and SI-19 are local points from those three Channels. ST-36 and LI-10 tonify *Qi* to nourish the face. LI-4 is the Master point for any facial problem. GV-26, *Fen-shui* and CV-24 are local points.

Herbal Medicine
- Facial P Formula:[a] 15 to 30 g twice daily for 1 to 2 months. This herbal formula clears Wind, invigorates *Qi*/Blood to relieve Stagnation.

Case Example:
A 10 year old mare sustained traumatic injuries to the left side of her face 6 weeks ago. She was in-foal, had a 4-month foal, with a history of 4 other successful births. A referring veterinarian diagnosed her with left facial paralysis. The major clinical complaints were drooping lips and ear on the left side. After three bi-weekly electro-acupuncture treatments (30 minutes each session) at ST-4, ST-5, ST-6, ST-7, SI-18, SI-19 and dry needle at LI-4 and LI-10, the mare showed a clinical complete recovery.

SUPRASCAPULAR, RADIAL NERVE AND BRACHIAL PLEXUS INJURY
Trauma is often the cause of suprascapular, radial nerve and brachial plexus injury. Traumatic injury is often caused by the horse running into an object such as a fence, tree or another horse or being kicked by another horse. Damage to the suprascapular nerve alone often leads to suprascapular and infrascapular muscle atrophy ("sweeney"). A loss of extensor function to the muscles of the forelimb with a dropped elbow indicates damage to the radial nerve.[11]

TCVM Etiology and Pathology:
Traumatic injury damages local nerves and other tissues, leading to local *Qi*-Blood Stagnation. The chronic blockage of *Qi*-Blood will cause *Qi* Deficiency, leading to muscle atrophy. Weakness, lack of function and muscle atrophy are significant signs of *Qi* Deficiency.

Clinical Signs:
- May be painful on palpation
- Muscle atrophy
- Paresis or paralysis
- Tongue: purple or pale
- Pulse: weaker on right, wiry

TCVM Diagnosis: Local *Qi*-Blood Stagnation with *Qi* Deficiency

Acupuncture treatment:
- Dry-needling: *Bai-hui*, LI-1, LI-3, LI-4, TH-1, TH-3, SI-1 and SI-3
- Aqua-puncture or Electro-acupuncture (alternately): BL-11, TH-15, SI-9, SI-10, TH-14, LU-1, *Yan-zhou, Cheng-deng*, LI-14, LI-15, LI-10, LI-11
- Pneumo-acupuncture: *Gong-zi* or any other atrophied area(s) if muscle atrophy is presented.

Herbal Medicine
- Acute Stage (painful on palpation):Equine Chest Formula,[a] 15 g, twice daily for 1 to 2 months
- Chronic Stage (non-painful on palpation and Sweeney): *Qi* Performance,[a] 15 g, twice daily for 1 to 3 months

Case example:

A 10 year old Dutch warmblood grey filly exhibited left front lameness because another horse ran into her left shoulder one year ago. Since then, she always has had a problem with her left front limb. Radiographic and scintigraphic findings were within normal limits. Nerve blocks did not clear the soreness. No conclusive conventional diagnosis was made. The lameness was non-responsive to stall rest and conventional medications including analgesics and nonsteroidal anti-inflammatory agents. She had a 3/5 lameness of left thoracic limb. The TCVM examination revealed strong acupoint sensitivities on the left TH-14, LI-15, LI-16, *Yan-zhou* and *Cheng-deng*. Her left shoulder was atrophied around SI-9 to SI-12. Her tongue was purple, and her pulse was deep and weak. Thus, *Qi* Deficiency and *Qi*-blood Stagnation of the left shoulder was the TCVM diagnosis.

The lameness and muscle atrophy was completely gone after six bi-weekly acupuncture treatments with dry needle (TH-1, LI-3 and SI-3), electro-acupuncture (bilateral GB-21, left SI-9 + LI-16, left TH-14 + LI-15 and left Yan-zhou + SI-10), and pneumo-acupuncture at *Gong-zi* and SI-9 (about 500 cc per point), along with the Chinese herbal medicine, *Qi* Performance, given for three months at a dose of 15 grams twice daily.

ENCEPHALOMYELITIS

Encephalomyelitis is an inflammation of the brain and spinal cord. It is often caused by Eastern equine encephalomyelitis (EEE) virus, Western equine encephalomyelitis (WEE) virus, Venezuelan equine encephalomyelitis (VEE) virus and West Nile (WN) virus. Most often, the body's immune system is able to contain and defeat an infection. But if *Wei Qi* is deficient, the infection passes into the blood stream and then into the cerebrospinal fluid that surrounds the brain and spinal cord. Finally the viruses can affect the nerves and travel to the brain and/or surrounding tissues, causing inflammation. The resulting inflammation and swelling can harm or destroy nerve cells and cause hemorrhages in the brain. West Nile Virus (WNV) and Eastern equine encephalomyelitis viruses (EEEV) are mosquito-borne viruses that causes encephalitis (inflammation of the brain) and/or meningitis (inflammation of the coverings of the brain and spinal cord). The WEE and VEE viruses are related, but genetically distinct alpha viruses. The EEE and VEE viruses are lethal in up to 90% of recognized equine cases, whereas the WEE virus is less virulent in horses. [18-19]

TCVM Etiology and Pathology:

The *Zheng Qi* protects the body from external pathogens including viruses and bacteria. When *Zheng Qi* is weak the body is at risk. The strength of the *Zheng Qi* is dependent on the strength of the *Yuan Qi, Gu Qi, Ying Qi* and *Wei Qi*. A weakness of *Zheng Qi* stems from a Deficiency in the component parts, so the best way to protect the body is to keep all forms of *Qi* strong.

1) Invasion of Heat Toxin

The external pathogen is able to invade because the *Zheng Qi* is not strong enough to protect the body. It is mostly seen in very young, very old or weakened animals. Once the pathogen has entered the body it causes excessive Heat Toxin.

2) *Yin* Deficiency

After Heat Toxin enters the body, it consistently consumes Body Fluids and damages *Yin*, gradually leading to *Yin* Deficiency (low-grade fever, chronic inflammation, red and dry tongue and thin/fast pulse).

3) *Qi* and Blood Deficiency

During any viral infections, the body tries to clear the invasion of the pathogen, and in the end, it becomes depleted in *Qi* and Blood, leading to general *Qi*-Blood Deficiency.

Pattern Differentiation and Treatment

1) Heat Toxin

Clinical Signs:
- Acute onset
- Fever
- Tongue: red
- Pulse: fast and strong
- Ears and body feel warm or hot

Acupuncture Treatment:
- *Er-jian, Wei-jian, Tai-Yang, Da-feng-men*, LI-4, LI-11, GB-20, KID-1, GV-14, GB-39

Herbal Medicine:
- *Pu Ji Xiao Du Yin* clears Heat and removes toxins for high fever cases

2) *Yin* Deficiency with Residual Heat

Clinical Signs:
- Prolonged low-grade fever
- Loss of consciousness, paresis, or seizures
- Warm ears/body
- Tongue: red and dry
- Pulse: thin and fast or weaker on the left side

Acupuncture Treatment:
- LI-4/10/11, GV-14, BL-23, SP-6, SP-9, KID-3, KID-6, KID-10

Herbal Medicine:
- *Qing Ying Tang* nourishes *Yin*, clears false Heat.

3) *Qi* Deficiency

Clinical Signs:

- Lethargy
- Poor recovery after exercise, lack of stamina
- Paresis or paralysis
- Tongue: pale
- Pulse: deep and weak

Acupuncture Treatment:
- BL-17, BL-18, BL-20, BL-21, *Qi-hai-shu*, BL-24, *Shen-shu,* SP-10, ST-36, LI-10, ST-41, KID-1, PC-9

Herbal Medicine:
- *Bu Yang Huan Wu* tonifies *Qi* and resolves Stagnation

Case example

An 11 year TB gelding was presented with four limb paralysis due to West Nile Virus infection 2 weeks ago. His rectal temperature was 101.5 – 102.5 °F. The TCVM Exam indicated that his *Shen* was depressed with decreased food intake and normal defecation. His pulse was thin and fast and tongue was pale purple. His TCVM diagnosis was *Qi* Deficiency with Residual Heat. His TCVM treatments included:

Acupuncture Treatment:
Dry needle: *Er-jian, Wei-jian*
Electro-acupuncture with 15 min 20 Hz + 15 min 80-120 Hz at the following points:
- BL-10 + *Jiu-wei*
- GV-14+ right TH-15
- GB-21 + PC-8
- Right LI-10+LI-11
- KID-1 + ST-36
- SI-3 + BL-62

Herbal Medicine:
i) *Qing Ying Tang*, 30 g, bid,
ii) *Bu Yang Huan Wu*, 30 g bid for 1 month.

Other Treatment:
Daily Physical Therapy

Outcome:
After 7 acupuncture treatments (1 session every 2 days), 2-week herbal medications and daily physical therapy, he was able to stand up by himself and his body temperature became normal. He was discharged from the hospital. *Qing Ying Tang* was discontinued. Acupuncture was given one session per month along with daily oral herbal medication of *Bu Yang Huan Wu* (15 g bid). He became pasture sound after 3 more monthly acupuncture treatments and 3 months of herbal medications.

Table 2: The most common neurological disorders of horses, the underlying TCVM pattern and specific treatments

Conventional Diagnosis	TCVM pattern	Acupuncture points	Herbal Medicine
Cervical Stenotic Myelopathy	Cervical *Qi* Stagnation	*Jing jia ji* points around cervical lesion BL-62, GV-14, LU-7, SI-3 KID-3, BL-23, BL-20, ST-36, SP-6, *Shen-shu*, GB-39, BL-67, GB-44, ST-45, TH-1, SI-1, LI-1 KID-7, *Chou-jin*, LIV-3, LI-10	Cervical Formula[a]
	Cervical Blood Stagnation		Cervical Formula[a] and Double P#2[a]
	Kidney *Jing* Deficiency		Epimedium Formula[a]
Equine Protozoal Myelitis	*Qi* Deficiency with *Qi* Stagnation	LI-4, LI-16, LI-10, ST-36, GV-14, *Yan-chi*, BL-25, BL-62, GB-39, *Qi-hai-shu*, SP-6, LIV-3, *Shen-shu*, BL-54	Qing Hao San
Laryngeal Hemiplegia	*Qi* Deficiency with *Qi* Stagnation	CV-23a, CV-23b, LI-18, *Hou-shu* a, *Hou-shu* b, SI-17, ST-9, GB-20, GB-21, LI-4, LU-7, SI-3, ST-36, LI-10, TH-17, KID-1 or KID-3, *Qi-hai-shu*	Four Gentlemen[a]
Facial Nerve Paralysis	Local *Qi*-Blood Stagnation with *Qi* deficiency	ST-4, ST-7, ST36, GB-20, SI-19, LI-4, LI10, TH-1, SI-1, *Qi-hai-shu*, BL-20, BL-21, BL-18	Facial P Formula[a]
Suprascapular, radial nerve	*Qi* deficiency with Local *Qi*-Blood Stagnation	TH-15, GB-21, LI-10, TH-5, PC-6, TH-1, SI-1, LI-1, *Gong-zi*, LI-11, LI-15 SI-9, SI-10, TH-14; If brachial plexus is involved, add HT-3, KID-24, KID-27	*Qi* Performance[a]
Encephalomyelitis	Heat Toxin	*Er-jian, Wei-jian, Tai-Yang, Da-feng-men*, LI-4, LI-16, GB-20, KID-1, GV-14, GB-39, LI-10, ST-36, *Qi-hai-shu*, BL-20, SP-6	Pu Ji Xiao Du Yin
	Yin Deficiency with Residual Heat		Qing Ying Tang
	Qi Deficiency		Bu Yang Huan Wu

Footnotes:

[a] (JT) = *Jing Tang* Herbal www.tcvmherbal.com; Reddick, FL

References:

1. Williams NM, Allen G, Powell D. Equine neurologic disease Journal of Equine Veterinary Science 2003; 23 (10): 431-4332.

2. Laugier C, Tapprest J, Foucher N, Sevin C. A necropsy survey of neurologic diseases in 4,319 horses examined in Normandy (France) from 1986 to 2006. Journal of Equine Veterinary Science 2009; 29(7):561-568
3. Chuan Yu. Traditional Chinese Veterinary Acupuncture and Moxibustion. Beijing, China:China Agricultural Press 1995:242-261.
4. Liu Z, Xie H, Xu J, Zhang K. Equine Acupuncture. Beijing, China: Beijing Agricultural University Press 1993:1-304.
5. Xie H, Preast V. Xie's Veterinary Acupuncture. Ames, IA:Blackwell Publishing 2006:1-359.
6. Xie H, Rimar T. Effect of a combination of acupuncture and herbal medicine on wobbler syndrome in dogs and horses. In: Yang and Xie (Ed): Traditional Chinese Veterinary Medicine-Empirical Techniques to Scientific Validation. Reddick, FL:Jing-tang Publishing 2010:101-112.
7. Kim MS, Xie H. Use of electroacupuncture to treat laryngeal hemiplegia in horses. Veterinary Record 2009; 165: 602-603.
8. Wang QL, Hu GL. Acupuncture for treatment of facial and radial paralysis in horses. Chinese Journal of Veterinary Medicine 1983; 10:33-35. (In Chinese).
9. Xiong SY Electro-acupuncture treatment for 2 cases with tetanus in horses. Chinese Journal of Veterinary Science and Technology 1981; 9: 53-54. (in Chinese).
10. Liu YM, Liu XJ, Bai SS et al. The effect of electroacupuncture on T cell responses in rats with experimental autoimmune encephalitis. J Neuroimmunol 2010; 220(1-2):25-33.
11. Ross M, Dyson S. Diagnosis and Management of Lameness in the Horse. Kennett Square, PA:Saunders 2003:566-570, 413-414.
12. Mi YQ, Wu YC, Chen Y. Effects of warm needle Moxibustion on nerve root local inflammatory factors (NOS and CGRP) in the lumbar root compress model in rats. Zhonggu Zhen Jiu 2009; 29(1);48-52.(in Chinese)
13. Xie H, Preast V. Chinese Veterinary Herbal Handbook 2nd ed. Reddick, FL:Chi Institute of Chinese Medicine 2008:1-598.
14. Hinchcliff K, Kaneps A, Geor R. Equine Sports Medicine and Surgery. Columbus OH: WB Saunders 2004: 579-584.
15. Kim MS, Xie H. Use of electroacupuncture to treat laryngeal hemiplegia in horses. Veterinary Record 2009; 165:602-603.
16. Shen TL. Clinical study on acupuncture intervention time for the treatment of peripheral facial paralysis. Zhongguo Zhen Jiu 2009; 29(5):357-60. (in Chinese)
17. Zeller HG, Schuffenecker I. West Nile virus: an overview of its spread in Europe and the Mediterranean basin in contrast to its spread in the Americas. Eur J Clin Microbiol Infect Dis 200; 23(3):147-56.
18. Pellegrini-Masini A, Livesey LC. Meningitis and encephalomyelitis in horses. Vet Clin North Am Equine Pract 2006; 22(2):553-89.
19. Franklin RP, Kinde H, Jay MT et al. Eastern Equine Encephalomyelitis Virus Infection in a Horse from California. Emerging Infectious Diseases 2002 ; 8 (3) :283-288.

TCVM Treatment of Suprascrapular Nerve Injury in a Dutch Warmblood Filly

Margaret Fowler, DVM, CVA, CVCH, CVTP, CVFT

Introduction

The suprascapular nerve courses around the cranial aspect of the scapular neck and in this relatively superficial position is vulnerable to acute trauma, often resulting from collision with a solid object. Neurogenic atrophy of the supraspinatus and infraspinatus muscles can occur within 7 days of injury and can result in an inability to extend the shoulder normally. If improvement is not seen within the first 6-8 weeks, the prognosis is not favorable.[1]

Background

A 10 month old Dutch warmblood filly was examined for injury of the suprascapular nerve which had occurred 3 months prior when the uncontrolled filly ran into a barn support pole. She had been examined and treated by a traditional veterinarian who referred her for evaluation and treatment at a major School of Veterinary Medicine. The expensive filly had been imported from Holland with hopes of becoming a high level dressage horse and the owner's goal was to return her to training. Unfortunately with over 90% muscle atrophy of the left shoulder, the owner was given a poor prognosis for this goal and was advised that the filly would likely become a lame broodmare. Unwilling to accept this outcome, the owner sought acupuncture therapy.

TCVM Evaluation

The filly was high-strung with little training and difficult to examine and treat. A TCVM evaluation revealed a Fire personality with excellent *Shen*, strong surging fast pulses, and a pale lavender tongue. No significant reactions were found at alarm and association points and overall temperature was normal. The filly had 5+ atrophy of the left shoulder and a hard painful warm swelling at the point of the shoulder. She was also underweight and had a shortened abnormal stride involving the left forelimb.

TCVM Patterns

Two TCVM patterns were identified. The first was an excess pattern of severe *Qi*/Blood Stagnation of the left shoulder as evidenced by the lavender tongue, forceful pulses, dysfunction of the suprascapular nerve, and a painful warm swelling at the shoulder point.[2] The second pattern was one of overall *Qi* Deficiency, despite her young age, as evidenced by the pale tongue, underweight body and profound muscle atrophy of the left shoulder.[3]

Treatment Principles

The treatment principles were to relieve the excess, re-establish the flow of *Qi* and Blood, and tonify the overall *Qi* Deficiency. To accomplish these treatment principles all branches of TCVM were utilized: acupuncture including electroacupuncture, aquapuncture, and pneumoacupuncture; *Tui-na*; Chinese herbal therapy; and nutrition (food therapy).

Treatment

The initial attempt to acupuncture was met with very limited success due to the high-strung Fire nature of the filly and her volatile and dangerous exaggerated reaction to needling attempts. It was then determined that heavy sedation would be necessary for future sessions. Although it is generally preferred not to sedate because it is thought to interfere with the effectiveness of acupuncture,[4] a reduced benefit is more effective than no treatment. The owner was instructed to administer 30 mg of Acepromazine orally to the filly 1 hour prior to treatment. Just prior to treatment 300 mg of Xylazine were administered IV with the help of a twitch. This sedation protocol proved effective in allowing future acupuncture sessions.

The owner, who had been restricting feed for over 2 months due to stall confinement and resulting anxiety, was instructed to provide increased amounts of a high quality feed to counteract the *Qi* deficiency, poor weight, and to aid in new muscle formation at the site of atrophy because correction of overall *Qi* Deficiencies begins with the Earth element.[5] *Ba Zhen Tang* modification (*Qi* Performance, manufactured by Jing Tang Herbal), was prescribed at a dose of 7.5 grams twice daily for 8-12 months to relieve the *Qi*/Blood Stagnation, aid in new muscle growth, and reduce the psychogenic stress of stall confinement in a young fire personality.[6] Relief Salve, also manufactured by Jing Tang Herbal, was prescribed with the instruction to apply topically to the swelling at the point of the shoulder every 48 hours for 1 month. Relief Salve is designed to relieve inflammation, swelling and pain due to traumatic soft tissue injuries.[7]

The owner was then instructed in the use of *Tui-na*. *Rou-fa* (Rotary Kneading) over the atrophied area and swollen shoulder point was selected as the initial technique because it is soothing and calming and unblocks stagnated *Qi* and Blood. *Yi-zhi-chan* (Single Thumb) was then performed on the Shoulder Diamond points for more intense stimulation of these acupuncture points, but not exceeding the level of comfort. *Dou-fa* (Shaking) of the left forelimb was chosen as the last technique for its ability to help with nerve damage and muscle atrophy.[8] Each technique was performed 10 minutes 3-5 times weekly.

Acupuncture was performed 9 times over the next 8 months. Electro acupuncture, the acupuncture technique of choice for nerve injury, was performed each session with the following protocol: 10 minutes at 80 plus 120 hertz, and 10 minutes at 0 plus 200 hertz. Points were chosen from the following list and paired in different combinations in different sessions: SI-9 (master point for the foreleg), remaining shoulder diamond points of *Jian-zhen*, *Tiang-zong*, and *Chong-tian* (alternates for SI-9), *Fei-men*, *Fei-pan*, *Bo-jian*, *Bo-lian*, *Bo-zhong*, and *Gong-zi* (classic points for suprascapular nerve injury and shoulder atrophy), LI-15 and TH-14 (close approximation to the course of the suprascapular nerve), GB-21 (major shoulder point), and LI-10 (substitute for the *Qi* tonification point ST-36). Sterile filiform 2 and 3 inch 28 gauge needles were chosen. Additionally, aquapuncture with 10cc of 1000 mcg per ml of Vitamin B12 was performed at one of the Shoulder Diamond points and at LI-10 each session for longer lasting stimulation. Pneumoacupuncture, the acupuncture technique of choice for muscle atrophy, was performed each time at the classical pneumo point *Gong-zi* and nearby area with approximately 250cc of air.[9]

Table 1: Ingredients and Actions of *Ba Zhen Tang* modification (*Qi* Performance)

English Name	Chinese *Pin-Yin*	Action
Paeonia	*Bai Shao Yao*	Tonify Blood and soothe Liver

Angelica	*Dang Gui*	Tonify and move Blood, resolve stagnation, relieve pain
Astragalus	*Huang Qi*	Tonify *Qi*
Condonopsis	*Dang Shen*	Tonify *Qi*
Apis	*Feng Hua Fen*	Tonify *Qi* and *Yin* Tonic
Moutan	*Mu Dan Pi*	Cool and move Blood, relieve pain
Crataegus	*Shan Zha*	Strengthen Stomach, promote appetite
Polygonum	*He Shou Wu*	Tonify Blood
Glycyrrhiza	*Gan Cao*	Harmonize

Manufactured by Jing Tang Herbal

Table 2: Ingredients and Actions of Relief Salve

English Name	Chinese *Pin-Yin*	Action
Clematis	*Wei Ling Xian*	Clear Wind-Damp, move *Qi*, relieve pain
Olibanum	*Ru Xiang*	Invigorate Blood, relieve pain, repair tissue
Myrrh	*Mo Yao*	Invigorate Blood, relieve pain, repair tissue
Draconis	*Xue Jie*	Dissipate stagnation, relieve pain, promote healing
Angelica	*Dang Gui Wei*	Invigorate Blood and relieve pain
Angelica	*Bai Zhi*	Clear the surface, relieve pain, promote healing
Corydalis	*Yan Hu Suo*	Invigorate Blood, relieve pain
Rheum	*Da Huang*	Break down stasis, dissipate swelling, cool Blood
Momordica	*Mu Bie Zi*	Dissipate swelling and nodules, relieve pain
Carthamus	*Hong Hua*	Move Blood, disperse swelling
Gardenia	*Zhi Zi*	Clear Heat, detoxify, cool Blood, dissipate stagnation
Erythinia	*Hai Tong Pi*	Dispel Damp, invigorate Channels
Sophora	*Hua Jiao*	Warm the middle, dispel Cold, relieve pain, dry up Damp
Camphora	*Zhang Nao*	Open the orifice, kill parasites, relieve pain
Borneol	*Bing Pian*	Open the orifice, dissipate stagnation, clear Heat, relieve pain
Beewax	*Feng La*	Carrier
Olive Oil	*Zhi Wu You*	Carrier

Manufactured by Jing Tang Herbal

After just 2 acupuncture sessions approximately 50% of the area above the scapular spine and 15% below the spine had filled in with new muscle. The hard swelling at the shoulder point has lost its heat and reduced in size by 25%. The pale lavender tongue had resolved to a normal pink color and the pulses were now the typically strong non-surging pulses of a filly. After 2 more sessions the swelling had resolved, 75% of the muscle atrophy over the scapular spine and 35% below the spine had been replaced by new muscle growth. The filly had also gained weight. *Ba Zhen Tang* modification (Qi Performance) and *Tui-na* were continued and at this time the owner was instructed to turn the filly out in a small paddock for several hours daily and hand walk her for 5-15 minutes daily.

Outcome

When the filly was re-evaluated at the 9th and final acupuncture session, over 90% of the atrophied muscle had returned and the filly walked and trotted with a normal full stride. Her body weight had also returned to normal. After this session *Tui-na* was discontinued; however, *Ba Zhen Tang* modification (*Qi* Performance) was continued another 2 months. The owner reported that the filly returned to training with no issues.

Conclusion

This case demonstrates how effective all branches of TCVM are in resolving peripheral nerve injury with profound dysfunction and muscle atrophy when traditional veterinary options are limited. It also demonstrates that acupuncture can still be very effective, although increased numbers of sessions may be required, even when heavy sedation is necessary.

References:
1. Ross, Mike, DVM and Dyson, Sue, VetMB. Diagnosis and Management of Lameness in the Horse. Saunders, 2003, pg 413-414, 1066.
2. Shoen, Allen, DVM. Veterinary Acupuncture, 2nd Edition. Mosby, 2001, pg 81-82, 221.
3. Shoen, Allen, DVM. Veterinary Acupuncture, 2nd Edition. Mosby, 2001, pg 81-82, 221.
4. Xie, Huisheng, DVM. Advanced Equine Acupuncture Techniques Class Notes. Chi Institute of Chinese Medicine, 2006, pg 140.
5. Clemmons, Roger, DVM. North American Veterinary Conference Postgraduate Institute, Acupuncture Course Notes. Chi Institute of Chinese Medicine, 2005, pg 154-155.
6. Xie, Huisheng, DVM and Preast, Vanessa, DVM and Liu, Wen, PhD. Chinese Herbal Handbook, 2nd Edition. Chi Institute of Chinese Medicine, 2008, pg 51-52.
7. Xie, Huisheng, DVM and Preast, Vanessa, DVM and Liu, Wen, PhD. Chinese Herbal Handbook, 2nd Edition. Chi Institute of Chinese Medicine, 2008, pg 285.
8. Xie, Huisheng, DVM and Ferguson, Bruce, DVM and Deng, Xiaolin, OMD. Application of *Tui-na* in Veterinary Medicine, 2nd Edition. Chi Institute of Chinese Medicine, 2007, pg 16, 9, 47.
9. Xie, Huisheng, DVM. Advanced Equine Acupuncture Techniques Class Notes. Chi Institute of Chinese Medicine, 2006, pg 38-42, 148-149, 154.

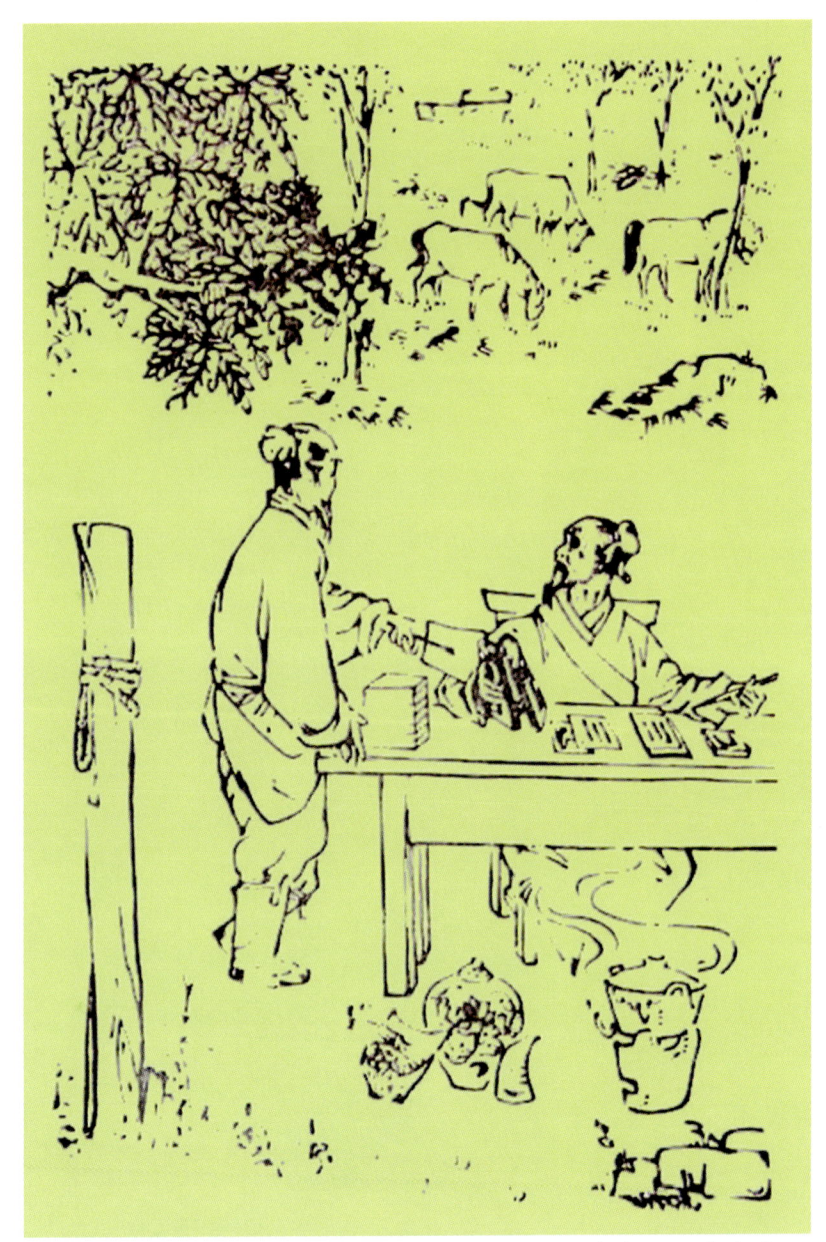

YU BEN YUAN AND YU BEN HENG, 喻本元, 喻本亨

Yu Ben Yuan and Yu Ben Heng were the most popular veterinarians during Ming Dynasty (1368-1644 CE). They were brothers, thus sometime called Yu Brothers. They were born in Liu-an County, Anhui Province. They started to write a very important ancient TCVM text called *Yuan Heng Liao Ma Ji* (Yuan-Heng's Therapeutic Treatise of Horses) in 1547 CE, and finally the text was published in 1608 CE. This book is a collection of detailed TCVM fundamental principles, herbal formulas and acupuncture points and stimulation techniques. In addition to detailed descriptions of 159 acupuncture points in horses, 33 bovine acupoints were listed. It was a well-respected TCVM work and became widely spread in China and other parts of Asia.

CHAPTER 8

Wei Syndrome, *Tan-Huan* Syndrome and Others

How I Treat *Wei* Syndrome

Bruce Ferguson, DVM, MS, CVA, CVCH, CVTP, CVFT
and Linda Boggie, DVM, CVA

Introduction

The Chinese character, *Wei*, means withered or wilting. This can eventually result in paresis and paralysis of the limbs. Pain is not a clinical sign of *Wei* Syndrome. Wei Syndrome refers to clinical signs which may include flaccid muscles, weak tendons and ligaments, numbness, and/or limb atrophy with diminished motor function. This can eventually result in paresis and paralysis of the limbs. Pain is not a clinical sign of *Wei* Syndrome.

In terms of modern understanding of diseases *Wei* Atrophy Syndrome can be the result of damage at several different levels: central nervous system – including brain and spinal cord, the peripheral nervous system, neuromuscular junction and the muscle itself. Various systemic disease processes can create these lesions including diseases of the central nervous system, peripheral nervous system, muscular disease, cardiovascular disease, metabolic or orthopedic diseases. *Wei* Atrophy Syndrome (also referred to as *Wei* Flaccidity) can result from dysfunction in both sensory and motor nervous systems. The clinical diseases seen often have to do with lack of proprioceptive function. Western biomedical diseases that may present as *Wei* Syndrome include nerve avulsion, fibrocartilagenous embolism, degenerative myelopathies, IVDD, brain infarcts, GME, sequelae to chronic disease, and aging[2].

Acupuncture and Moxibustion, Herbal Medicine, and *Tui-na* (TCVM) is able to help these conditions through their effects on the peripheral sensory nervous system, the spinal cord itself, the motor nervous system and its effects on blood flow.

TCVM is such an effective medical system because it is both integrative and individuated. By integrative, I mean that we commonly combine acupuncture, herbal medicine, *Tui-na*, and food therapies into a treatment regimen. Individuation implies that we seek the actual energetic disharmony in our patients before choosing treatment strategies rather than merely treating a broad disease "name" in all patients with the same strategies without considering their unique status[1].

Causes and Diagnosis

Causes involve External Pathogenic Factors as well as Internal Pathogenic factors, especially deficiencies in the Fundamental Substances. The primary cause described is Heat as a Pathogenic Factor. Heat dries the body fluids (*Jin-ye*) and leads to withering of the skin, muscles, blood vessels, sinews and bones. The tissue affected depends on which *Zang* Organ is most affected. The resulting clinical signs not only include atrophy and weakness of the muscles and sinews but can also involve dryness, weakness and a lack of neurologic function due to the body's inability to nourish the muscles and tissues. In general there is an excess condition or a condition with excess signs and symptoms followed by a mixture of excess and deficiency. Eventually the result is a deficiency state and this leads to atrophy and weakness as the body is unable to nourish the muscles and tissues. Characteristic to all patterns is deficiency, weakness, loss of muscle and flesh, ± lack of neurologic function, ± dryness, and a lack of pain. Common clinical diseases seen in modern veterinary practice will be given as examples of these disease patterns. Table 1 gives a list of various Western medical diseases that can be consistent with a Chinese medical pattern of *Wei* Atrophy Syndrome.

Table 2 delineates diagnostic criteria for the most common *Wei* Syndromes. Deficiency patterns like most *Wei* Syndromes typically take more time to resolve than the Bi Syndromes which are mostly Excess patterns. The positive changes between sessions are also less dramatic, which may discourage some clients from continuing a course of treatment.

Table 1: Western diseases correlated with *Wei* Atrophy Syndrome

Brain: 　Granulomatous Meningoencephalitis (GME) 　Neoplasia 　Toxoplasmosis 　Equine Encephalitis	**Primary Muscle Disease:** 　Immune Mediated Myositis 　Hyperkalemic Periodic Paralysis 　Nutritional Myopathies 　Lyme Disease 　Strains and sprains
Upper Motor Neuron Disease: 　Intervertebral Disk Disease (IVDD) 　Degenerative Myelopathy 　Diskospondylitis 　Neoplasia 　Fibrocartilagenous Embolism (FCE) 　Trauma 　Cervical Vertebral Instability (CVI) 　Equine Protozoal Myelitis (EPM)	**Cardiovascular Disease:** 　Any heart disease which results in decreased cardiac output 　Thromboembolic Disease
Lower Motor Neuron Disease: 　Facial Paralysis 　IVDD 　Lumbosacral Instability 　Trauma 　Neoplasia 　Peripheral Nerve Degeneration (Krabbe's Syndrome)	**Metabolic Disease:** 　Atrophy of Chronic Renal Failure 　Cancer cachexia 　Hypothyroidism 　Protein losing enteropathy 　End-stage hepatic disease 　Hypoadrenocorticism 　Hyperadrenocorticism
Neuromuscular Junctional Disease: 　Myasthenia Gravis 　Hypothyroidism	**Orthopedic Disease**: 　Atrophy secondary to arthritis 　Atrophy secondary to fractures, luxations, ligament rupture

Table 2: Diagnostic Criteria for Most Common *Wei* Syndromes

Wei Type	Damp-Heat	Spleen *Qi* Deficiency	Kidney *Qi* and/or *Yang* Deficiency	*Qi* and *Yin* dual Deficiency
Diagnostic Indicator	Excess pattern	Deficiency pattern	Deficiency pattern	Deficiency pattern
Clinical signs	Obesity, chronic skin problems, edema	Weak limbs, flaccid tissues, anorexia, loose stools	Weak and cold lumbus and hind end, difficulty rising	Emaciation, weak hindend, dry skin
Tongue	Greasy, moist	Pale, swollen	Pale, moist	Pale or red and dry
Pulse	Rapid, slippery	Deep, weak	Very deep/weak	Weak and thin

TCM Patterns:
There are Six primary etiologies; 3 excess and 3 deficiency patterns:[1]

1. Wind-Heat following a febrile disease
   - Due to an infectious pathogenic factor, affects the Lungs
   - Same as Lung Heat leading to Skin *Wei*
2. External Dampness
   - Living in a Damp environment will affect Spleen function
3. Diet
   - Consumption of greasy food, raw food
   - Food with poor nutritional content
   - Affects Spleen function

   Etiologies 2 and 3 are seen as Invasion of Damp-Heat or Damp-Cold
   - Excess patterns that can lead to deficiency of Spleen and Stomach *Qi*
   - Similar to Spleen Heat leading to Muscle Tissue *Wei*
   *Note that poor diet can lead directly to Spleen and Stomach Deficiency

4. Excessive sexual activity or overwork
   - Depletes Kidney and Liver *Qi* and Blood, eventually the *Yin*
   - Similar to Kidney Heat and Liver Heat patterns
   - May also lead to Blood Stasis (Liver influence)
5. Traumas
   - Lead to stagnation of *Qi* and Blood in channels
   - Atrophy is distal to sight of Stagnation
6. Shock
   - Emotional shocks deplete the Heart and Spleen[1]
   - TCM pattern of Heart and Spleen Collapse[1]
   - Rarely seen in animals

Pathophysiology
Zang Organ Pathology – Classic etiology with Heat or Dampness as Pathogenic Factors[3]

First there will be a discussion on the patterns as they were classically discussed in the *Nei Jing Su Wen*. These patterns would begin as excess patterns that may or may not be seen clinically but then develop to the deficient patterns which are often seen.

1) Lung Heat – Skin *Wei*/ Flaccid Syndrome

In TCM terminology this would be seen as Heat in Lungs Injuring *Yin*. There is invasion of the lungs by a Heat External Pathogenic Factor and the signs can develop during or shortly after this invasion. This can include such things as infection leading to bronchitis or pneumonia or traumatic invasion such as smoke inhalation or chest trauma. In addition the emotional Internal Pathogenic factor of Grief can also induce this pattern. Signs can be latent in onset, occurring 1-2 months post infection and recovery. Since the Lungs Govern the Skin and Body hair signs such as dry skin and brittle hair can be seen. The Lungs distribute *Wei Qi* and fluids (the *Jin*) to the surface of the body and to the extremities. The Heat consumes the Fluids, the lung lobes become atrophied and the LU *Qi* Function and quality of LU *Yin* is disturbed. There is a lack of nourishment (due to lack of *Jin*) to the tendons and ligaments and the suppleness of these structures declines. It is a Dry *Wei* Condition.

Clinical signs include dry and cracked skin, brittle body hair, pale skin, rapid respiration, mental restlessness, increased thirst, dry stools, scanty brown urine due to lack of LU *Yin* circulating downward to lower *jiao*. Sings are typical of LU impairment due to chronic consumptive disease. The forelimbs may be more affected as the LU and LI channels course along this limb; the hind limbs may be more affected than the forelimbs as the LU *Qi* and *Yin* is unable to fully descend. The metal constitution may be more prone to this pattern. The tongue will be red and dry, possibly with a yellow or dried white coating. If there is concurrent Blood Deficiency it may also be pale and dry. The pulse will be weak, and rapid. In the acute stages it may be full as the *Wei Qi* battles the Heat pathogen on the surface.

Veterinary diseases as causes of Skin *Wei* include any URI leading to pneumonia, feline asthma or feline allergic bronchitis, COPD (RAO disease) in horses, Bordetella sp., and neoplasia.

The *Yangming* channels are indicated for any *Wei* Syndrome pattern. In the *Nei Jing Su Wen*, Chapter 44, it is stated by Qi Bo: "*Yangming* is the source of nourishment for all the *Zang-fu* viscera. Only with this nourishment can the tendons, bones and joints be lubricated."

2) Spleen Heat – Muscle *Wei*/ Flaccid Syndrome

The TCM etiology of this pattern is Invasion of Damp-Heat or Cold-Damp which affects the Spleen function. Spleen is the Organ most affected by Damp thus Damp-Heat can directly affect SP Function. Cold-Damp can enter the body and over time transforms into Damp-Heat as the Cold and Damp create stagnation which will lead to the generation of internal Heat as the body tries to move *Qi* and Blood against the blockage. As the Spleen function is affected the muscles and tendons are damaged leading to flaccidity.

Clinical signs include thirst with a lack of body fluids, numbness of muscles and flesh, poor appetite (secondary to the Damp creating fullness in the epigastrium), diarrhea, edema, a general heaviness or heavy head due to Damp, overall lethargy, and dark yellow or brown urine with painful urination due to Damp-Heat. The tongue will be red due to Heat invasion or creation, with a thick coating and/ or thick slimy saliva due to Damp. The pulse is often soft and rapid due to the Heat; it may be more slippery and deep if Cold is still present.

The cause of this pattern is often internal and is due to eating foods high in fat or inappropriate foods for particular constitutions. A patient that is prone to SP *Qi* deficiency should not be fed a raw diet as this engenders Damp and the body's system is already challenged with suboptimal SP Function. Foods that are high in carbohydrates for carnivores are also taxing to the SP and potentially damaging. A common disease seen in veterinary patients is pancreatitis – either in its acute or chronic presentations. There may also be a history of inflammatory bowel disease or chronic problems with Damp-Heat skin conditions.

3) Spleen *Qi* Deficiency – Muscle *Wei*/ Flaccid Syndrome

Stomach and Spleen *Qi* Deficiency can result from the above two Excess patterns over time. It can also occur directly as a result of a poor nutritional diet. Due to the poor nutrition the body's inability to produce good *Qi* and Blood results directly in muscle weakness and fatigue. The Spleen function is damaged and there is a poor appetite, emaciation, edema, loose lips, loose stools and generalized malaise. The tongue would be pale and moist; the pulse weak and possibly thin. With geriatric patients this can occur with age as SP and KI *Qi* decline.

Veterinary diseases that can be seen related to this pattern include chronic pancreatitis, inflammatory bowel disease and pancreatic insufficiency syndrome.

4) Heart Heat – Vessel *Wei* / Flaccid Syndrome

The Heart is responsible for the flow of blood through the vessels and is susceptible to Heat as a Pathogenic Factor. In most instances the Pericardium or the Small Intestine will protect the Heart from Heat as a pathogenic factor but in instances of overwhelming climatic heat, intense fevers or strong emotions the Heart may be affected. As the Heart is attacked by Heat the Blood flows upwards and leads to a pattern of Excess in the upper *jiao* and Deficiency in the lower *jiao*. The Deficiency below produces "hollow" vessels with a lack of circulation to the joints and limbs. This is also a dry form. The primary cause classically was felt to be emotional insult.

Clinical signs include red color in the face with visible capillaries, panting, restlessness, the joints become stiff and the tendons become loose and flaccid, the muscles atrophy. The tongue is red and dry; the pulse can be full and rapid or weak, rapid and hollow depending on stage of presentation.

Veterinary diseases can include the acute stage of heat stroke or other infectious diseases that lead to extreme fever that affects the Heart. Of course emergency treatment is provided for these patients but acupuncture can be used to support the Organs and more importantly used to balance these patients after the initial insult has passed. Some of the patients present after the emergency for weakness and failure to completely recover. Chronic emotional stress is an underlying cause that can lead to this pattern.

5) Liver Heat – Musculotendinous *Wei* / Flaccid Syndrome

The Liver governs the tendons and ligaments. When Heat attacks the Liver bile flows upwards causing a bitter taste in the mouth, the tendons become dry, contracted and atrophic, the nails are dry and brittle. Heat consumes and damages the Blood and *Yin* leading to Liver Blood and/ or *Yin* Deficiency Pattern. These can be the patients with active hepatitis in the acute phase or patients that are recovering from infectious hepatitis. These patients may even present months after an episode but continue to have problems with weakness and lack of supple movements in their joints due to the dry nature of the sinew tissue. Depending on the time of presentation the pulse may be full and wiry or deficient and tight. The tongue as well will vary: perhaps red, dry and swollen in the acute stages or dry, red and small in chronic condition if the *Yin* is most damaged or pale and dry if Liver Blood is most damaged.

6) Kidney Heat – Bone *Wei* / Flaccid Syndrome

The Kidney governs the bones and bone marrow. It was stated in the *Nei Jing Su Wen* that when Kidney is attacked by Heat "the *jing* is exhausted and the marrow decreases. This leads to dry bones and weakness of the spine. The back becomes so weak that the patient cannot support himself in an upright position. This is a *Wei* condition of the bones." The etiology of heat attacking the kidney was described as being internally generated due to over taxation: "overtiredness from traveling through severe heat leads to thirst. The heat is excessive internally." This Heat attacks the Kidney which can no longer balance this fire and the *Jing* is consumed.

Clinical signs include dry bones, weakness of the spine, a weak back, atrophy and flaccidity of the muscles (primarily the hind limbs), the patient is unable to stand or stretch due to weakness and pain, the coat is dry and lusterless and there is premature aging of the teeth. The tongue is pale red and dry, the pulse weak and rapid.

7) Liver and Kidney Heat – *Yin* Deficiency *Wei* Flaccidity

This is primarily a pattern seen in geriatric patients where there is a combination of signs from Liver and Kidney *Yin* Deficiency patterns. It is said that the Liver and the Kidney have the same source and often when one is deficient in *Yin* the other is as well. They can also be used to nourish each other when one is replete and the other deficient. The Heat is a result of a *Yin* deficiency which has evolved over time.

Clinical signs can include poor vision, dry mouth, insomnia, lumbago, pain in the stifles, false heat in the joints as well as weakness and muscle atrophy. The pulse is rapid and thready and the tongue will be small, red and dry. Veterinary diseases seen include chronic renal failure, end stage hyperthyroidism, chronic hepatitis, or chronic emotional heat such as anger and frustration.

Recap of Generalized *Wei* Atrophy due to *Zang* Organ Dysfunction

The most common patterns seen in veterinary medicine involve Heat in the Lung, Damp-Heat, Spleen Deficiency, Deficiency of Liver and Deficiency of Kidney.[5] Deficiency of Kidney is often seen with either a deficiency of Kidney *Qi* and *Yang* or a Deficiency of Kidney *Qi* and *Yin*.[5] Refer to table 5 for more detailed comparison. What should be remembered with each of these patterns is that there is often an Excess process at the beginning, be it an invasion of Heat or Dampness as a pathogenic factor or generation of Internal Heat or Dampness due to emotions, lifestyle or the constitution of the patient. As the Excess process consumes *Qi*, Blood and *Yin*, the Deficiency pattern becomes predominant. Many patients present to the veterinary acupuncturist for weakness or "lameness" that is non-responsive to western anti-inflammatory medications. This lameness or weakness is no longer an active inflammatory process thus common western medications cannot help. However, acupuncture can.

Trauma Induced *Wei Bi*

Perhaps one of the most common *Wei* conditions veterinary acupuncturists are asked to treat is *Wei Bi* following a traumatic incident. This can be trauma following an accident such as being hit by an automobile and sustaining nerve injury or as sequelae to a ruptured intervertebral disc. Repetitive stress injuries, such as carpal tunnel syndrome seen in people or the joint injuries seen in many of the agility dogs, can also induce *Wei Bi*. The traumatic incident, either acute or chronic in nature, sets up a stagnation of *Qi* and Blood flow through the channels such that there is a lack of *Qi* and Blood flow distal to the injury. Due to the lack of nourishment to the tissues there is weakness, muscle atrophy, tendon and ligament laxity and sometimes lack of sensation (nerve function) as is often seen with injuries to the spinal cord or peripheral nerves.

In patients with traumatically induced *Wei Bi* the tongue will often be lavender to purple due to the stagnation that is present and the pulse will have a wiry or sometimes choppy quality to it. Depending on the individual's concomitant state of Fundamental Substances the tongue may be pale or red, moist or dry and the pulse may be thin, rapid, slippery or slow. In the acute stages the tongue is most often purple and the pulse quality is wiry and full. The treatment principle for these patients is to Move the *Qi* and Blood in the Channels, Support the Sinews and address any other underlying deficiencies of the Fundamental Substances.

Wei Bi as progression from Chronic Bony *Bi*

Wei Bi can also develop in patients with chronic Bony *Bi* Syndrome with significant arthritis and joint deformities. Due to the stagnation in the channels around the joints the *Qi* and Blood are not able to nourish the tissues distally or caudally leading to localized areas of *Wei* Atrophy which leads to further weakness and instability. As weakness of one of more limbs develops this puts further strain on the other limbs and postural muscles of the back and abdomen and can create a more generalized *Wei* Atrophy due to *Qi* Deficiency. Acupuncture can do nothing for the chronic degenerative joint changes but it can reduce the pain associated with the arthritis, aid the nervous system in functioning better (partially via direct effects but also by decreasing inflammation and swelling locally). Through its effects on mediating the circulatory system via neurotransmitters and vascular mediators the blood circulation to the supporting muscles, tendons and ligaments is improved. Through this improvement of circulation to and surrounding the peripheral nerves they are also able to function better. As the limbs that are most predominantly affected improve the rest of the body musculature is able to function more normally and the patients overall health condition improves.

Veterinary patients seen most commonly include dogs with advanced hip dysplasia or elbow dysplasia (Bony *Bi*), patients with spinal injury that develop neurologic deficits and muscle atrophy caudal to the lesion (e.g. IVDD, CVI, lumbosacral stenosis) and many competition animals that develop arthritis in a particular joint and develop tissue atrophy distally.

Treatment principles for these patients not only involve moving *Qi* and Blood stagnation in the channels of the affected area but also supporting the manufacture and circulation of the Fundamental Substances and improving the circulation of *Qi* and Blood throughout the entire body. In the case of chronic *Bi* Syndromes that are caused by the invasion of External Pathogenic Factors it is also important to support the production and circulation of *Wei Qi* and include *Shu*-Stream or *Jing*-well points in the acupuncture prescription to aid the body in ridding the pathogenic factor and prevent it from traveling deeper and possibly affect the *Zang*-Fu Organs.

HOW TO TREAT *WEI* WITH DRY NEEDLING

I use acupuncture to treat *Wei* with great success integrating aspects of Dr. Tan's Balance Method[3], Channel Clearing Technique, Governing Vessel Focus[4], and Trigger Point therapy. Dr. Tan's Balance Method has at least five subsystems that treat a few, select acupuncture points far from the primary lesion and gets rapid clinical results. The first and most commonly used subsystem for clearing blockages, in limbs for example, is treating the same Chinese-name channel on diagonally opposite areas which "mirror" one another. Channel-clearing techniques focus on using distal, mostly metacarpal/metatarsal and phalangeal points. Electroacupuncture is particularly important as it tonifies *Qi* and Blood (e.g. releases nerve growth factors) to reverse atrophy[7].

Source points on both the *Yang* (e.g. LI-4, GB-40) and *Yin* (e.g. LIV-3, LU-9) channels may be acupunctured to access *Yuan* or Source *Qi* in *Wei* Syndrome deficiency patterns. Further, *Shu*-stream points such as SP-3 and LU-9 may be used to treat disharmonies of the muscles and flesh[5]. Extraordinary vessels are reservoirs for *Qi* and Blood and I tend to use GB-41 (Dai Mai) coupled with TH-3 (small quadruped variation of TH-5) to treat the *Dai Mai* or Girdle Vessel. Since the *Dai Mai* "wraps" other longitudinal acupuncture channels, *Dai Mai* disharmonies may lead to weakness distal to the thoracolumbar junction.

HOW TO TREAT *WEI* WITH HERBS

Some herbal formulas such as *Si Miao San* are used to drain pathogenic Damp and Heat from the body and should be discontinued when the pathogenic influence is gone. Herbal formulas used as tonics may be given for extended periods of time, sometimes for the remainder of the patient's life. Food therapy is of primary importance in treating *Wei* Syndrome; foods are the ultimate daily tonics for deficiency. It is also common for species- or constitution-inappropriate diets to be at least partially causative in *Wei* Syndrome.

HOW TO TREAT *WEI* WITH MOXABUSTION AND ELECTROACUPUNCTURE

Moxibustion is a method by which moxa punk or other herbs are burned on or above the skin near acupuncture points. The heat and herbal essence warms the *Qi* and Blood in the channels and collaterals and thus increases the flow during times of Stasis. Moxibustion also invigorates the *Yang Qi* and dispels internal Cold and Dampness as well as eliminates some forms of local Heat Toxin[2]. Moxibustion according to Wang Le-Ting: "Acupuncture and moxibustion each have their limits and abilities and therefore should mutually assist and mutually support each other". According to Dr. Wang, moxibustion has the following functions: Warming action and supports *Yang*, Course and free the flow of the channels and network vessels, Move the *Qi* and quicken the Blood, Dispel Dampness and expel Cold, Disperse swelling and scatter nodulation, and Secure *Yang* and stem counterflow[1].

Electroacupuncture is the use of electrical current passed through the acupuncture needles that have already been inserted into acupuncture points. There are many types of electroacupuncture units available with the ultimate goal of strengthening and altering the needle stimulation. Electroacupuncture was first used in China in the 1930's and has become common in veterinary practices throughout the world.

The advantages that electroacupuncture offers over hand-needling are primarily the following. First, electroacupuncture stimulation can at some level mimic the manual needle stimulation offered by the therapist thus eliminating time spent manipulating needles by the acupuncturist. Second, the amount of needle stimulation can be accurately measured by known frequencies, amplitudes and duration of treatment. This enables the acupuncturist to rigorously assess a treatment session and more exactly replicate effective treatments in the future. Lastly, electroacupuncture allows the acupuncturist to deliver a higher and more continuous level of needle stimulation than by hand thus facilitating special treatments for pain and neurodegenerative disorders.

Although the exact settings of an electroacupuncture device will vary with its type and manufacture, the following general guidelines are common to all treatments. First, since electroacupuncture is similar but stronger than manual acupuncture, the patient should have demonstrated prior tolerance and response to dry needle therapy. Second, the machine should have all of its leads turned to zero amplitude as well as be completely turned off before connecting to the needles. Third, stimulation should always start at the lowest amplitude and gradually be increased until there is an obvious *de qi* response and then lowered slightly from that amplitude. Since tolerance and habituation to the stimulus occurs, the amplitude or the frequency may be slightly increased or changed every 5-10 minutes.

Electroacupuncture may be used to tonify or sedate acupuncture points as with manual therapies. It is especially useful for neuralgia and nervous system injury and degeneration. Many veterinary acupuncturists believe that continuous, regular high frequency (80-120 Hz) mediates endorphin release and is best for treating pain and muscle spasms. Lower frequency (5-20 Hz) and intermittent, alternating or discontinuous stimulation may be best to re-educate the motor neurons in paresis and paralysis. This is akin to saying the regular high frequencies drain excess and stagnation while intermittent low frequencies tonify deficiency.

HOW TO TREAT *WEI* WITH *TUI-NA*

Tui-na is also very important to treat *Wei* Syndrome; indeed it seems to be the one most important treatment modality in some of my cases. In TCM terminology, *Tui-na* or *An-mo* can regulate meridians, soothe joints and sinews, promote circulation of *Qi* and Blood, balance *Zang-Fu* organs and strengthen the body's resistance. "Regulate meridians" means that these manual therapy techniques can regulate the functions of meridians or channels which include: transporting *Qi* and Blood throughout the body, protecting the body, and transmitting *Qi* to diseased areas[3]. "Soothe joints and sinews" means that *Tui-na* can soften the local tissues, reduce pain in and possibly lead to realignment/restructuring of dense connective tissue[4]. Increased *Qi* and Blood circulation leads to a reduction of pain and increase in nutritional factors to tissues[5]. Balancing the function of the primary organs of the body, the *Zang-Fu*, refers to increasing individual organ function when they are sub-optimal and normalizing the interactions between these organs[6]. Strengthening the body's resistance refers to the positive benefit that *Tui-na* has on immune system function.

These techniques of manual therapy have been successfully used for treatment of musculoskeletal conditions[7], *Bi* syndrome (painful obstruction) and osteoarthritis, disc problems such as IVDD[8], peripheral nerve paralysis, *Wei* syndrome (wasting and general weakness)[9] and internal diseases such as organ hypofunction[10]. Although any non-fractious patient may benefit, both geriatric and pediatric patients may be especially good candidates for *Tui-na* therapy due to its potential for gentle application. Pediatric diseases amenable to treatment include enuresis[11], viral infections, cough, fever, diarrhea, infantile malnutrition, awareness deficits[12], torticollis, infantile paralysis, tendon contracture and bursitis. Geriatric disorders include those found in adult animals with an emphasis on organ hypofunction[13] and pain[14]. There are few western biomedical treatments for organ hypofunction[16], further, *Tui-na* application may preclude some of the effects seen with the common use of analgesic drugs used to treat pain[15].

Table 3 summarizes some treatment strategies for the most common *Wei* syndromes.

Table 3: Treatment Strategies for Most Common *Wei* Syndromes

Wei Type	Damp-heat	Spleen *Qi* Deficiency	Kidney *Qi* and/or *Yang* Deficiency	*Qi* and *Yin* Dual Deficiency
Acupuncture	LI 4, LI 11, SP 9, GV 14, GV 8, GB 34	BL 20, BL 21, ST 36, LI 10, GV 5, GV 6	GV 3, GV 4, BL 23, *Shen Shu*, KID 7	SP 3, LU 9, CV 4, GV 3, *Shen Shu*
Herbal Formula	*Si Miao San*	*Bu Zhong Yi Qi Tang*	*You Gui Wan*	*You Gui Wan* *Zuo Gui Wan*
Food Therapy	Mung beans, barley	Sweet potato, chicken	Black beans, mutton	Sweet potato, sea vegetables
Tui-na	*An-fa*	*Rou-fa*	*Ca-fa*	*Nie-fa*

Conclusion

Wei Bi can be very rewarding to treat or very difficult to treat depending upon the presenting pattern and the duration of clinical symptoms. *Wei Bi* secondary to acute trauma or as sequelae to progressive *Bi* Syndrome can in fact be very rewarding as western medications are not designed to help build tissue and help with circulation to the tissues. They are targeting inflammation and can be very powerful and useful medications in the acute phases but are of little help with chronic conditions where atrophy is present. In cases of demyelinating disease, acupuncture can slow the process but usually cannot stop the disease. In cases of severe trauma to the nervous system, as in brachial plexus avulsion, acupuncture can be helpful in balancing the patient structurally, supporting the other limbs and optimizing *Zang-fu* Organ function, but it is not able to re-grow severed axons. Herbal and dietary support can be important adjunctive therapies in these patients (see table 3). It is well worth pursuing additional training in these modalities as they are an integral part of the Chinese medical system.

Wei and *Bi* Syndromes subsume a large proportion of patient disharmonies commonly seen in veterinary practice. With proper Pattern Differentiation and integrative use of acupuncture, herbal medicine, food therapy, and *Tui-na*, we can relieve suffering and prolong life. What can be more rewarding than this?

References:
1. Yu Hui-chan and Han Fu-ru. Golden Needle Wang Le-Ting: A 20th Century Master's Approach to Acupuncture, Blue Poppy Press, 2001 Boulder, CO, USA.
2. Ferguson, B. Acupuncture and Moxibustion Techniques, in Traditional Chinese Veterinary Medicine, Volume 2, Elesevier, edited by Xie, Huisheng. 2007.
3. Deadman, P., Al-Khafaji, M. (1998). A Manual of Acupuncture. Journal of Chinese Medicine Publications, East Sussex, England.
4. Vachiramon, A., Wang, W.C. (2005). Acupuncture and acupressure techniques for reducing orthodontic post-adjustment pain. J Contemp Dent Pract. Feb 15;6(1):163.

5. Barker, R., Kober, A., Hoerauf, K., Latzke, D., Ade,l S., Kain, Z.N., Wang, S.M. (2006). Out-of-hospital auricular acupressure in elder patients with hip fracture: a randomized double-blinded trial. Acad Emerg Med. 2006 Jan;13(1):19-23.
6. Goidenko, V.S., Komarova, I.B. (2003). [Efficacy of acupressure therapy in combined treatment of psycho-autonomic neurotic disorders in children]. Zh Nevrol Psikhiatr Im S S Korsakova. 103(8):23-8.
7. Hsieh, L.L, Kuo, C.H., Lee, L.H., Yen, A.M., Chien, K.L., Chen, T.H. (2006). Treatment of low back pain by acupressure and physical therapy: randomised controlled trial. BMJ, 332:696-700.
8. Huang, S.R., Shi, Y.Y., Shi, G.T. (2003). [Pathogenic factors of blood circulation disturbance in lumbar intervertebral disc herniation and mechanism of Tuina manipulation in promoting circulation]. Zhong Xi Yi Jie He Xue Bao. Nov;1(4):255-8.
9. McDougall, G. (2005). The effect of acupressure with massage on fatigue and depression in patients with end-stage renal disease. Geriatric Nursing, Volume 26, Issue 3, Pages 164-165.
10. Jeon, S.Y., Jung, H.M. (2005). [The effects of abdominal meridian massage on constipation among CVA patients]. Taehan Kanho Hakhoe Chi. Feb;35(1):135-42.
11. Harris, R.E., Jeter, J., Chan, P., Higgins, P., Kong, F.M., Fazel, R., Bramson, C., Gillespie, B. (2005). Using acupressure to modify alertness in the classroom: a single-blinded, randomized, cross-over trial. J Altern Complement Med. Aug;11(4):673-9.
12. Yuksek, M.S., Erdem, A.F., Atalay, C., Demirel, A. (2003). Acupressure versus oxybutinin in the treatment of enuresis. J Int Med Res. Nov-Dec;31(6):552-6.
13. Yang, H. (2004). Dan zhi xiao yao yin combined with auricular-point-pressing for treatment of optic atrophy--a clinical observation of 51 cases. J Tradit Chin Med. Dec;24(4):259-62.
14. Trentini, J.F. 3rd, Thompson, B., Erlichman, J.S. (2005). The antinociceptive effect of acupressure in rats. Am J Chin Med. ;33(1):143-50.
15. Reed, S.K., Messer, N.T., Tessman, R.K., Keegan, K.G. (2006). Effects of phenylbutazone alone or in combination with flunixin meglumine on blood protein concentrations in horses. American Journal of Veterinary Research, Vol. 67, No. 3, Pages 398-402
16. Wu, B., He, J., and GAO, B. Q.; Effect of electroacupuncture on nerve growth factor in regeneration chamber after facial nerve injury. Chinese Journal of Clinical Rehabilitation 2006, Vol. 10(07) p.186-188.

How to Use Acupuncture to Treat Downer Cow Syndrome

Huisheng Xie, DVM PhD

Downer cow syndrome is a commonly fatal condition of dairy cows that are unable to get up for no apparent reason. Downer cow refers to any cow that remains in sternal recumbency for more than 24 hours after initial recumbency and after treatment of primary medical problems.[1] Downer cow syndrome is often caused by metabolic diseases such as hypocalcemia, milk fever and trauma during calving, fractured pelvis, dislocated hip, or nerve paralysis. There are two conventional approaches to the management of downer cows: 1) lifting like flotation, 2) providing good bedding such as sand or grass along with adequate nursing care such as rolling. The overall success is limited.

TCVM Pattern Differentiation

In TCVM, the downer cow syndrome belongs to *Wei* syndrome (too weak to get up), which is primarily associated with *Qi* Deficiency (muscle atrophy, body weight loss, pale tongue and weak pulse) and local *Qi*-Blood Stagnation around the hindquarter. In some case, it may be combined with *Yin* Deficiency if the patient shows warm ears/body, dry stool, red tongue, or fast pulse. In other case, it may be combined with *Yang* Deficiency if the patient has cold ears/body/feet, pale/swollen/purple tongue and deep/weak/slow pulse.

TCVM Treatment

Acupuncture:
>Basic Acupoints: BL-20/21, *Bai-hui, Shen-shu, Shen-peng, Shen-jiao, Ba-jiao*, BL-54/40, KID-1, ST-36
>*Yin* Deficiency: Add GV-14
>*Yang* Deficiency: Add GV-3/4

>-Methods: Dry needle, Aqu, Moxibustion or Electro-acupuncture

Herbal Medicine: *Bu Yang Huan Wu*, 30 grams bid for 1 to 2 months.

Case Example

A 6 year old Holstein Female was presented with sternal recumbency for 60 days after parturition. She was alert, had normal food/water intake and stool. She had pale tongue, weak pulse. Her TCVM Pattern was *Wei* syndrome due to *Qi* Deficiency.

Electro-acupuncture was performed with 30 Hz 15 min + 200 Hz 15 min for a total of 30 minutes at the following pairs of acupoints:
Shen-shu, left to right;
Bai-hui + GV-1;
Si-liao + KID-1;
ST-36, left to right.

Outcome

After the end of the first electro-acupuncture treatment, she was able to get up by herself and stood for 15 minutes. Three more weekly electro-acupuncture treatments were given. Her recumbent condition resolved.

Reference:

1. http://www.cvm.umn.edu/Academics/Current_student/Notes/Downer%20cow%20lecture%20juniors%20112001.pdf

Suggested Changes in Location and Function and Pairing of Eight Distal Limb Acupoints in Dogs and Cats

Bruce Ferguson, DVM, MS, CVA, CVCH, CVTP, CVFT

Reprinted with permission from AJTCVM volume 6, number 2, August 2011

From: The School of Veterinary and Biomedical Sciences, Murdoch University, Murdoch, Western Australia

ABSTRACT

The locations and functions of many acupoints in animals have been transposed from humans. Using mirror imagery and altering acupoint locations to achieve symmetry, changes in acupoint locations are suggested. Acupoints LIV-3 and LI-4, the "four gates", are located in symmetrical mirror locations in humans. To achieve symmetry with LIV-3 in dogs and cats, it is proposed that LI-4 always be located between the 2nd and 3rd metacarpal bones. Acupoints LU-9 and SP-3 are suggested to be located on the medial side of the second metacarpal or metatarsal bone just proximal to the metacarpophalangeal and metatarsophalangeal joints respectively to achieve symmetry and become a balancing pair. It is also proposed that TH-3 function as the *Yang-Wei* confluent point instead of TH-5, as TH-3 has anatomic symmetry with GB-41, the *Dai-Mai* confluent point and the two acupoints can be paired together to balance the Extraordinary Vessels. Slight alterations in the locations of BL-65 and SI-3 are suggested to achieve anatomic symmetry, so that they can also be combined as pairs to achieve balance through the Extraordinary Vessels. The acupoint pairs LU-9/SP-3, TH-3/GB-41 and BL-65/SI-3 are all *Shu*-Stream acupoints and located on the same level Channel (e.g. LU-9/SP-3 *Tai Yin* Channels; TH-3/GB-41 *Shao Yang* Channels; BL-67/SI-3 *Tai Yang* Channels). Anatomically the suggested changes are rational. However it has been the author's positive clinical experiences using these new acupoint locations and functions that motivated beginning this dialogue. Successful clinical use by other acupuncturists will determine the validity of these suggested changes.

Key words: Traditional Chinese veterinary medicine, acupuncture, acupoint pairs, transpositional acupoints, acupoint symmetry, global balancing, Extraordinary Vessels

In order to use acupuncture effectively, the practitioner must know the accurate acupoint locations and functions.[1-4] Many of the locations and functions of acupoints in animals have been based on the anatomical transposition from humans.[1-4] Experiential clinical results by veterinary acupuncturists support many of the transpositional acupoint locations and functions. Channels in animals that are similar to those found in humans have been demonstrated in experimental studies.[5]

According to the morphogenetic singularity theory, acupoints originate from organizing centers during morphogenesis.[6,7] Dr. Charles Shang proposed the morphogenetic singularity theory in the late 1980s. He applied the singularity theory of mathematics to explain the origin, distribution and nonspecific activation phenomena of the Channel (*Jing Luo*) system. In development, the fate of a larger region is frequently controlled by a small group of cells called an organizing center. Both organizing centers and acupoints are areas of high electrical conductance, have a high density of gap junctions that allows for direct electrical communication between cells and can be activated by nonspecific stimuli. Acupuncture points are suggested to originate from these organizing centers. Shang concludes that based on the morphogenetic singularity theory, the Channel system originates from a network of organizing centers and the evolutionary origin of the Channel system is likely to have preceded all the other physiological systems including the nervous, circulatory and immune systems. The genetic blueprint of the Channel system might have served as a template from which the newer systems evolved. He further postulates that the Channel system overlaps and interacts with other systems, but is distinct from them.[6,7]

Acupoint location and function may vary due to differences in developmental and embryological relationships, local nerves, blood, lymphatic vessels and connective tissue and regional and whole body tissue function in each animal species. Limb anatomy and function differ between bipedal humans and quadrupeds. For example, LI-10 is non-weight bearing in humans, so has a different function than in quadrupeds, where LI-10 is weightbearing.[1-4]

Balancing Techniques and Acupoint Symmetry and Pairing

Basically "Balancing Techniques" are used to treat pain and chronic and complex (multifocal) diseases and detailed descriptions of these are beyond the scope of this text. Acupoints located at similar locations on different limbs are selected for balance and in some situations may be paired.[7,8] The appropriate limb acupoints to treat are selected using mirror imaging and anatomic imaging. In mirror imaging, the thoracic limb digits mirror the pelvic limb digits, the carpi mirror the tarsi, the elbows mirror the stifles and the shoulders mirror the hips. When disease affecting the limbs occurs, acupoints in the area that mirrors the location of the diseased tissues are treated. Anatomic imaging is used to select limb acupoints to treat, when disease is not located on the limbs, but instead occurs on another part of the body.[8] Each limb can be viewed as an anatomical image of the head and trunk. The digits and metacarpal region can be viewed as analogous to the head, the carpus or tarsus analogous to the neck, the radius and ulnar or tibia and fibular regions analogous to the thorax, the elbow or stifle analogous to the abdomen and the shoulder or hip analogous to the pubis and genital region. A mirror acupoint contralateral to the site of the lesion is often selected for treatment in focal unilateral lesions.

Along with the mirror and anatomic image acupuncture techniques, acupoints are also chosen based on five subsystems: 1) Anatomical Image System Based on the Chinese Channel Name, 2) *Bie Jing* or Branching Channel System, 3) The Interior/Exterior Relationship System, 4) The Chinese Clock: Opposite System and 5) The Chinese Clock: Neighbor System.[7,8] In these microsystems of acupuncture, many acupoints have functions (proposed below) that are not found in current veterinary acupoint function descriptions. An example of an acupuncture treatment using mirror imaging and the first subsystem "Anatomical Image System based on the Chinese Channel Name" is as follows: a right anterolateral stifle injury with disease located on the right Stomach Channel (a *Yang Ming* Channel) would be treated with a mirror acupoint at the left anterolateral elbow on the Large Intestine Channel (the *Yang Ming* Channel). In this case, an *Ah-shi* point around the left LI-10 to LI-11 would be treated and provide immediate relief from the stifle pain. An example of anatomic imaging using the first subsystem would be as follows: abdominal pain at the level of the umbilicus on the Spleen Channel (*Tai Yin*) is treated by choosing an acupoint on the Lung Channel (*Tai Yin*) around the elbow (the anatomic image of the abdominal area), treating the same Chinese Channel name where the disease is located. In this case, an *Ah-shi* point in the area of LU-5 on one side would be treated to give abdominal pain relief. In all the "Balancing Techniques", only unilateral needling of acupoints is proposed.

Current acupuncture experts have suggested that symmetrical bilateral needling of acupoints on the limbs leads to a reduction in efficacy due to some form of energetic "waveform" cancellation.[9] With regard to Global or Dynamic Balancing, the unilateral needling seems to set into effect an energetic directional activity. Global or Dynamic Balancing involves selecting specific acupoint pairs based on similar locations, level of the *Yin or Yang* Channel (*Tai Yin, Shao-Yin or Jue Yin* and *Yang Ming, Tai Yang or Shao Yang*) or functions.

Changes in Acupoint Locations and Pairing Based on the Concept of Anatomic Symmetry

Regional anatomy and symmetry and experientially and experimentally derived functions have been used to localize acupuncture points in dogs and cats.[2-4] Developmental and functional species-specific regional anatomy results in potentially important variations that may effect acupoint location and function. Human feet are plantigrade and contact with the earth is first made with the calcaneous, when walking.[1] This contrasts with dogs and cats that contact the earth first with their metacarpal and metatarsal soft tissues and bones, when walking.

Anatomical symmetry has been proposed to be important in acupoint location, acupoint pairing and acupoint function.[7] The acupoints LI-4 and LIV-3, known as "the four gates", are commonly used as a pair during acupuncture treatment. It has been suggested that the *Yuan*-Source points of the six *Yang* Channels emerge at the four gates.[1-4,7-8] Deadman and Al-Khafaji state the following about human LI-4 and LIV-3: "This is an elegant combination [LI-4 and LIV-3]. *Hegu* LI-4 on the upper extremity lies in the wide valley between the first and second metacarpals, whilst *Taichong* LIV-3 on the lower extremity lies in the wide valley between the first and second metatarsals."[1]

With the evolutionary diminution of digits in animals, the acupoints beginning or ending near the finger tips of humans tend to migrate proximally, especially evident in horses. The widest spaces between the medial metacarpals and metatarsals result in the strongest *De Qi* and tend to relieve pain most effectively.[8] In humans the widest space is between the 1st and 2nd metacarpal and metatarsals, but in dogs and cats, the widest gaps are between the 2nd and 3rd metacarpals.[2] The front feet of dogs and cats commonly have vestigial first metacarpals and the reduced structure tends to have a weaker *De Qi* and clinical responses.[2] Some veterinary atlases place LI-4 between the 1st and 2nd metacarpal bones exactly transposed from humans, while other sources place it between the 2nd and 3rd metacarpal bones.[2-4] If LI-4 is placed between the 2nd and 3rd metacarpals, then LI-4 and LIV-3 become in homologous regions of the thoracic and pelvic limb feet respectively and appear visually symmetrical (Table 1). The acupuncture practitioner will thus find that this proposed acupoint location for LIV-3 and LI-4 could be used as a symmetrically balanced pair for treating pain as well as a wide range of disorders.

The 2nd through the 5th digits and metacarpals of the human hand are roughly the same length and parallel with one another.[1] The 1st digit and metacarpal (thumb) is only about 2/3 the length of the other digits and metacarpals. Acupoint LU-9 is on the thoracic limb *Tai Yin* Channel and in humans is located at the wrist in a depression between the radial artery and the abductor pollicis longus muscles.[1] The LU-9 acupoint is the Lung Channel *Shu*-stream point, *Yuan*-Source point and the *Hui*-meeting point of the blood vessels and its powerful actions are in part due to its location at the base of the large human first digit or thumb.[1] Since most dogs and cats do not have an active first digit (thumb) and only a vestigial first metacarpal, LU-9 may actually be in a slightly different location (Table 1). The Spleen Channel is the *Tai Yin* Channel of the pelvic limb and SP-3 is the *Shu*-stream and *Yuan* Source point. To achieve symmetry in the homologous locations, it is suggested that LU-9 and SP-3 are located on the medial side of the second metacarpal or metatarsal bone just proximal to the metacarpophalangeal and metatarsophalangeal joints respectively (Table 1).

Table 1: Published small quadruped distal acupoint locations and proposed new location

Acupuncture Point	Reference A[4]	Reference B[2]	Suggested Acupoint Location	Difference in Location or Function
LI-4	Between the 1st and 2nd metacarpal bones at the level of the head of the first metacarpus	On the medial side of the thoracic limb between the 2nd and 3rd metacarpal bones at the midpoint of the 3rd metacarpal bone	Same as Reference B	Point moved laterally one metacarpal space from Reference A
LIV-3	On the dorsomedial aspect of the hind paw, in the middle of the 2nd metatarsal bone	On the medial side of the pelvic limb, proximal to the metatarsophalangeal joint between the 2nd and 3rd metatarsal bones	Same as Reference B	Point moved laterally from Reference A
LU-9	On the medial aspect of the carpus, cranial to the tendon of the flexor carpi radialis and immediately distal to the radial styloid process	On the medial aspect of the radiocarpal joint just cranial to the radial artery, at the level of HT-7	On the medial side of the thoracic limb proximal and slightly ventromedial to the 2nd metacarpo-phalangeal joint	Moved distal and slightly medial to References A and B due to anatomical differences between the hand and the paw and to achieve symmetry with new SP-3 location (below)
SP-3	Due to the lack of the first digit in the hindpaw, location of SP-3 is at best uncertain. The point may be midpoint on the medial side of the second metatarsal.	On the medial side of the pelvic limb just proximal to the metatarsophalangeal joint on the medial side of the 2nd metatarsal bone	Similar to Reference B but proximal and slightly ventro-medial to the 2nd metatarso-phalangeal joint	Paired with new proposed LU-9 to achieve symmetry between the two acupoints

TH-3	On the dorsum of the forepaw, in a depression between the 4th and 5th metacarpal bones, next to the head (distal end) of the 5th metacarpal bone	Just proximal to the metacarpophalangeal joint on the lateral side of the 4th metacarpal bone on the dorsum of the foot of the thoracic limb	Same as Reference A and B	New function suggested: TH-3 proposed as *Yang-Wei* confluent point to achieve symmetry with GB-41
GB-41	On the dorsum of the foot, in the depression distal to the base of the 4th and 5th metatarsal bones	On the lateral side of the pelvic limb distal to the hock, on the dorsum of the foot proximal to the metatarsophalangeal joint, just distal the junction of the 4th and 5th metatarsal bones	Same as Reference A and B	*Dai-Mai* confluent point. Suggested to be paired with TH-3 to achieve symmetry
BL-65	Not described	On the lateral aspect of the pelvic limb caudal to the distal end of the 5th metatarsal bone at the metatarsophalangeal joint	Similar to Reference B but slightly ventral to the 5th metatarsophalangeal joint	BL-65 is suggested as the new *Yang-Qiao* confluent point to achieve symmetry with SI-3
SI-3	On the lateral side of the 5th metacarpophylangeal joint, proximal to the head of the 5th metacarpal bone	Proximal to the metacarpophalangeal joint on the lateral side of the 5th metacarpal	Similar to References A and B but proximal and slightly ventrolateral to the 5th metacarpophalangeal joint	Governing Vessel confluent point; suggest pairing with with BL-65 to achieve symmetry

According to the classical Traditional Chinese Medicine (TCM) text, the *Spiritual Pivot*, distal acupoints clear obstruction from Channels, so LU-9 and SP-3 are two good medial Channel (myofascial) clearing points.[1] Since the *Shu*-stream, third level acupoints are used to treat Stagnation, both LU-9 and SP-3 are recommended for pain in the joints of their respective limbs.[2,3] Pairing LU-9 and SP-3 may be an effective treatment for *Bi* Syndrome pain commonly seen in veterinary patients.

Changes in Extraordinary Vessel Acupoint Functions and Pairing Based on the Concept of Anatomic Symmetry

Important acupoint functions may also be incorrect for some quadruped acupoints or omitted from others especially for the confluent (opening) points to the Extraordinary Channels. The Eight Extraordinary Channels include the Governing Vessel (*Du* Channel), the Conception Vessel (*Ren* Channel) and the *Chong, Dai, Yang-Qiao, Yang-Wei, Yin-Qiao* and *Yin-Wei* Channels.[3] The Extraordinary Channels coordinate and balance the *Qi* and Blood flow in all the 12 regular Channels and are used to achieve global balance of the body. Except for the Governing Vessel and Conception Vessel Channels, the Extraordinary Channels share acupoints with the 12 regular Channels.

Extraordinary Channel acupoint point pairing based on the suggested changes in acupoint function may result in better treatment responses especially in chronic conditions and complex diseases. Acupoints TH-3 and GB-41 are *Shu*-stream acupoints on the *Shao Yang* Channels of the thoracic and pelvic limbs respectively.[1-3] Currently, TH-3 is placed just proximal to the metacarpophalangeal joint on the lateral side of the 4th metacarpal bone on the dorsum of the thoracic limb feet in dogs and cats.[2-4] The transpositional functional uses for TH-3 are for tonification of Deficiency disease patterns, otitis, auditory dysfunction, fever, metacarpophalangeal joint pain and thoracic limb paresis or paralysis.[2-4] Acupoint GB-41 is located on the dorsum of the paw just distal to the junction the 4th and 5th metatarsals and is the confluent point of the *Dai* Channel and is known to treat pain among other disorders. Acupoint TH-5 is located 3 cun proximal to the carpus and has been described as the confluent point of the *Yang-Wei* Channel.[2] If this function is correct TH-5 could be paired with GB-41 to open both *Dai* and *Yang-Wei* Channels and globally balance the *Qi* and Blood flow. However since symmetry is suspected to enhance treatment effects, then pairing GB-41 and TH-3 would be more logical. Acupoints GB-41 and TH-3 are *Shu*-stream points located on *Shao Yang* Channels and both located between the 4th and 5th metatarsals and metacarpals respectively. If GB-41 and TH-3 are paired, they produce greater symmetry and better balance between the pelvic and thoracic limbs. It is therefore suggested that TH-3, not TH-5, is most likely the confluent point for *Yang-Wei* and thus the pairing of TH-3 and GB-41 could more effectively open both *Dai* and *Yang-Wei* Channels and globally balance the *Qi* and Blood flow than pairing TH-5 and GB-41.

Similarly the acupoints BL-65 and SI-3 are both third level, *Shu*-stream points on the *Tai Yang* Channels of the pelvic and thoracic limbs respectively. They are located on the fifth metatarsal or metacarpal bones respectively and although BL-65 is usually described as slightly more proximal than SI-3, if the positions of each were shifted slightly they could represent symmetrical balancing acupoints between the thoracic and pelvic limbs (Table 1).[2-4] Both acupoints are used to treat pain among other functions. Acupoint SI-3 is the confluent point for the Governing Vessel Channel. Currently BL-62 is described as the confluent point of the *Yin-Qiao* Channel.[2] Again, since symmetry is suspected to enhance treatment effects it is proposed that BL-65 not BL-62 is really the confluent point for the *Yang-Qiao* Channel and pairing acupoints BL-65 and SI-3 can create symmetry and together function as opening points of the Extraordinary Vessels achieve gloal balance and better treat chronic disease in dogs and cats.

The clinical application of acupoint symmetry and pairing can be illustrated with the following case. A 14-year-old female neutered Border Collie had been receiving Traditional Chinese Veterinary Medicine (TCVM) treatment over the last 3 years for pelvic limb weakness and urinary incontinence and suddenly developed left pelvic limb collapse. On examination the dog exhibited bilateral pelvic limb muscle atrophy and weak ambulation, but conscious proprioception was normal. A cool and moist nose, cool ears, pale-pink tongue, deep weak pulse and depressions at BL-23 through BL-25 were found on the TCVM examination. The TCVM pattern diagnosis was a Kidney *Qi* Deficiency *Wei* Syndrome. Each limb was treated with only one needle. The left GB-41 and right TH-3 (pelvic and thoracic limb *Shu-stream* acupoints on *Shao Yang* Channels) were paired and right SP-3 and left LU-9 (pelvic and thoracic limb *Shu-stream* acupoints on *Tai Yin* Channels) were also paired and treated with dry needles to achieve dynamic or global *Yang Yin* balance. The midline acupoints *Bai-hui* (midline between L7-S1), GV-3 and GV-4 were also treated. The clients telephoned the following day to say that, not only was the dog moving normally, but had pulled out toys from a storage bin and was playing like a puppy.

Challenges with New Acupoint Locations

There are problems when transpositional acupoints are changed to new locations. First, many practitioners may continue to use and name the acupoints in the locations where they first learned them. This leads to miscommunication between those practitioners and other acupuncturists who use the points at the new suggested locations. To avoid miscommunications, acupoint nomenclature must be changed or the location of the acupoints clarified. A simple way to rename these acupoints is to add the word "alternative" or "alt" before the point name (e.g. new LI-4 becomes alt LI-4) to imply that this point is related to the transpositional acupoint LI-4, but has an alternative placement. Another possibility is to use a point location prefix to alert the acupuncturist of an alternative placement, but this might lead to a cumbersome acupoint name (e.g. "PSIMCS" LI-4 = the LI-4 in the proximal second inter-metacarpal space). It might be easier to simply put the location in parentheses, if it is different than the typical transpositional location, as is done for classical points when the name is the same but the location is different.

Conclusion

If anatomical differences between bipedal humans and quadripedal dogs and cats are considered, the changes suggested in this commentary are rational. However it has been the author's positive clinical experiences using these new acupoint locations and functions that were the motivation for sharing this information. These suggested alternative locations and functions are meant to begin a dialogue and encourage further study of the concepts of mirror and anatomic images, acupuncture subsystems, acupoint symmetry and pairing acupoints to achieve dynamic global balance in veterinary acupuncture. The clinical application and successful use by other veterinary acupuncturists will be necessary to determine the validity of these suggested changes.

References:
1. Deadman P, Al-Khafaji M. A Manual of Acupuncture. East Sussex, England: Journal of Chinese Medicine Publications 1998: 111-112, 477-479.
2. Xie H, Preast V. Xie's Veterinary Acupuncture. Ames Iowa: Blackwell Publishing 2007:139, 138, 156, 177-178, 189, 137.
3. Xie H, Preast V. Traditional Chinese Veterinary Medicine. Reddick, FL:Jing Tang 2002:69-74, 151, 169.
4. Hwang HC, Limehouse JB. Canine Acupuncture Atlas. Veterinary Acupuncture 2nd Ed, Schoen AM (ed) 2001;129,131.
5. Luo CY, Zheng JF, Wang YX et al. Detection of acoustic emission signals propagated along 14 Meridians in sheep" Amer Journal of Traditional Chinese Vet Med 2006;

1(1):5-13.
6. Shang C. Electrophysiology of growth control and acupuncture. Life Sci 2001; 68(12):1333-42.
7. Matsumoto K, Birch S. Hara Diagnosis: Reflections on the Sea, Brookline, MA: Paradigm Publications 1988:131-153.
8. Ross J. Acupuncture Point Combinations. Edinburgh Scotland:Churchill, Livingstone 1995:1-457.
9. Lee M. Master Tong's Acupuncture: An Ancient Alternative Style in Modern Acupuncture Practice. Boulder, CO:Blue Poppy Press 2002:1-7.

INDEX

INDEX

A

Ah-shi, 17, 22, 27, 243, 470
Ah-shi points, 17, 22, 27, 243
Atlantoaxial malformation, 4, 24, 225

B

Ba Zhen Tang, 424, 448, 449, 450
Bi Syndrome, 130, 271, 272, 295, 298, 301, 304, 424, 461, 464, 473
Blood Deficiency, 23, 25, 53, 54, 55, 77, 85, 87, 100, 104, 113, 114, 115, 126, 130, 143, 169, 170, 173, 174, 180, 198, 199, 206, 247, 248, 271, 272, 314, 341, 424, 442, 458
Body Sore, 102, 105, 107, 109, 238, 239, 241, 242, 256, 259, 262, 264, 358, 359, 367, 370, 382, 401, 409, 413, 432, 437
Bo Le, 351
Brachial plexus, 21, 24, 400, 403
Brain tumor, 4, 41, 42, 44, 49, 62, 63, 76, 109, 112
Breathe Easier B, 393
Bu Qi Zi Yin Tang, 218, 219
Bu Yang Huan Wu, 97, 102, 217, 218, 219, 238, 239, 240, 241, 242, 254, 256, 259, 268, 276, 279, 288, 296, 331, 333, 335, 358, 359, 370, 375, 382, 420, 434, 443, 444, 467
Bu Yong Yi Qi, 158, 204
Bue Xue Xi Feng, 74, 86

C

Cancer Diet, 123
CAT scans. *computer-assisted tomography*
Cauda equina injury, 4, 411
Cerebral Hemorrhage, 130
Cervical Formula, 237, 238, 239, 240, 241, 250, 252, 254, 256, 259, 262, 265, 268, 274, 276, 279, 281, 282, 285, 288, 308, 400, 404, 405, 434
Cervical spondylomyelopathy, 4, 14, 24, 225, 243, 269, 270, 274, 277, 279, 282, 285
Clostridium tetani, 387
Cognitive dysfunction, 4, 14, 25, 41, 42, 43, 45, 49, 50, 51, 115, 118
Computer-assisted tomography, 121
Congenital hydrocephalus, 4, 14, 24, 25, 71, 73, 90
Cryptococcus neoformans, 56

D

Dandruff Formula, 130, 131
Deafness, 4, 13, 24, 149, 150, 152, 189, 190, 191, 192, 194, 196, 418, 423
Degenerative myelopathy, 4, 12, 14, 24, 225, 231, 243, 293, 295, 297, 298, 299, 301, 302, 304, 305, 322, 347, 350, 456
Dementia, 12, 13, 14, 16, 41, 42, 47, 116, 311
Di Er You, 156, 157, 177, 188, 196
Di Gu Pi, 237, 238, 239, 252, 262, 265
Di Huang Yin Zi, 241, 285, 305, 349, 350
Di Tan Tang, 44, 45, 48, 59, 61, 65, 67, 74, 79, 81, 84, 86, 88, 92, 96, 99, 109, 110
Ding Xian Wan, 44, 61, 96, 99
Diskospondylitis, 4, 225, 290
DM. *Degenerative Myelopathy*
Double P II, 237, 238, 239, 240, 241, 242, 243, 250, 252, 254, 256, 259, 262, 264, 265, 268, 274, 276, 279, 282, 285, 288, 308, 357, 358, 362, 365, 400, 401, 404, 405, 409, 413
Dysmyelinogenesis, 95

E

Electro-acupuncture, 46, 115, 214, 321, 328, 337, 339, 342, 343, 344, 345, 388, 433, 434, 436, 438, 439, 440, 443, 445, 467
Electroencephalography, 117, 118
Electromyography, 117, 399
Encephalitis. *Meningoencephalitis*
Epimedium Formula, 43, 74, 81, 92, 156, 157, 158, 182, 192, 200, 239, 241, 274, 296, 308, 434
Equine Chest Formula, 440
Equine protozoal myeloencephalitis, 431
Erhlichia canis, 56

F

Facial P Formula, 155, 156, 173, 175, 440
Facial paralysis, 4, 23, 24, 149, 150, 151, 153, 168, 169, 170, 172, 174, 176, 178, 187, 195, 209, 388, 431, 435, 439, 440, 445
Fang Fen San, 155, 162
Fibrocartilaginous embolism, 4, 12, 14, 225, 226, 243, 244, 286, 289, 321
Four Gentlemen. *Si Jun Zi Tang*

G

Geriatric tremors, 4
GME. *Granulomatous meningoencephalomyelitis*
Granulomatous meningoencephalomyelitis, 139
Gui Pi San, 143
Gui Pi Tang, 420

H

Han Lian Cao, 143
Head injury, 4, 24, 41, 42, 43, 45, 46, 49, 75, 90
Heart Qi Deficiency, 23, 25
Hindquarter Weakness Formula, 115
Hu Qian Wan, 240, 241, 282, 302, 349
Hua Tuo, 427
Huang Di, 37
Huang Qi Tang, 331
Hydrocephalus, 73, 74, 92, 117, 118, 119
Hypocalcemia, 95, 467

Hypoglycemia, 14, 16, 25, 41, 42, 43, 71, 95

I

Idiopathic epilepsy, 4, 12, 14, 49, 60, 62, 71, 73, 75, 76, 77
Idiopathic tremors, 4, 23, 24, 95, 96, 97
Intervertebral disk disease, 4, 11, 14, 226, 234, 242, 243, 244, 245, 246, 269, 293, 320, 321, 331, 333, 339, 340, 341, 343, 344, 346, 392, 411

J

Jia Wei Xiao Yao, 211, 212, 213
Jiang Tang Cha, 358, 367
Jue Ming San, 155, 164

L

Laryngeal paralysis, 4, 210
Liu Wei Di Huang Wan, 137, 331, 423
Liver Happy, 109, 110
Long Dan Xie Gan, 74, 79, 156, 157, 177, 188, 196
Lumbosacral degeneration, 4, 293, 411

M

Ma Shi Huang, 145
Magnetic resonance imaging, 41, 117, 129, 338, 431
Masticatory myopathy, 4
Max's Formula, 241, 242, 316
Meningoencephalitis, 4, 11, 12, 14, 22, 24, 41, 42, 45, 56, 57, 58, 60, 62, 71, 75, 95, 149, 150, 159, 205, 310, 456
Meningomyelitis, 4, 225, 310, 311
Milk thistle, 124
Moxibustion, 249, 254, 258, 278, 284, 298, 304, 335, 336, 358, 364, 445, 455, 462, 464, 467
MRI. *Magnetic resonance imaging*
Mu Dan Pi San, 142
Myasthenia gravis, 4, 355, 376

N

Neospora caninum, 56, 376

O

Ophiopogon Powder, 142
Optic neuritis, 4, 149, 151, 159, 160, 165, 166, 169

P

Peanut Hydrocephalus Formula, 74
Polymyositis, 4, 24, 25, 205, 355, 372, 374, 376, 377, 378, 380, 381, 383, 385

Polyneuropathy, 4, 24, 25, 34, 149, 151, 198, 355, 359, 360, 369
Polyradiculoneuritis, 355, 359, 363, 366
Portosystemic Liver shunt, 42
Portosystemic shunt, 43
Pu Ji Xiao Du Yin, 155, 158, 159, 167, 171, 202, 208, 357, 362, 419, 432, 442, 444

Q

Qi Performance, 158, 200, 400, 401, 405, 409, 413, 440, 441, 448, 449, 450
Qing Hao San, 436, 437, 444
Qing Ying Tang, 142, 240, 291, 292, 442, 443, 444

R

Radioablative surgery, 121
Rehmannia 14, 107, 108
Rehmannia 6. *Liu Wei Di Huang Wan*
Relief Salve, 107, 108, 448, 449

S

Sang Zhi San, 107, 108
Sciatic nerve, 21, 24, 400, 401, 408
Sciatic nerve injury, 4, 407
Seizures, 71
Shen disturbance, 76, 218
Shen Nong, 7
Shu Jin Huo Lou, 358, 365
Si Jun Zi Tang, 438
Spinal cord trauma, 4, 225, 233, 242, 266, 271, 272
Spinal cord tumor, 4
Stasis in the Mansion of Mind, 43, 44, 45, 48, 52, 55, 64, 67, 109, 110, 111, 112, 114, 115, 129, 130, 131, 135, 136, 156, 157, 182, 184, 186, 211, 213, 217, 218

T

Tan-Huan Syndrome, 453
Tao Hong Si Wu Tang, 331, 419, 424
Tendon Ligament Formula, 97, 105
Tian Ma Bai Zhu, 43, 111
Tian Ma Plus II, 74, 88
Tian Wan Bu Xin Dan, 420
Toxicity, 7, 41, 95, 124, 190
Toxoplasma gondii, 56, 376
Tremors, 95
Trigeminal neuritis, 4, 23, 24, 149, 151, 165, 166, 168, 169

V

Vestibular disease, 4, 23, 178, 179, 211, 217, 218

W

Wei Qi Booster, 130, 131, 135, 136, 241, 242, 316, 318
Wei Syndrome, 453, 455, 458, 462, 463, 475
Wen Dan Tang, 43, 52, 114
West Nile virus, 431, 445
Wu Wei Xiao Du Yin, 241, 312, 358, 359, 379, 401, 432

X

Xue Fu Zhu Yu Tang, 331, 417, 419, 420, 423

Y

Yang Yin Xi Feng, 74
Yu brothers, 451

Z

Zhang Zhongjing, 395
Zhao fu, 221
Zi Xue Dan, 419